MDCT: From Protocols to Practice

M.K. Kalra • **S. Saini** • **G.D. Rubin** *(Eds.)*

MDCT

From Protocols to Practice

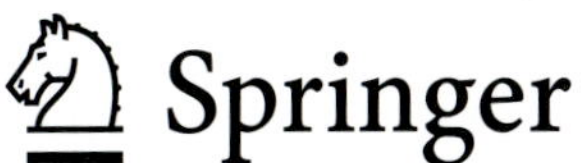
Springer

Mannudeep K. Kalra
Department of Radiology
Massachusetts General Hospital
Boston, MA, USA

Sanjay Saini
Department of Radiology
Emory University School of Medicine
Emory University Hospital
Atlanta, GA, USA

Geoffrey D. Rubin
Department of Radiology
Stanford University School of Medicine
Stanford, CA, USA

*MDCT: **From Protocols to Practice***
is the updated edition of
MDCT: A Practical Approach (2006)
edited by S. Saini, G.D. Rubin and M.K. Kalra

Library of Congress Control Number: 2008921923

ISBN 978-88-470-0831-1   Springer Milan Berlin Heidelberg New York
e-ISBN 978-88-470-0832-8

Springer is a part of Springer Science+Business Media
springer.com
© Springer-Verlag Italia 2008
Printed in Italy

Typesetting: Compostudio, Cernusco s/N (Milan), Italy
Printing and binding: Arti Grafiche Nidasio, Assago (Milan), Italy

Springer-Verlag Italia S.r.l., Via Decembrio 28, I-20137 Milan, Italy

Preface to the new edition

MDCT: A Practical Approach is back, with updated and expanded contents. At the time of its publication, we knew that the book's success and popularity would dictate our efforts to publish a new edition. What we did not realize was that, because of the constant and almost relentless progress in the technology of multi-detector-row computed tomography, it would be necessary to improve the contents and publish the updated edition, *MDCT: From Protocols to Practice,* so soon.

In the new edition, we update the chapter on radiation dose to include the results of recent investigations and technological developments, and the chapter on reactions to contrast media is thoroughly revised by Dr. Solomon. In addition, the content is expanded by the inclusion of a number of new chapters, all from leaders and experts in the field. For example, the chapter on dual-source CT technology and its applications is new. Dr. Thomsen, an international expert on contrast-media use in medical imaging, reflects on the concepts and risks associated with the use of contrast medium in pregnancy. Dr. Uppot provides his unique expertise to highlight the important issues related to MDCT imaging of obese patients. Drs. Moore and Blake enrich the book with their chapter on the role of PET/CT in abdominal malignancies. Drs. Rogers and Hoffmann share their tremendous experience and expertise in imaging acute coronary artery syndrome with state-of-the MDCT. Dr. Donald Frush, a renowned expert in pediatric MDCT technology, including protocols and radiation dose, contributes a detailed chapter on the pediatric applications of MDCT. Drs. Sirineni, Tigges, and Stillman do a remarkable job in their chapter on the role of MDCT for coronary-stent evaluation. Drs. Ramesh and Sahani, international experts on pancreatic imaging, contribute a highly informative chapter on the status of MDCT in pancreatic imaging. The important topic of CT urography is the subject of the excellent chapter by Drs. McSweeney, O'Connor, and Maher.

In keeping with the global standards of publishing, international standards (S.I.) units were used over conventional units, such as use of kilogram for weight rather than pounds. Therefore, to avoid any potential confusion, readers are strongly cautioned to pay close attention to the units before applying them in their practice or research.

This new edition of our textbook would not have been possible without help from our contributing coauthors. We thank those from the previous edition for their invaluable contributions, without which neither the previous nor the present edition would have been complete. In this respect, we are grateful to Drs. Bae, Solomon, Sahani, Singh, Schindera, Nelson, Shah, Wang, Rybicki, Sheth, Kavanagh, Lake, Costello, Enterline, Shetty, Lev, Halvorsen, Sebastian, and Salamipour.

We also extend our heartfelt gratitude to James Waples, at Bracco Diagnostics, for his untiring help and encouragement for an updated edition.

Also, we are grateful to Springer Verlag's editorial staff, notably, Antonella Cerri, Alessandra Born, and Angela Vanegas, for their help in acquiring manuscripts and the publication of this book.

Last not least, we thank our supportive readers, who motivated us in our endeavor to publish this expanded edition, and we hope they will receive it with the same enthusiasm as granted the previous edition.

March 2008

Mannudeep K. Kalra
Sanjay Saini
Geoffrey D. Rubin

Contents

Contributors

Kyongtae Ty Bae
School of Medicine
Washington University
St. Louis, MO, USA

Michael A. Blake
Division of Abdominal Imaging
Radiology Department
Massachusetts General Hospital
Boston, MA, USA

Philip Costello
Division of Thoracic Imaging
Department of Radiology
Medical University of South Carolina
Charleston, SC, USA

David S. Enterline
Divisions of Neuroradiology and
Interventional Neuroradiology
Duke University Medical Center
Durham, NC, USA

Donald P. Frush
Department of Radiology
Duke University Medical Center
Durham, NC, USA

Robert A. Halvorsen
Department of Radiology
MCV Hospitals/VCU Medical Center
Richmond, VA, USA

Udo Hoffmann
Department of Radiology
Massachusetts General Hospital
Harvard Medical School
Boston, MA, USA

Mannudeep K. Kalra
Department of Radiology
Massachusetts General Hospital
Boston, MA, USA

Joseph J. Kavanagh
Division of Thoracic Imaging
Department of Radiology
Medical University of South Carolina
Charleston, SC, USA

Douglas R. Lake
Division of Thoracic Imaging
Department of Radiology
Medical University of South Carolina
Charleston, SC, USA

Michael H. Lev
Emergency Neuroradiology and
Neurovascular Lab
Massachusetts General Hospital
Boston, MA, USA

Michael M. Maher
Department of Radiology
Cork University Hospital
Mercy University Hospital and
University College Cork
Cork, Ireland

Sean E. McSweeney
Department of Radiology
Cork University Hospital
Mercy University Hospital and
University College Cork
Cork, Ireland

Christine O. Menias
School of Medicine
Washington University
St. Louis, MO, USA

Zaheerabbas Momin
Division of Abdominal Imaging
Department of Radiology
Emory University School of Medicine
Atlanta, GA, USA

Michael Moore
Division of Abdominal Imaging
Department of Radiology
Massachusetts General Hospital
Boston, MA, USA

Rendon C. Nelson
Division of Abdominal Imaging
Duke University Medical Center
Durham, NC, USA

Owen J. O'Connor
Department of Radiology
Cork University Hospital
Mercy University Hospital and
University College Cork
Cork, Ireland

Avinash R. Kambadakone
Division of Abdominal
Imaging and Intervention
Department of Radiology
Massachussets General Hospital
Boston, MA, USA

Ian S. Rogers
Division of Cardiology and
Department of Radiology
Massachusetts General Hospital
Harvard Medical School and
School of Public Health
Boston, MA, USA

Geoffrey D. Rubin
Department of Radiology
Stanford University School of Medicine
Stanford, CA, USA

Frank J. Rybicki
Cardiovascular Imaging Section
Applied Imaging Science Laboratory
Brigham & Women's Hospital Radiology
Harvard Medical School
Boston, MA, USA

Dushyant V. Sahani
Department of Radiology
Massachusetts General Hospital
Boston, MA, USA

Sanjay Saini
Department of Radiology
Emory University School of Medicine
Emory University Hospital
Atlanta, GA, USA

Hamid Salamipour
Department of Radiology
Massachusetts General Hospital
Boston, MA, USA

Sebastian T. Schindera
Division of Abdominal Imaging
Duke University Medical Center
Durham, NC, USA

Sunit Sebastian
Department of Radiology
Emory University School of Medicine
Atlanta, GA, USA

Zarine K. Shah
Department of Abdominal Imaging and
Intervention
Massachusetts General Hospital
Boston, MA, USA

Tarang Sheth
Department of Diagnostic Imaging
Trillium Health Centre
Mississauga, ON, Canada

Sanjay K. Shetty
Division of Musculoskeletal Radiology
Department of Radiology
Massachusetts General Hospital
Boston, MA, USA

Anandkumar H. Singh
Abdominal Imaging
Massachusetts General Hospital
Depatment of Abdominal Imaging
Boston, MA, USA

Gopi K.R. Sirineni
Department of Radiology
Emory University School of Medicine
Emory University Hospital
Atlanta, GA, USA

William C. Small
Division of Abdominal Imaging
Department of Radiology
Emory University School of Medicine
Atlanta, GA, USA

Richard Solomon
Division of Nephrology
University of Vermont College of
Medicine
Burlington, VT, USA

Arthur E. Stillman
Department of Radiology
Emory University School of Medicine
Emory University Hospital
Atlanta, GA, USA

Henrik S. Thomsen
Department of Diagnostic Radiology
54E2
Copenhagen University Hospital
Herlev, Denmark

Stefan Tigges
Department of Radiology
Emory University School of Medicine
Emory University Hospital
Atlanta, GA, USA

Unni K. Udayasankar
Division of Abdominal Imaging
Department of Radiology
Emory University School of Medicine
Atlanta, GA, USA

Raul N. Uppot
Department of Radiology
Harvard Medical School and
Division of Abdominal Imaging and
Interventional Radiology
Department of Radiology
Massachusetts General Hospital
Boston, MA, USA

Lisa L. Wang
School of Medicine
Washington University
St. Louis, MO, USA

SECTION I

Physics and Techniques of MDCT

1

A Practical Approach to MDCT

Mannudeep K. Kalra, Sanjay Saini

Introduction

Over the past 8 years, computed tomography (CT) technology has developed tremendously with the introduction of multi-detector row CT (MDCT) scanners to the clinical radiology practice [1]. Use of CT scanning has increased immensely over the last decade with the introduction of newer applications. Demand for better technology continues to propel vendors to develop further innovations in very short time periods. As a result, it has become difficult for many radiologists, physicists, and technologists to keep up with the pace of development. This chapter outlines growth patterns in MDCT application and use and the history of CT technology and describes the fundamentals of MDCT technology.

MDCT: Explosive Growth Patterns

It is estimated that there are more than 25,000 CT scanners in the world, and since 1998, worldwide CT sales have doubled. In 2002, the CT market was reported to be worth in excess of US$2.6 billion [1]. A recent survey indicates that every year, about 90 million CT examinations are performed globally, which corresponds to a frequency of 16 CT examinations per 1,000 inhabitants [1, 2]. According to the 2000–2001 Nationwide Evaluation of X-ray Trends (NEXT) – a survey of patient radiation exposure from CT, performed under the auspices of the United States Food and Drug Administration – approximately 58 million (± 9 million) CT studies are performed annually in 7,800 CT facilities in the United States [1]. As regards CT applications, during 1991–2002, vascular and cardiac applications of CT showed the highest growth rates (over 140%), followed by much smaller increments in abdominal, pelvic, thoracic, and head and neck applications (7–27%).

MDCT: Chronology of Technological Advances

- **1971:** The Nobel laureate Sir Godfrey Neobold Hounsfield at the Electrical and Musical Industries, London, a British electronics and music company, developed the first conventional CT scanner. It took 15 h to scan the first patient using this CT instrument and 5 min to acquire each image.

- **1971–1976:** During this period, four generations of conventional CT scanners were developed, and the scan time for each image dropped manyfold to 1–2 s. These conventional scanners revolved a single X-ray tube and detector array on a gantry assembly around the patient. Following each revolution, the X-ray tube and/or detector array returned to their initial position to "unwind" their attached wires and prepare for the next revolution after table movement.

- **Early 1990s:** Just as magnetic resonance imaging (MRI) threatened to make inroads into several "CT applications," introduction of slip-ring or spiral or helical CT technology marked the beginning of a resurgence of CT scanning in clinical practice. Helical scanning obviated the need for wires and hence the "unwinding" time by using innovative slip rings on the gantry assembly. An increase in temporal resolution (decrease in scan time) to subsecond durations and acquisition of contiguous volumetric scan data with helical CT scanners improved dynamic contrast-enhanced studies and three-dimensional (3-D) rendering of axial source data.

- **Late 1990s to 2005:** During this period, different vendors offered MDCT scanners with several different slice options from 2, 4, 6, 8, 10, 16, 32, 40, and 64 slices per revolution. The addition of multiple detector rows to the detector array of helical CT scanners in the scanning direction or Z-axis allowed acquisition of more than one image per revolution of X-ray tube and detector array around the patient and led to development of multidetector or multisection, multichannel, multislice, or multidetector-row helical CT scanners. MDCT scanners offer several advantages over the prior helical and nonhelical CT scanners. In addition, there are several differences in the hardware and software components of single-slice helical CT and MDCT scanners. Depending on the detector configuration, MDCT scanners have multiple detector rows in the scanning direction or Z-axis. The number of detector rows in MDCT scanners can be less than the number of slices reconstructed per rotation (Siemens Sensation 64 with double Z-sampling), equal to the number of slices per rotation (LightSpeed VCT, General Electric Healthcare Technologies), or more than the number of reconstructed slices (LightSpeed QXi, General Electric Healthcare Technologies). For most MDCT scanners, the smallest reconstructed slice thickness is equal to the thickness of an individual detector row. For example, with 64 × 0.625 detector configuration (LightSpeed VCT), minimum slice thickness is 0.625 although it is possible to generate images with 1.25-, 2.5-, 3.75-, 5-, and 10-mm slice thickness also. However, one vendor (Siemens Medical Solutions) provides scanners that can acquire 0.4-mm slices with 0.6-mm detector width, due to double Z-sampling that occurs due to dynamic, online motion of the focal spot (Z-flying focal spot) and X-ray beam projections over adjoining detector rows.

Compared with single-slice CT, MDCT permits image reconstruction at various slice thicknesses different from the one chosen prior to the scan. Also, MDCT scanners allow faster scan times (330–350 milliseconds), wider scan coverage, and thinner section thickness. Higher temporal resolution helps in vascular and cardiac scanning, better utilization of contrast medium injection bolus, as well as scanning of uncooperative, breathless, or pediatric patients (less need for sedation or shorter duration of sedation). Wider scan coverage with MDCT scanners helps in vascular studies over longer regions, such as chest, abdomen, pelvis for aortic aneurysms or dissection workup, and peripheral CT angiography from origins of renal arteries to feet. Along with wider coverage, MDCT can also acquire "isotropic" scan data, which helps create exquisite 3-D or orthogonal multiplanar images. In addition, due to the wider detector configuration and use of cone-shaped X-ray, more complex cone-beam reconstruction techniques are used for MDCT compared with single-slice CT scanners. These cone-beam reconstruction techniques help reduce streak artifacts, particularly at the site of inhomogeneous objects in the scanning direction, such as ribs.

- **2005:** At 330–350 ms gantry revolution time, MDCT scanners are approaching the engineering limits of the gantry to withstand the mechanical forces from gantry components, so further improvements in scan time appear challenging. For cardiac or coronary CT angiography studies, however, a higher temporal resolution may imply better quality examinations in patients with higher or irregular heart rates. In this respect, dual-source MDCT scanners (Siemens Medical Solutions), with two X-ray tubes (both 80 kW) and two detector arrays (both with 64-slice acquisition per rotation with double Z-axis sampling), may prove beneficial by decreasing single-segment reconstruction scan time to 83 ms [3, 4]. However, patient studies are needed to validate the findings of initial phantom studies. Another recent innovation in MDCT technology is the introduction of the "sandwich" detector array (Philips Medical Systems), which can enable acquisition of images with characteristics of dual-energy spectra. The dual-source MDCT can also acquire dual kilovoltage peak (kVp) or energy image data when different kVp are selected for the two sources. However, rigorous studies will be required to assess the clinical potential of dual-energy CT scanning.

MDCT: Practical Approach to Building Scan Protocols

Several important considerations apply when building an "optimum" scanning protocol (Table 1). An "optimum" scanning protocol may be defined as one that provides adequate diagnostic information with an appropriate amount of contrast media and as low as reasonably achievable radiation dose (Table 2). Important aspects of a diagnostic CT study that must be considered while making a protocol are summarized in Figure 1 and include [5]:

- **Diagnostic indication:** Will help determine the number of phases (one or more, arterial, venous, delayed), scan area of interest, need for contrast (oral and/or rectal and/or intravenous), contrast administration protocol, scanning parameters, and appropriate radiation dose required to generate images to answer the diagnostic query. Development of specific scanning protocols for different clinical indications can help in optimizing workflow and managing radiation dose [6, 7].

- **Scan area of interest and scan direction:** It is important to predetermine the appropriate region of interest based on clinical indication [6, 8], for example, scanning of regions such as abdomen only, abdomen-pelvis, or chest-abdomen-pelvis. Concerns have been raised about "overextending" the scan area of interest, as faster MDCT scanners re-

Table 1. Important scanning parameters and contrast considerations that must be addressed during development of scanning protocols for a given diagnostic indication

Computed tomography (CT) scanning parameters	Contrast consideration
Scan area of interest	Contrast versus noncontrast
Scan direction	Route
Localizer radiograph	Concentration
Scan duration	Volume
Gantry revolution time	Rate of injection
Table speed, beam pitch, beam collimation	Trigger-fixed, automatic tracking, or test bolus
Reconstructed section thickness	
Extent of overlap	
Reconstruction algorithms	
Tube potential	
Tube current and automatic exposure control	
Radiation dose	

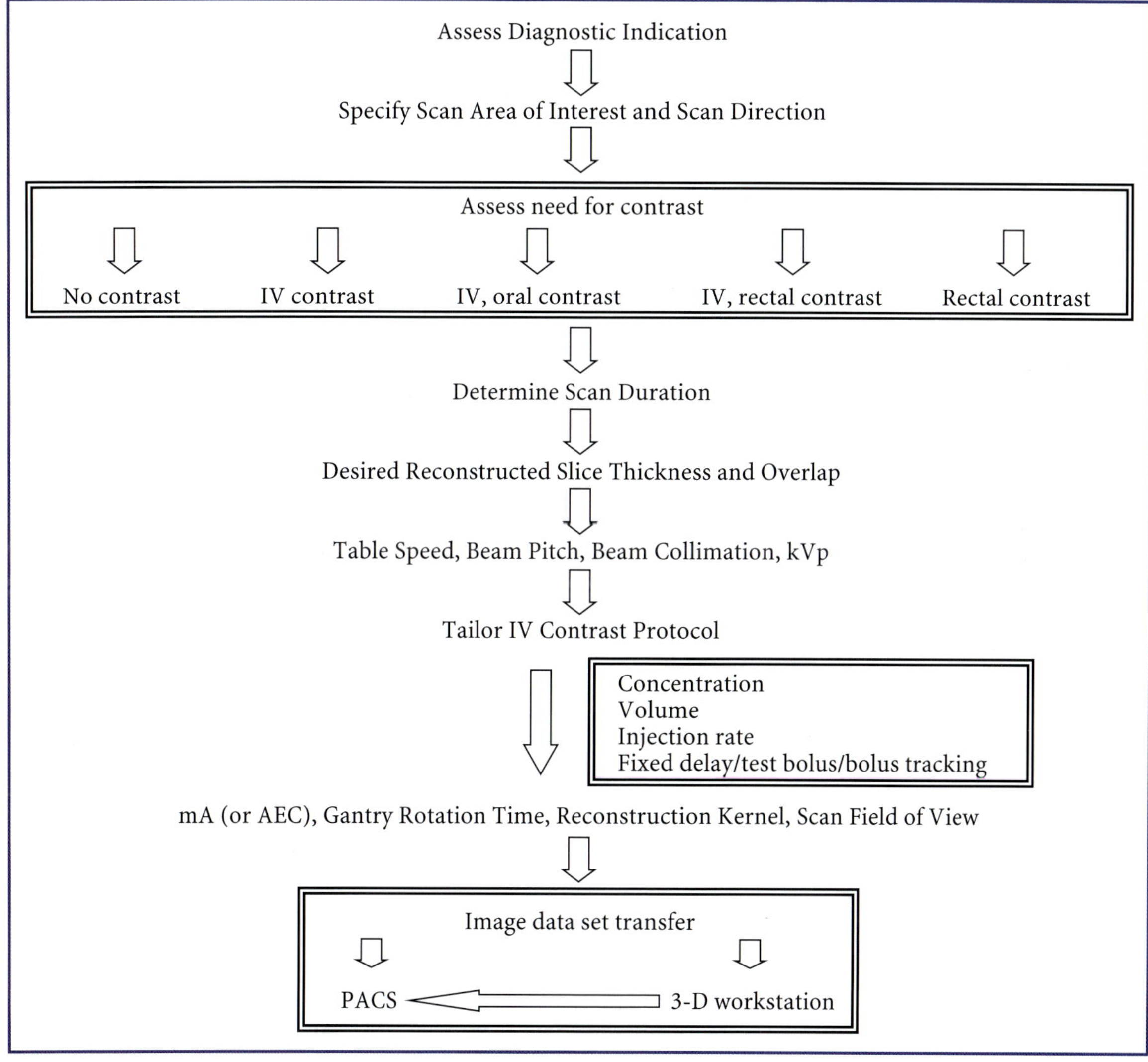

Fig. 1. Building blocks for scanning protocols. *IV* intravenous, *kVp* kilovolt peak, *mA* milliampere, *AEC* automatic exposure control, *PACS* picture archiving and communication system

Table 2. Salient features of multidetector-row computed tomography (MDCT) scanners

Features	Details
X-ray tube	80–100 kW
	Higher tube current output (up to 800 mA)
	Less issues with tube cooling
	Z-flying focal spot (double Z-sampling)[a]
X-ray filters	Prepatient beam filters – to improve dose efficiency
	Bowtie filters – to reduce dose (especially cardiac applications)
Detector array	> one detector row in scanning direction (Z-axis)
	Effective detector widths: may be constant or variable
	Effective detector-row width (64-MDCT): 0.5, 0.6, or 0.625 mm
	Most scanners: effective detector width = section width
	Double Z-sampling: effective detector width ⩾ section width[a]
DAS	Represents data acquisition system or data channels
	Determines slice profiles (number of slices per rotation)
	Example: 4 data channels: 16 detector rows for 4-slice MDCT
	64 data channels: 64 detector rows for 64-slice MDCT
Detector configuration	Describes number of data channels and effective detector-row width
	Example: 16×1.25 mm = 16 data channels; 1.25-mm row width
Beam collimation	Refers to X-ray beam width
	Cone-shaped beam leads to "overbeaming" (penumbra effect)
	= number of data channels × effective detector-row width
	Example: 16-slice MDCT
	a. 16 data channels × 1.25-mm row width = 20 mm
	b. 16 data channels × 0.625-mm row width = 10 mm
	Radiation dose: b > a
Beam pitch	Table speed in mm per gantry revolution/beam collimation in mm
	Smaller effect on image quality for MDCT than for SSCT
	> 1: nonoverlapping, interspersed acquisition
	= 1: nonoverlapping, contiguous acquisition
	< 1: overlapping acquisition
	Low-contrast lesions (liver): prefer beam pitch <1
	High contrast lesions (CT colonography): prefer beam pitch >1
Table speed	Closely related to beam pitch and beam collimation
	Usually described as table travel in mm per gantry revolution
	For mm/s: multiply with number of revolutions per second
	Compared with SSCT, MDCT provides higher table speed, allows faster scanning
	for thinner sections with dose savings

[a] Siemens 64-slice MDCT
MDCT multi-detector row computed tomography
SSCT single-slice CT

quire very little extra time to cover extended scan length. Determination of scan area of interest or scan length (which also depends upon patient length or height) can help to determine scanning parameters, scan duration, and contrast administration protocol. Scan direction is an important determinant of vascular contrast enhancement. In general, direction of scanning is similar to the direction of blood flow in the area of interest in order to follow the contrast flow column (for example, peripheral MDCT angiography – craniocaudal) with few exceptions (for example, MDCT angiography of pulmonary embolism to avoid streaks from contrast in systemic veins – caudocranial).

• **Localizer radiograph:** With availability of automatic exposure control techniques and bowtie filters (a hardware component of the scanner), it is important to emphasize to technologists that patients must be centered appropriately in the scanner. Acquisition of localizer radiograph with miscentering of patient in the gantry isocenter can lead to erroneous calculation of tube current with use of automatic exposure control technique, and this can affect resulting image quality [9, 10]. Likewise, localizer radiograph length must also include the entire scan area of interest, as some automatic exposure control techniques (Z-axis and XYZ-axis modulation) require these radiographs to estimate tube current [9].

- **Contrast consideration:** This aspect of scanning protocol is discussed elsewhere in the textbook.

- **Scan duration:** State-of-the-art MDCT scanners cover most routine CT studies of chest, abdomen, and/or pelvis in a single breath-hold, fast acquisition (less than 15 s). Further reduction in scan duration with MDCT will also be helpful to avoid or reduce the need for sedation in uncooperative patients or children. Estimation of scan duration with MDCT scanning is most critical for catching the peak contrast enhancement over the scan length. Thus, estimation of scan duration can help optimize contrast media injection duration. Scan duration depends on several factors, such as gantry revolution time, table speed, and pitch, as well as scan area(s) of interest.

- **Gantry revolution time:** In general, the shortest gantry revolution time (such as 0.4–0.5 s) must be used for most CT studies. An exception to this rule is CT evaluation of a large patient, where use of longer gantry rotation time helps increase total tube current – time product [milliampere second (mAs)].

- **Table speed, beam pitch, and beam collimation:** For MDCT scanners, change in these parameters affects scan duration and radiation dose more than image quality. However, there are some exceptions to this rule. In the liver, use of higher pitch (>1:1 beam pitch) and faster table speed has been shown to be inferior to lower pitch and slower table speed for detection of small metastatic lesions [11]. Conversely, in high-contrast situations, such as CT colonography and CT angiography, use of higher pitch (>1:1 beam pitch) and faster table speed does not affect image quality [2].

From scan length and scan duration, table speed can be estimated. For example, a 350-mm scan length for abdomen-pelvis in 10 s can be covered with a table speed of 35 mm/s or 17.5 mm per gantry revolution (at 0.5-s gantry revolution time). For a given MDCT scanner, desired table speed can then be achieved by selecting beam pitch, number of data channels, effective detector-row width, and gantry revolution speed. Thus, for an 8-slice MDCT scanner, a table speed of 35 mm/s can be achieved with 0.875:1 beam pitch, 8 data channels with 2.5-mm effective detector-row width (detector configuration of 8 × 2.5 mm = 20 mm beam collimation), and 0.5-s gantry revolution time. When selecting the detector configuration and beam pitch – most notably, the effective detector-row width – one must take into account the required reconstructed section thickness. For example, if 1.25-mm section thickness is required for an 8-slice MDCT scanner, one must select 8 × 1.25-mm detector configuration (effective detector-row width = 1.25 mm) and not 8 × 2.5-mm detector configuration (effective detector-row width = 2.5mm). This becomes redundant for MDCT scanners with matrix array detector configuration, such as 64 × 0.625 mm (LightSpeed VCT) since users select the same detector configuration (64 × 0.625 mm) to obtain any section thickness (0.625, 1.25, 2.5, 3.75, or 5 mm).

- **Reconstructed section thickness:** Compared with single detector-row CT scanners, MDCT (≥4-slice scanners) allows acquisition of thinner section thickness in shorter duration and with less radiation exposure. However, an increase in indications for thinner sections with MDCT scanners can lead to overall increase in radiation dose contributions from these scanners. In such circumstances, radiation dose can be reduced by acquiring thicker sections and reconstructing thinner images from the volumetric raw data. Thinner sections have more noise content but higher spatial resolution and less partial volume averaging so that greater noise can be tolerated. Whereas thinner sections can now be acquired in a short duration, this also poses interpretation and archiving challenges to radiologists and their departments. Therefore, scanning protocols must define use of thinner sections- for interpretation or 3-D postprocessing on picture archiving and communication system (PACS) or dedicated, stand-alone, image postprocessing workstations.

In general, for most routine abdominal CT studies, a section thickness of 2.5–5 mm is preferred for diagnostic interpretation. For these studies, multiplanar reconstructions can be performed at the scanner console from thinner reconstructions or directly from the volumetric raw data. Thinner sections are generally acquired for imaging of other regions of the body, including CT angiography studies of the abdomen.

- **Extent of overlap:** With isotropic scan data from most modern MDCT scanners, need for overlapping intersection distance is limited and can be avoided.

- **Reconstruction algorithms:** Reconstruction algorithms are an important component of scanning protocols. Selection of higher spatial resolution kernels (or sharper kernels) is necessary for viewing bones and lungs but can lead to unacceptably noisy images for soft tissues. Therefore, appropriate algorithms must be selected for specific regions of interest. A softer kernel (or a kernel with lower spatial resolution) provides smoother images and can help in decreasing noise content for low-contrast lesions, lower-dose studies, obese patients, or thinner sections.

- **Tube potential:** Most CT studies in adults are performed at 120 kVp. Tube potential (kVp) has a complex relationship with image noise, CT attenuation values (contrast), and radiation dose. A decrease in kVp increases noise and decreases radiation dose if other parameters are held constant but leads to higher attenuation values (except for water) and image contrast irrespective of other scanning parameters. The latter can help reduce the volume of intravenous contrast media administered for CT scanning. Low kVp CT can help in dose and contrast media volume reduction. Low kVp CT studies are especially well suited for high-contrast regions of interests, such as chest CT and CT angiography. To avoid inadvertently high image noise with low kVp CT studies, tube current may be raised. Several pediatric CT examinations can also be performed at lower kVp in order to reduce associated dose. However, kVp reduction in obese or large patients must be avoided to ensure adequate signal-to-noise ratio for acceptable diagnostic interpretation.

- **Tube current:** Unlike kVp, a change in tube current [milliampere (mA)] does not affect image contrast or CT attenuation values. However, reduction in mA is the most common method of reducing radiation dose. Either fixed tube current or automatic exposure control techniques can be used for maintaining adequate image quality and for managing radiation dose associated with MDCT [9, 12]. These techniques have been discussed in detail in the chapter on radiation dose. Automatic exposure control techniques can help optimize tube current and dose irrespective of other scanning parameters. As automatic exposure control techniques allow dose optimization during each gantry revolution (XY-axes) and from one to the next gantry revolution (Z-axis), it may be more dose efficient to use automatic exposure control over fixed tube-current protocols [10, 13].

- **Radiation-dose consideration:** This aspect of scanning protocols is described comprehensively elsewhere in this textbook.

MDCT: Are there Disadvantages to the Technology?

Used appropriately, most state-of-the-art MDCT scanners can help reduce overall radiation dose compared with the prior single-slice or conventional CT scanners. Although each technological breakthrough in MDCT has contributed to improved resolution and coverage with expansion of its clinical applications, recent trends in radiation dose contribution from MDCT scanners are alarming. CT scanning contributes the most radiation dose among all medical radiation-based imaging procedures. Several experts have raised concerns over potential overuse and inappropriate use of MDCT scanners. Several vendors have introduced sophisticated techniques, such as automatic exposure control, detectors with better dose efficiency, improved reconstruction kernels, and noise-reduction filters, but much remains to be accomplished for optimization of radiation dose. Most importantly, the definition of "optimum image quality at lowest possible dose" for different-sized patients in different body regions for different clinical indications remains elusive. In the absence of these guidelines, users must employ strategies for dose reduction, when indicated.

Summary

In summary, understanding the fundamentals of MDCT helps adequate planning of scanning protocols.

References

1. Kalra MK, Maher MM, D'Souza R, Saini S (2004) Multidetector computed tomography technology: current status and emerging developments. J Comput Assist Tomogr 28 [Suppl 1]:S2–6
2. Kalra MK, Maher MM, Toth TL et al (2004) Strategies for CT radiation dose optimization. Radiology 230(3):619–628
3. Kalra MK, Schmidt B, Flohr TG et al (2005) Can dual-source MDCT technology provide 83 millisecond temporal resolution for single segment reconstruction of coronary CT angiography? 91st Annual Meeting and Scientific Assembly of Radiological Society of North America, November 27–December 2, 2005
4. Kalra MK, Schmidt B, Flohr TG (2005) Coronary stent imaging with dual source MDCT Scanner: an in vivo study with an ECG synchronized moving heart phantom. 91st Annual Meeting and Scientific Assembly of Radiological Society of North America, November 27–December 2, 2005
5. Saini S (2004) Multi-detector row CT: principles and practice for abdominal applications. Radiology 233(2):323–327

6. Campbell J, Kalra MK, Rizzo S (2005) Scanning beyond anatomic limits of the thorax in chest CT: findings, radiation dose, and automatic tube current modulation. AJR Am J Roentgenol 185(6):1525–1530

7. Jhaveri KS, Saini S, Levine LA et al (2001) Effect of multislice CT technology on scanner productivity. AJR Am J Roentgenol 177(4):769–772

8. Kalra MK, Maher MM, Toth TL et al (2004) Radiation from "extra" images acquired with abdominal and/or pelvic CT: effect of automatic tube current modulation. Radiology 232(2):409–414

9. Kalra MK, Maher MM, Toth TL et al (2004) Techniques and applications of automatic tube current modulation for CT. Radiology 233(3):649–657

10. Kalra MK, Maher MM, Kamath RS et al (2004) Sixteen-detector row CT of abdomen and pelvis: study for optimization of Z-axis modulation technique performed in 153 patients. Radiology 233(1): 241–249

11. Abdelmoumene A, Chevallier P, Chalaron M et al (2005) Detection of liver metastases under 2 cm: comparison of different acquisition protocols in four row multidetector-CT (MDCT). Eur Radiol 15(9):1881–1887

12. Kalra MK, Prasad S, Saini S et al (2002) Clinical comparison of standard-dose and 50% reduced-dose abdominal CT: effect on image quality. AJR Am J Roentgenol 179(5):1101–1106. Erratum in: AJR Am J Roentgenol 179(6):1645

13. Kalra MK, Rizzo S, Maher MM et al (2005) Chest CT performed with z-axis modulation: scanning protocol and radiation dose. Radiology 237(1):303–308

2

Principles of Contrast Medium Delivery and Scan Timing in MDCT

Kyongtae T. Bae

Introduction

The advent of multidetector-row computed tomography (MDCT) technology has brought substantial advantages over single-detector-row CT (SDCT) in terms of image quality and clinical practice. The dramatically improved spatial and temporal resolution achievable on MDCT permits previously highly technically demanding clinical applications such as CT angiography (CTA) and cardiac CT to be practiced routinely.

Another major advantage of MDCT over SDCT is that contrast medium can be used more efficiently and flexibly. However, in order to fully appreciate the benefits of MDCT, certain technical challenges involving scan timing and optimization of contrast enhancement need to be overcome. This chapter aims to review the numerous factors associated with contrast medium delivery and scan timing. Moreover, modifications to protocol design that are necessary for optimized contrast enhancement in MDCT are discussed, along with clinical considerations for CTA and hepatic imaging.

Scan Timing and Factors Affecting Contrast Medium Delivery

The principal factors affecting contrast medium enhancement in CT imaging can be grouped into three broad categories: the patient, the injection of contrast medium, and the CT scan. Whereas factors associated with the former two categories determine the contrast enhancement process itself (independently of the CT scan), factors associated with the latter category (i.e., image acquisition parameters) play a critical role in permitting optimal visualization of the resulting contrast enhancement at specific time points. Whereas patient and injection factors involved in contrast enhancement are highly interrelated, some factors more closely affect the magnitude of contrast enhancement while others more closely affect the timing of contrast enhancement.

Patient Factors

The principal patient-related factors that influence contrast enhancement are body weight and cardiac output (cardiovascular circulation time). Other factors that can be considered of less significance include height, gender, age, venous access, renal function, and various pathological conditions.

Body Weight

The most important patient-related factor affecting the magnitude of vascular and parenchymal contrast enhancement is body weight [1–4]. Since large patients have larger blood volumes than small patients, contrast medium administered into the blood compartment of a large patient is diluted more than that administered to a small patient. The result is a reduced magnitude of contrast enhancement. Patient weight and the magnitude of enhancement are inversely related in a nearly one-to-one linear fashion. For a given administered dose of contrast medium, the magnitude of contrast enhancement is reduced proportionally to patient weight (Fig. 1). However, whereas the magnitude of contrast enhancement is strongly affected by patient weight, the timing of enhancement is largely unaffected by this parameter due to the concomitant proportional increase in both blood volume and cardiac output [3, 5, 6]. The result is a largely unaltered contrast medium circulation time that is independent of patient weight.

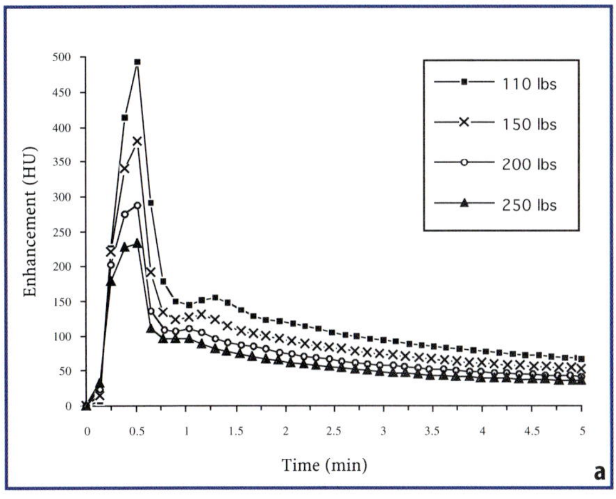

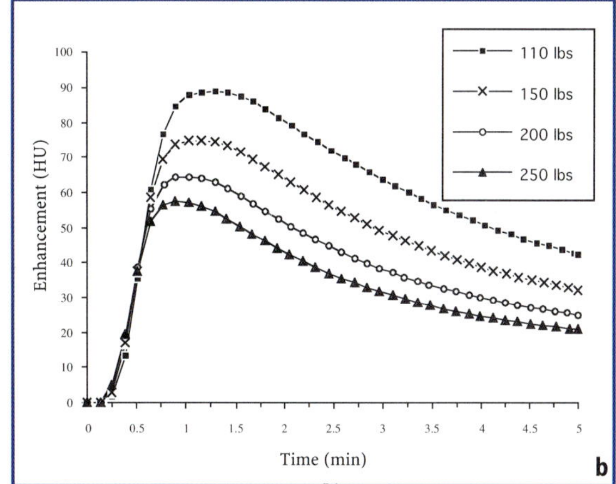

Fig. 1a, b. Simulated contrast enhancement curves with four different body weights. Simulated enhancement curves of the **a** aorta and **b** liver based on a hypothetical adult male with a fixed height (5′8″ or 173 cm) and varying body weight (110, 160, 200, and 260 lbs, or 49.8, 72.5, 90.7, and 117.9 kg), subjected to injection of 125 ml of contrast medium at 5 ml/s (14). The magnitude of contrast enhancement is inversely proportional to body weight. Reprinted from [53]

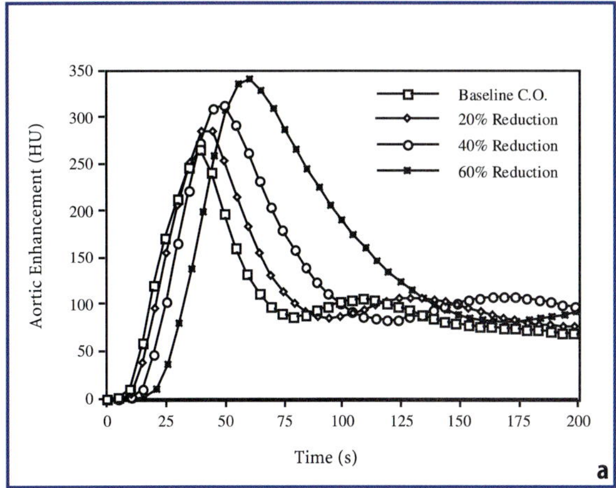

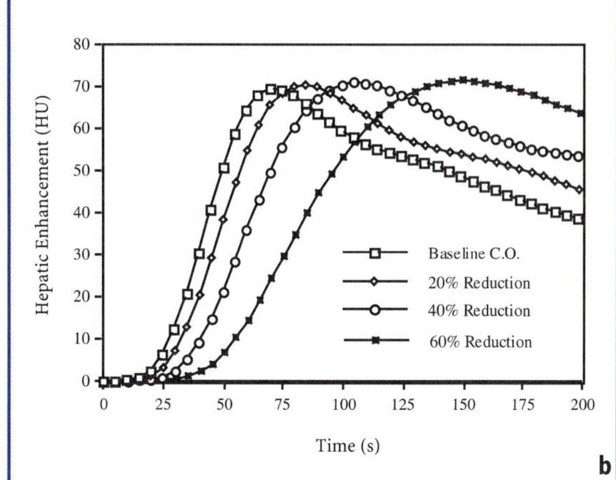

Fig. 2a, b. Simulated contrast enhancement curves at baseline and reduced cardiac outputs. Simulated enhancement curves of the **a** aorta and **b** liver based on a hypothetical adult male with a fixed height (5′8″, or 173 cm) and body weight (150 lbs, or 68 kg), subjected to injection of 120 ml of contrast agent at 4 ml/s. A set of aortic and hepatic contrast enhancement curves was generated by reducing the baseline cardiac output, i.e., 6,500 ml/min, by 20%, 40%, and 60%. Reprinted from [53]

Practical Tips

1. To maintain a constant degree of contrast enhancement in larger patients, one should consider increasing the overall iodine dose by increasing contrast medium volume and/or concentration. Increasing injection rate also increases the magnitude of vascular contrast enhancement (and hepatic enhancement in limited circumstances).
2. The timing of enhancement is largely unaffected by patient weight.

Cardiac Output

The most important patient-related factor affecting the timing of contrast enhancement is cardiac output (or cardiovascular circulation time) [7]. As cardiac output is reduced, the circulation of contrast medium slows, resulting in delayed contrast bolus arrival and delayed peak arterial and parenchymal enhancement (Fig. 2). The time delay between injection of the contrast medium bolus and the arrival of peak enhancement in the aorta and liver is highly correlated with, and linearly proportional to, cardiac output. Thus, in patients with reduced cardiac output, once the contrast bolus arrives in the central blood compartment, it is cleared more slowly, resulting in a higher, prolonged enhancement.

A consequence of the slower contrast bolus clearance in patients with reduced cardiac output is an increased magnitude of peak aortic and parenchymal enhancement. The rate of increase, however, is different in the aorta and liver. Whereas the magnitude of peak aortic enhancement increases substantially in patients with reduced cardiac output, the magnitude of peak hepatic enhancement increases only slightly.

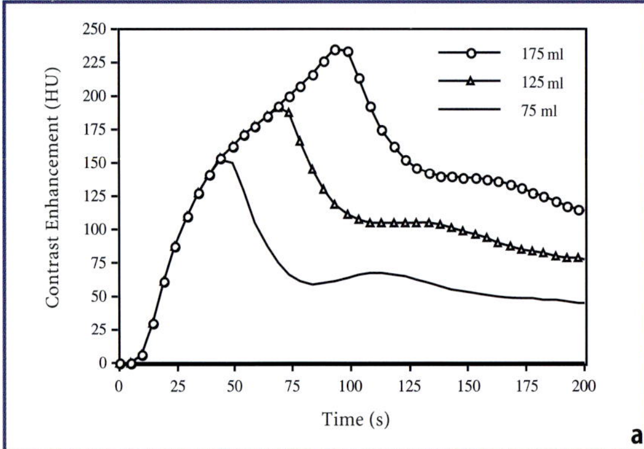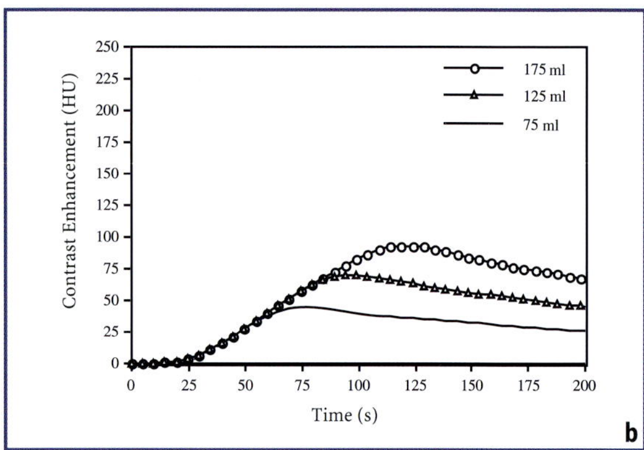

Fig. 3a, b. Simulated contrast enhancement curves with three different contrast medium volumes. Simulated enhancement curves of the **a** aorta and **b** liver based on a hypothetical adult male with a fixed height (5′8″, or 173 cm) and body weight (150 lbs, or 68 kg), subjected to injection of 75, 125, and 175 ml of contrast medium at 2 ml/s. Time-to-peak and magnitude of enhancement peak increases with contrast medium volume. Reprinted from [53]

Practical Tips

1. When scan timing is critical, it is important to individualize the scan delay to account for variations in cardiac output among patients. Scan delay can be individualized by using a test bolus or a bolus tracking technique.

Contrast Injection Factors

Key factors related to the injection of contrast medium include injection duration, injection rate, contrast medium volume (injection duration × rate), concentration, and use of a saline flush.

Injection Duration

Injection duration, which is determined by the volume of contrast medium and the rate at which it is administered (injection duration = contrast volume ÷ injection rate), critically affects both magnitude and timing of contrast enhancement [8–13]. Increased injection duration at a fixed rate of injection leads to greater deposition of iodine mass. This results in increased magnitude of vascular and parenchymal enhancement, which is proportional to injection duration (Fig. 3).

The appropriate injection duration is determined by scanning conditions and the clinical objectives of the examination. Injection duration should be prolonged for a long CT scan to maintain good enhancement throughout image acquisition. An injection duration that is too short leads to insufficient contrast enhancement. On the other hand, too long an injection duration results in a waste of contrast medium and the generation of undesirable tissue and venous contrast enhancement. Pertinent clinical factors to be considered in determining injection duration include body size,

the vessel or organ of interest, and the desired level of enhancement [14].

A sufficiently long injection is particularly crucial in portal-venous phase imaging of the liver because the principal determinant of hepatic enhancement is total iodine dose administered [9–11, 13, 15–21]. Thus, for a fixed injection rate, the injection duration for a large patient should be longer than that for a small patient. On the other hand, for a fixed injection duration and contrast medium concentration, the injection rate should be adjusted according to the patient's body size to deliver the appropriate amount of iodine mass. In this case, larger patients require faster injections.

The duration of contrast medium injection is the most important technical factor that affects scan timing. In patients with normal cardiac output, peak arterial contrast enhancement is achieved shortly after termination of a contrast medium injection [20]. As the volume of contrast medium increases, so too does the time required to reach the peak of arterial or parenchymal contrast enhancement (Fig. 3). Conversely, a shorter time-to-peak enhancement is noted for a fixed volume of contrast medium injected at a faster injection rate (Fig. 4).

Practical Tips

1. The use of a higher contrast medium concentration or a faster injection rate facilitates faster delivery of the total iodine load, allowing use of a shorter injection to achieve the desired degree of contrast enhancement.
2. A rapid contrast delivery rate and short injection duration are desirable for arterial enhancement with MDCT but are much less important for parenchymal or venous enhancement.
3. A short injection duration (i.e., low volume

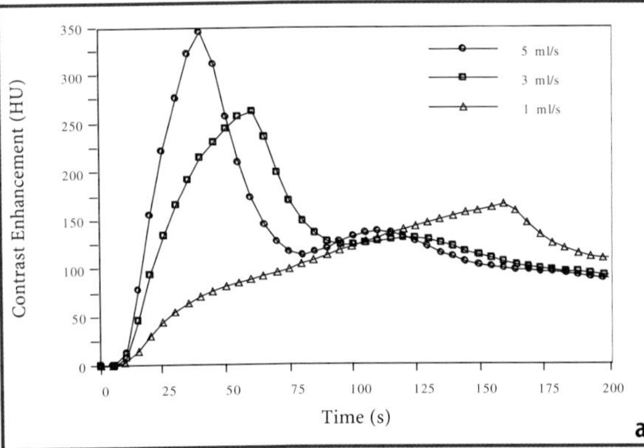

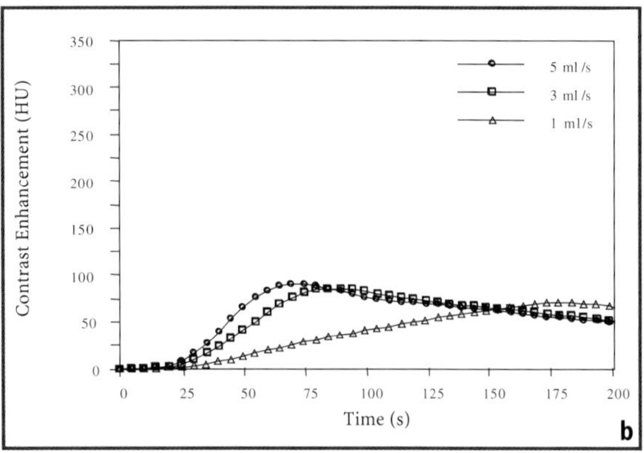

Fig. 4a, b. Simulated contrast enhancement curves with three different contrast medium injection rates. Simulated enhancement curves of the **a** aorta and **b** liver based on a hypothetical adult male with a fixed height (5'8", or 173 cm) and body weight (150 lbs, or 68 kg) subjected to 150 ml of contrast medium injected at 1, 3, and 5 ml/s. The curves show that for a fixed volume of contrast medium, as the rate of injection increases, the magnitude of contrast enhancement increases and the duration of high-magnitude contrast enhancement decreases. Figure 4a reprinted with permission of Anderson Publishing from Bae KT. Technical aspects of contrast delivery in advanced CT. Appl Radiol. 32 (12) (Suppl): 12-19. © Anderson Publishing

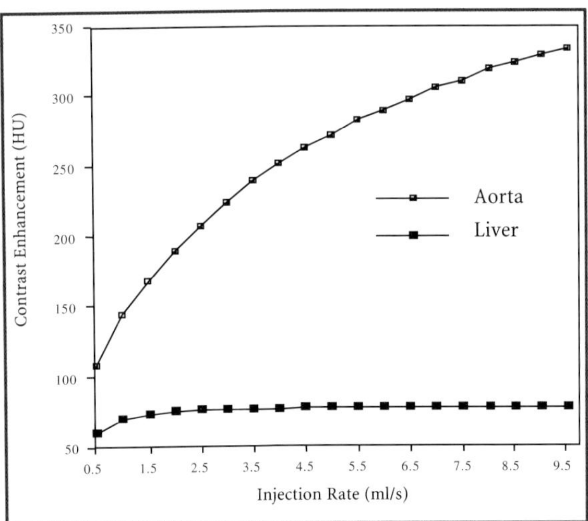

Fig. 5. Effect of contrast medium injection rate on the magnitude of peak contrast enhancement. Simulation of peak aortic and hepatic contrast enhancement at different injection rates based on a hypothetical adult male with a fixed height (5'8", or 173 cm) and body weight (150 lbs, or 68 kg) subjected to injection of 120 ml of contrast medium. Reprinted with permission from Bae KT, Heiken JP, Brink JA (1998) Aortic and hepatic peak enhancement at CT: effect of contrast medium injection rate-pharmacokinetic analysis and experimental porcine model. Radiology 206:455-464

desired contrast enhancement. On the other hand, when the injection rate is increased at a fixed volume of contrast medium, the peaks of enhancement increase in magnitude and occur earlier and the duration of high-magnitude enhancement decreases (Fig. 4). However, for a given increase in injection rate, the rate of increase in the magnitude of aortic contrast enhancement is substantially greater than that of the liver (Fig. 5) [22–24].

To obtain a fast arterial CT scan (e.g., for MDCT angiography applications), an increased injection rate resulting in a shortened but elevated magnitude of arterial enhancement is beneficial. On the other hand, a longer injection duration resulting in more prolonged vascular enhancement is preferable for slower CT scans. Faster injection rate and shorter injection duration result in a longer interval between peak arterial enhancement and hepatic parenchymal equilibrium enhancement. Thus, a faster injection rate results not only in a higher magnitude of arterial enhancement but also in a greater temporal separation between the arterial and venous phases of hepatic enhancement (Fig. 6).

Practical Tips

1. The magnitude of peak aortic enhancement increases almost linearly with increases of injection rate (up to 8–10 ml/s), while peak hepatic enhancement increases much more gradually and is apparent only at relatively low injection rates (<3 ml/s).

2. A fast injection rate improves the separation of contrast-enhancement phases and thus is beneficial for multiphase examinations of the liver, pancreas, and kidneys, as optimized enhancement during each contrast enhancement phase may improve lesion detection and characterization.

and/or high injection rate) results in earlier peak arterial and parenchymal enhancement and requires a short scan delay. A long injection duration (i.e., high volume and/or low injection rate) results in later peak enhancement, and thus a longer scan delay is preferable.

Injection Rate

Both rate of delivery and total delivered mass of iodine are increased when the injection rate is increased at a fixed duration of injection. The magnitude of peak vascular and parenchymal enhancement increases with a wider temporal window of

Table 1. Contrast enhancement times and proposed scan delays in different applications

	Pulmonary CTA	Coronary thoracic aorta CTA	Abdominal aorta/peripheral runoff	Hepatic parenchyma/portal vein
Contrast arrival time (s)[a]	$Tarr = 7$–10	$Tarr = 12$–15	$Tarr = 15$–18	30–40 ($Tarr = 15$–18)
Peak time (s)[a]	From 15 to ID (peak reaches a plateau rapidly)	$ID + (0 \text{ to } 5)$[b]	$ID + (5 \text{ to } 10)$[b]	$ID + (25 \text{ to } 40)$[b]
Fixed scan delay (s)	15 (20 for slow injection)	20	30 (20-25 for slow scan)	60–70
Variable scan delay (s)	15 (20 for slow injection)	$ID + 5 - SD/2$	$ID + 5 - SD/2$	$ID + 35 - SD/2$
Circulation-adjusted delay	$Tarr + 5$	$ID + (Tarr - 10) - SD/2$	$ID + (Tarr - 10) - SD/2$	$ID + (Tarr \times 2 + 5) - SD/2$

CTA computed tomography angiography, *Tarr* contrast arrival time, *ID* injection duration (s), *SD* scan duration (s)
For CTA, ID = "15 s + $^1/_2$ SD" (with saline flush) or "20 s + $^1/_2$ SD" (without saline flush) is suggested with the injection rate of 4 ml/s
For the liver, ID is determined by considering the total iodine load of 0.5 gI/kg
Peak time increases by 3–5 s with the use of saline flush
Tarr: **a** for pulmonary CTA, 100 HU threshold over the pulmonary artery with the first scan at 10 s after the start of the injection; **b** for aorta and hepatic phases, 50 HU threshold over the aorta with the first scan at 10 s after the start of the injection
[a] Assuming normal cardiac circulation, body weight of 60–80 kg, and the injection rate of 3–5 ml/s via the antecubital vein
[b] A larger number is used for a shorter injection duration

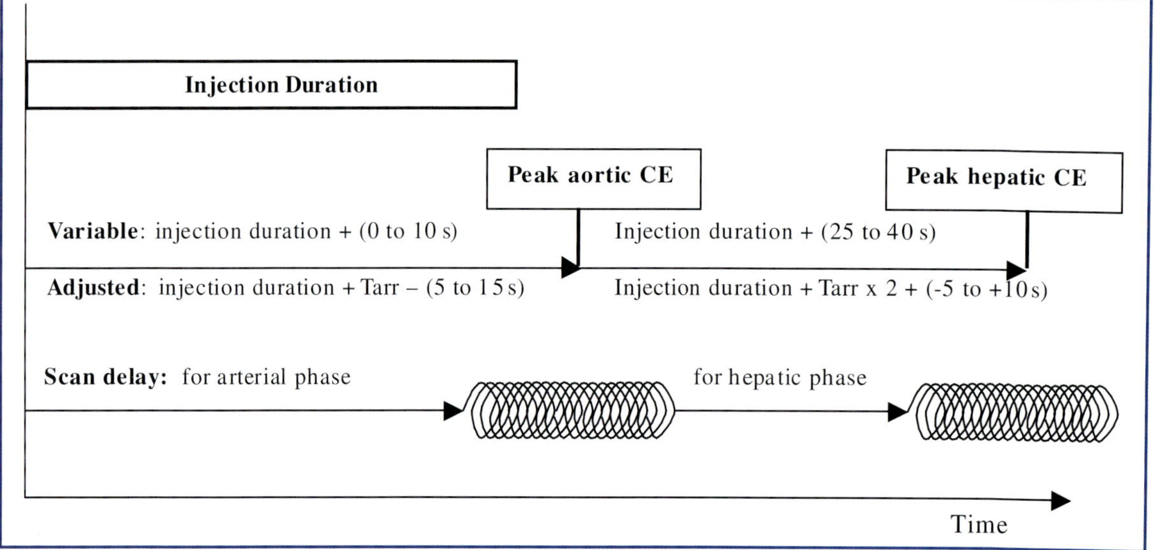

Fig. 9. Schematic diagram describing the times-to-peak aortic and hepatic contrast enhancement (CE) and associated scan delays for a given injection duration. Times-to-peak enhancement of the arterial and hepatic phases are estimated from injection durations and contrast arrival times. We propose two approaches of estimating time-to-peak enhancement: variable (contrast arrival time is empirically estimated assuming normal circulation) and circulation-adjusted (contrast arrival time is measured using a test-bolus or bolus-tracking technique). From estimated peak time, scan delay can be calculated by subtracting one-half of the scan duration

Practical Tips

1. Three factors should be considered when determining a scan delay for CTA: (1) contrast medium injection duration, (2) *Tarr*, and (3) scan duration.

2. Traditionally, for slow CTA studies, the scan delay was chosen to equal a patient's *Tarr*. Because this approach does not provide precise scan timing with faster MDCT scanners and shorter injection durations, an additional diagnostic delay must be included to determine the

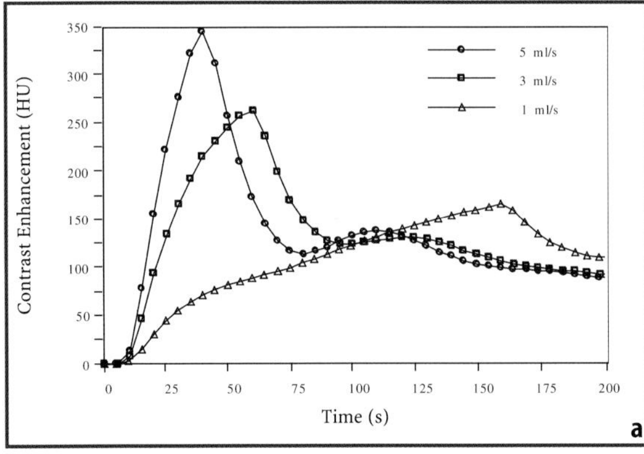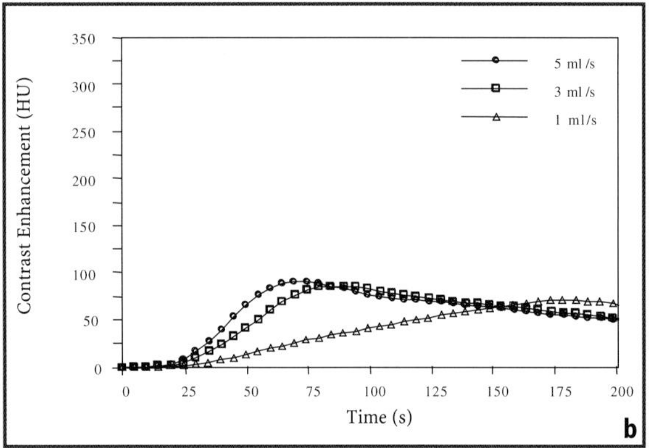

Fig. 4a, b. Simulated contrast enhancement curves with three different contrast medium injection rates. Simulated enhancement curves of the **a** aorta and **b** liver based on a hypothetical adult male with a fixed height (5'8", or 173 cm) and body weight (150 lbs, or 68 kg) subjected to 150 ml of contrast medium injected at 1, 3, and 5 ml/s. The curves show that for a fixed volume of contrast medium, as the rate of injection increases, the magnitude of contrast enhancement increases and the duration of high-magnitude contrast enhancement decreases. Figure 4a reprinted with permission of Anderson Publishing from Bae KT. Technical aspects of contrast delivery in advanced CT. Appl Radiol. 32 (12) (Suppl): 12-19. © Anderson Publishing

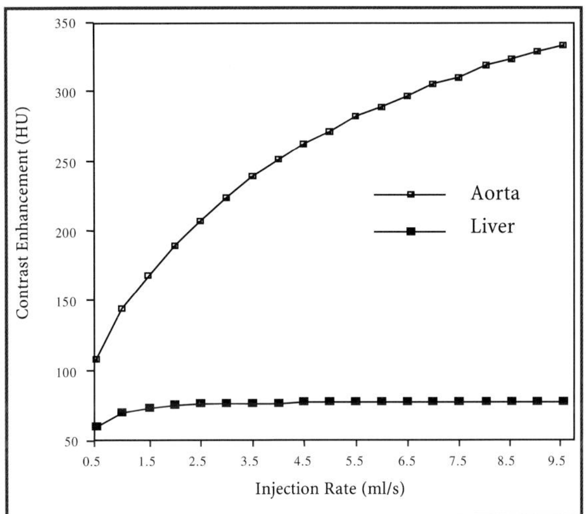

Fig. 5. Effect of contrast medium injection rate on the magnitude of peak contrast enhancement. Simulation of peak aortic and hepatic contrast enhancement at different injection rates based on a hypothetical adult male with a fixed height (5'8", or 173 cm) and body weight (150 lbs, or 68 kg) subjected to injection of 120 ml of contrast medium. Reprinted with permission from Bae KT, Heiken JP, Brink JA (1998) Aortic and hepatic peak enhancement at CT: effect of contrast medium injection rate-pharmacokinetic analysis and experimental porcine model. Radiology 206:455-464

and/or high injection rate) results in earlier peak arterial and parenchymal enhancement and requires a short scan delay. A long injection duration (i.e., high volume and/or low injection rate) results in later peak enhancement, and thus a longer scan delay is preferable.

Injection Rate

Both rate of delivery and total delivered mass of iodine are increased when the injection rate is increased at a fixed duration of injection. The magnitude of peak vascular and parenchymal enhancement increases with a wider temporal window of

desired contrast enhancement. On the other hand, when the injection rate is increased at a fixed volume of contrast medium, the peaks of enhancement increase in magnitude and occur earlier and the duration of high-magnitude enhancement decreases (Fig. 4). However, for a given increase in injection rate, the rate of increase in the magnitude of aortic contrast enhancement is substantially greater than that of the liver (Fig. 5) [22–24].

To obtain a fast arterial CT scan (e.g., for MDCT angiography applications), an increased injection rate resulting in a shortened but elevated magnitude of arterial enhancement is beneficial. On the other hand, a longer injection duration resulting in more prolonged vascular enhancement is preferable for slower CT scans. Faster injection rate and shorter injection duration result in a longer interval between peak arterial enhancement and hepatic parenchymal equilibrium enhancement. Thus, a faster injection rate results not only in a higher magnitude of arterial enhancement but also in a greater temporal separation between the arterial and venous phases of hepatic enhancement (Fig. 6).

Practical Tips

1. The magnitude of peak aortic enhancement increases almost linearly with increases of injection rate (up to 8–10 ml/s), while peak hepatic enhancement increases much more gradually and is apparent only at relatively low injection rates (<3 ml/s).
2. A fast injection rate improves the separation of contrast-enhancement phases and thus is beneficial for multiphase examinations of the liver, pancreas, and kidneys, as optimized enhancement during each contrast enhancement phase may improve lesion detection and characterization.

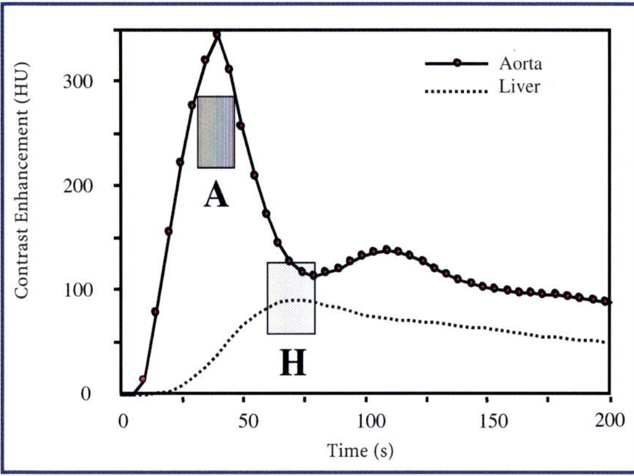

Fig. 6. Simulated aortic and hepatic contrast enhancement curves with a high contrast injection rate. Aortic (*solid line*) and hepatic (*dashed line*) contrast enhancement curves are simulated using a physiologically based compartment model (body weight 150 lbs, or 68 kg, and height 5′8″, or 173 cm) subjected to a high injection rate protocol (150 ml of contrast medium injected at 5 ml/s) (14). A high injection rate not only increases the magnitude of arterial enhancement, but it also provides greater temporal separation between the arterial (*A*) and venous (*H*) phases of enhancement. This distinct phase separation is beneficial for multiphase scanning of the liver, pancreas, and kidneys. Reprinted from [94]

Concentration

The availability of contrast media with high iodine concentrations (350 mgI/ml and above) has attracted a great deal of interest recently for MDCT applications [21, 25–39]. For injections of fixed duration, rate, and volume, a contrast medium with a high iodine concentration will deliver a larger total iodine load more rapidly. The resulting magnitude of peak contrast enhancement is increased, and the temporal window at a given level of enhancement is wider. Conversely, time-to-peak enhancement is unaffected because duration and rate of injection remain constant.

On the other hand, when the need is to maintain a constant total iodine mass and injection rate, injection volume and duration vary with contrast medium concentration. Under these conditions, the injected volume of a contrast medium with high iodine concentration is smaller than that of a contrast medium with low iodine concentration. The duration of enhancement is shorter with the higher concentration agent because of reduced contrast medium volume. Nevertheless, contrast medium with a higher iodine concentration delivers more iodine mass per unit time and thus results in earlier and greater peak aortic enhancement (Fig. 7). The effect is the same as that seen with the use of a high injection rate.

Practical Tips

1. For a fast MDCT scan, a high iodine delivery rate is desirable to maximize arterial enhancement for CTA and to depict hypervascular tumors.
2. Use of a contrast medium with high iodine concentration is an alternative approach to using an increased injection rate to increase iodine delivery rate.

Saline Flush

A saline flush "pushes" the tail of the injected contrast medium bolus into the central blood volume and thus makes use of contrast medium that

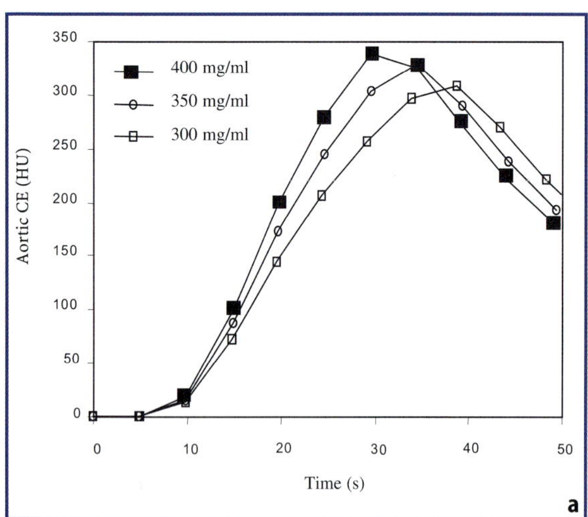

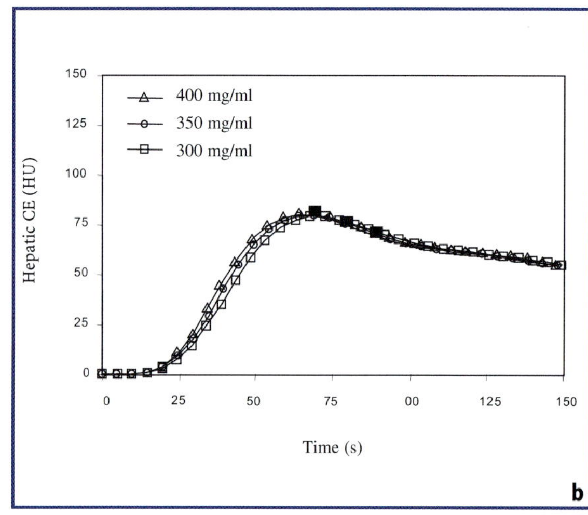

Fig. 7a, b. Simulated contrast enhancement curves with a fixed amount of iodine mass but three different contrast medium concentrations injected at a constant rate. Simulated enhancement curves of the **a** aorta and **b** liver based on a hypothetical adult male with a fixed height (5′8″, or 173 cm) and body weight (150 lbs, or 68 kg) subjected to 5 ml/s injection of the same amount of iodine mass but at three different concentrations and volumes: 300 mgI/ml, 140 ml; 350 mgI/ml, 120 ml; and 400 mgI/ml, 105 ml. The aortic time-enhancement curves demonstrate that the use of high-concentration contrast material is associated with earlier and greater peak aortic enhancement. The effect of high iodine concentration contrast material on liver enhancement is minimal if iodine mass is unchanged. Reprinted with permission of Anderson Publishing from Bae KT. Technical aspects of contrast delivery in advanced CT. Appl Radiol 32 (12) (Suppl):12-19. © 2003 Anderson Publishing

would otherwise remain unused in the injection tubing and peripheral veins. A saline flush therefore increases both the level of contrast enhancement and the efficiency of contrast medium utilization [40–47]. Additional advantages of a saline flush include improved bolus geometry due to reduced intravascular contrast medium dispersion and, on thoracic CT studies, reduced streak artifact from dense contrast material in the brachiocephalic vein and superior vena cava. A saline flush is particularly beneficial when a small volume of contrast medium is used. For this reason, a saline flush is commonly used for gadolinium-enhanced magnetic resonance imaging (MRI) but has not been widely used in CT, in part because a double-barrel CT contrast injector has not been commercially available until recently. With the increasing use of MDCT and the increasing clinical application of CTA, use of a saline flush is rapidly becoming accepted in clinical practice to compensate for the use of smaller contrast medium volumes.

The volume of contrast medium that can be substituted by saline flush without affecting the degree of contrast enhancement depends on the "dead-space" volume of the injection tubing and the peripheral venous blood volume between the brachial vein and the superior vena cava. The peripheral venous blood volume is in turn related to patient size or weight. In a typical clinical setting, the amount of contrast medium saving may be anything between 12 ml and 20 ml.

Practical Tips

1. A saline flush improves contrast enhancement, the efficiency of contrast medium use and reduces artifacts; this is particularly beneficial when a small total amount of contrast medium is used.
2. Twenty to 30 ml of saline flush may be sufficient, and injection of a larger quantity might not further improve contrast enhancement.

Arterial CT Angiography

MDCT readily permits acquisition of images with high spatial and temporal resolution. The benefits of MDCT angiography are such that most conventional catheter-based diagnostic angiography examinations have been replaced by this technique.

For example, pulmonary CTA is now the most commonly practiced CTA application in the routine clinical setting. Improved spatial resolution on MDCT permits excellent delineation of peripheral pulmonary arteries and detection of small emboli. Improved temporal resolution deriving from increased scan speeds on the more recent 16- and 64-slice MDCT scanners permits a pulmonary CTA examination to be performed within a few seconds. Moreover, better temporal resolution results in reduced motion artifacts, with improved contrast enhancement and image quality. Advances in MDCT and electrocardiogram (ECG)-gating technology enable acquisition of high-resolution, motion-free images of the heart and coronary CTA within a single short breath hold. Aortic CTA and peripheral run-off CTA are additional routine applications with MDCT.

Contrast Enhancement Magnitude

As discussed above, the magnitude of arterial contrast enhancement for CTA depends on a number of patient-related and injection-related factors, including body weight and cardiac output, contrast medium volume and concentration, injection rate, type of contrast medium, and saline flush. The magnitude of arterial enhancement increases in direct proportion to the rate of iodine delivery, which is dependent on injection rate and contrast medium concentration (Figs. 4 and 7). In addition, when contrast medium is injected at a constant rate, enhancement increases continuously over time, with increasing injection duration due to the cumulative effects of new incoming contrast medium and recirculated contrast medium. Without recirculation, contrast enhancement reaches a steady-state plateau. The use of a contrast medium with a higher iodine concentration results in a greater magnitude of aortic contrast enhancement, even if the total iodine dose and injection rate are unchanged. This is due to the increased rate of iodine delivery into the vascular system.

The amount of contrast medium required for CTA is determined by the desired level of enhancement, vessels of interest, and scan duration. Although the magnitude of hepatic enhancement needed to detect focal lesions has been investigated extensively, to date, only a few studies have addressed the minimum degree of enhancement needed for CTA. Becker et al. [26] considered an attenuation of 250–300 HU to be optimal for coronary CTA, since this attenuation permitted adequate differentiation of low-density coronary artery atherosclerotic lesions (which typically have a density of approximately 40 HU), intermediate fibrous plaque (approximately 90 HU), and calcified plaque (>350 HU) without obscuring coronary calcifications. However, when imaging is performed to identify significant stenoses, visualization of the lumen is more important, and higher vascular attenuation (>300 HU) may improve visualization of small coronary vessels [39]. In our opinion, for most CTA applications, contrast enhancement of 250–300 HU (i.e., attenuation of

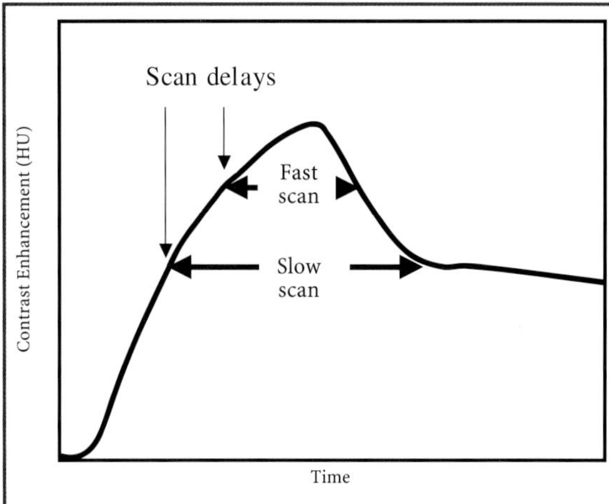

Fig. 8. Simulated aortic contrast enhancement curve with two different scan delays designated for the fast and the slow scans. For given duration of contrast enhancement or injection, the shorter the scan duration, the longer the additional delay needed to ensure that imaging takes place during the peak of aortic enhancement

300–350 HU) is adequate for the diagnosis of a wide range of vascular pathology.

In a coronary CTA study performed on a 4-row MDCT scanner, Becker et al. [26] reported that 40 g iodine (gI) (equivalent to 114 ml of a 350 mgI/ml concentration) injected at a flow rate of 1 gI/s (equivalent to 3.3 ml/s of a 350 mgI/ml concentration) resulted in an attenuation of 250–300 HU, although no information was given about patient weight. In a similar but more elaborate comparative coronary CTA study with 16-row MDCT, Cademartiri et al. [39] reported that 42–49 gI at an injection rate of 1.2–1.4 gI/s generated a mean coronary artery attenuation of 273–333 HU (average patient weight 72–74 kg). In our experience, with a 64-row MDCT scanner, a volume of approximately 1.2 ml/kg of 350 mgI/ml contrast medium injected at a rate of 4 ml/s (i.e., 0.4 gI/kg of contrast medium injected at 1.4 gI/s) yields a contrast enhancement of approximately 250 HU in the pulmonary artery. Based on these observations, we thus estimate that diagnostically adequate coronary artery enhancement may be obtained for a 70-kg patient with (1) 45 gI injected at 1.2 gI/s (e.g., 128 ml of 350 mgI/ml concentration @ 3.3 ml/s) over 40 s for 4-row MDCT, (2) 42 gI injected at 1.4 gI/s (e.g., 120 ml of 350 mgI/ml concentration @ 4 ml/s) over 30 s for 16-row MDCT, and (3) 35 gI injected at 1.4 gI/s (e.g., 100 ml of 350 mgI/ml concentration @ 4 ml/s) over 25 s for 64-row MDCT. With these contrast medium administration schemes, a mean coronary artery attenuation of 300–350 HU can be expected for a 70-kg patient. A saline flush may further reduce the contrast medium requirement by 15–25 ml as well as helping to reduce the level of artifact in the superior vena cava and right heart. In order to maintain an equivalent degree of contrast enhancement, larger patients require a larger iodine dose while smaller patients require a smaller iodine dose.

For peripheral run off CTA, the amount of contrast medium required for adequate enhancement of the abdominal aorta and peripheral arteries depends on patient weight and scan duration. For a patient with a body weight of 60–80 kg, an injection rate of 1.4 gI/s (4 ml/s of a 350 mgI/ml concentration) is probably sufficient. This is similar to the scheme for pulmonary and coronary CTA described above. The rate can be increased or decreased depending on the patient's body weight and the concentration of contrast medium used.

A common approach to selecting the injection duration for a CTA examination with a long scan time (>25 s) is to keep injection duration identical to scan duration. This approach, however, does not work with a short scan time (<15 s). If scan time and injection duration are equally short, then the result will be poor overall enhancement. Although enhancement can be improved by using a faster injection rate or a higher iodine concentration, there are clear practical restrictions on the extent to which these parameters can be increased to compensate for a short injection duration or low contrast volume.

Practical Tips

1. When contrast medium volume is reduced for CTA with MDCT, an increased injection rate and high contrast medium concentration can compensate for the somewhat decreased magnitude of aortic enhancement achieved with the smaller contrast medium volume.
2. One approach to estimating the injection duration for a short scan may be to add a constant factor to the scan duration. For a patient with body weight of 60–80 kg who receives contrast medium injected at 1.4 gI/s (e.g., 4 ml/s of 350 mgI/ml concentration), our proposed injection duration is "15 s + $^1/_2$ scan duration" with a saline flush or "20 s + $^1/_2$ scan duration" without a saline flush. The injection rate can be increased or decreased depending on body weight and the concentration of contrast medium used.

Scan Timing

Three factors should be considered for determination of scan delays for CTA or parenchymal imaging: (1) contrast medium injection duration, (2) contrast arrival time (*Tarr*), and (3) scan duration.

In patients with normal cardiac output, peak arterial contrast enhancement is achieved shortly after termination of the contrast medium injection [20, 23]. Thus, in general, an injection of short duration (i.e., low volume and/or high injection rate) results in earlier peak arterial and parenchymal enhancement. In such cases, a short scan delay is required for CTA. On the other hand, an injection of long duration (i.e., high volume and/or low injection rate) results in later peak enhancement, and thus a longer scan delay is needed for CTA (Figs. 3 and 4).

In addition to injection duration, variation among patients in cardiac output (cardiovascular circulation time) should be taken into account when individualizing the scan delay for CTA studies. *Tarr* is related to the patient's cardiac output and can be measured using a test-bolus or bolus-tracking method. In our experience, the bolus-tracking method is a more efficient and practical approach, although some radiologists prefer the test-bolus method because it provides an additional opportunity to "test" the integrity of the venous access prior to injecting the full bolus of contrast medium. With both techniques, a region of interest (ROI) is usually placed just proximal to the organ of interest, e.g., on the main pulmonary artery or right ventricle for pulmonary CTA or on the ascending aorta or left ventricle for coronary CTA.

Traditionally, for slow CTA studies (single-row and 4-detector-row scanners), the scan delay was chosen to equal a patient's *Tarr*. However, this approach does not provide precise scan timing when faster MDCT scanners and shorter injection durations are utilized. This is because *Tarr* merely represents time of contrast arrival rather than optimal scan delay. For fast (i.e., 16- and 64-row) MDCT scanners, an "additional or diagnostic delay" must be included to determine the appropriate scan delay [20, 28]. The significance of the additional delay for optimal enhancement has been demonstrated both empirically [48] and theoretically [49]. Determination of the appropriate additional delay, which is related to scan speed and injection duration, is critical for fast MDCT. The shorter the scan duration, the longer the additional delay needed to ensure that imaging takes place during the peak of aortic enhancement (Fig. 8), unless the injection duration is shortened to match the reduced scan duration.

For the majority of pulmonary CTA studies, well-designed fixed scan delays (typically 15 s) are usually adequate because contrast enhancement in the pulmonary arteries increases rapidly with fast injections of contrast medium. However, precise timing in pulmonary CTA is crucial when a "tight" contrast bolus is used with fast MDCT because pulmonary artery enhancement can be delayed considerably in patients with cardiac dysfunction, pulmonary artery hypertension, or compromised central or peripheral venous flow [50, 51]. The need to individualize the scan delay for cardiac and coronary artery CTA is well recognized. For peripheral run-off CTA, it is crucial that the scan delay is long enough that the scan does not outpace the contrast bolus but is completed when the bolus reaches the pedal arteries. One approach is to reduce scan speed and to use a longer injection to match scan duration; this may be particularly appropriate for imaging diseased peripheral vessels [52].

Our proposed approach to determining a scan delay involves: (1) estimating time-to-peak contrast enhancement from injection duration and *Tarr*, and (2) calculating scan delay by subtracting one-half of the scan duration from the estimated peak enhancement time (Table 1, Fig. 9). Time-to-peak enhancement may be estimated using either a "variable" approach, in which *Tarr* is estimated assuming normal circulation, or a "circulation-adjusted" approach, in which *Tarr* is measured using a test-bolus or bolus-tracking technique.

For the variable scan delay approach, time-to-peak aortic enhancement is determined as "injection duration + (x s)," in which "x" is larger for shorter injection durations but is typically a number between 0 and 10 [23]. For example, for a 30-s injection, the peak aortic enhancement would occur at "30 + 5=35 s" (a 5-s additional delay is used in this example because a 30-s injection is considered to be of intermediate duration). Using this estimated peak time, scan delay for the arterial phase for a 20-s scan would be calculated as "35 – 20/2=25 s". Likewise, the scan delay for a 10-s scan would be "35 – 10/2=30 s".

For the circulation-adjusted delay approach, either a test-bolus or a bolus-tracking technique is used to measure *Tarr*. If 15 s is taken as the normal default value for *Tarr* (i.e., a typical value in a patient with normal circulation), time-to-peak aortic enhancement corresponds to "injection duration + (*Tarr* – 15) + (0 to 10 s)" or " injection duration + *Tarr* – (5 to 15 s)." Thus, at *Tarr* = 15, the circulation-adjusted and variable delay approaches are equivalent. The scan delay can be computed from this equation using the same steps as for the variable delay approach: for example, for a 10-s scan with a 30-s injection, the scan delay would be "30 + (*Tarr* – 15) + (5) – (10/2)" or "*Tarr* +15". Thus, when a test-bolus method is used, the scan delay is determined by adding 15 s to the measured *Tarr*. On the other hand, when a bolus-tracking method is used, *Tarr* is not estimated prior to the injection of a full bolus of contrast medium. In this case, the scan will start at "*Tarr* + 15": i.e., after 15 s of additional "diagnostic delay" once the 50-HU enhancement threshold is reached [53].

Table 1. Contrast enhancement times and proposed scan delays in different applications

	Pulmonary CTA	Coronary thoracic aorta CTA	Abdominal aorta/peripheral runoff	Hepatic parenchyma/portal vein
Contrast arrival time (s)[a]	$Tarr = 7–10$	$Tarr = 12–15$	$Tarr = 15–18$	30–40 ($Tarr = 15–18$)
Peak time (s)[a]	From 15 to ID (peak reaches a plateau rapidly)	ID + (0 to 5)[b]	ID + (5 to 10)[b]	ID + (25 to 40)[b]
Fixed scan delay (s)	15 (20 for slow injection)	20	30 (20-25 for slow scan)	60–70
Variable scan delay (s)	15 (20 for slow injection)	ID + 5 – SD/2	ID + 5 – SD/2	ID + 35 – SD/2
Circulation-adjusted delay	$Tarr$ + 5	ID + ($Tarr$ – 10) – SD/2	ID + ($Tarr$ – 10) – SD/2	ID + ($Tarr$×2+5) – SD/2

CTA computed tomography angiography, *Tarr* contrast arrival time, *ID* injection duration (s), *SD* scan duration (s)
For CTA, ID = "15 s + ¹/₂ SD" (with saline flush) or "20 s + ¹/₂ SD" (without saline flush) is suggested with the injection rate of 4 ml/s
For the liver, ID is determined by considering the total iodine load of 0.5 gI/kg
Peak time increases by 3–5 s with the use of saline flush
Tarr: **a** for pulmonary CTA, 100 HU threshold over the pulmonary artery with the first scan at 10 s after the start of the injection; **b** for aorta and hepatic phases, 50 HU threshold over the aorta with the first scan at 10 s after the start of the injection
[a]Assuming normal cardiac circulation, body weight of 60–80 kg, and the injection rate of 3–5 ml/s via the antecubital vein
[b]A larger number is used for a shorter injection duration

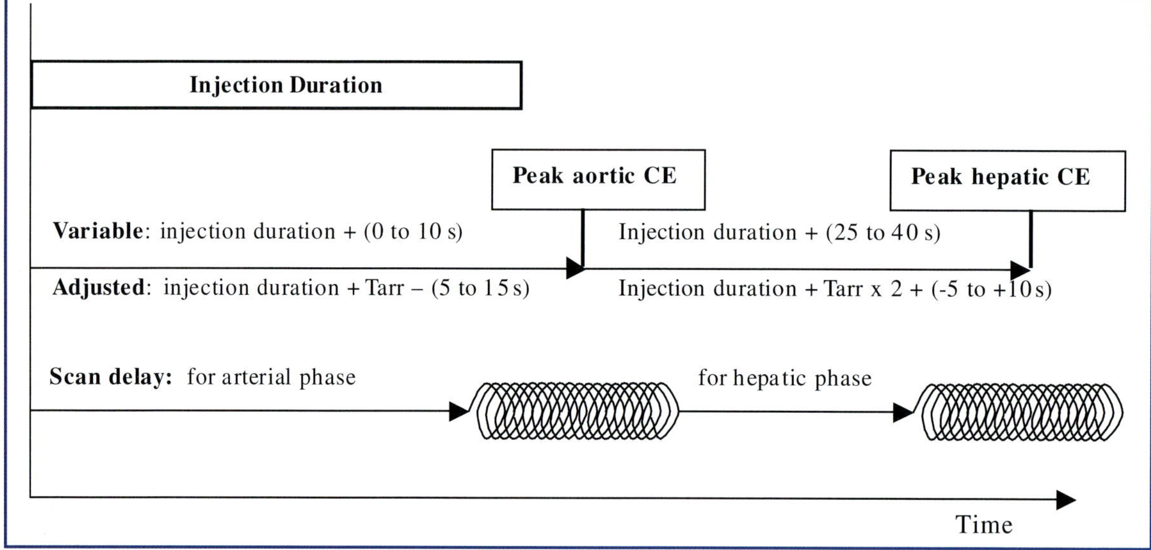

Fig. 9. Schematic diagram describing the times-to-peak aortic and hepatic contrast enhancement (CE) and associated scan delays for a given injection duration. Times-to-peak enhancement of the arterial and hepatic phases are estimated from injection durations and contrast arrival times. We propose two approaches of estimating time-to-peak enhancement: variable (contrast arrival time is empirically estimated assuming normal circulation) and circulation-adjusted (contrast arrival time is measured using a test-bolus or bolus-tracking technique). From estimated peak time, scan delay can be calculated by subtracting one-half of the scan duration

Practical Tips

1. Three factors should be considered when determining a scan delay for CTA: (1) contrast medium injection duration, (2) *Tarr*, and (3) scan duration.

2. Traditionally, for slow CTA studies, the scan delay was chosen to equal a patient's *Tarr*. Because this approach does not provide precise scan timing with faster MDCT scanners and shorter injection durations, an additional diagnostic delay must be included to determine the

appropriate scan delay.

3. The shorter the scan duration, the longer the additional delay needed to ensure that imaging takes place during the peak of aortic enhancement.

4. The scan delay can be calculated by subtracting one-half of the scan duration from time-to-peak enhancement time. The time-to-peak enhancement in turn is estimated from the injection duration and *Tarr* using either a variable approach or a circulation-adjusted approach.

Hepatic Imaging

Among the many clinical applications for MDCT in hepatic imaging are: detection and characterization of primary or metastatic hepatic lesions, diagnosis of diffuse liver diseases, assessment of vascular and biliary patency or obstruction, tumor staging, monitoring treatment response, and preoperative evaluation for surgical resection. The high temporal resolution of MDCT permits the liver to be imaged during multiple, precisely defined phases of contrast enhancement.

Multiphasic Hepatic Imaging

Approximately 20% of the blood supply to the liver derives from the hepatic artery, while the remaining 80% derives from the portal vein. Injected contrast medium initially reaches the liver via the hepatic artery; in patients with normal circulation, the typical hepatic artery arrival time is approximately 15 s after the start of the injection. During the next 10–20 s, contrast medium from the splanchnic venous return enters the portal vein and hepatic parenchyma. However, whereas contrast medium from the splenic and pancreatic circulation arrives in the portal vein earlier than that from the intestinal circulation, the contribution of the portal vein to hepatic enhancement is usually very small within the first 30 s after initiation of the contrast injection [54, 55].

For routine abdominal CT or as part of a thoracoabdominal and pelvic imaging survey, the liver is scanned once during the hepatic phase, i.e., during the phase of maximal liver parenchyma enhancement. However, to detect hypervascular liver lesions or to evaluate the hepatic vascular anatomy, it is highly desirable to scan during at least one phase prior to the hepatic phase. When optimizing multiphasic hepatic imaging, the goal is to scan during maximal enhancement for each phase and to minimize the influence of other enhancement phases.

For dedicated hepatic CT imaging, the three contrast-enhancement phases of interest are early arterial phase, late arterial/portal vein inflow phase, and hepatic parenchymal phase [56]. The early arterial phase begins with the arrival of contrast medium in the hepatic artery and ends prior to portal vein enhancement. The diagnostically useful early arterial phase begins about 10 s after contrast arrival and lasts for approximately 10 s (20–30 s from the start of contrast medium injection with a typical injection protocol and normal circulation). Prior to this, at the time of earliest contrast arrival in the hepatic artery, enhancement is too weak for adequate early arterial phase imaging. The late arterial/portal vein inflow phase (referred to simply as the late arterial phase in this chapter) corresponds to the time of maximum aortic enhancement. This occurs shortly (typically 0–10 s) after completion of injection, with the optimal temporal window lasting approximately 10 s. The hepatic parenchymal phase occurs when the peak contrast bolus has traveled through the splanchnic circulation and has returned to the portal venous system. This occurs typically at 25–40 s after completion of the injection and corresponds to the phase of maximum hepatic parenchyma enhancement.

The early arterial phase of enhancement is useful primarily for acquisition of a pure arterial data set for CTA and has only a limited role in imaging the liver. For detection of hypervascular primary or metastatic neoplasms, the late arterial phase is the preferred imaging phase [25, 57–67]. During this phase, hypervascular hepatic lesions enhance maximally while the hepatic parenchyma remains relatively unenhanced, commensurate with the relatively small contribution of the hepatic artery to the total hepatic blood supply. The hepatic parenchymal phase, the period of peak hepatic enhancement, is the phase used for routine abdominal CT imaging. Most hepatic lesions, including most metastases, are hypovascular and are therefore best depicted against the maximally enhanced hepatic parenchyma during this phase. The delayed imaging phase (>3 min after the start of contrast injection) is useful for detecting and characterizing some hepatocellular carcinomas [68] and for characterizing cholangiocarcinomas [69]. During this phase, hepatocellular carcinomas typically appear hypoattenuating whereas cholangiocarcinomas often demonstrate delayed contrast enhancement relative to the background hepatic parenchyma.

Contrast Enhancement Magnitude

The magnitude of hepatic enhancement is affected by numerous factors, such as contrast medium volume and concentration, rate and type of injection, scan delay time, and body weight [2, 7–10, 13–15,

22, 23, 25, 32, 33, 70–78]. The magnitude of hepatic parenchymal enhancement is directly and almost linearly related to the amount of total iodine mass administered (i.e., total contrast medium volume × concentration) [2, 8, 10, 15, 22, 23, 70–73, 75, 77, 78] (Fig. 3b). The most important patient-related factor affecting the magnitude of hepatic enhancement is body weight, which demonstrates a linear inverse relationship with the magnitude of enhancement: as body weight increases, the magnitude of hepatic parenchymal enhancement decreases [1, 2, 73] (Fig. 1b). As a consequence, the total iodine load should be increased when imaging large patients in order to achieve a constant degree of hepatic enhancement. The iodine load can be increased by increasing contrast medium concentration, volume injected, or injection rate [13, 23, 78].

Insufficient hepatic parenchymal enhancement results in diminished lesion conspicuity [16, 17, 73]. The minimum level of hepatic enhancement acceptable for adequate liver imaging has variously been reported to be 30 HU [79], 40 HU [80–82], or 50 HU [9, 33, 74, 77, 83, 84]. In a multicenter study, Megibow et al. [19] found that 30 HU was the lowest limit of acceptable hepatic enhancement and that no definite clinical gain was achieved with hepatic enhancement greater than 50 HU. The iodine mass required to achieve this enhancement can be estimated on the basis of patient weight [2, 77]. In this regard, Heiken et al. [2] found that the maximum hepatic enhancement calculated as a function of patient weight was 96±19 HU per gram of iodine per kilogram of body weight. Thus, approximately 0.5 gI/kg is needed to achieve the maximum hepatic enhancement of 50 HU; i.e., 35 gI for a 70-kg patient. A similar weight-adjusted dose conversion ratio was reported in later studies [37, 67, 73, 78, 85].

Hepatic parenchymal enhancement increases mildly with an increase in injection rate although this is apparent only at relatively low injection rates (<3 ml/s) [22, 23, 74] (Figs. 4 and 5). Although the magnitude of hepatic parenchymal enhancement may not increase substantially at high injection rates (e.g., 4– 6 ml/s) compared with intermediate injection rates (e.g., 2–3 ml/s), a fast injection rate increases the magnitude of hepatic arterial enhancement and thus better separates the peaks of hepatic arterial and hepatic parenchymal enhancement [23, 62, 86]. As a result, fast injection rates are desirable in multiphase hepatic imaging and for detection of hypervascular liver masses [62, 73–75, 86, 87] (Fig. 6). Likewise, recent studies [25, 33, 35, 37, 38] that compared contrast media with different iodine concentrations for dual-phase MDCT liver imaging found that high-concentration contrast medium increases detection of hypervascular lesions by increasing the iodine delivery rate (Fig. 7a).

Practical Tips

1. The magnitude of hepatic parenchymal enhancement is directly and almost linearly related to the total administered iodine mass per body weight. When imaging large patients, the total iodine load should be increased to achieve a constant degree of hepatic enhancement.
2. Approximately 0.5 gI/kg is needed to achieve the maximum hepatic enhancement of 50 HU; i.e., 35 gI for a 70-kg patient.
3. Although increasing the delivery rate of iodine (i.e., use of high injection rate or high-concentration contrast medium) may not substantially increase the magnitude of hepatic parenchymal enhancement, it is desirable in multiphase hepatic imaging and for detection of hypervascular liver masses because it increases the magnitude of hepatic arterial enhancement and better separates the peaks of hepatic arterial and hepatic parenchymal enhancement.

Scan Timing

Fixed scan delays from the initiation of contrast medium injection are commonly used for hepatic imaging. The typical scan delay for arterial phase imaging for a 30-s contrast medium injection is 20–30 s for SDCT [58] and 30–35 s for MDCT. For both SDCT and MDCT, the scan delay for hepatic parenchymal phase imaging is approximately 55–70 s. Note that the scan delay required for arterial phase imaging on MDCT is longer than that on SDCT because the shorter image acquisition time of MDCT permits scanning to be performed more closely to the peak of aortic enhancement.

Whereas the hepatic enhancement phase lasts 20–30 s, with gradual changes in enhancement, the arterial phase lasts for only 10-15 s, with abrupt changes in enhancement [88]. Thus, it is more critical to accurately determine the scan delay for the arterial phase. The time to aortic contrast arrival varies widely, from 10–36 s [64, 66, 86, 89], due to interindividual variations in circulation time. It is therefore necessary to use a test-bolus or bolus-tracking technique to acquire images during individualized enhancement phases.

Both test-bolus [13, 25, 37, 64, 66, 78] and bolus-tracking methods [11, 32, 34, 86, 89–92] have been used to determine the arterial phase scan delay for dual-phase hepatic imaging studies. Typically, an ROI is placed over the descending thoracic aorta just above the diaphragmatic dome at the same level as the start of the diagnostic scan. *Tarr* in the aorta is measured from the peak timing of a test bolus (15–20 ml of contrast) or, when using a bolus-tracking program, from the time to reach a contrast enhancement threshold of 50–100 HU above baseline attenuation. In order to avoid the early arterial phase and to scan during the late arterial phase, a further 5- to 15-s delay is added to determine scan delay. As discussed above, the magnitude of this additional delay depends on injection duration and scan speed.

Scan delays for both the arterial and hepatic phases can be determined by considering injection duration, *Tarr*, and scan duration. The time-to-peak enhancement of the arterial and hepatic phases can be estimated from injection duration and arterial *Tarr* (Table 1, Fig. 9). The scan delay can be calculated from the estimated peak enhancement time by subtracting one-half of the scan duration. Again, both variable and circulation-adjusted approaches can be used.

Time-to-peak aortic enhancement is estimated as described previously in the section on CTA. For the variable scan delay approach, using an estimated peak time derived as "injection duration + (0 to 10 s)" [23], the scan delay for the arterial phase for a 20-s scan with a 30-s injection would be "30 + 5 – 20/2=25" s, while that for a 10-s scan would be "30 + 5 – 10/2 = 30 s". For the circulation-adjusted scan delay approach, the time-to-peak aortic enhancement corresponds to "injection duration + (*Tarr* – 15)+(0 to 10 s)" or "injection duration + *Tarr* – (5 to 15 s)." For a 10-s scan with a 30-s injection, the scan delay would be "30 + (*Tarr* – 15) + (5) – (10/2)" or "*Tarr* + 15". When a bolus-tracking method is used, the scan will start at "*Tarr* + 15," i.e., after 15 s of additional diagnostic delay once the 50 HU enhancement threshold is reached [53].

Time-to-peak hepatic enhancement for the variable scan delay approach is estimated as "injection duration + (25 to 40 s)" [23, 73, 93]. Again, a longer additional delay is added for injections of shorter duration. For example, for a 30-s injection, peak hepatic enhancement would occur at "30 + 35 = 65" s. The scan delay for the hepatic phase for a 20-s scan would then be "65 – 20/2=55 s", while that for a 10-s scan would be "65 – 10/2=60 s". Using arterial *Tarr* measured over the abdominal aorta, for the circulation-adjusted scan delay approach, time-to-peak hepatic enhancement can be estimated as "injection duration + *Tarr*×2 + (–5 to +10 s)." When *Tarr* is 15 s, this equation is again identical to that of a delay determined using the variable approach. For a 10-s scan with 30-s injection, the scan delay would be "30 + *Tarr*×2 + (5) – (10/2)" s, or "*Tarr* × 2 + 30 s". At a *Tarr* of 15 s, the scan delay for the hepatic phase would be 60 s.

Practical Tips

1. Three factors should be considered when determining scan delays for hepatic imaging: (1) contrast medium injection duration, (2) *Tarr*, and (3) scan duration.
2. For multiphase hepatic imaging, it is more crit-

ical to accurately determine the scan delay for the arterial phase than for the hepatic phase. A test-bolus or bolus-tracking technique is used to acquire images during individualized enhancement phases.

3. Time-to-peak enhancement of the arterial and hepatic phases can be estimated from injection duration and arterial *Tarr*. From the estimated peak enhancement time, the scan delay can be calculated by subtracting one-half of the scan duration. Just as with CTA, both the variable and circulation-adjusted approaches to estimating the times-to-peak enhancement are possible for hepatic imaging.

Summary

A variety of patient-related and injection-related factors can affect the magnitude and timing of intravenous contrast medium enhancement. Although these factors are interrelated, some (body size, contrast volume, iodine concentration, saline flush) have more of an effect on enhancement magnitude, while others (cardiac output, contrast injection duration, contrast injection rate) have more of an effect on the temporal pattern of contrast enhancement.

MDCT, with its dramatically shorter image acquisition times, permits images with high spatial resolution to be acquired at multiple, precisely defined phases of contrast enhancement. However, to make full use of the benefits that MDCT provides, protocols for contrast administration and scan timing must be modified to take into account the specific objectives of each clinical imaging application and the different MDCT scanners available. For example, a faster injection rate or a contrast medium with high iodine concentration may be desirable for many MDCT applications to improve arterial enhancement and tumor-to-parenchyma attenuation difference during the hepatic arterial phase. Injection duration should be considered for determinations of scan delay because it critically affects time-to-peak enhancement. Individualized scan delay is more critical with MDCT than with SDCT. The contrast arrival time (*Tarr*) measured using test-bolus or bolus-tracking techniques can be integrated with injection duration to predict peak enhancement time. The scan delay is then estimated such that the center of the scan is timed to the peak of contrast enhancement.

References

1. Kormano M, Partanen K, Soimakallio S, Kivimaki T (1983) Dynamic contrast enhancement of the upper abdomen: effect of contrast medium and body

weight. Invest Radiol 18:364–367

2. Heiken JP, Brink JA, McClennan BL et al (1995) Dynamic incremental CT: effect of volume and concentration of contrast material and patient weight on hepatic enhancement. Radiology 195:353–357

3. Platt JF, Reige KA, Ellis JH (1999) Aortic enhancement during abdominal CT angiography: correlation with test injections, flow rates, and patient demographics. AJR Am J Roentgenol 172:53–56

4. Bae KT (2003) Technical aspects of contrast delivery in advanced CT. Applied Radiology 32 [Suppl]:12–19

5. van Hoe L, Marchal G, Baert AL et al (1995) Determination of scan delay time in spiral CT-angiography: utility of a test bolus injection. J Comput Assist Tomogr 19:216–220

6. Kirchner J, Kickuth R, Laufer U (2000) Optimized enhancement in helical CT: experiences with a real-time bolus tracking system in 628 patients. Clin Radiol 55:368–373

7. Bae KT, Heiken JP, Brink JA (1998) Aortic and hepatic contrast medium enhancement at CT. Part II. Effect of reduced cardiac output in a porcine model. Radiology 207:657–662

8. Dean PB, Violante MR, Mahoney JA (1980) Hepatic CT contrast enhancement: effect of dose, duration of infusion, and time elapsed following infusion. Invest Radiol 15:158–161

9. Heiken JP, Brink JA, McClennan BL et al (1993) Dynamic contrast-enhanced CT of the liver: comparison of contrast medium injection rates and uniphasic and biphasic injection protocols. Radiology 187:327–331

10. Chambers TP, Baron RL, Lush RM (1994) Hepatic CT enhancement. Part I. Alterations in the volume of contrast material within the same patients. Radiology 193:513–517

11. Kopka L, Rodenwaldt J, Fischer U et al (1996) Dual-phase helical CT of the liver: effects of bolus tracking and different volumes of contrast material. Radiology 201:321–326

12. Han JK, Kim AY, Lee KY et al (2000) Factors influencing vascular and hepatic enhancement at CT: experimental study on injection protocol using a canine model. J Comput Assist Tomogr 24:400–406

13. Awai K, Hiraishi K, Hori S (2004) Effect of contrast material injection duration and rate on aortic peak time and peak enhancement at dynamic CT involving injection protocol with dose tailored to patient weight. Radiology 230:142–150

14. Bae KT, Heiken JP, Brink JA (1998) Aortic and hepatic contrast medium enhancement at CT. Part I. Prediction with a computer model. Radiology 207:647–655

15. Berland LL, Lee JY (1988) Comparison of contrast media injection rates and volumes for hepatic dynamic incremented computed tomography. Investigative Radiology 23:918–922

16. Small WC, Nelson RC, Bernardino ME, Brummer LT (1994) Contrast-enhanced spiral CT of the liver: effect of different amounts and injection rates of contrast material on early contrast enhancement. AJR Am J Roentgenol 163:87–92

17. Freeny PC, Gardner JC, von Ingersleben G et al (1995) Hepatic helical CT: effect of reduction of iodine dose of intravenous contrast material on hepatic contrast enhancement. Radiology 197:89–93

18. Han JK, Choi BI, Kim AY, Kim SJ (2001) Contrast media in abdominal computed tomography: optimization of delivery methods. Korean J Radiol 2:28–36

19. Megibow AJ, Jacob G, Heiken JP et al (2001) Quantitative and qualitative evaluation of volume of low osmolality contrast medium needed for routine helical abdominal CT. AJR Am J Roentgenol 176:583–589

20. Bae KT (2003) Peak contrast enhancement in CT and MR angiography: When does it occur and why? Pharmacokinetic study in a porcine model. Radiology 2003; 227:809–816

21. Roos JE, Desbiolles LM, Weishaupt D et al (2004) Multi-detector row CT: effect of iodine dose reduction on hepatic and vascular enhancement. Rofo 176:556–563

22. Garcia PA, Bonaldi VM, Bret PM et al (1996) Effect of rate of contrast medium injection on hepatic enhancement at CT. Radiology 199:185–189

23. Bae KT, Heiken JP, Brink JA (1998) Aortic and hepatic peak enhancement at CT: effect of contrast medium injection rate – pharmacokinetic analysis and experimental porcine model. Radiology 206:455–464

24. Garcia P, Genin G, Bret PM et al (1999) Hepatic CT enhancement: effect of the rate and volume of contrast medium injection in an animal model. Abdom Imaging 24:597–603

25. Awai K, Takada K, Onishi H, Hori S (2002) Aortic and hepatic enhancement and tumor-to-liver contrast: analysis of the effect of different concentrations of contrast material at multi-detector row helical CT. Radiology 224:757–763

26. Becker CR, Hong C, Knez A et al (2003) Optimal contrast application for cardiac 4-detector-row computed tomography. Invest Radiol 38:690–694

27. Brink JA (2003) Use of high concentration contrast media (HCCM): principles and rationale-body CT. Eur J Radiol 45 [Suppl 1]:S53–58

28. Fleischmann D (2003) High-concentration contrast media in MDCT angiography: principles and rationale. Eur Radiol 13 [Suppl 3]:N39–43

29. Fleischmann D (2003) Use of high-concentration contrast media in multiple-detector-row CT: principles and rationale. Eur Radiol 13 [Suppl 5]:M14–20

30. Fleischmann D (2003) Use of high concentration contrast media: principles and rationale-vascular district. Eur J Radiol 45 [Suppl 1]:S88–93

31. Shinagawa M, Uchida M, Ishibashi M et al (2003) Assessment of pancreatic CT enhancement using a high concentration of contrast material. Radiat Med 21:74–79

32. Awai K, Inoue M, Yagyu Y et al (2004) Moderate versus high concentration of contrast material for aortic and hepatic enhancement and tumor-to-liver contrast at multi-detector row CT. Radiology 233:682–688

33. Furuta A, Ito K, Fujita T et al (2004) Hepatic enhancement in multiphasic contrast-enhanced MDCT: comparison of high- and low-iodine-concentration contrast medium in same patients with chronic liver disease. AJR Am J Roentgenol 183:157–162

34. Suzuki H, Oshima H, Shiraki N et al (2004) Comparison of two contrast materials with different iodine concentrations in enhancing the density of the the aorta, portal vein and liver at multi-detector row CT: a randomized study. Eur Radiol 14:2099–2104

35. Yagyu Y, Awai K, Inoue M et al (2005) MDCT of hypervascular hepatocellular carcinomas: a prospective study using contrast materials with different iodine concentrations. AJR Am J Roentgenol 184:1535–1540

36. Schoellnast H, Deutschmann HA, Fritz GA et al (2005) MDCT angiography of the pulmonary arteries: influence of iodine flow concentration on vessel attenuation and visualization. AJR Am J Roentgenol

184:1935–1939

37. Marchiano A, Spreafico C, Lanocita R et al (2005) Does iodine concentration affect the diagnostic efficacy of biphasic spiral CT in patients with hepatocellular carcinoma? Abdom Imaging 30:274–280

38. Itoh S, Ikeda M, Achiwa M (2005) Multiphase contrast-enhanced CT of the liver with a multislice CT scanner: effects of iodine concentration and delivery rate. Radiat Med 23:61–69

39. Cademartiri F, Mollet NR, van der Lugt A et al (2005) Intravenous contrast material administration at helical 16-detector row CT coronary angiography: effect of iodine concentration on vascular attenuation. Radiology 236:661–665

40. Hopper KD, Mosher TJ, Kasales CJ et al (1997) Thoracic spiral CT: delivery of contrast material pushed with injectable saline solution in a power injector. Radiology 205:269–271

41. Dorio PJ, Lee FT Jr, Henseler KP et al (2003) Using a saline chaser to decrease contrast media in abdominal CT. AJR Am J Roentgenol 180:929–934

42. Haage P, Schmitz-Rode T, Hubner D et al (2000) Reduction of contrast material dose and artifacts by a saline flush using a double power injector in helical CT of the thorax. AJR Am J Roentgenol 174:1049–1053

43. Irie T, Kajitani M, Yamaguchi M, Itai Y (2002) Contrast-enhanced CT with saline flush technique using two automated injectors: how much contrast medium does it save? J Comput Assist Tomogr 26:287–291

44. Schoellnast H, Tillich M, Deutschmann HA et al (2003) Abdominal multidetector row computed tomography: reduction of cost and contrast material dose using saline flush. J Comput Assist Tomogr 27:847–853

45. Cademartiri F, Mollet N, van der Lugt A et al (2004) Non-invasive 16-row multislice CT coronary angiography: usefulness of saline chaser. Eur Radiol 14:178–183

46. Schoellnast H, Tillich M, Deutschmann MJ et al (2004) Aortoiliac enhancement during computed tomography angiography with reduced contrast material dose and saline solution flush: influence on magnitude and uniformity of the contrast column. Invest Radiol 39:20–26

47. Schoellnast H, Tillich M, Deutschmann HA et al (2004) Improvement of parenchymal and vascular enhancement using saline flush and power injection for multiple-detector-row abdominal CT. Eur Radiol 14:659–664

48. Cademartiri F, Nieman K, van der Lugt A et al (2004) Intravenous contrast material administration at 16-detector row helical CT coronary angiography: test bolus versus bolus-tracking technique. Radiology 233:817–823

49. Bae KT (2005) Test-bolus versus bolus-tracking techniques for CT angiographic timing. Radiology 236:369–370 (Author reply 370)

50. Yankelevitz DF, Shaham D, Shah A et al (1998) Optimization of contrast delivery for pulmonary CT angiography. Clin Imaging 22:398–403

51. Washington L, Gulsun M (2003) CT for thromboembolic disease. Curr Probl Diagn Radiol 32:105–126

52. Fleischmann D, Rubin GD (2005) Quantification of intravenously administered contrast medium transit through the peripheral arteries: implications for CT angiography. Radiology 236:1076–1082

53. Bae KT, Heiken JP (2000) Computer modeling approach to contrast medium administration and scan timing for multislice CT. In: Marincek B, Ros PR, Reiser M, Baker ME, eds. Multislice CT: a practical guide: Springer, Berlin, Heidelberg, New York, pp 28–36

54. Leggett RW, Williams LR (1995) A proposed blood circulation model for Reference Man. Health Phys 69:187–201

55. Frederick MG, McElaney BL, Singer A et al (1996) Timing of parenchymal enhancement on dual-phase dynamic helical CT of the liver: how long does the hepatic arterial phase predominate? AJR Am J Roentgenol 166:1305–1310

56. Foley WD, Kerimoglu U (2004) Abdominal MDCT: liver, pancreas, and biliary tract. Semin Ultrasound CT MR 25:122–144

57. Hollett MD, Jeffrey RB Jr, Nino-Murcia M et al (1995) Dual-phase helical CT of the liver: value of arterial phase scans in the detection of small (< or = 1.5 cm) malignant hepatic neoplasms. AJR Am J Roentgenol 164:879–884

58. Oliver JH 3rd, Baron RL (1996) Helical biphasic contrast-enhanced CT of the liver: technique, indications, interpretation, and pitfalls. Radiology 201:1–14

59. Oliver JH 3rd, Baron RL, Federle MP et al (1997) Hypervascular liver metastases: do unenhanced and hepatic arterial phase CT images affect tumor detection? Radiology 205:709–715

60. Oliver JH 3rd, Baron RL, Federle MP, Rockette HE Jr (1996) Detecting hepatocellular carcinoma: value of unenhanced or arterial phase CT imaging or both used in conjunction with conventional portal venous phase contrast-enhanced CT imaging. AJR Am J Roentgenol 167:71–77

61. Paulson EK, McDermott VG, Keogan MT et al (1998) Carcinoid metastases to the liver: role of triple-phase helical CT. Radiology 206:143–150

62. Mitsuzaki K, Yamashita Y, Ogata I et al (1996) Multiple-phase helical CT of the liver for detecting small hepatomas in patients with liver cirrhosis: contrast-injection protocol and optimal timing. AJR Am J Roentgenol 167:753–757

63. Baron RL, Oliver JH 3rd, Dodd GD 3rd et al (1996) Hepatocellular carcinoma: evaluation with biphasic, contrast-enhanced, helical CT. Radiology 199:505–511

64. Foley WD, Mallisee TA, Hohenwalter MD et al (2000) Multiphase hepatic CT with a multirow detector CT scanner. AJR Am J Roentgenol 175:679–685

65. Lee KH, Choi BI, Han JK et al (2000) Nodular hepatocellular carcinoma: variation of tumor conspicuity on single-level dynamic scan and optimization of fixed delay times for two-phase helical CT. J Comput Assist Tomogr 24:212–218

66. Murakami T, Kim T, Takamura M et al (2001). Hypervascular hepatocellular carcinoma: detection with double arterial phase multi-detector row helical CT. Radiology 218:763–767

67. Kanematsu M, Goshima S, Kondo H et al (2005) Optimizing scan delays of fixed duration contrast injection in contrast-enhanced biphasic multidetector-row CT for the liver and the detection of hypervascular hepatocellular carcinoma. J Comput Assist Tomogr 29:195–201

68. Lim JH, Choi D, Kim SH et al (2002) Detection of hepatocellular carcinoma: value of adding delayed phase imaging to dual-phase helical CT. AJR Am J Roentgenol 179:67–73

69. Lacomis JM, Baron RL, Oliver JH 3rd et al (1997) Cholangiocarcinoma: delayed CT contrast enhancement patterns. Radiology; 203:98–104

70. Claussen CD, Banzer D, Pfretzschner C et al (1984)

Bolus geometry and dynamics after intravenous contrast medium injection. Radiology 153:365–368
71. Harmon BH, Berland LL, Lee JY (1992) Effect of varying rates of low-osmolarity contrast media injection for hepatic CT: correlation with indocyanine green transit time. Radiology 184:379–382
72. Chambers TP, Baron RL, Lush RM (1994) Hepatic CT enhancement. Part II. Alterations in contrast material volume and rate of injection within the same patients. Radiology 193:518–522
73. Tello R, Seltzer SE, Polger M et al (1997) A contrast agent delivery nomogram for hepatic spiral CT. J Comput Assist Tomogr 21:236–245
74. Kim T, Murakami T, Takahashi S et al (1998) Effects of injection rates of contrast material on arterial phase hepatic CT. AJR Am J Roentgenol 171:429–432
75. Tublin ME, Tessler FN, Cheng SL et al (1999) Effect of injection rate of contrast medium on pancreatic and hepatic helical CT. Radiology 210:97–101
76. Hanninen EL, Vogl TJ, Felfe R et al (2000) Detection of focal liver lesions at biphasic spiral CT: randomized double-blind study of the effect of iodine concentration in contrast materials. Radiology 216:403–409
77. Yamashita Y, Komohara Y, Takahashi M et al (2000) Abdominal helical CT: evaluation of optimal doses of intravenous contrast material – a prospective randomized study. Radiology 216:718–723
78. Awai K, Hori S (2003) Effect of contrast injection protocol with dose tailored to patient weight and fixed injection duration on aortic and hepatic enhancement at multidetector-row helical CT. Eur Radiol 13:2155–2160
79. Bluemke DA, Fishman EK, Anderson JH (1994) Dose requirements for a nonionic contrast agent for spiral computed tomography of the liver in rabbits. Invest Radiol 29:195–200
80. Baker ME, Beam C, Leder R et al (1993) Contrast material for combined abdominal and pelvic CT: can cost be reduced by increasing the concentration and decreasing the volume? AJR Am J Roentgenol 160:637–641
81. Herts BR, Paushter DM, Einstein DM et al (1995) Use of contrast material for spiral CT of the abdomen: comparison of hepatic enhancement and vascular attenuation for three different contrast media at two different delay times. AJR Am J Roentgenol 164:327–331
82. Herts BR, O'Malley CM, Wirth SL et al (2001) Power injection of contrast media using central venous catheters: feasibility, safety, and efficacy. AJR Am J Roentgenol 176:447–453
83. Walkey MM (1991) Dynamic hepatic CT: how many years will it take 'til we learn? Radiology 181:17–18
84. Brink JA, Heiken JP, Forman HP et al (1995) Hepatic spiral CT: reduction of dose of intravenous contrast material. Radiology 197:83–88
85. Takeshita K (2001) Prediction of maximum hepatic enhancement on computed tomography from dose of contrast material and patient weight: proposal of a new formula and evaluation of its accuracy. Radiat Med 19:75–79
86. Shimizu T, Misaki T, Yamamoto K et al (2000) Helical CT of the liver with computer-assisted bolus-tracking technology: scan delay of arterial phase scanning and effect of flow rates. J Comput Assist Tomogr 24:219–223
87. Schoellnast H, Brader P, Oberdabernig B et al (2005) High-concentration contrast media in multiphasic abdominal multidetector-row computed tomography: effect of increased iodine flow rate on parenchymal and vascular enhancement. J Comput Assist Tomogr 29:582–587
88. Bader TR, Prokesch RW, Grabenwoger F (2000) Timing of the hepatic arterial phase during contrast-enhanced computed tomography of the liver: assessment of normal values in 25 volunteers. Invest Radiol 35:486–492
89. Kim T, Murakami T, Hori M et al (2002) Small hypervascular hepatocellular carcinoma revealed by double arterial phase CT performed with single breath-hold scanning and automatic bolus tracking. AJR Am J Roentgenol 178:899–904
90. Mehnert F, Pereira PL, Trubenbach J et al (2001) Biphasic spiral CT of the liver: automatic bolus tracking or time delay? Eur Radiol 11:427–431
91. Sandstede JJ, Tschammler A, Beer M et al (2001) Optimization of automatic bolus tracking for timing of the arterial phase of helical liver CT. Eur Radiol 11:1396–1400
92. Itoh S, Ikeda M, Achiwa M et al (2004) Late-arterial and portal-venous phase imaging of the liver with a multislice CT scanner in patients without circulatory disturbances: automatic bolus tracking or empirical scan delay? Eur Radiol 14:1665–1673
93. Irie T, Kusano S (1996) Contrast-enhanced spiral CT of the liver: effect of injection time on time to peak hepatic enhancement. J Comput Assist Tomogr 20:633–637
94. Bae KT (2004) Contrast injection techniques and CT scan timing. In: Claussen CD, Fishman EK, Marincek B, Reiser M (eds.) Multislice CT: a practical guide. Springer, Berlin, Heidelberg, New York, pp 121–128

3

Contrast Media Safety and Managing At-Risk Patients: Update 2008

Richard Solomon

Introduction

The use of iodinated contrast media (CM) for radiological and cardiological applications continues to increase. An estimated 50 million computed tomography (CT) exams are performed annually, with almost 50% involving the use of contrast material. Additionally, 500,000 procedures are done annually for peripheral arterial interventions, and 3 million coronary diagnostic and/or therapeutic procedures are done each year in the USA alone. In this chapter, we review recent developments in the field of contrast-induced nephrotoxicity (CIN).

Definition of Contrast-Induced Nephrotoxicity

There continues to be confusion and controversy surrounding the most appropriate definition of acute kidney injury (AKI), including CIN. At the individual patient level, small changes in serum creatinine are associated with adverse outcomes in hospitalized patients [1]. Data from large cardiology databases also confirm that an absolute (≥ 0.5 mg/dl) or relative ($\geq 25\%$ over baseline) change in serum creatinine predicts adverse outcome [2, 3]. For patients with a baseline creatinine <2.0 mg/dl, more patients will be identified as having AKI/CIN when defined by a relative increase of $\geq 25\%$ rather than by an absolute increase of ≥ 0.5 mg/dl. The former definition is also preferred for clinical trials because: (a) the greater identification of cases increases the power of the study and (b) this definition, by adjusting for baseline level of creatinine, reflects similar quantitative changes in renal function for comparisons across groups of patients [4].

Who is At Risk?

A number of patient and procedure characteristics have been identified as contributing to a greater risk of CIN in patients receiving intra-arterial contrast. These include: (1) a baseline decrease in glomerular filtration rate (GFR $<$ 60 ml/min), (2) increasing age, (3) female gender, (4) intravascular volume depletion, such as might occur with chronic use of diuretics, (5) diabetes, congestive heart failure, or cirrhosis, and (6) the concomitant administration of drugs that diminish renal function, such as NSAIDs, cyclosporine, and cisplatin [5]. However, patients with these risk factors are not the only ones who will have a decrease in renal function. Studies using accurate and sensitive markers of GFR in 'low-risk' patients indicate that most patients, not the minority, have significant falls in GFR following contrast-medium injection, both intravenous and intra-arterial [6]. However, the clinical significance of such changes in this population is unknown.

Renal insufficiency remains the most significant risk factor. The risk is inversely proportional to the number of nephrons, best reflected in the GFR. With fewer nephrons, the load of contrast medium to be excreted per nephron is higher, therefore exposing each nephron to a greater toxic potential. Serum creatinine alone is a poor marker of GFR; however, a more accurate estimate of GFR can be obtained by using the serum creatinine together with age, gender, and race to calculate the GFR according to the validated MDRD (Modification of Diet in Renal Disease) equation [7]. Obtaining a serum creatinine prior to contrast-medium injection is necessary in patients identified to be potentially at high risk by virtue of a history of kidney disease, heart failure, diabetes, and some additional features. Point-of-services devices for measuring serum creatinine will be available soon and should permit outpatient imaging facilities and emergency departments to rapidly screen patients prior to contrast injection. Patients identified as high risk should receive prophylaxis (see below) and a follow-up serum creatinine should be measured 48–72 h after contrast injection.

What are the Characteristics of the Contrast-Enhanced Exam itself that Enhance the Risk of CIN?

In addition to patient-specific risk factors, there are independent risk factors related to the procedure itself. These are: (1) the dose of contrast administered for which gI/ estimated GFR (eGFR) rather than volume is the preferred metric; (2) the route of administration, intra-arterial vs intravenous; (3) multiple contrast studies within 72 h; (4) the type of contrast used; and (5) concurrent procedures such as percutaneous coronary intervention (PCI).

Many of these factors can be controlled in the imaging department through the use of protocols that diminish the dose of contrast. Contrast dose can be decreased by a higher initial injection rate with subsequent variable flow rates, saline flushing, and appropriate timing of the acquisition of images after contrast administration. Use of a contrast agent with the highest amount of iodine per unit volume will not reduce the dose (gI/eGFR) but will allow a smaller volume to be given in a shorter period of time. Strategies for protocol building are beyond the scope of this chapter but are covered elsewhere in this volume.

It appears that the risk of CIN is less with intravenous injection than with intra-arterial injection [8] (Table 1). This may be a consequence of the lower dose of contrast material typically used in intravenous studies. Based upon data from recent clinical trials, patients with eGFRs < 60 ml/min/$1.73m^2$ have approximately a 5% incidence of CIN (defined as a $\geq25\%$ increase in serum creatinine) [16, 17]. This is approximately one half the incidence reported with intra-arterial injection in a similar high-risk patient group. However, it should be remembered that there are ~ten times as many intravenous contrast exams as intra-arterial ones. A second contrast exposure within 72 h also increases the risk of nephropathy significantly. Thus, a second exposure should be delayed whenever possible and contrast should not be administered twice within 72 h unless it is urgently needed for patient management.

The specific contrast agent used may affect the incidence of CIN. The physical characteristics of the contrast have been hypothesized to explain renal toxicity. For example, the osmolality of the contrast medium has been suggested as a mediator of the toxic effect. Support for the role of osmolality comes from experimental animal data as well as clinical experience. Many of the immediate adverse effects observed with high osmolality contrast medium (HOCM), such as nausea, vomiting, arrhythmia, and heat sensation, were significantly diminished with the use of low osmolality contrast medium (LOCM). It was a logical extension of these observations to attribute renal toxicity to a similar mechanism. A meta-analysis of prospective randomized trials comparing HOCM

Table 1. Prospective randomized trials of intravenous administration of contrast media in patients at high risk of contrast-induced nephrotoxicity (CIN)

Author	Date	Number	Exam	Contrast	CIN (%)
Heller et al. [9]	1991	187	CT	LOCM	12
Carraro et al. [10]	1998	32	Urography	Iodixanol	3
Carraro et al. [10]	1998	32	Urography	Iopromide	0
Lundqvist et al. [11]	1998	63	Urography	Iohexol	2
Tepel et al. [12]	2000	42	CT, abd	Iopromide	21
Kolehmainen et al. [13]	2003	25	CT, head/abd	Iobitridol	17
Kolehmainen et al. [13]	2003	25	CT, head/abd	Iodixanol	17
Garcia-Ruiz et al. [14]	2004	50	CTA	Iopromide	4
Becker and Reiser [15]	2005	100	CTA	Iodixanol	9
Barrett et al. [16]	2006	76	MDCT	Iodixanol	4
Barrett et al. [16]	2006	77	MDCT	Iopamidol	4
Erley et al. [17]	2007	76	MDCT	Iomeprol	5
Erley et al. [17]	2007	72	MDCT	Iodixanol	7

CT computed tomography, *LOCM* low-osmolality contrast media, *CTA* computed tomography angiography, *abd* abdomen, *MDCT* multidetector CT

Table 2. Summary of prospective randomized trials comparing iso-osmolality contrast media to low-osmolality contrast media in high-risk patients receiving intra-arterial contrast

Study	Year	Number	LOCM	Result
Chalmers and Jackson [21]	1999	102	Iohexol	NS
Aspelin et al. [19]	2003	129	Iohexol	LOCM inferior
Jo et al. [22]	2006	275	Ioxaglate	LOCM inferior
Solomon et al. [23]	2007	414	Iopamidol	NS
Rudnick [24]	2005	259	Ioversol	NS
Mehran [25]	2006	145	Ioxaglate	NS

NS no significant difference between iso-osmolality and low-osmolality contrast media, *LOCM* low-osmolality contrast media

(>1,500 mOsm/kg) to LOCM (600–900 mOsm/kg) in the early 1990s found risk reduction (RR) in the incidence of CIN with the use of LOCM (RR=0.50) [18]. However, the RR was statistically significant only in patients with a GFR < 55 ml/min and only following intra-arterial but not intravenous injection. The recent availability of iso-osmolality contrast media (290 mOsm/kg) has quite naturally raised the question of whether these agents are less nephrotoxic than LOCM agents. A trial of an iso-osmolality contrast medium (iodixanol) compared with a specific LOCM (iohexol) in 129 patients with both diabetes and renal insufficiency (mean creatinine 1.55 mg/dl) indeed found a lower incidence of CIN with the use of the iso-osmolality contrast material [19]. The incidence of CIN in this trial, however, was probably underestimated because of the use of the more conservative definition of CIN (increase ≥0.5 mg/dl). A systematic review of data from prevention trials in high-risk patients that involved LOCM and iso-osmolality contrast media did not support a benefit of iso-osmolality contrast medium over *all* other LOCM [20]. In particular, the data showed comparable rates of CIN with the use of iodixanol and iopamidol, another nonionic monomer contrast agent. Recently, a number of prospective randomized trials with larger numbers of patients have compared LOCM and iso-osmolality contrast media (Table 2). These trials included patients given intra-arterial and intravenous contrast, high-risk and low-risk patients, and a variety of different LOCM. If osmolality were the physical characteristic that determined nephrotoxicity, a lower incidence of CIN would be expected with iso-osmolality contrast media. This is not observed when the LOCM is iopamidol or ioversol but is found in trials including iohexol or ioxaglate. A recent meta-analysis of 16 trials in the database of one of the contrast media manufacturers confirmed a higher incidence of CIN with iohexol and ioxaglate but not with other LOCM [26]. The inescapable conclusion is that some other property of contrast media rather than osmolality plays the primary role in causing kidney injury.

Are there Strategies to Minimize Contrast-Induced Nephropathy?

A number of strategies to reduce the incidence of CIN have been studied in prospective randomized trials. The trials were conducted almost exclusively in high-risk patients, such as those with renal insufficiency or undergoing emergency PCI, because the expected incidence of CIN was higher. This allowed for a smaller trial to generate statistical power. Such trials use a variety of CIN definitions and are most often conducted in patients receiving intra-arterial contrast medium. The trial strategies can be grouped into those that make the kidney less vulnerable to contrast material (hydration or IV volume infusion), those that attempt to produce renal vasodilation, those that use antioxidants to protect the kidney, and those that attempt to remove contrast from the body before it can harm the kidney.

Reducing the Vulnerability of the Kidney

Two prospective randomized trials have addressed the role of IV fluid with intravenous contrast administration (Table 3). A study in patients with renal insufficiency found that IV 0.9% saline given for 6 h before contrast injection was as effective as oral salt tablets given for 2 days before the study, and more effective than furosemide with IV saline [27]. Another study in a smaller group of patients with normal renal function found a smaller fall in true GFR with IV fluid before and after contrast injection than with a bolus of IV fluid (300 ml) at the time of contrast injection [6]. However, there were no long-term outcome data in this small trial and therefore it was not possible to determine whether these changes are of any clinical significance.

Two multi-center trials comparing different contrast media found an incidence of CIN of only 5% using the ≥25% increase definition in patients with eGFR < 60 ml/min who underwent MDCT [16, 17]. Neither study mandated IV hydration; indeed, the minority of patients received intravenous

Table 3. Prospective randomized trials of different CIN-prophylactic hydration protocols in patients receiving intravenous contrast

Reference	Patients (n)	Renal function[a]	CM	Control	Experi-mental	Outcome at 48 h	Result
Bader et al. [6]	CT/DSA (39)	SCr 0.9, GFR 110 ml/min	LOCM	0.9% saline (1 ml/kg/h, 12 h pre-CM, 12 h post-CM)	0.9% saline (bolus of 300 ml at CM)	↓GFR (50%)	5 vs 20% (NS); ↓GFR (18 vs 35 ml/min>; $p < 0.05$)
Dussol et al. [27]	Cardiac CT (312)	SCr 2.27, GFR 33 ml/min	iLOCM, nLOCM	0.9% saline (15 ml/kg over 6 h pre-CM)	0.9% saline (15 ml/kg over 6 h pre CM + 3 mg F/kg)	↑SCr (0.5 mg/dl)	5.2 vs 15.2% ($p < 0.05$)
Dussol et al. [27]	Cardiac CT (312)	SCr 2.27, GFR 33 ml/min	iLOCM, nLOCM	0.9% saline (15 ml/kg over 6 h pre-CM)	Oral NaCl tablets (1 g/10 kg body weight × 2 days pre-CM)	↑SCr (0.5 mg/dl)	5.2 vs 6.6% ($p = NS$)

[a]Mean data for SCr (serum creatinine) and CrCl (creatinine clearance) or GFR (glomerular filtration rate).
CT computed tomography, *DSA* digital subtraction angiography, *LOCM* low-osmolality contrast media, *CM* contrast medium, *NS* not significance difference between iso-osmolality and low-osmolality, *iLOCM* ionic low-osmolality contrast medium (600 mOsm/kg), *F* furosemide, *nLOCM* non-ionic low-osmolality contrast medium (750–850 mOsm/kg), *NaCl* sodium chloride, *HOCM* high-osmolality contrast medium (>1,500 mOsm/kg), *IOCM* iso-osmolality contrast medium (290 mOsm/kg), *D* dopamine

fluids. The observation in these two studies of a relatively low incidence of CIN in patients with an average GFR of 45 ml/min suggests that IV fluid may not be necessary for those with only moderate renal insufficiency. Further studies regarding IV fluid administration are clearly needed.

Prophylaxis with Antioxidants

The use of anti-oxidants for IV contrast injections is limited to a single trial. Patients with renal insufficiency (mean creatinine 2.5 mg/dl) undergoing abdominal CT with 75 ml of LOCM were randomized to IV saline 12 h before and after contrast injection or the same IV saline plus *N*-acetylcysteine (NAC) 600 mg twice daily starting the day before contrast injection. A significant benefit in favor of NAC was found [12]. This therapy was widely adopted for intra-arterial contrast injection but with inconsistent results [28], perhaps because the dose of NAC was inadequate for the higher dose of contrast usually administered during intra-arterial studies. Currently, the administration of intravenous NAC in patients with moderate renal insufficiency (eGFR 30–60 ml/min/1.73m^2) is not recommended.

Sodium bicarbonate infusion before and after contrast injection has also been reported to reduce the incidence of CIN in patients receiving intra-arterial injections [29]. Alkalinization of the urine is proposed to have an antioxidant effect. This therapy has not been validated in all trials with intra-arterial contrast nor has it been studied in patients receiving IV contrast.

Use of Vasodilators

Randomized controlled trials of theophylline, dopamine, fenoldopam, prostaglandin E2, atrial natriuretic peptide, and calcium-channel blockers have all failed to identify a clear advantage for such interventions. In many cases, therapeutic efficacy may have been confounded by systemic hypotension resulting from the high doses of the vasodilator used in the trial. More recent attempts have focused on targeted renal therapy (TRT), in which a vasodilator drug is delivered directly into the renal vascular bed via a bifurcating catheter placed in the renal arteries. Clinical trials are planned for 2008–2009.

Removal of Contrast Material

Multiple attempts to remove contrast material, including hemodialysis before, during, and after contrast administration, in order to prevent CIN have failed. However, in patients with severe renal insufficiency (eGFR < 30 ml/min) a single center found that hemofiltration before and after contrast administration was associated with a reduced need for subsequent dialysis and improved hospital survival [30]. Confirmation of these exciting results from other centers is awaited.

Conclusion

As the number of contrast-enhanced CT procedures continues to increase, together with the growing prevalence in the patient population of comorbidities contributing to a higher risk of CIN, the importance of the renal toxicity of contrast media will grow. Prevention of AKI depends upon adequate screening of patients for risk factors and the use of a hydration protocol in those with risk factors. This creates a logistical problem for a busy CT service. While intravenous fluid administration is at least feasible in hospitalized patients, it is much more difficult in the outpatient arena. The following recommendations represent the opinion of the author and are based upon all of the currently available data (Fig. 1).

Recommendations

1. Screen patients for renal insufficiency by history and calculation of eGFR using the serum creatinine and the MDRD formula.
2. For all patients, regardless of eGFR, encourage a liberal intake of water before and after CM injection. Ideally, patients should start drinking water the night before the CT exam and continue until the night after the exam.
3. For patients with eGFR < 40 ml/min/1.73 m^2, administer one ampule of sodium bicarbonate (50 ml, 1M) intravenously over 10–15 min prior to contrast-medium injection.
   a. For outpatients, give a second ampule following the completion of the imaging study before removing the IV line.
   b. For inpatients, follow the CT exam with 1 ml isotonic sodium bicarbonate/kg/h for 6 h.

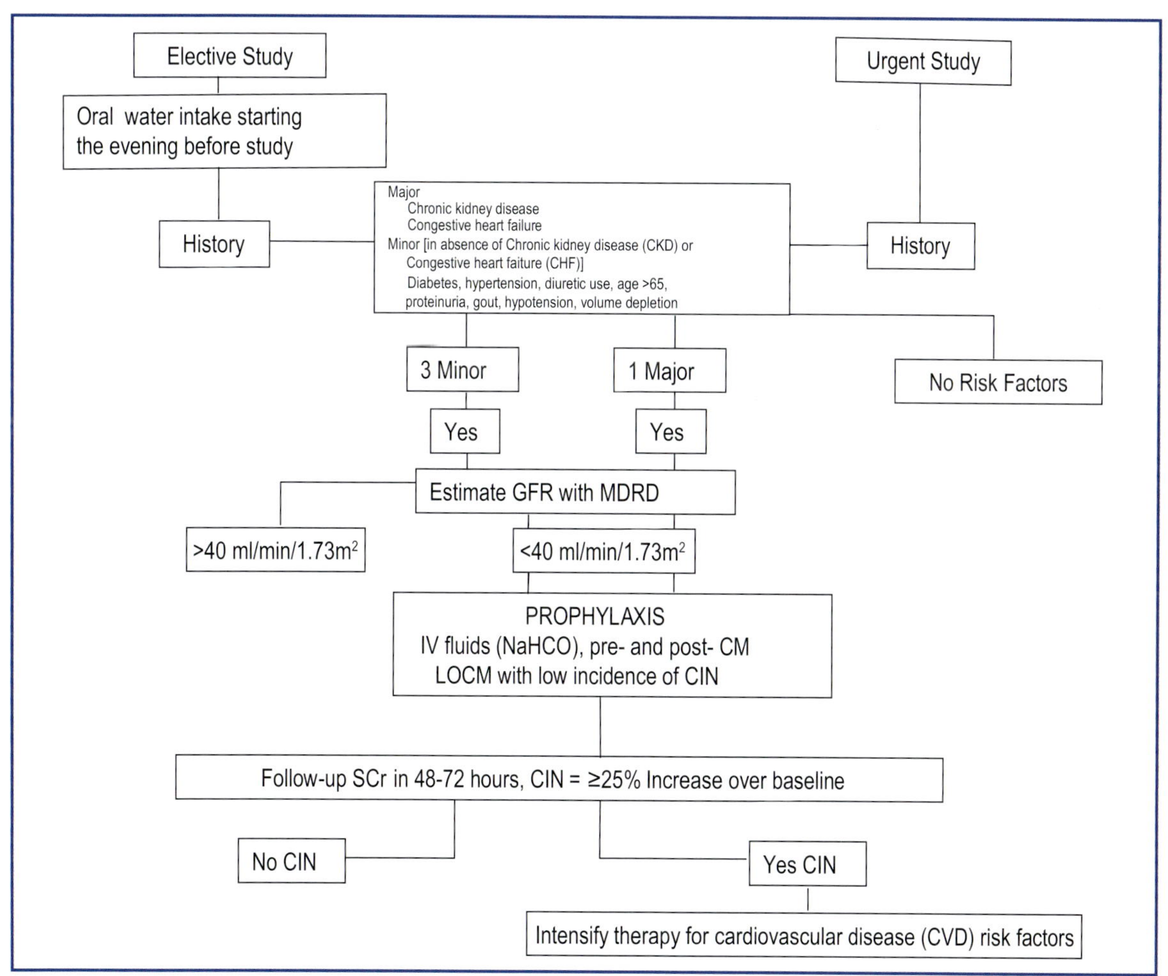

Fig. 1. Algorithm for the management of patients receiving intravenous contrast medium

References

1. Chertow G, Soroko SH, Paganini EP et al (2006) Mortality after acute renal failure: models for prognostic stratification and risk adjustment. Kidney Int 70:1120-1126
2. Gruberg L, Mintz GS, Mehran R et al (2000) The prognostic implications of further renal function deterioration within 48 h of interventional coronary procedures in patients with pre-existent chronic renal insufficiency. J Am Coll Cardiol 36:1542-1548
3. McCullough P, Wolyn R, Rocher LL et al (1997) Acute renal failure after coronary intervention: incidence, risk factors, and relationship to mortality. Am J Med 103:368-375
4. Solomon R, Barrett B (2006) Follow-up of patients with contrast-induced nephropathy. Kidney Int 69:S46-S50
5. Solomon R (1998) Contrast-medium-induced acute renal failure. Kidney Int 53:230-242
6. Bader B, Berger ED, Heede MB (2004) What is the best hydration regimen to prevent contrast media-induced nephrotoxicity? Clin Nephrol 62:1-7
7. Levey A, Bosch JP, Lewis JB (1999) A more accurate method to estimate glomerular filtration rate from serum creatinine: A new prediction equation. Ann Intern Med 130:461-470
8. Katzberg R, Barrett BJ (2007) Risk of iodinated contrast material-induced nephropathy with intravenous administration. Radiology 243:622-628
9. Heller C, Knapp J, Halliday J et al (1991) Failure to demonstrate contrast nephrotoxicity. Med J Aust 155:329-332
10. Carraro M, Malalan F, Antonione R et al (1998) Effects of a dimeric vs a monomeric nonionic contrast medium on renal function in patients with mild to moderate renal insufficiency: a double-blind, randomized clinical trial. Eur Radiol 8:144-147
11. Lundqvist S, Holmberg G, Jakobsson G et al (1998) Assessment of possible nephrotoxicity from iohexol in patients with normal and impaired renal function. Acad Radiol 39:362-367
12. Tepel M, Van Der Giet M, Schwarzfeld C et al (2000) Prevention of radiographic-contrast-agent-induced reductions in renal function by acetylcysteine. N Engl J Med 343:180-184
13. Kolehmainen H, Soiva M (2003) Comparison of Xenetrix 300 and Visipaque 320 in patients with renal failure. Eur Radiol 13:B32
14. Garcia-Ruiz C, Martinez-Vea A, Sempere T et al (2004) Low risk of contrast nephropathy in high-risk patients undergoing spiral computed tomography angiography with the contrast medium iopromide and prophylactic oral hydration. Clin Nephrol 61:170-176
15. Becker C, Reiser MF (2005) Use of iso-osmolar nonionic dimeric contrast media in multidetector row computed tomography angiography for patients with renal impairment. Invest Radiol 40:672-675
16. Barrett B, Thomsen H, Katzberg R (2006) Nephrotoxicity of low-osmolar iopamidol vs iso-osmolar iodixanol in renally impaired patients: the IMPACT study. Invest Radiol 41:815-821
17. Erley C, Thomsen HS, Morcos S et al (2007) Contrast-induced nephropathy (CIN) after iomeron-400 or iodixanol-320 in patients with moderate-to-severe chronic kidney disease. J Am Soc Nephrol 18:795A
18. Barrett B, Carlisle EJ (1993) Metaanalysis of the relative nephrotoxicity of high- and low-osmolality iodinated contrast media. Radiology 188:171-178
19. Aspelin P, Aubry P, Fransson S et al (2003) Nephrotoxic effects in high-risk patients undergoing angiography. N Engl J Med 348:491-499
20. Solomon R (2005) The role of osmolality in the incidence of contrast induced nephropathy: a systematic review of angiographic contrast media in high risk patients. Kidney Int 68:2256-2263
21. Chalmers N, Jackson RW (1999) Comparison of iodixanol and iohexol in renal impairment. Br J Radiol 72:701-703
22. Jo S, Youn TJ, Koo BW et al (2006) Renal toxicity evaluation and comparison between Visipaque (Iodixanol) and Hexabrix (Ioxaglate) in patients with renal insufficiency undergoing coronary angiography: The RECOVER study: a randomized controlled trial. J Am Coll Cardiol 48:924-930
23. Solomon R, Natarajan MK, Doucet S et all (2007) The CARE (Cardiac Angiography in REnally Impaired Patients) Study: A randomized, double-blind trial of contrast-induced nephropathy in high risk patients. Circulation 115:3189-3196
24. Rudnick M (2005) Contrast media induced nephrotoxicity. ASN Clinical Nephrology Conferences Nov 8-13:343-353
25. Mehran R, for the ICON Investigators (2006) Ionic versus non-ionic contrast to obviate worsening nephropathy after angioplasty in chronic renal failure patients. Abstract TCT meeting, Washington, DC
26. McCullough P, Bertrand ME, Brinker JA, Stacul F (2006) A meta-analysis of the renal safety of isosmolar iodixanol compared with low-osmolar contrast media. J Am Coll Cardiol 48:692-699
27. Dussol B, Morange S, Loundoun A et al (2006) A randomized trial of saline hydration to prevent contrast nephropathy in chronic renal failure patients. Nephrol Dial Transplant 21:2120-2126
28. Zagler A, Azadpour M, Mercado C, Hennekens CH (2006) N-acetylcysteine and contrast-induced nephropathy: A metaanalysis of 13 randomized trials. Am Heart J 151:140-145
29. Merten G, Burgess WP, Gray LV et al (2004) Prevention of contrast-induced nephropathy with sodium bicarbonate: a randomized controlled trial. JAMA 291:2328-2334
30. Marenzi G, Lauri G, Campodonico J et al (2006) Comparison of two hemofiltration protocols for prevention of contrast-induced nephropathy in high-risk patients. Am J Med 119:155-162

4

MDCT Radiation Dose: Recent Advances

Mannudeep K. Kalra

Introduction

The emergence of multi-detector-row computed tomography (MDCT) scanners in radiology practice has increased the number of CT studies being performed for different clinical applications. This has raised concerns about the risk of radiation-induced cancer following low-dose exposure associated with CT scanning. In order to optimize the radiation dose necessitated by MDCT scanning, it is important to understand the basic dose quantities and scanning parameters that can be modified to optimize radiation exposure. These aspects, together with the strategies for CT dose reduction, are discussed in this chapter. In addition, radiation dose considerations for cardiac CT are examined.

Radiation Dose Quantities

The absorbed dose is the energy deposited in tissue/organ per unit mass, measured in Gy (Gray). It is the basic quantity used for assessing the relative radiation risk to the tissue or organ. Effective dose represents a calculated quantity that accounts for the difference in radiosensitivity of different tissues. It compares relative radiation risk from different radiological procedures and is expressed in Sv (Sievert) [1, 2]. However, the principal dosimetric quantities that are displayed on the CT user-interface are CT dose index, volume (CTDI vol) and dose length product (DLP) [3]. Both of these quantities can be applied to sequential or helical scanning, for single- or multi-slice scanners. CTDI integrates the radiation dose delivered both within and beyond the scan volume. Weighted CT dose index (CTDIw) represents average absorbed dose across the field of view for contiguous CT acquisitions. This measurement takes into account regional variations in the absorbed dose. When CT scanning is performed with either a gap or an overlap between sequential scans (based on pitch values), the CTDIw is scaled accordingly and results in the dose descriptor CTDI vol (mGy). While CTDI does not provide the dose to any specific patient, it is a standardized index of the average dose delivered from the scan series. DLP represents the integrated dose and is equal to the average dose within the scan volume (mGy.cm).

In fact, most scanners provide CTDI vol and DLP values prior to patient scanning. These dose quantities can be used to compare radiation doses for different CT examinations, equipment, or imaging centers.

Radiation Risks Associated with CT Scanning

Given the fact that the radiation associated with most diagnostic CT examinations is generally considered to be a low-dose exposure, the principle concern is that of stochastic effects leading to radiation-induced carcinogenesis. Stochastic effects do not have a threshold level below which they do not occur; thus, any dose, however small, can be associated with these effects. Although this association is somewhat controversial, the United States National Toxicology Program: Carcinogens Report, Eleventh Edition labels low levels of X-ray radiation as "known human carcinogens" based on human studies suggesting that radiation exposure causes many types of cancer, including leukemia and cancers of the thyroid, breast, and lung. Furthermore, the report declares that children are at particularly high risk for leukemia and thyroid cancer compared with adults.

Mutagenesis in the offspring of irradiated patients, also a stochastic effect, has not been demonstrated in humans, although it has been documented in animals and plants at much higher doses than those associated with CT scanning [4].

Deterministic effects of radiation, such as skin reactions (erythema, necrosis, burns), cataracts, infertility, and sterility, do not occur below a certain threshold dose. In pregnancy, deterministic effects can lead to fetal death, mental and growth retardation, and congenital abnormalities. Fortunately, the radiation dose associated with most CT examinations is several-fold lower than the threshold for deterministic effects.

Strategies for Dose Reduction

There are several scanning parameters that affect the radiation dose associated with multi-slice CT (MSCT) scanning [5]. These include parameters that can be modified by users and those that cannot be adjusted. CT scanning parameters that can be adjusted to optimize radiation dose include tube potential, tube current, gantry rotation time, automatic exposure control, detector configuration, pitch, table speed, slice collimation, scan length, scan modes, scan region of interest, scanning phases, post-processing image-based filters, metal-artifact reduction software, and shielding devices. The scan features that users cannot change include scanner geometry, X-ray beam filters, pre-patient tracking of the X-ray-tube focal spot, and projection-adaptive reconstruction filters. We focus on the scanning parameters that users can adjust to optimize dose.

Although there is an inverse relationship between image noise, an important component of image quality, and radiation dose, several studies have shown that diagnostic information can be achieved with substantial dose reduction [3]. Hence, efforts to reduce the radiation dose must be preceded by an evaluation of the effect of dose reduction on the diagnostic requirements for a specific indication or region of interest and for a patient of specific size or age.

Scanner Geometry

There is a considerable difference between the geometry of single-slice CT and MSCT scanners. This difference is related to the distance between the focal spot of the X-ray tube and the isocenter of the scanner. Also, it is not uncommon for large medical centers to have two or more scanner types. If all scanning parameters are kept constant, both the interaction between the radiation dose and the patient and the amount of image noise will be lower with a short-geometry scanner than with a long-geometry one. Thus, when scanning protocols are prepared for MSCT scanners, care must be taken in assuming the transfer of scanning parameters from one scanner type to another. Careful transfer of protocols helps in maintaining image quality with identical or reduced radiation dose depending on scanner geometry and other features (such as reconstruction algorithms) [5].

Tube Current and Tube Current-Time Product

Tube current (mA) reduction is the most frequently used method of reducing the radiation dose. Tube current-time product (mAs) settings are proportional to the number of photons within a defined exposure time. There is a linear relationship between mA and radiation dose. Thus, a 50% mAs reduction results in a radiation dose that is reduced by half. However, the mAs should be reduced carefully, as it leads to an increase in image noise, which can adversely affect diagnostic image quality.

Reduction in gantry rotation time (scan time) has been the main focus of MSCT developments aimed at improved temporal resolution. Fast scan times imply shorter exposure time and lower radiation dose if all other MSCT parameters are kept constant. To allow a shorter exposure time, X-ray tubes are designed to give better radiation output, improved heat capacity, and heat dissipation. With the development of MSCT scanners, problems arising from tube cooling have been eliminated, thus allowing a substantially higher mA with a fast scan time.

Despite improved temporal resolution with MSCT, the radiation dose can be higher than that used for single-slice CT due to the increase in overall mAs. In MSCT, this increase may be explained on the basis of increasing applications for thinner slices, which require higher mAs to maintain a similar noise level. Also, the improved temporal resolution of MSCT allows multi-phase acquisition protocols with high spatial resolution, which are otherwise associated with a higher dose. Furthermore, unlike single-slice CT, considerably higher mAs (about 800 mA at half-second rotation) can be used with MSCT scanners for single- or multi-phase CT studies.

Unfortunately, to date, there are no data to limit increasing mAs with decreasing reconstructed slice thickness. Multi-institutional studies are needed to determine the optimum section thickness for various clinical applications and to define the maximum level of image noise that can be tolerated for these applications. It is important to remember that MSCT allows volumetric data acquisition, which can be used to retrospectively reconstruct thinner sections, albeit with higher noise. To avoid higher image noise, several institutions prospectively acquire thin sections by using a smaller pitch and slower table speed. In such circumstances, a relatively higher noise level may be acceptable, as thinner sections have higher spatial resolution and less partial volume artifacts. However, in regions with low inherent contrast, such as the abdomen, a small increase in noise can affect the conspicuity of small, low-contrast liver lesions.

Several studies have recommended mAs reduction for MSCT scanning [6, 7]. For example, mAs can be reduced for small patients (children and small adults), under conditions of high inherent contrast in which the diagnostic quality of MSCT is not affected by higher noise (CT colonography, CT for kidney stone, routine chest CT, pelvic CT, maxillofacial CT, CT of the bony skeleton), and for applications in which lower resolution is acceptable (CT perfusion). Adaptation schemes for adjusting mAs and kVp to the age, weight or size of a child have been evaluated for dose reduction with MSCT scanners [8]. As dose requirements in CT of the chest are much smaller than those for the abdomen, because of low X-ray absorption in the lungs, the tube current for CT scanning of the chest is lower than that needed for abdominal examinations. For MSCT of the chest [9], acceptable image quality with a 50% reduction in tube current has been reported. Scans performed with reduced tube current (20–80% reduction) have been reported to be as effective as standard-dose scans obtained at higher tube current for evaluation of acute lung in-

jury, follow-up of malignant lymphoma and extra-pulmonary primary tumors, lung-cancer screening, calcium screening of the coronary arteries, pulmonary nodules, benign asbestos-related pleural-based plaques, benign diseases in young patients, and guided lung biopsy [3]. A similar reduction of the tube current has been reported for routine MSCT examinations of the head, paranasal sinuses, neck, abdomen, and pelvis [3].

Automatic Exposure Control

Automated tube-current modulation (ATCM) refers to techniques that enable automatic adjustment of tube current in the x, y plane (angular modulation) (Fig. 1), along the z-axis (z-axis modulation) (Fig. 2), or both (combined modulation) (Fig. 3) to the size and attenuation of the body part being scanned. This approach allows constant image quality in the CT examination at a lower radiation dose. There have been several studies that have shown 20–70% dose reduction with use of these automated exposure control (AEC) techniques depending on body region and patient size. Electrocardiographically (ECG) controlled tube-current modulation is also a type of AEC technique for coronary CT examinations.

Dose reduction with AEC has been reported in several MSCT applications, including the neck, chest, abdomen, pelvis, and extremities. Further-

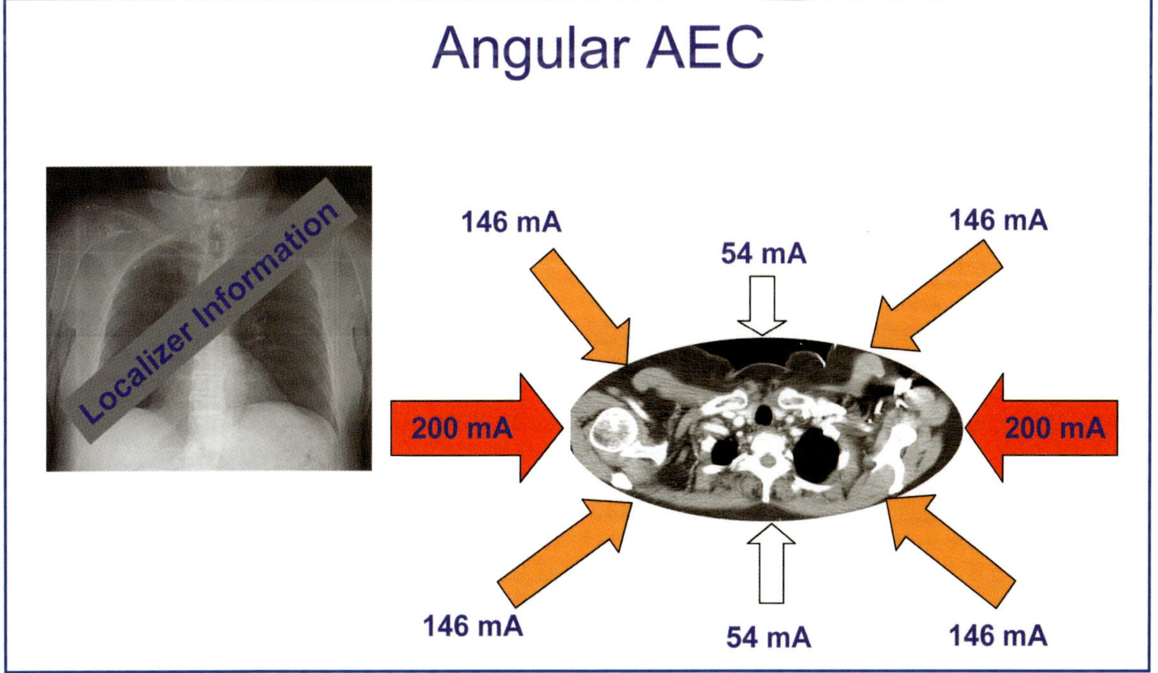

Fig. 1. In localizer image-based angular AEC (automated exposure control; smart mA, GE Healthcare), modulation of the tube current is based on the patient's attenuation profile at different projection angles around the patient. Thus, projections with a lower attenuation profile receive a lower dose of radiation than projections with a higher attenuation profile

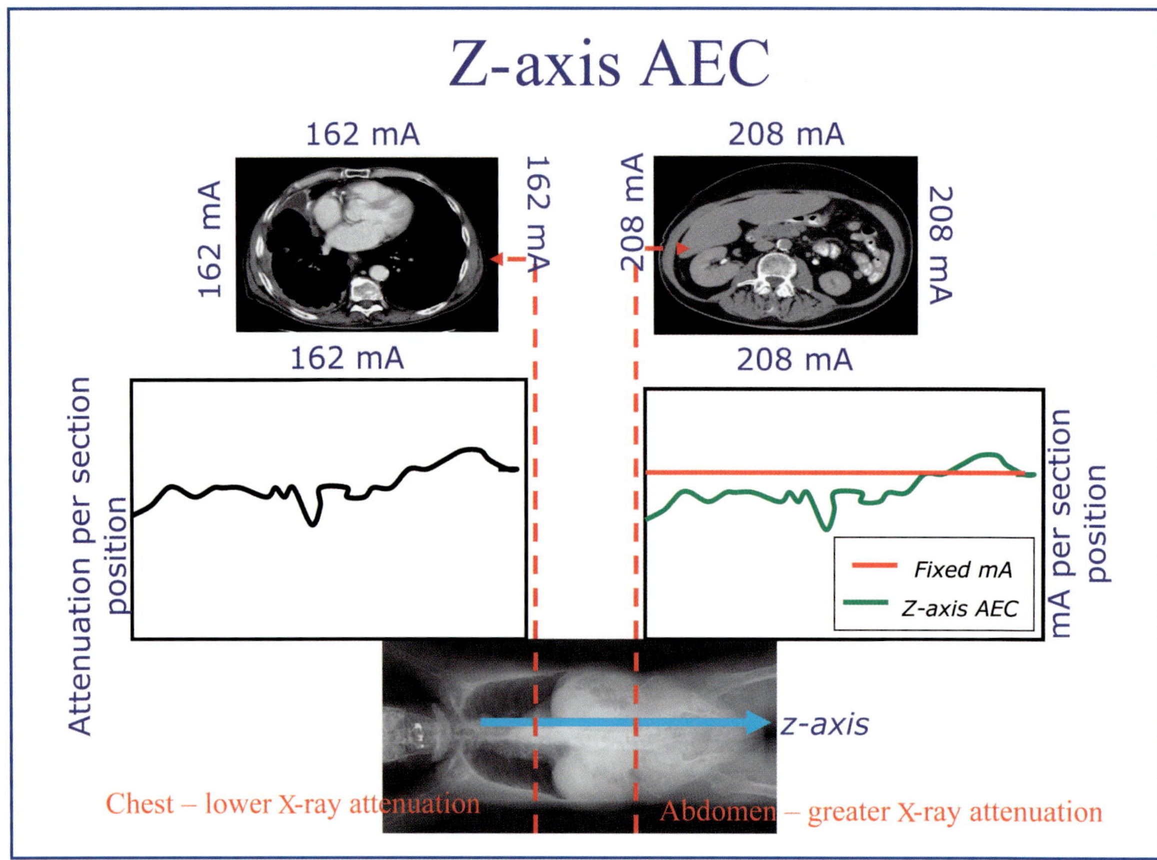

Fig. 2. In z-axis automated exposure control (AEC), the tube current is adapted based on the patient's attenuation profile along the scan length. Thus, section positions with a lower attenuation profile (such as of the chest) receive a lower radiation dose than those with a greater attenuation profile (such as of the abdomen in chest-abdomen computed tomography)

more, recent studies have reported that combined dose modulation techniques provide substantially higher dose savings than angular dose modulation for MSCT of the neck, chest, abdomen, and pelvis [10-13].

Compared with fixed tube current, AEC techniques can help in homogenizing MSCT scanning protocols for different scanners and applications. This is made possible by replacing fixed, current values with the selection of the required or desired image quality (for example, noise index with Auto mA, GE Healthcare, and reference effective mAs with CARE Dose 4-D, Siemens Medical Solutions) using AEC techniques. In addition, some vendors allow the user to control the extent of dose reduction to avoid an excessive drop in mA. Users can select the desired image quality for AEC based on the patient's study indications, irrespective of patient size. In fact, initial AEC studies have shown that selection of a fixed tube current for scanning was associated with a higher dose for small patients and a lower dose for large patients [10, 14]. For clinical applications (such as CT angiography, kidney-stone CT) that can tolerate higher image noise, the user can select a lower image-quality re-

quirement with AEC to achieve a further dose reduction.

Despite several encouraging reports on AEC techniques, there are, nonetheless, several limitations. Notably, the desired image quality for AEC must be selected carefully, as higher quality can lead to higher radiation exposure. Further studies are necessary to define reference image quality requirements for different clinical applications of MSCT so that AEC techniques can then be applied in a more scientific manner.

Tube Potential

Tube potential (kVp) determines the energy of the incident X-ray beam. Variation in the tube potential causes a substantial change in CT dose as well as image noise and contrast. Reduction in kVp leads to dose reduction and an increase in both image noise and image contrast. Most MSCT examinations are performed at either 120 or 140 kVp. Recent reports suggested a substantial dose reduction with the use of low kVp (80–100 kVp) for CT angiography studies of the head, chest, and

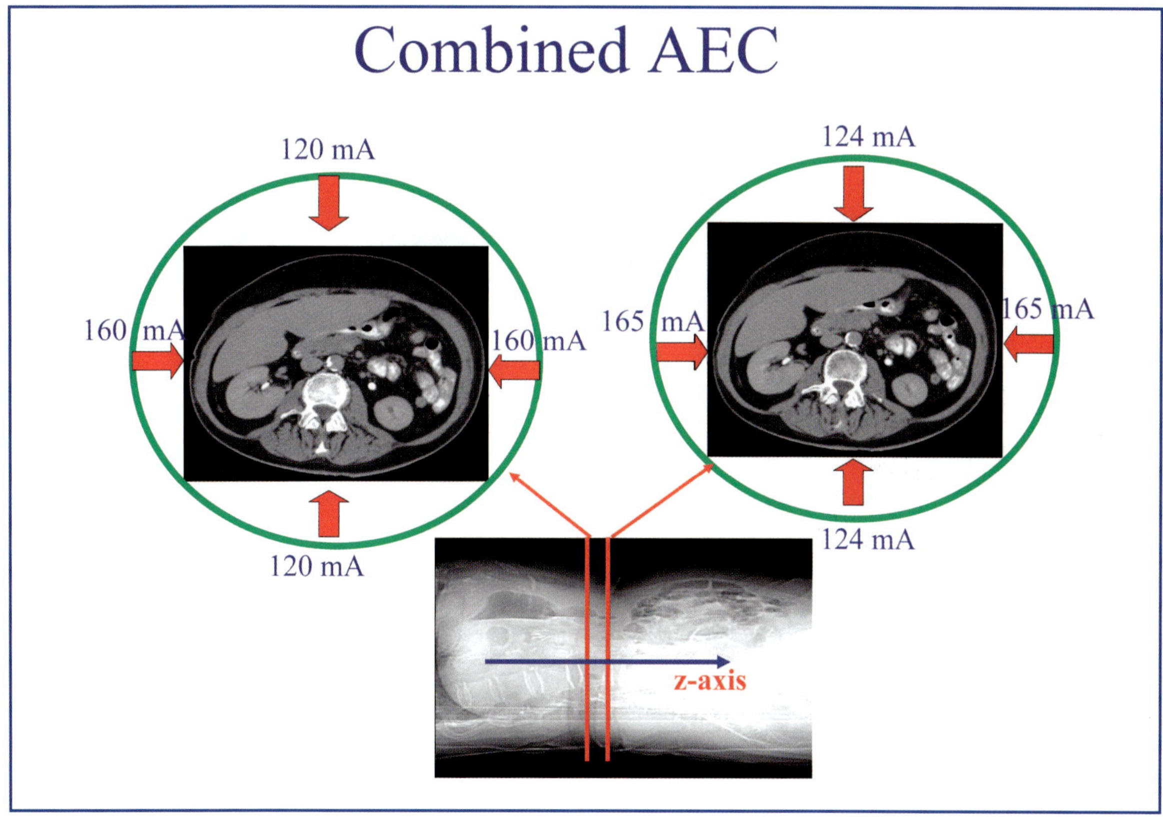

Fig. 3. In combined modulation, there is adaptation of tube current both within each section position at different projection angles [angular automated exposure control (AEC) and at different section positions along the scan length (z-axis AEC)]

abdomen [15-17]. In the abdomen, the use of a 100-kVp protocol resulted in a dose reduction of about 37% compared with a 120-kVp procedure for MSCT angiography of the abdominal aorta and iliac arteries [17]. Likewise, a substantial dose reduction (30–56%) was also reported in cerebral and pulmonary MSCT angiography studies with use of a lower tube potential (80 kVp). Dose reduction with a lower kVp (80-100) has also been recommended for chest and abdominal MSCT in newborns and infants [8]. Since a reduction in kVp can result in a substantial increase in image noise, it may impair image quality if the patient is very large or if the tube current is not appropriately increased to compensate for the lower tube voltage. Thus, for such patients, a higher tube voltage is generally more appropriate.

Scanning Modes

For MSCT scanners, over-ranging of the X-ray beam with helical scanning leads to some amount of unused radiation extending beyond the beginning and end of the region of interest. Consequently, in the absence of over-riding clinical considerations for the patient, such as breathing movements, to achieve greater dose efficiency, efforts must be directed toward the use of a single helical acquisition rather than multiple helical scans. The use of multiple contiguous helical acquisitions should be restricted with modern high-speed MSCT scanners. However, this may be unavoidable in multi-region MSCT studies, such as simultaneous neck and chest CT (position of arm) or simultaneous chest and abdomen CT (differential delay time for contrast enhancement).

Scan Length

With the rapid improvements in the temporal resolution of MSCT, there has been a tendency to increase the scan length, including to regions beyond the actual area of interest in the neck, chest, abdomen, or pelvis (Fig. 4); however, this increases the effective radiation dose to the patient [3]. The proliferation of whole-body-screening CT studies must therefore be restricted. It is also essential to draw physicians' attention to the dose consequences of increasing scan length and to establish guidelines to restrict the examination to what is absolutely essential. In this regard, technologists or monitoring radiologists should restrict the acqui-

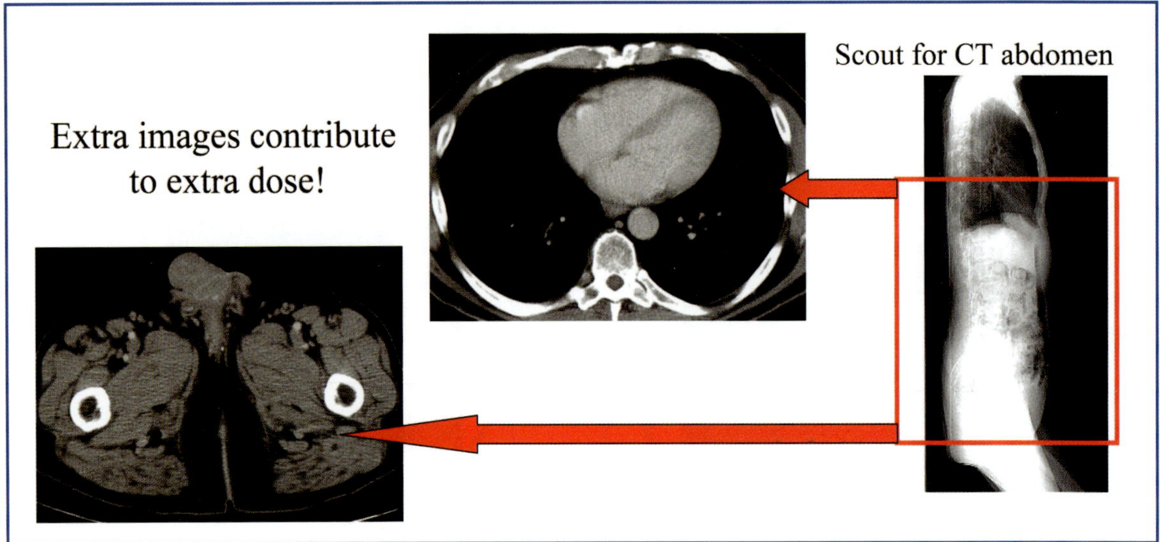

Fig. 4. Extra slices beyond the area of specified scan length increase radiation dose and should thus be avoided unless clinical indications necessitate an extension of scan coverage

sition of any "extra images" beyond the actual area of interest [18].

Scan Overlap

Multi-region CT protocols obtained in a single imaging session have become common. Most frequently, these include neck-chest, chest-abdomen, or neck-chest-abdomen CT studies. For these multi-region studies, generally, separate sets of acquisitions are planned with overlapping scan volume. Thus, in a neck-chest CT, the lower neck is scanned once during the acquisition of neck CT images, and again during the chest CT. Likewise, the lower chest and upper abdomen are scanned twice during a chest-abdomen CT. Namasivayam et al. have shown that this overlapping of scan volume increases the radiation dose by 17% for neck-chest CT and by 18% for chest-abdomen CT without contributing any significant findings (Fig. 5) [19]. Thus, when possible, the extent of overlapping scan volumes should be minimized.

Scanning Phases

Radiation dose is related to the number of phases acquired with a study protocol. If all parameters are kept constant, the radiation dose with bi- or tri-phase protocols is two or three times greater than for a single-phase scan protocol. Therefore, indications for multi-phase CT protocols must be well defined and limited. The overall radiation dose for multi-phase CT can be reduced by decreasing the dose of one or more phases by adjust-

ing tube current, tube potential, or scan length. Alternatively, elimination of one or more phases may also help in dose reduction. For example, Namasivayam et al. reported that modification of contrast-injection protocols allows the information derived from a three-phase renal-donor protocol to be obtained from a single-phase protocol, thereby reducing the dose substantially (Fig. 6) [20].

Scan Collimation, Table Speed, and Pitch

These factors are interlinked to each other as well as to the detector configuration used for MSCT scanning. For helical CT scanners, pitch was defined as the ratio of table feed per gantry rotation to the nominal width of the X-ray beam. With MDCT, two terminologies were introduced for pitch: slice or volume pitch (ratio of table feed per gantry rotation to the nominal slice width) and beam pitch (ratio of table feed per gantry rotation to the beam width or effective detector thickness). The latter terminology is preferred. A beam-pitch of 1.0:1 implies acquisition without overlap or gap, a beam-pitch of less than 1.0:1 implies an overlapping acquisition, and a beam-pitch of greater than 1.0:1 facilitates an interspersed acquisition. An increase in the pitch decreases the duration of exposure received by the anatomical part being scanned. Faster table speed for a given collimation results in higher pitch, shorter exposure time, and lower dose. A narrow collimation with slow table travel speed results in lower pitch, longer exposure time, and a higher dose.

This relationship between exposure and pitch is not true for scanners that use effective mAs and

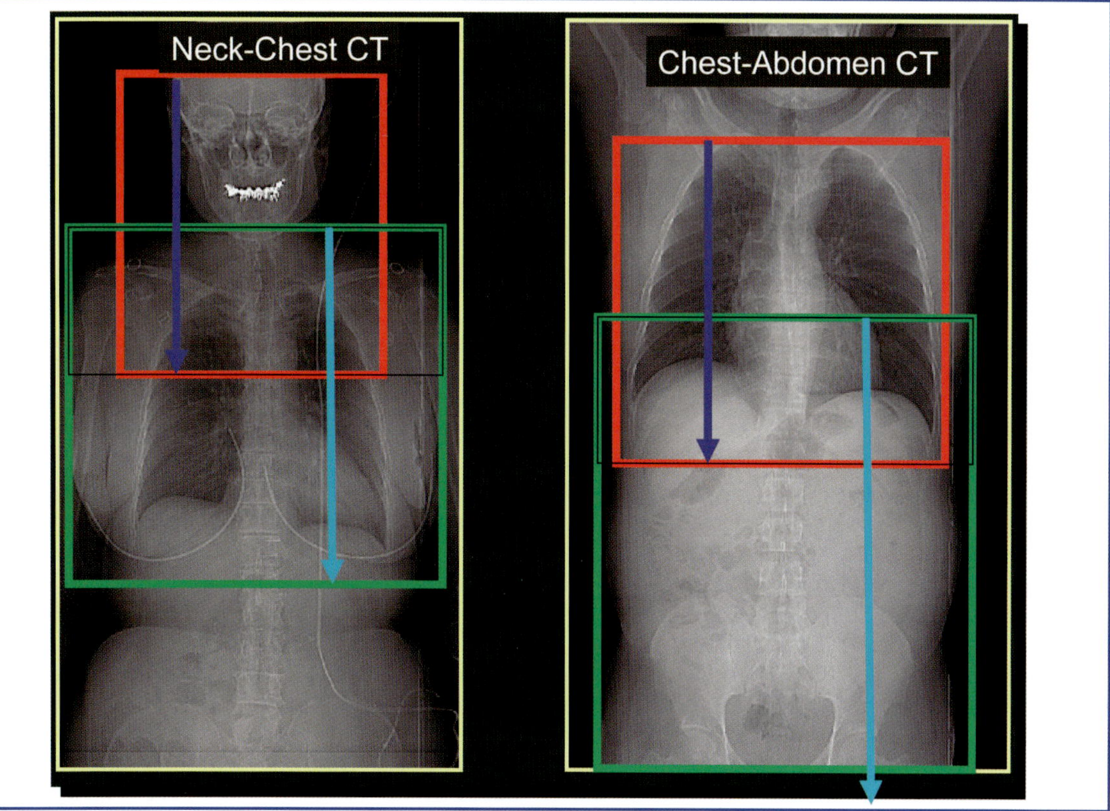

Fig. 5. Effect of overlapping scan volume: for neck-chest and chest-abdomen computed tomography studies, the extent of the scan-volume overlap must be reduced to decrease radiation to, respectively, the thyroid and the lower chest-upper abdomen [19]

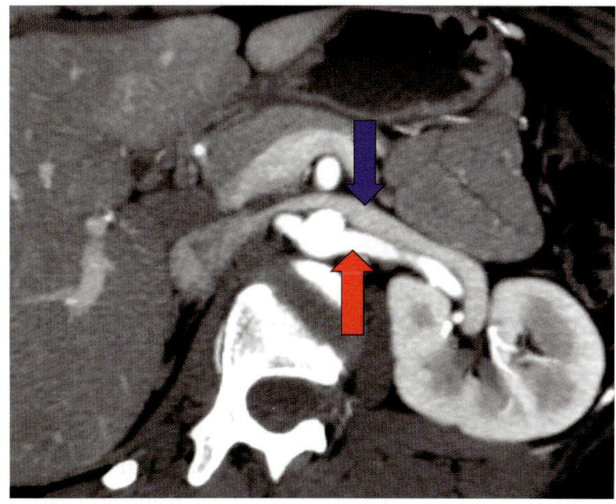

Fig. 6. The radiation dose for multi-phase protocols can be reduced by adjusting the scan parameters or reducing the number of phases. In this example of a renal donor evaluation computed tomography (CT), the contrast injection protocol was modified such that the desired information was obtained with a single-phase CT protocol with simultaneous renal arterial and venous enhancement rather than from a multi-phase CT protocol [20]

maintain a constant value of effective mAs irrespective of pitch value, so that the dose does not vary when the pitch is changed. Many MSCT scanners automatically recommend or make the appropriate tube-current adjustment to maintain a constant image noise for a change in pitch. Pitch has less effect on image quality of MSCT scanners than on single-slice CT scanners. A higher pitch is generally more dose efficient but tends to cause helical artifacts, degradation of the section sensitivity profile (slice broadening), and a decrease in spatial resolution [21]. Alterations in pitch can have varying effects on image quality in different situations. For instance, in CT colonoscopy and CT angiography studies, image quality and reconstruction artifacts are less affected by the pitch value than by beam collimation, so that a higher pitch with narrow beam collimation may be preferable in order to reduce the radiation dose [22, 23]. However, in situations such as imaging of metastatic liver lesions or pancreatic lesions, which generally require thin collimation, an increased pitch may affect detectability since lesions may be missed due to degradation of the section sensitivity profile [24].

Generally, thicker beam collimation in MSCT results in more dose-efficient examinations, as overbeaming constitutes a smaller proportion of the detected X-ray beam. However, a wider collimation can limit the thinnest reconstructed sections. Conversely, although thin beam collimation increases overbeaming X-rays, it allows reconstruction of thinner sections. Hence, beam collimation and pitch must be carefully selected to address specific clinical requirements. For instance, a wider collimation and pitch greater than 1:1 are usually sufficient for CT angiography studies and screening CT examinations such as CT colonography and renal calculus examinations.

In-plane Shielding

In-plane shielding devices can be used to protect radiosensitive organs such as the breast, eye lenses, and gonads in pediatric patients and young adults, as these structures frequently lie in the beam pathway. With lead shields, thyroid and breast radiation doses can be reduced by an average of 45% and 76%, respectively, in patients undergoing routine head CT [25]. The use of a shield for radioprotection of the eye lenses in paranasal sinus CT has also been found to be a suitable and effective means of reducing skin radiation by 40%. Recently, thinly layered bismuth-impregnated radioprotective latex shields have been used to reduce the surface dose to the breast, thyroid, and lens when these structures lie in the area of interest. However, the use of gonadal shielding during CT examinations is controversial. A testis capsule (shield) can reduce the absorbed dose to the testes in abdominal CT, whereas a lead apron is not appropriate for dose reduction to the ovaries (due to their frequently irregular position).

Recent studies suggested that although the use of in-plane bismuth shields can reduce exposure to important parts of the body, such as thyroid, breasts, and lens, they also lead to changes in the image noise and CT attenuation values or Hounsfield units [26]. Geleijns et al. therefore recommended that the use of these shields should be avoided by achieving dose reduction with tube-current reduction [26].

Patient Centering

As patients generally have an elliptical cross-section, that is, they are thinner in the periphery and thicker in the center, identical image noise over the area can be obtained with a lower dose to the peripheral thinner parts than to the thicker central parts. Bowtie or beam-shaping filters are thicker in the periphery and thinner in the center, thus allowing more X-rays or radiation through the thicker center and less X-rays through the thinner periphery (Fig. 7). Most modern CT scanners are equipped with beam-shaping or bowtie filters to maintain constant image quality while reducing radiation dose. However, these filters function best when the patient is centered at the gantry isocenter. With off-centering of the patient, less X-rays pass through the patient's thicker central part, resulting in greater noise in the center of the images, while more X-rays pass through the peripheral portion of the body cross-section, increasing the radiation dose to it. This increase in image noise can be especially problematic when patients are scanned with low-dose or AEC techniques.

Li et al. have shown that most patients (almost 95%) undergoing chest or abdominal CT are off-centered in the CT gantry [27]. In fact, off-centering increased the peripheral and surface CTDI val-

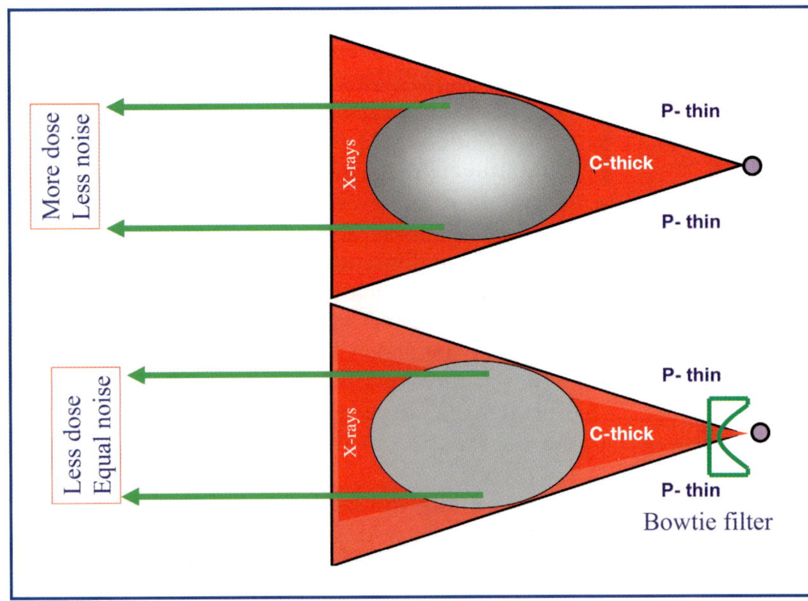

Fig. 7. Bowtie filters require that patients be centered in the gantry isocenter for an optimal reduction of peripheral radiation dose and uniform distribution of image noise

ues by 12–18% and 4–49%, respectively, at off-center distances of 3 and 6 cm. The authors used automatic centering to facilitate appropriate patient centering and to reduce the peripheral radiation dose by up to 30% [27].

Metal-Artifact Reduction Algorithm

Streak or starburst artifacts from metallic implants, such as joint replacement prosthesis, dental implants, or surgical clips, can affect CT image quality. Often, a second series of images are acquired (for face or neck CT in the case of dental implants) to reduce the loss of information from these artifacts, or the tube current is increased in an attempt to lessen the effects of these artifacts. Linear interpolation of re-projected metal traces and multi-dimensional adaptive filtering of the raw data have been developed to reduce starburst artifacts from metallic implants, which act as high-attenuation objects [28, 29]. Metal-artifact reduction (MAR) algorithms reduce starburst artifacts from metallic implants and help in reducing the radiation dose. These algorithms are expected to be released for clinical applications in the near future.

Noise-Reduction Filters

Noise in images obtained with a reduced radiation dose or in thin images can be reduced by noise-reduction filters (NRFs). Several approaches, such as linear low-pass filters, non-linear smoothing and non-linear, three-dimensional (3-D) filters, have been used to reduce noise in scan datasets.

NRFs are based on the principle that any image consists of a set of structural pixels representative of the structures of interest and a set of non-structural pixels representative of non-structural regions. The filters perform isotropic filtering of non-structured regions with a low-pass filter and directional filtering of the structured regions with a smoothing filter, operating parallel to the edges and with an enhancing filter operating perpendicular to the edges. Two-dimensional (2-D), non-linear NRF reduce noise in low-radiation-dose CT images but adversely affect image contrast and sharpness [30-32]. A recent report documented a 3-D NRF technique (3D optimized reconstruction algorithm or 3-D ORA, Siemens Medical Solutions) that generalizes the 2-D non-linear smoothing technique in all three directions (x, y, and z axes) in order to avoid the loss of image contrast and sharpness [33]. These NRFs may improve image noise without affecting contrast and lesion conspicuity in low-dose CT [33].

Radiation Dose Considerations with Coronary CT Angiography

Although coronary CT angiography offers a rapid and non-invasive technique to evaluate patients with coronary artery disease, the associated radiation dose is generally regarded to be greater than that associated with diagnostic coronary catheterization. Thus, several strategies have been developed that address this problem [34-36]. These include the use of lower tube current, lower tube potential, and prospective electrocardiography triggering for coronary-artery calcium quantification.

In prospective ECG triggering, scanning is done only within a pre-defined phase of the cardiac cycle. Thus, the X-ray tube is triggered to deliver X-rays only during a pre-specified phase of the cardiac cycle. With prospective ECG triggering, the radiation dose for CT-guided coronary-artery calcium quantification can be reduced to 1–2 mSv [37].

Some vendors (GE Healthcare) advocate the use of prospective ECG triggering for coronary CT angiography in order to reduce the radiation dose in selected patients with regular or slow heart rates. However, in patients with irregular heart rates, this can lead to erroneous estimation of the trigger point from the average of the previous three consecutive cardiac cycles. In such cases, the absence of raw data in the remaining phases of cardiac cycles may result in a limited study and necessitate a repeat CT. Also, prospective ECG triggering does not allow for the evaluation of cardiac function and the cardiac valves.

Compared with prospective triggering, ECG-controlled tube-current modulation or ECG pulsing (an AEC technique) maintains tube current at a specified level during a specific cardiac phase, and decreases tube current by up to 80% for the remainder of the cardiac cycle [37, 38]. Either the duration of the cardiac cycle or the heart rate determines the duration for which scanning will be performed, with an 80% dose reduction. The greater the duration for which low tube current is used, the greater is the dose reduction with ECG pulsing. So, at slower heart rates with a longer cardiac cycle, there will be a greater dose reduction with ECG pulsing and vice versa. Administration of β-blockers reduces heart rates and therefore allows for a greater reduction of the radiation dose. Some vendors (for example, GE Healthcare and Philips Medical Solutions) allow users to control the extent of the tube-current reduction as well as the cardiac phases for which full tube current is desired. As data are continuously acquired during the entire cardiac cycle, albeit at different tube currents, the user can reconstruct images in any or all phases of the cycle. Although images acquired at a lower tube current have much higher noise, they are generally sufficient for evaluating cardiac function and valves, particularly if reconstructed at thicker slices. For coronary evaluation, however, images reconstructed at cardiac phases scanned at low tube current may be substantially impaired due to greater noise in thin slices. Therefore, it is important for the user to observe the patient's ECG tracing before using ECG pulsing. This will help to determine whether the patient is a suitable (slow and regular heart rate) or unsuitable (high or irregular heart rate, premature ventricular contractions) candidate for ECG pulsing. Based on the heart rate, ECG pulsing can save 20–50% of the radiation dose compared with fixed non-modulated scan protocols. In addition, some vendors also adapt the pitch to the heart rate. Thus, for faster heart rates, a higher pitch is used to lower the radiation dose.

Radiation dose reduction with dual-source CT of the heart is described elsewhere in the textbook.

Conclusion

Several recent surveys have shown considerable variation in radiation dose with MSCT, which can lead to a higher radiation exposure from this type of imaging [39, 40]. Appropriate selection of scanning protocols and use of the newer dose-reduction techniques can help to optimize the radiation dose.

References

1. McNitt-Gray MF (2002) AAPM/RSNA Physics Tutorial for Residents: Topics in CT. Radiation dose in CT. Radiographics 22:1541-1553
2. Rehani MM, Berry M (2000) Radiation doses in computed tomography. The increasing doses of radiation need to be controlled. BMJ 320:593-594
3. Kalra MK, Maher MM, Toth TL et al (2004) Strategies for CT radiation dose optimization. Radiology 230:619-628
4. NAS/NRC (1990) National Academy of Sciences/National Research Council. Health effects of exposure to low levels of ionizing radiation. Committee on the Biological Effects of Ionizing Radiation. BEIR V. Washington, DC. National Academy Press
5. Hamberg LM, Rhea JT, Hunter GJ, Thrall JH (2003) Multi-detector row CT: radiation dose characteristics. Radiology 226:762-772
6. Kalra MK, Prasad S, Saini S et al (2002) Clinical comparison of standard-dose and 50% reduced-dose abdominal CT: effect on image quality. AJR Am J Roentgenol 179:1101-1106
7. Kalra MK, Maher MM, Prasad SR et al (2003) Correlation of patient weight and cross-sectional dimensions with subjective image quality at standard dose abdominal CT. Korean J Radiol 4:234-238
8. Frush DP, Soden B, Frush KS, Lowry C (2002) Improved pediatric multidetector body CT using a size-based color-coded format. AJR Am J Roentgenol 178:721-726
9. Prasad SR, Wittram C, Shepard JA et al (2002) Standard-dose and 50%-reduced-dose chest CT: comparing the effect on image quality. AJR Am J Roentgenol 179:461-465
10. Kalra MK, Maher MM, Toth TL et al (2004) Techniques and applications of automatic tube current modulation for CT. Radiology 233:649-657
11. Kalra MK, Maher MM, D'Souza RV et al (2005) Detection of urinary tract stones at low-radiation-dose CT with z-axis automatic tube current modulation: phantom and clinical studies. Radiology 235:523-529
12. Rizzo S, Kalra MK, Schmidt B et al (2007) Combined modulation and angular modulation techniques in CT scanning of abdomen and pelvis. AJR Am J Roentgenol (in press)
13. Mulkens TH, Bellinck P, Baeyaert M et al (2005) Use of an automatic exposure control mechanism for dose optimization in multi-detector row CT examinations: clinical evaluation. Radiology 237:213-223
14. Kalra MK, Maher MM, Kamath RS et al (2004) Sixteen-detector row CT of abdomen and pelvis: study for optimization of Z-axis modulation technique performed in 153 patients. Radiology 233:241-249
15. Bahner ML, Bengel A, Brix G et al (2005) Improved vascular opacification in cerebral computed tomography angiography with 80 kVp. Invest Radiol 40:229-234
16. Sigal-Cinqualbre AB, Hennequin R, Abada HT, Chen X, Paul JF (2004) Low-kilovoltage multi-detector row chest CT in adults: feasibility and effect on image quality and iodine dose. Radiology 231:169-174
17. Wintersperger B, Jakobs T, Herzog P et al (2005) Aorto-iliac multidetector-row CT angiography with low kV settings: improved vessel enhancement and simultaneous reduction of radiation dose. Eur Radiol 15:334-341
18. Kalra MK, Maher MM, Toth TL et al (2004) Radiation from "extra" images acquired with abdominal and/or pelvic CT: effect of automatic tube current modulation. Radiology 232:409-414
19. Namasivayam S, Mittal P, Small WC, Kalra MK (2006) radiation exposure and diagnostic usefulness of "duplicate" CT images. Scientific paper presented at the 87th Annual meeting of the Radiological Society of North America, Chicago, IL
20. Namasivayam S, Kalra MK, Waldrop S et al (2006) single phase mesenteric MDCT angiography using a split-bolus contrast injection technique: comparison with biphasic MDCT protocol using single bolus contrast injection. Scientific paper presented at the 87th Annual meeting of the Radiological Society of North America, Chicago, IL
21. Abdelmoumene A, Chevallier P, Chalaron M et al (2005) Detection of liver metastases under 2 cm: comparison of different acquisition protocols in four row multidetector-CT (MDCT). Eur Radiol 15:1881-1887
22. Power NP, Pryor MD, Martin A et al (2002) Optimization of scanning parameters for CT colonography. BJR 75:401-408
23. Laghi A, Iannaccone R, Mangiapane F et al (2003) Experimental colonic phantom for the evaluation of the optimal scanning technique for CT colonography using a multidetector spiral CT equipment. Eur Radiol 13:459-466
24. Rehani MM, Bongartz G, Kalender W et al (2000)) Managing X-ray dose in computed tomography. ICRP Special Task Force Report. Annals of the ICRP 30:7-45
25. Beaconsfield T, Nicholson R, Thornton A, Al-

Kutoubi A (1998) Would thyroid and breast shielding be beneficial in CT of the head? Eur Radiol 8:664-667

26. Geleijns J, Salvado Artells M, Veldkamp WJ et al (2006) Quantitative assessment of selective in-plane shielding of tissues in computed tomography through evaluation of absorbed dose and image quality. Eur Radiol 16:2334-2340

27. Li J, Udayasankar UK, Toth TL, et al (2007) Automatic patient centering for MDCT: effect on radiation dose. AJR 188:547-552

28. Mahnken AH, Raupach R, Wildberger JE et al (2003) A new algorithm for metal artifact reduction in computed tomography: in vitro and in vivo evaluation after total hip replacement. Invest Radiol 38:769-775

29. Watzke O, Kalender WA (2004) A pragmatic approach to metal artifact reduction in CT: merging of metal artifact reduced images. Eur Radiol 14:849-856

30. Kalra MK, Maher MM, Blake MA et al (2004) Detection and characterization of lesions on low-radiation-dose abdominal CT images postprocessed with noise reduction filters. Radiology 232:791-797

31. Kalra MK, Maher MM, Sahani DV et al (2003) Low-dose CT of the abdomen: evaluation of image improvement with use of noise reduction filters plot study. Radiology 228:251-256

32. Kalra MK, Wittram C, Maher MM et al (2003) Can noise reduction filters improve low-radiation-dose chest CT images? Pilot study. Radiology 228:257-264

33. Rizzo SM, Kalra MK, Schmidt B et al (2005) CT images of abdomen and pelvis: effect of nonlinear three-dimensional optimized reconstruction algorithm on image quality and lesion characteristics. Radiology 237:309-315

34. Thomas CK, Muhlenbruch G, Wildberger JE et al (2006) Coronary artery calcium scoring with multi-slice computed tomography: in vitro assessment of a low tube voltage protocol. Invest Radiol 41:668-673

35. Takahashi N, Bae KT (2003) Quantification of coronary artery calcium with multi-detector row CT: assessing interscan variability with different tube currents pilot study. Radiology 228:101-106

36. Rosol M, Sachdev K, Enzweiler CN et al (2006) A novel model to test accuracy and reproducibility of MDCT scan protocols for coronary calcium in vivo. Int J Cardiovasc Imaging 22:111-118

37. Paul JF, Abada HT (2007) Strategies for reduction of radiation dose in cardiac multislice CT. Eur Radiol [Epub ahead of print]

38. Deetjen AG, Mollmann S, Conradi G et al (2007) Use of Automatic exposure control in multislice computed tomography of the coronaries: Comparison of 16-slice and 64-slice scanner data with conventional coronary angiography. Heart [Epub ahead of print]

39. Hollingsworth C, Frush DP, Cross M, Lucaya J (2003) Helical CT of the body: a survey of techniques used for pediatric patients. AJR Am J Roentgenol 180:401-406

40. Cohnen M, Poll LJ, Puettmann C et al (2003) Effective doses in standard protocols for multi-slice CT scanning. Eur Radiol 13:1148-1153

5

Dual-Source CT: Practical Aspects of Techniques and Applications

Mannudeep K. Kalra

Introduction

The quest for non-invasive imaging of cardiac maladies began with conventional radiography and continues today. Echocardiography has established itself as the screening and diagnostic modality of choice for a variety of cardiac ailments. Since the early 1990s, cardiac magnetic resonance imaging (MRI) has also become an imaging standard of reference for a variety of cardiac pathologies, including cardiac tumors, myocarditis, cardiomyopathies, viability, complex congenital heart diseases, and valvular heart diseases. However, up until the development of multi-detector computed tomography (MDCT) scanners, the imaging of coronary artery diseases with a noninvasive imaging test was a largely elusive approach; instead, invasive conventional coronary catheterization remained and, to date, firmly remains, the imaging modality for most coronary artery diseases.

With the introduction of MDCT scanning into clinical practice, perhaps no other CT application has grown as much as coronary CT angiography (CTA) [1]. The speed and resolution of modern MDCT scanners has made it possible to obtain "acceptable quality" studies for those subjects with slow and regular heart rates. The development of dual-source CT scanners (Definition, Siemens Medical Solutions, Erlangen, Germany) further improved the temporal resolution of MDCT scanners by the addition of a second X-ray source and detector array to the single-source 64-slice MDCT scanners [2, 3]. This chapter reviews the techniques and applications of dual-source MDCT (DS-MDCT) scanners.

Faster Imaging

The earliest CT "step-and-shoot" conventional scanners were encumbered by the wires attached directly to the X-ray tube and detector array panel, with the consequent need to rewind. These scanners also had smaller z-axis coverage per gantry rotation. The slip-ring technology in helical CT scanners allowed engineers to attach these wires to a ring and then mount the tube and the detector array panels onto the ring, thus avoiding the need for rewinding. Thus, helical CT scanners allowed rapid continuous acquisition, whereas the multi-detector-row helical CT scanners made single-detector-row helical scanners truly volumetric, with extended z-axis coverage. Sub-second X-ray tube rotation times of MDCT scanners allowed the rapid acquisition of image data with multiple submilimeter detector elements arranged in multiple rows, enabling acquisition of a near-isotropic image data set.

The 4-slice MDCT scanners allowed subjects with slow and steady heart rates to be imaged with sufficient-quality images of the coronary arteries and reasonable sensitivities and specificities for proximal coronary segments [4]. However, these 4-slice scanners had several limitations. Due to the relatively thin beam collimation and use of small overlapping pitch, image quality in patients with rapid or irregular heart rates was limited, as was the evaluation of more distal segments of coronary arteries. Likewise, these factors also mandated acquisition of a large number of rotations, which were associated with greater slab artifacts and longer breath-hold durations. Most 4-slice scanners were also limited by poor radiation-dose efficiency compared with their predecessors, the conventional non-helical and single-slice-single-detector row helical scanners. Introduction of 8-, 16-, 32-, and 64-slice MDCT scanners with improved detector geometry, wider beam collimation, and efficient online pre-patient beam collimations led to substantially better radiation dose efficiency and speed of acquisition for coronary imaging than obtained with the 4-slice scanners.

Based on MRI experience, it has become clear that temporal resolution, for at least the functional part of cardiac analysis, needs to be less than 50 ms. Depending on the vendor type, 64-slice MDCT scanners have beam collimations of 2–4 cm and a single-segment temporal resolution of 165–200 ms. Although with multi-segment reconstructions it is possible to reduce the 165- to 200-ms duration to 83–100 ms for two-segment reconstructions and to around 50 s for four-segment reconstructions, the use of such techniques requires that the patient have a regular heart rate and that data are averaged over more than one cardiac cycle. Furthermore, such multi-segment reconstruction of a cardiac data set requires the use of extremely small, overlapping pitch, which increases radiation dose and scan duration. The latter, in turn, requires a slower contrast medium injection rate and volume as well as longer breath-holds.

Also, 2- to 4-cm beam collimation requires multiple gantry rotations over several heartbeats to image the entire heart, which can lead to stair-step and slab artifacts.

Another limitation of current single-source MDCT scanners is in the imaging of large patients [5]. Increased image noise due to large body habitus can substantially drop the contrast-to-noise ratio and lead to suboptimal studies. Although the power of modern X-ray tubes is better, allowing use of higher tube current, as for scanning of other body regions, coronary imaging with these scanners may not provide the required information in very large or obese patients [5, 6].

Evaluation of coronary stents and calcified plaques with single-source MDCT scanners is also hampered due to blooming artifacts, which can lead to overestimation of the degree of vessel-lumen stenosis or even to a non-evaluable study [7, 8]. Likewise, evaluation of the distal coronary arteries and collateral circulation is also affected by the limited spatial resolution of the currently available CT scanners.

Efforts to improve the temporal resolution of MDCT scanners could have involved improving the X-ray tube rotation speed. However, as the force on the gantry components increases in proportion to the square of the angular velocity, it was difficult to improve the gantry rotation speed [1]. Therefore, the concept of using two X-ray tubes and detector assemblies with the same gantry rotation time (330 ms) in order to improve temporal resolution, was pursued [2, 3]. In order to reconstruct the images, data from about 180° or a half-gantry rotation (plus the fan angle of the X-ray beam) are needed. Thus, with single-source CT scanners, one-segment reconstruction needs at least one-half of the gantry rotation time. However, for dual-source CT scanners, a single-segment reconstruction of at least one-half gantry rotation

can be obtained by fusing data from quarter rotations of two X-ray tubes, thereby improving the single-segment reconstruction time to about 83 ms. With dual-segment reconstruction, dual-source CT has a temporal resolution of 60 ms (with a minimum of 42 ms) [2]. It is interesting to note that multiple X-ray source design is not new to CT scanning. Almost three decades earlier, a multiple X-ray source CT scanner, the high temporal resolution cylindrical scanning computerized tomographic system (Dynamic Spatial Reconstructor), was developed to image the heart. It consisted of 14 X-ray tubes mounted on a single semicircular arch [9, 10]. Unfortunately, use of this scanner was limited to research purposes due to the poor signal-to-noise ratio and computational power for image reconstructions required for human use.

While the DS-MDCT scanner attempts to improve temporal resolution, its beam collimation and spatial resolution are identical to those of its corresponding predecessor, the single-source 64-slice MDCT scanner.

Practical Physical Aspects of the Dual-Source Scanner

A dual source scanner is basically a 64-slice MDCT scanner with two X-ray sources and two detector arrays (Table 1).

X-Ray Tubes

Dual-source MDCT scanners have two X-ray tubes, each with a power equal to a single-source 64-slice MDCT scanner. Thus, the combined power of the X-ray tubes in dual-source scanners is two-fold greater than that of a single-source scanner (160 kW compared with 80 kW) [3]. These X-ray tubes are mounted orthogonally from each other on the same gantry assembly (Fig. 1). They can be operated at similar or different kilovoltage (kVp) and milliamperage (mA). For cardiac imaging, the best temporal resolution can only be obtained at similar kVp for the two tubes. With different kVp or dual energy, a single-segment temporal resolution of 165 ms is achievable, which is identical to that of a 64-slice MDCT scanner. Like its predecessor 64-slice single-source CT scanner, both X-ray tubes have z-flying focal spots, which enable the acquisition of 64 slices from a 32-slice detector assembly. Also, to reduce the radiation dose, an additional targeted field-of-view (FOV) cardiac beam-shaping or bowtie filter is used. McCollough et al. showed that the addition of this filter reduces radiation dose by 17% compared with the body beam-shaping filter only [11]. It is also important to re-

Table 1. Similarities and differences between single- and dual-source 64-slice multi-detector row computed tomography (MDCT) scanners

Features	Dual-source CT	Single-source 64-slice CT
X-ray tubes	2	1
z-flying focal spot	Present in both tubes	Present
Additional targeted field-of-view beam-shaping filter	Present	-
X-ray power	80 + 80 = 160 kW	80 kW
Detector arrays	2	1
Field of view		
Detector array A	50 cm	50 cm
Detector array B	26 cm	Not applicable
Detector configuration	32 × 0.6 mm or 24 × 1.2 mm	32 × 0.6 mm or 24 × 1.2 mm
Gantry rotation time	330 ms	330 ms
Dual energy	In same rotation	With separate gantry rotations
Cross scattering	Present	Not applicable
Pitch for gated scanning	0.2–0.5:1	0.2–0.33:1
Temporal resolution		
Single segment	~ 83 ms	~ 165 ms
Dual segment	~ 60 ms (minimum up to 42 ms)	~ 83 ms

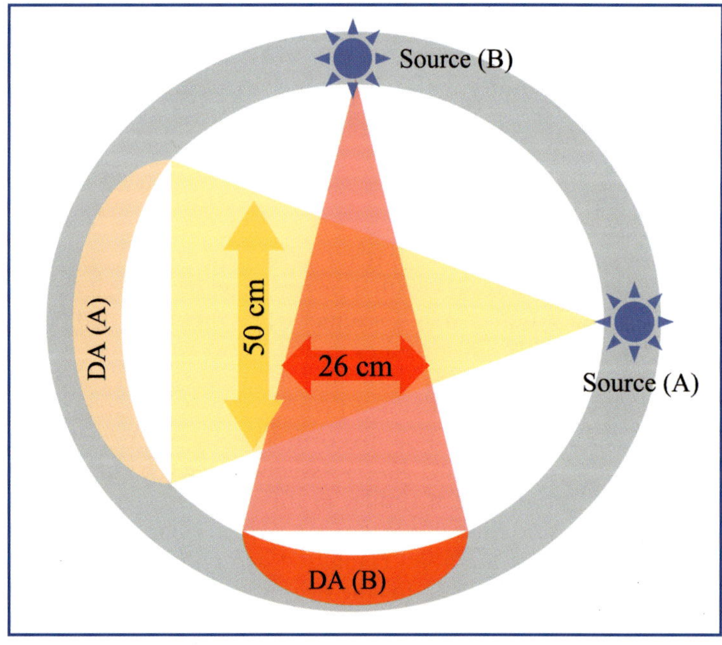

Fig. 1. Dual-source computed tomography (CT) system design with two identical X-ray tubes (sources A and B) mounted orthogonally to each other on the same gantry assembly and dissimilar detector arrays, one larger [DA(A)] and one smaller [DA(B)]

member that the reduced FOV of the second X-ray tube (corresponding to the smaller detector array) also restricts radiation dose to some extent.

Detector Arrays

To capture X-ray beam attenuation data, there are two detector arrays in a dual-source CT scanner. These are mounted on the same gantry assembly opposite to their respective X-ray sources. Each detector array has a detector geometry (32×0.6 mm = 19.2 cm or 24×1.2 mm = 28.8 cm) identical to that of a 64-slice CT scanner, with a single exception. Due to space constraints, one detector array (50 cm) is larger than the other (26 cm). The smaller detector array is generally sufficient for small FOV imaging, as performed for coronary imaging. This small FOV underscores the importance of some scanning fundamentals. Firstly, it is important to center the subjects appropriately in the gantry isocenter for optimum temporal resolution. Secondly, for dual-energy applications, the region of interest must lie within the 26-cm FOV of the smaller detector array.

Scatter Correction Algorithm

The data from the two detector arrays are combined to generate a single image data set. However, the two X-ray tubes and two detector arrays give rise to the important issue of cross scatter; that is, the scattering of X-ray photons from one source to the detector array of other source. Drs. Kyriakou and Kalender have shown that cross scatter in dual-source CT scanners is not negligible and special cross-scatter correction methods help to reduce the resulting artifacts [12]. In fact, the dual-source CT scanners employ scatter correction algorithms to circumvent the adverse effects of cross scattering.

Adaptive Three-Dimensional Noise-Reduction Filters

To reduce image noise and help in radiation dose reduction, adaptive 3-D noise-reduction filters are used in dual-source CT scanners [11]. These filters are applied in tandem with certain reconstruction kernels of dual-source CT scanners for noise reduction and/or edge enhancement.

Specific Applications of Dual-Source CT

From the above discussions, it is clear that the DS-MDCT scanner has three distinct features regarding its imaging applications: (1) combined X-ray tube power, (2) dual energy or dual kVp, and (3) scanning speed or temporal resolution. The applications of dual-source CT are discussed below in detail.

Combined X-Ray Tube Power

Uppot et al. reported that imaging of obese or very large patients is an ever more common problem in radiology. The authors note that 0.25–0.4% of chest and abdominal CT studies are diagnostically limited due to large patient body habitus [5].

As mentioned above, DS-MDCT scanners have two X-ray tubes, each with the power of an X-ray tube of a 64-slice MDCT scanner. Thus, the combined X-ray tube power of a dual-source CT scanner is 160 kW. Although the vendor of this scanner claims that greater combined X-ray tube power coupled with greater table-load capacity (up to 615 lb) should enable optimal scanning of obese or large subjects, no patient study to support this claim has been published thus far [2, 3]. However, in a phantom study with single-source MDCT and DS-MDCT, it was reported that the latter, with its combined X-ray tube power, decreased image noise about 25% compared with the single-source MDCT (Fig. 2) [13]. It is unclear, however, whether

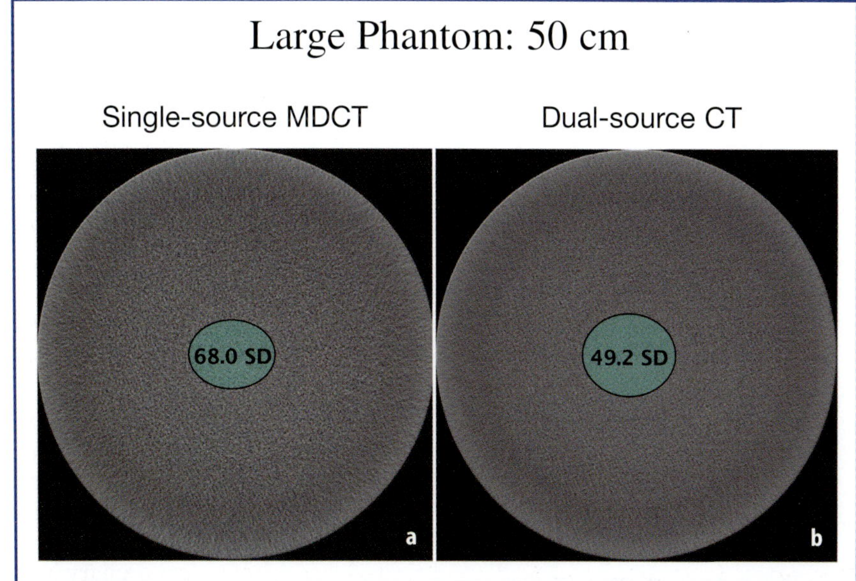

Fig. 2. Single (**a**) and dual-source (**b**) 64-slice multidetector row computed tomography (MDCT) images of a large phantom measuring 50 cm in diameter. Compared with the single-source 64-slice MDCT, the dual-source CT images of the large phantom have less (22–27%) image noise. There are, however, few patient data to support the use of dual-source CT in large patients. *SD* Standard deviation

the noise reduction noted in phantom studies with dual-source CT scanners will translate into improved diagnostic acceptability in patient studies. Other vendors have also introduced MDCT scanners with wider bore gantry and greater table-load capacity for imaging obese subjects. Nonetheless, presently, there are no clinical data to support the advantage of these scanners over other MDCT scanners.

Dual-Energy or Dual-Kilovoltage Scanning

The rationale for the application of dual-energy or dual-kVp CT scanning for tissue characterization is the differential attenuation properties of tissues and materials to different energy spectra of X-ray energies at different kVp. For example, iodine and calcium attenuate more photons of low-energy beam and consequently have much higher CT attenuation numbers at lower kVp than at higher kVp [14]. Most soft tissues, with the exception of fat, are near water density; therefore, due to the system calibration of most CT scanners, these tissues show no change in attenuation numbers at different kVp. The attenuation numbers of fat-rich tissues, however, are lower at lower kVp than at higher kVp scanning.

Table 2 summarizes the applications of dual-energy CT that have been evaluated to date. Most of these studies were performed without the use of dual-source CT scanners.

Presently, there are few data to support any of the dual-energy applications of dual source CT, with the exception of fatty liver quantification in living related liver donors. Prior studies have shown that dual-kVp CT is not helpful in differentiating benign from malignant pulmonary nodules [15]. However, recent studies for kidney-stone differentiation and adrenal-mass characterization showed promising results [16-18]. Accurate determination of the chemical composition of urinary

stones is still in the experimental stage, with most data coming from phantom studies using the dual-kVp CT technique [16]. Prior studies with single-slice helical CT showed that dual-kVp CT can help to differentiate the composition of uric acid, struvite, and calcium oxalate stones [19]. In a recent study with an anthropomorphic phantom model with multiple stone types, it was reported that dual-energy CT accurately discriminated uric acid stones from other stone types [16]. The use of dual-energy CT images to obtain virtual unenhanced CT images from dual-energy post-contrast CT images has also been described [20]. Scheffel et al. assessed the use of virtual unenhanced images obtained from a dual-energy post-contrast nephrographic phase for the detection of renal calculi [20].

Patient studies conducted by Kalra et al. and Udayasankar et al. showed that unenhanced dual-energy CT can help differentiate a fat-containing benign adenoma from malignant adrenal lesions [17, 18]. These investigators employed 16- and 64-slice MDCT scanners to image adrenal lesions at 80 and 140 kVp [17, 18]. At 80 kVp, they noted a substantial decrease in the CT attenuation values of the fat-containing adrenal adenomas but not in the malignant adrenal lesions. However, further validation studies are needed to establish this application and to avoid the administration of contrast medium and the need for additional radiation exposure through a multi-phase adrenal CT protocol for characterizing adrenal lesions.

Although dual-kVp or dual-energy CT scanning is useful in several circumstances involving lesion characterization, currently, there are insufficient data about the use of dual-source or dual-energy CT to quantify coronary artery calcium or to characterize coronary plaques or myocardial perfusion abnormalities [14]. Flohr et al. reported that the use of dual-energy CT and special 3-D image post-processing filters reduced the extent of blooming artifacts from calcified coronary plaques

Table 2. Applications of dual-energy computed tomography (CT)

Applications	Bottom-line inference
Pulmonary nodule characterization	Not useful
Fatty liver quantification for liver donors	Useful, present application
Characterization of liver lesions	Limited data
Characterization of an adrenal mass	Useful (more validation needed)
Coronary in-stent stenosis	Further data needed
Bone subtraction for CTA post-processing	Few data available
Kidney-stone differentiation	Useful results from initial patient studies
	More data needed
Iron deposition in liver	MRI is superior to CT in this respect
Bone densitometry	Better tests are available

CTA computed tomography angiography, *MRI* magnetic resonance imaging

by 42% and image noise by 30% [21]. From the cardiac-imaging standpoint, the use of dual energy in electrocardiography (ECG)-gated coronary angiography through a dual-source CT scanner implies that each tube must contribute half-scan (plus the fan angle) data; for a single segment, the temporal resolution is about 165 ms.

Cardiac Applications: Effect of Improved Temporal Resolution and Other Features

Clearly, the most dominant implication of dual-source CT has been on coronary CTA. Some features of dual-source CT scanners contribute to these positive implications. For example, the 83-ms single-segment reconstruction time for dual-source CT is less than that of the single-source MDCT scanners currently on the market (Fig. 3). Generally, for patients being examined without a single-source 64-slice MDCT scanner, intravenous beta-blockers are administered to bring the heart rate to 60–65 beats per min (bpm). For the dual-source CT scanner, beta-blockers are not administered. With dual-source CT, Scheffel et al. showed that neither beta-blockers nor heart rate control is necessary for subjects with an average heart rate of 70 bpm (range: 47–102) [22]. In this small clinical study ($n = 30$), the authors reported a sensitivity, specificity, and positive and negative predictive values for evaluating coronary artery disease in all segments with diameter ≥1.5 mm of 96.4, 97.5, 85.7, and 99.4%, respectively. Johnson et al. reported similar high accuracy for per patient analysis, with invasive coronary angiography as the standard of reference [23]. However, those authors

found that, for the detection of >50% coronary stenosis on a per-coronary segment basis (98% assessable segments with more than 50% coronary stenosis), dual-source CT had a sensitivity, specificity, and positive and negative predictive values of 88, 98, 78, and 99%, respectively. Likewise, in subjects with variable heart rates from atrial fibrillation, Oncel et al. reported similar sensitivity and specificity with a 99% negative predictive value for dual-source coronary CTA [24]. Nonetheless, Ropers et al. recently published that, although not statistically different, dual-source coronary CTA has better overall per segment evaluability at heart rates < 65 bpm than at higher heart rates [25]. Matt et al. also reported sufficient image quality for a wide range of mean heart rates, but some compromise in image quality was noted at heart rates that were both high and variable [26].

Rist et al. also documented acceptable image quality of the coronary arteries independent of the heart rate with dual-source CT scanners [27]. These authors and Busch et al. found good correlation for ejection fraction as well as end-systolic and end-diastolic volumes between MRI and dual-source CT scanners [27, 28].

A recent study from Groen et al. showed that, compared with 64-slice MDCT, the dual-source CT scanner with 0.6-mm reconstructed section thickness better approximates the electron beam for absolute calcium scores [29]. Furthermore, dual-source CT was about 50% less susceptible to cardiac motion than was the case with single-source 64-slice MDCT.

Dual-source coronary CTA was recently evaluated for coronary in-stent restenosis. Pugliese et al. reported that the technique is satisfactory for stents measuring 3.5 mm and greater (100% sensitivity, specificity, and positive and negative predic-

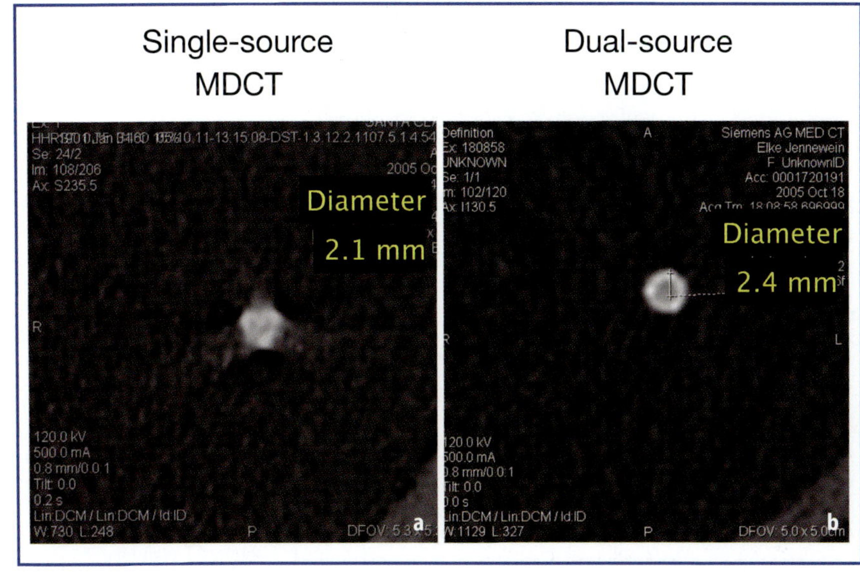

Fig. 3. Compared to the single source 64-slice MDCT images of the moving stent (3.5 mm) phantom-simulating heart rate of 90 (**a**) beats per minute, there is greater stent evaluability on dual-source CT images (**b**) at the corresponding heart rate

tive values) but leads to frequent false-positive diagnosis of in-stent restenosis in stents ≤2.75 mm [30]. Although image quality with dual-source CT of a robotic device simulating cardiac motion was similar at 0 bpm (static) and 50–120 bpm, erroneous measurements were very frequent for stents < 3 mm (27–32%) [31].

The above-noted dual-source coronary CTA studies provide evidence for the advantages of dual-source CT in terms of fewer motion artifacts and greater coronary artery evaluability in distal segments and in patients with higher heart rates. These studies also highlight the need for further improvements in MDCT technology, with or without dual sources, in order to improve the accuracy and reproducibility of coronary CTA, especially for evaluation of distal coronary artery segments and stents <3 mm. Presently, there are few data on the extent of blooming artifacts with dual-source CT compared with other single-source MDCT scanners (Fig. 4).

The improved temporal resolution of dual-source CT has also enabled more aggressive adaptation of pitch to heart rate than is possible with single-source MDCT scanners. For ECG-gated studies, whereas single-source CT scanners allow pitch adaptation from about 0.2 to 0.3:1, dual-source CT adapts pitch to between 0.2 and 0.5 based on heart rate.

Flohr et al. reported that as the heart rate increases, the dual-source CT scanners use greater pitch and faster table speed [2, 3]. For example, at heart rates of 50, 60, 70, 80, and 90 bpm, dual-source CT employs pitches of 0.21, 0.27, 0.32, 0.37, and 0.43, respectively, and table feeds (mm/s) of 12.8, 16.0, 19.2, 22.4, and 25.6, respectively [2]. McCollough et al. reported substantial dose reduction with dual-source CT with adaptation of pitch to the heart rate. Compared with a volume CT dose index of 61.2 mGy at 0.2 pitch, the authors documented corresponding dose values of 46.2, 34.0, and 26.6 mGy at pitch values of 0.265, 0.36, and 0.46, respectively [11]. In general, with dual-source CT, the greater the heart rate, the higher the pitch and the lower the resulting radiation dose. Thus, pitch adaptation helps in radiation dose reduction with dual-source CT studies involving subjects with faster heart rates. The scanner determines the pitch automatically from the average heart rate over the previous ten cardiac cycles. Since in some patients heart rate can change due to breath-hold, the vendor recommends checking the effect of breath-hold on heart rate and overwriting the automatically selected pitch value in patients with large changes in heart rate upon breath-hold.

Radiation dose reduction with ECG-controlled tube-current modulation depends on the pulsing window (duration for which full non-modulated

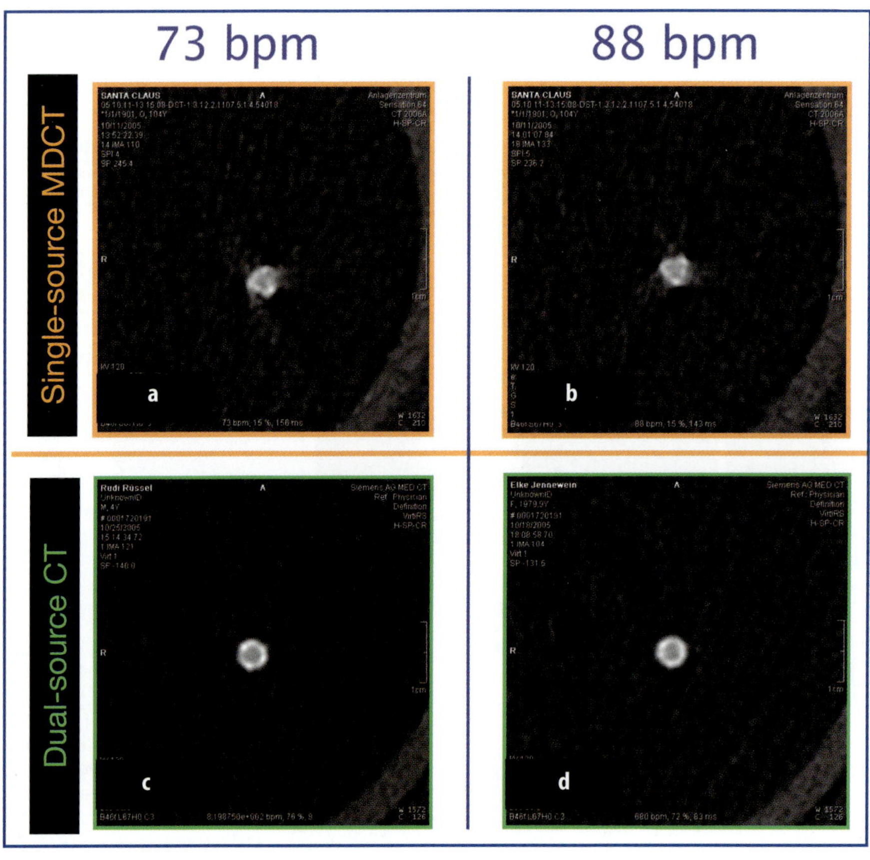

Fig. 4. Moving phantom with coronary stent simulating cardiac motion at 70 and 90 beats per minute was scanned at single (**a**, **b**) and dual-source (**c**, **d**) 64-slice multi-detector row computed tomography (MDCT) scanners. The images show fewer motion artifacts at different heart rates with the dual-source CT scanner

tube current is used), the selected full non-modulated tube current value, and the extent of tube-current modulation [11]. In addition to the benefits of a cardiac beam-shaping filter, noise-reduction filters, pitch adaptation, and restricted collimation of the X-ray source corresponding to the smaller detector array, the dual-source CT scanner, due to its 83-ms single-segment reconstruction time, allows specific adjustment of ECG-controlled tube current modulation based on patients' heart rates. For example, the tube current can be reduced to up to 4% of the full non-modulated value for the desired R-R interval of the cardiac cycle. Furthermore, not only is it possible to select a lower tube current for non-critical portions of the R-R interval, the higher temporal resolution of dual-source CT allows the selection of a narrower pulsing windows of as little as 110 ms [11]. Users have an option of employing pre-set pulsing windows based on the vendor's default setting or specifying their own preferences (a feature also available on some single-source 64-slice MDCT scanners). It is important, however, to remember all the caveats about the use of ECG pulsing that are applicable to single-source CT scanners. The pulsing windows can be set at relatively narrow width with dual-source CT for patients with slow and steady heart rates, whereas a wider pulsing window is more appropriate for patients with higher or variable heart rates. McCollough and colleagues documented dose reduction for dual-source coronary CTA. Based on the heart rate, ECG-controlled tube-current modulation with dual-source CT reduces the volume CT dose index to 9.1–25.1 mGy at temporal pulsing windows of 110, 210, and 310 ms [11].

Thus, at faster heart rates, pitch adaptation with dual-source CT is an important way of reducing the dose. At slower heart rates, users can select a narrow pulsing window with ECG-controlled tube current modulation for dose reduction.

Level of Evidence

Presently, most data supporting use of dual-source CT come from small studies from single institutions. There are few data to support use of the dual-energy capabilities of the scanner for tissue and plaque characterization.

Pursuit of the "Third Kind"

Unrelenting progress in CT technology continues (Table 3). Currently, there are indications that pur-

Table 3. The pursuit of a "third kind" of computed tomography (CT) scanner

Target (improved alternate imaging)	Available vs. in development	Benefits

Better temporal resolution: 4-7 ms (ICA)	DSCT: 83 ms (single segment), 60 ms (up to 42 ms: dual segment)	Rapid or irregular heart rate
		Better evaluation of
		  - Distal coronary arteries
		  - ? Calcified plaques
		  - ? Stents
		  - Cardiac functions
		  - Less need for beta blockers

Better spatial resolution	DSCT: 0.4–0.6 mm 0.1 mm (ICA) HDCT < 0.4 mm (in development) Flat-panel CT ~0.2 mm (in development)	Better evaluation of: Distal coronary arteries Calcified plaques Stents Collaterals ? Plaque characterization ? Better quantification of stenosis
Better z-axis coverage	256 or 320 slice CT: 12.8–16 cm (in development) ? Superior function assessment ? Smaller contrast volume ? Smaller dose ? Shorter breath-hold	Fewer slab artifacts ? Cardiac perfusion studies
Radiation dose: 4-6 mSv (diagnostic ICA)	1-15 mSv (available and in development)	Less risk for radiation-induced cancer

ICA invasive coronary angiography, *DSCT* dual-source CT, *HDCT* high-definition CT (GE Healthcare)

suit of a "third kind" of MDCT scanner, i.e., beyond the dual-source scanner, is underway. As discussed above, the beam collimation of current dual-source CT scanners is still < 3 cm per rotation, and overlapping scan volumes necessitate multiple rotations of the X-ray tubes and detector arrays around the patient for the 15–20 cm of coverage required for routine coronary CTA and many more rotations for the extended coverage needed to evaluate coronary artery bypass grafts [32, 33]. Therefore, some vendors, notably Toshiba and Philips, have taken the route of developing scanners with broader beam width (up to 16 cm) with capabilities of acquiring 320 or 256 slices per gantry rotation [32, 33]. Although the idea of imaging the entire heart and coronary arteries in a single gantry rotation is attractive and may usher in new applications for studies of the heart and other organs, these scanners are work-in-progress concepts. Furthermore, although the beam collimation of these scanners will be wider than that of dual-source CT scanners, the spatial resolution of these scanners is not much better than the presently available 64-slice MDCT scanners.

Another vendor, GE Healthcare, has released plans for improving the spatial resolution of its "new generation" of MDCT scanners while maintaining the beam collimation identical of their 64-slice scanners (about 4 cm).

Given the successful resume of CT vendors in bringing out a new "slice-and-source scanner" almost every other year, it is expected that vendors will now devote more time and resources to clinical trials aimed at defining and, more importantly, limiting, the clinical applications to those in which true benefits can be established while taking into account the undesired effect of increasing health costs and collective radiation doses.

Conclusion

Dual-source MDCT offers advantages over single-source MDCT scanners in terms of superior temporal resolution for cardiac CT. Although initial phantom and patient studies are encouraging, the applications of dual-energy scanning need further research.

References

1. Kalra MK, Maher MM, D'Souza R, Saini S (2004) Multidetector computed tomography technology: current status and emerging developments. J Comput Assist Tomogr 28(Suppl 1):S2-6
2. Flohr TG, McCollough CH, Bruder H et al (2006) First performance evaluation of a dual-source CT (DSCT) system. Eur Radiol 2006 16(2):256-68. Epub 2005 Dec 10. Erratum in: Eur Radiol 2006 16(6):1405
3. Flohr TG, Schoepf UJ, Ohnesorge BM (2007) Chasing the heart: new developments for cardiac CT. J Thorac Imaging 22(1):4-16
4. Marano R, Storto ML, Maddestra N, Bonomo L (2004) Non-invasive assessment of coronary artery bypass graft with retrospectively ECG-gated four-row multi-detector spiral computed tomography. Eur Radiol 14(8):1353-1362
5. Uppot RN, Sahani DV, Hahn PF et al (2006) Effect of obesity on image quality: fifteen-year longitudinal study for evaluation of dictated radiology reports. Radiology 240(2):435-439
6. Uppot RN (2007) Impact of obesity on radiology. Radiol Clin North Am (2):231-246
7. Sirineni GK, Kalra MK, Pottala K et al (2007) Effect of contrast concentration, tube potential and reconstruction kernels on MDCT evaluation of coronary stents: an in vitro study. Int J Cardiovasc Imaging 23(2):253-263
8. Schlosser T, Scheuermann T, Ulzheimer S et al (2007) In vitro evaluation of coronary stents and in-stent stenosis using a dynamic cardiac phantom and a 64-detector row CT scanner. Clin Res Cardiol 96(12):883-890
9. Ritman EL, Kinsey JH, Robb RA et al (1980) Physics and technical considerations in the design of the DSR: a high temporal resolution volume scanner. AJR Am J Roentgenol 134:369-374
10. Ritman EL (2003) Cardiac computed tomography imaging: a history and some future possibilities. Cardiol Clin 21:491-513
11. McCollough CH, Primak AN, Saba O et al (2007) Dose performance of a 64-channel dual-source CT scanner. Radiology 243(3):775-784
12. Kyriakou Y, Kalender WA (2007) Intensity distribution and impact of scatter for dual-source CT. Phys Med Biol 52(23):6969-6989
13. Kalra MK, Schmidt B, Suess C et al (2005)Comparison of single and dual source 64-channel MDCT scanners for evaluation of large patients: A phantom study. 91st Annual Meeting of the Radiological Society of North America, Chicago, IL (Hot topic)
14. Johnson TR, Krauss B, Sedlmair M et al (2007) Material differentiation by dual energy CT: initial experience. Eur Radiol 17(6):1510-1517
15. Swensen SJ, Yamashita K, McCollough CH et al (2000) Lung nodules: dual-kilovolt peak analysis with CT—multicenter study. Radiology 214(1):81-85
16. Primak AN, Fletcher JG, Vrtiska TJ et al (2007) Noninvasive differentiation of uric acid versus non-uric acid kidney stones using dual-energy CT. Acad Radiol 4(12):1441-1447
17. Kalra MK, Blake MA, Sahani DV et al (2007) Dual energy CT for characterization of adrenal adenoma. 93rd Annual Meeting of the Radiological Society of North America (RSNA), Chicago, IL
18. Udayasankar U, Li J, Nye J, Small W (2007) Effect of Tube Potential on CT Histogram Analysis of Adrenal Masses. 93rd Annual Meeting of the Radiological Society of North America (RSNA), Chicago, IL
19. Deveci S, Coflkun M, Tekin MI et al (2004) Spiral computed tomography: role in determination of chemical compositions of pure and mixed urinary stones—an in vitro study. Urology 64(2):237-240
20. Scheffel H, Stolzmann P, Frauenfelder T et al (2007) Dual-energy contrast-enhanced computed tomography for the detection of urinary stone disease. Invest Radiol 42(12):823-9
21. Flohr T, Raupach R, Bruder H (2006) Reduction of the Blooming Effect for Calcified Plaques in CT An-

giographic Examinations by Means of dual energy CT. Radiological Society of North America , IL (Scientific paper presented on November 28, 2006)

22. Scheffel H, Alkadhi H, Plass A et al (2006) Accuracy of dual-source CT coronary angiography: First experience in a high pre-test probability population without heart rate control. Eur Radiol 16(12):2739-2747

23. Johnson TR, Nikolaou K, Busch S et al (2007) Diagnostic accuracy of dual-source computed tomography in the diagnosis of coronary artery disease. Invest Radiol 42(10):684-691

24. Oncel D, Oncel G, Tastan A (2007) Effectiveness of dual-source CT coronary angiography for the evaluation of coronary artery disease in patients with a trial fibrillation: initial experience. Radiology 245(3):703-711

25. Ropers U, Ropers D, Pflederer T et al (2007) Influence of heart rate on the diagnostic accuracy of dual-source computed tomography coronary angiography. J Am Coll Cardiol 50(25):2393-8

26. Matt D, Scheffel H, Leschka S et al (2007) Dual-source CT coronary angiography: image quality, mean heart rate, and heart rate variability. AJR Am J Roentgenol 189(3):567-73

27. Rist C, Johnson TR, Becker A et al (2007) Dual-source cardiac CT imaging with improved temporal resolution: Impact on image quality and analysis of left ventricular function. Radiologe 47(4):287-290, 292-294

28. Busch S, Johnson TR, Wintersperger BJ et al (2007) Quantitative assessment of left ventricular function with dual-source CT in comparison to cardiac magnetic resonance imaging: initial findings. Eur Radiol [Epub ahead of print]

29. Groen JM, Greuter MJ, Vliegenthart R et al (2007) Calcium scoring using 64-slice MDCT, dual source CT and EBT: a comparative phantom study. Int J Cardiovasc Imaging [Epub ahead of print]

30. Pugliese F, Weustink AC, Van Mieghem C et al (2007) Dual-source coronary computed tomography angiography for detecting in-stent restenosis. Heart [Epub ahead of print]

31. Lell MM, Panknin C, Saleh R et al (2007) Evaluation of coronary stents and stenoses at different heart rates with dual source spiral CT (DSCT). Invest Radiol (7):536-541

32. Mori S, Endo M, Nishizawa K et al (2006) Comparison of patient doses in 256-slice CT and 16-slice CT scanners. Br J Radiol 79(937):56-61

33. Funabashi N, Yoshida K, Tadokoro H et al (2005) Cardiovascular circulation and hepatic perfusion of pigs in 4-dimensional films evaluated by 256-slice cone-beam computed tomography. Circ J 69(5):585-589

6

Contrast Considerations in Pregnancy

Henrik S. Thomsen

Introduction

Radiological investigations using iodinated contrast media are not often carried out in pregnant patients in order to avoid exposing the foetus to ionising radiation [1]. Occasionally, however, investigations such as CT head scan or CT pulmonary angiogram may be necessary to protect the mother's health, and the potential additional hazard posed by the contrast medium has to be considered. In addition, the fear of causing foetal harm or even death through medications used in pregnancy has meant that there has been no clinical research about the safety of drugs in pregnancy. Instead, medication safety information has only become available from case reports, epidemiological studies and animal studies, all of which have limitations that make determining the risks of using a particular drug during pregnancy difficult. For these reasons, the pharmaceutical industry discourages the use of medications during pregnancy and lactation. Likewise, the administration of contrast media is off-label, but not contraindicated, in this group of patients [2].

The potential hazards of radiography for a pregnant woman stem not only from the contrast agent but also from the radiation and the procedure itself, particularly image-guided interventions. Before a pregnant woman undergoes an imaging procedure, the examination must be justified based on her clinical symptoms and signs. The over-riding decision regarding the use of iodinated contrast agents in the pregnant patient usually relates to the amount of radiation necessary to generate the image and the subsequent risk to the foetus. The mother may receive direct benefit while the foetus may be exposed without direct benefit. If the mother's medical problem is life threatening, imaging of the mother may lead to her survival, which directly benefits the foetus.

Water-soluble iodinated contrast media when given intravascularly to a pregnant woman cause only brief foetal exposure, and any associated free iodide is short-lived. Concerns about the effects of contrast media are mainly related to the early and late stages of pregnancy.

In a lactating mother who is given an iodinated contrast medium, the amount of the agent that reaches the infant's blood is tiny compared with the amount that reaches the foetus.

Pregnancy

Placental Transfer and Foetal Circulation

In the human placenta, there is only a single layer of chorionic epithelium separating maternal blood from foetal connective tissue [3]. Most drugs traverse the chorionic epithelium by diffusion. Iodinated non-ionic monomeric contrast agents that are water-soluble and have molecular masses of 500–850 Daltons would be expected to traverse the placenta less easily than lipid-soluble or smaller water soluble molecules [4]. Only small amounts of iobitridol, a non-ionic iodinated agent, crossed the placenta of rabbits in the 24 h following injection [5].

Iodinated contrast agents that cross the placenta into the foetal blood are excreted by the kidneys into the bladder. When the bladder empties, these compounds enter the amniotic fluid, which, when swallowed, causes the contrast media to reach the foetal gut (Fig. 1). It has been known for many years that intravenous contrast media given to the mother could result in a neonatal pyelogram or opacification of the neonatal gut [6-11]. Contrast media injected into the amniotic fluid have been used to opacify the foetal gut before intrauterine transfusion [12]. Assays of amniotic fluid for iodine when amniocentesis was done following maternal intravenous urography showed large

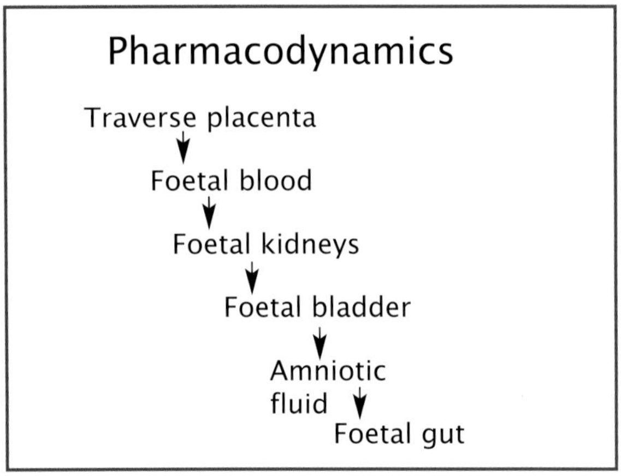

Pharmacodynamics

Traverse placenta
↓
Foetal blood
↓
Foetal kidneys
↓
Foetal bladder
↓
Amniotic
fluid ↓
Foetal gut

Fig. 1. Foetal pharmacodynamics of contrast media administered to the mother

amounts of iodine 24 h after urography, and much lower amounts 22 days later [13]. This suggests that contrast media diffuse out through the placenta into the mother but also pass from the mother into the foetus.

Concerns during Pregnancy

Early Pregnancy
During early pregnancy, the potential mutagenicity and teratogenicity of contrast media are of concern. No mutagenic effects have been shown with ionic iodinated contrast media in vitro [14]. In animals, mutagenic or teratogenic effects of non-ionic iodinated contrast media tested in vivo have not been found [15-22]. In contrast, abnormal micronuclei indicating chromosomal damage were detected in lymphocytes following radiological investigations using iodinated ionic and non-ionic agents [23-25]. This effect, however, appears to be cytotoxic rather than genetic, and only cells circulating in the blood at the time of the examination are affected [23, 26].

Late Pregnancy
The most important potentially harmful effect of iodinated contrast media that cross the placenta is depression of the foetal thyroid. By week 12 of gestation, the foetal thyroid, under the influence of thyroid stimulating hormone (TSH), synthesises thyroxine (T4). From 30 weeks onwards, triiodothyronine (T3) levels increase until birth [27]. Foetal thyroid function is essential for the normal development of the central nervous system [28, 29]. For this reason, iodine-containing drugs are usually contraindicated during pregnancy, because they may depress iodide uptake by the foetal thyroid [4].

Amniography carried out using a mixture of Lipiodol (iodised ethyl esters of the fatty acids of poppy-seed oil) and water-soluble agents showed elevated TSH levels during the first week in most neonates examined [30]. Several infants subsequently developed hypothyroidism [30, 31]. Fat-soluble Lipiodol is deposited on the vermix, where it can be absorbed by the foetus over a long period. In rabbits, Lipiodol crosses the placenta and accumulates in the foetal thyroid [32]; it also persists in the body when given intramuscularly. These properties have led to its use in the treatment of iodine deficiency, with increased urinary iodine levels detectable for over 12 months following its administration [33].

When water-soluble iodinated contrast media were used alone for amniography, no abnormalities in cord blood T4 and T3 were detected [34]. The decline in amniotic-fluid iodine levels over time after water-soluble iodinated contrast agents were given to the mother indicates the diffusion of contrast agent, and thus of potentially harmful free iodide, back across the placenta into the mother [13, 35]. In a contrast agent with 300 mg I/ml, the upper level of free iodide allowed immediately after production of the compound is 50 mg/ml and at 3–5 years after production 90 mg/ml. In practice, the free iodide concentration is usually one tenth of these amounts [35]. If the free iodide content of a contrast agent is 50 mg/ml and if 150 ml of the agent is used for CT pulmonary angiography in a pregnant woman, the total free iodide dose is 7,500 mg. Although there are no data on the pharmacodynamics of free iodide, it likely traverses the placenta readily in both directions so that the foetal thyroid is exposed to the iodide for only a short period of time. In pregnant women with impaired renal function, blood levels of contrast medium and free iodide remain higher for longer, with concomitantly longer exposure of the foetus. The neonatal thyroid appears to tolerate high doses of non-ionic agents (e.g., 1,500 mg I/kg iopamidol) in the first month of life, as thyroid function is not usually affected [36]. Nonetheless, it is recommended that following exposure, neonatal thyroid function is checked during the first week of life [37]. Although in many countries this is standard paediatric practice [38], it is mandatory when the mother has received an iodinated contrast agent during pregnancy

Other Effects of Contrast Media
Other adverse effects of iodinated contrast media given during pregnancy have not been described. Similarly, harmful effects of arteriography and amniography undertaken with ionic agents have yet to be reported [12, 39, 40]. Thus, there are no differences between pregnant women and non-pregnant women regarding the incidence and

severity of acute non-renal adverse reactions, acute renal adverse reactions (contrast-induced nephropathy), and late and very adverse reactions. The precautions are the same.

Lactation

The excretion of drugs into breast milk is facilitated when the drugs are lipid soluble and bind readily to plasma and milk proteins [41]. Iodinated contrast media are water soluble with minimal protein-binding ability, suggesting that they are likely to enter milk only with difficulty. Nonetheless, the drug package inserts recommend that babies not be breast fed for 24-48 h after intravascular administration of iodinated contrast media to a lactating patient.

Early reports suggested that iodinated contrast media was excreted into breast milk in very low or undetectable amounts after the injection of intravenous ionic agents or an intrathecal non-ionic agent [42, 43]. Even after the injection of fat-soluble cholecystographic agents, iodine excretion in breast milk was very low [44]. A detailed study of larger doses (350 mg I/kg) of the non-ionic agent iohexol and the ionic agent metrizoate showed that small amounts of these contrast agents reached the milk [45]. It was calculated that with a breast-milk intake of 0.15 l/kg/day, the infant would have received 1.7 mg I/kg with iohexol and 0.7 mg I/kg with metrizoate, corresponding to 0.5% and 0.3% of the maternal dose, respectively [45]. For paediatric urography, the recommended dose is 900 mg I/kg for babies less than 6.5 kg and 600 mg I/kg for babies 7.0 kg or more [46]. The dose of iohexol received in the milk over 24 h is only 0.002% of the recommended intravenous dose for urography. Only very small amounts of iodinated contrast agents in the gut are absorbed into the blood. When the non-ionic agent metrizamide was administered as an oral contrast agent, 0.8% of the total dose was excreted into the urine by the end of the third day [47].

The very low risk to the neonate suggests that the potential disruption to mother and baby that is caused by stopping breast feeding for 24-48 h after the administration of contrast medium is not warranted. As with all drugs and foodstuffs, the baby may notice a change in the taste of the milk.

Conclusion

If multi-detector-row CT is justified, contrast medium should be given whenever it may benefit the mother.

References

1. Bury RF (2002) Radiation hazards in urological practice. BJU Int 89: 505-509
2. Raine JM (2006) Off-label use of medicines – Legal Aspects. In: Thomsen HS (ed.) Contrast media: Safety issues and ESUR Guidelines. Heidelberg, Springer, pp 5-8
3. Broughton-Pipkin F, Hull D, Stephenson T (1994) Foetal physiology. In: Lamming GE (ed) Marshall's Physiology of Reproduction, 4th edition. London, Chapman & Hall, 777
4. Bloomfield TH, Hawkins DF (1991) The effects of drugs on the human fetus. In: Philipp E, Setchell M (eds) Scientific Foundations of Obstetrics and Gynaecology, 4th edition. Oxford, Butterworth-Heinemann 320
5. Bourrinet P, Dencausse A, Havard P et al (1995) Transplacental passage and milk excretion of iobitridol. Invest Radiol 30:156-158
6. Thomas CR, Lang EK, Lloyd FP (1963) Fetal pyelography – a method for detecting fetal life. Obstet Gynecol 22:335-340
7. Kelleher J, Feczko PJ, Radkowski MA, Griscom NT (1979) Neonatal intestinal opacification secondary to transplacental passage of urographic contrast medium. AJR Am J Roentgenol 132:63-65
8. Moon AJ, Katzberg RW, Sherman MP (2000) Transplacental passage of iohexol. J Pediatr 136:548-549
9. Hill BJ, Saigal G, Patel S, Abdenour Jr. GE (2007) Transplacental passage of non-ionic contrast agnets resulting in fetal bowel opafication: a mimic of pneumoperitoneum in the newborn. Pediatr Radiol 37:396-398
10. Vanhaesebrouck P, Verstraete AG, De Praeter C et al (2005) Transplacental passage of a nonionic contrast agent. Eur J Pediatr 164:408-410
11. Saigal G, Abdenour GE (2007) Another case of transplacental passage of the non-ionic contrast agent ioversol. Pediatr Radiol 37:726-727
12. Raphael MJ, Gordon H, Schiff D (1967) Radiological aspects of intra-uterine blood transfusion. Br J Radiol 40:520-527
13. Etling N, Gehin-Fouque F, Vielh JP, Gautray JP (1979) The iodine content of amniotic fluid and placental transfer of iodinated drugs. Obstet Gynecol 53:376-380
14. Nelson JA, Livingstone GK, Moon RG (1982) Mutagenic evaluation of radiographic contrast media. Invest Radiol 17:183-185
15. Felder E (1984) Iopamidol toxicology. Invest Radiol 19 (Suppl):S168-S170
16. Shaw DD, Potts DG (1985) Toxicology of iohexol. Invest Radiol 20(Suppl 1):S10-S13
17. Ralston WH, Robbins MS, James P (1989) Reproductive, developmental and genetic toxicity of ioversol. Invest Radiol 24(Suppl 1):S16-S22
18. Morisetti A, Tirone P, Luzzani F, de Haen C (1994) Toxicological safety assessment of iomeprol, a new x-ray contrast agent. Eur J Radiol 18(Suppl 1):S21-S31
19. Fujikawa K, Sakaguchi Y, Harada S et al (1995) Reproductive toxicity of iodixanol, a new non-ionic, iso-tonic contrast medium in rats and rabbits (in Japanese). J Toxicol Sci 20 (Suppl 1):107-115
20. Heglund IF, Michelet AA, Blazak WF et al (1995) Preclinical pharmacokinetics and general toxicity of iodixanol. Acta Radiol Suppl 399:69-82
21. Donandieu AM, Idee JM, Doncet D et al (1996) Toxicologic profile of iobitridol, a new nonionic low osmolality contrast medium. Acta Radiol Suppl

400:17-24

22. Krause W, Schobel C, Press WR (1994) Preclinical testing of iopromide. 2nd communication: toxicological evaluation. Arzneimittelforschung 44:1275-1279
23. Norman A, Adams FH, Riley RF (1978) Cytogenetic effects of contrast media and tri-iodobenzoic acid derivatives in human lymphocytes. Radiology 129:199-203
24. Cochran ST, Khodadoust A, Norman A (1980) Cytogenetic effects of contrast material in patients undergoing excretory urography. Radiology 136:43-46
25. Cochran ST, Norman A (1994) Induction of micronuclei in lymphocytes of patients undergoing excretory urography with ioversol. Invest Radiol 29:210-212
26. Norman A, Cochran ST, Sayre JW (2001) Meta-analysis of increases in micronuclei in peripheral blood lymphocytes after angiography or excretory urography. Radiat Res 15:740-743
27. Ramsay I (1986) The thyroid. In: Philipp EE, Barnes J, Newton M (eds) Scientific Foundation of Obstetrics and Gynaecology, 3rd edition. London, Heinemann 463
28. Semba RD, Delange F (2001) Iodine in human milk: perspectives for infant health. Nutr Rev 59:269-278
29. Delange F, De Benoist B, Pretell B, Dunn JT (2001) Iodine deficiency in the world: where do we stand at the turn of the century? Thyroid 11:437-447
30. Rodesch F, Camus M, Ermans AM, Dodion J, Delange F (1976) Adverse effect of amniofetography on fetal thyroid function. Am J Obst Gynecol 126:723-726
31. Stubbe P, Heidermann P, Schumbraad P, Ulbrich R (1980) Transient congenital hypothyroidism after amniofetography. Eur J Pediatr 135:97-99
32. Bourrinet P, Dencausse A, Cochet P et al (1997) Secretion in milk and transplacental transfer of two iodised oils, Lipiodol UF and Oriodol, in rabbits. Biol Neonate 71:395-402
33. Leverge R, Bergmann JF, Simoneau G et al (2003) Bioavailability of oral vs intramuscular iodinated oil (Lipiodol UF) in healthy subjects. J Endocrinol Invest 26 (Suppl 2):2-6
34. Morrison JC, Boyd M, Friedman BI et al (1973) The effects of Renografin-60 on the fetal thyroid. Obstet Gynecol 42:99-103
35. van der Molen AJ, Thomsen HS, Morcos SK, members of Contrast Media Safety Committee of European Society of Urogenital Radiology (2004) Effect of iodinated contrast media on thyroid function in adults. Eur Radiol 14:902-907
36. Bona G, Zaffaroni M, Defilippe C et al (1992) Effects of iopamidol on neonatal thyroid function. Eur J Radiol 14:22-25
37. Webb JAW, Thomsen HS, Morcos SK Members of Contrast Media Safety Committee of European Society of Urogenital Radiology (ESUR) (2005) The use of iodinated and gadolinium contrast media during pregnancy and lactation. Eur Radiol 15:1234-1240
38. Klein RZ, Mitchell ML (2000) Hypothyroidism in infants and children. In: Braverman LE, Utiger RD (eds) The Thyroid: A Fundamental and Clinical Text, 8th edition. Philadelphia, Lippincott, Williams & Wilkins, pp 973-974
39. Wholey MH (1967) Evaluation of arteriography in obstetrics. Radiol Clin North Am 121-131
40. Blumberg ML, Wohl GT, Wiltchik S et al (1967) Placental localisation by amniography. AJR Am J Roentgenol 100:688-697
41. Wilson JT, Brown RR, Cherek DR et al (1980) Drug excretion in human breast milk: principles, pharmacokinetics and projected consequences. Clin Pharmacokinet 5:1-66
42. Fitzjohn TP, Williams DG, Laker MF, Owen JP (1982) Intravenous urography during lactation. Br J Radiol 55:603-605
43. Ilett KF, Hackett LP, Paterson JW, McCormick CC (1981) Excretion of metrizamide in milk. Br J Radiol 54:537-538
44. Holmdahl KH (1956) Cholecystography during lactation. Acta Radiol 45:305-307
45. Nielsen ST, Matheson I, Rasmussen JN et al (1987) Excretion of iohexol and metrizoate in human breast milk. Acta Radiol 28:523-526
46. Jorulf II (1983) Iohexol compared with diatrizoate in pediatric urography. Acta Radiol Suppl 366:42-45
47. Johansen JG (1978) Assessment of a non-ionic contrast medium (Amipaque) in the gastrointestinal tract. Invest Radiol 13:523-527

7

MDCT and Obesity

Raul N. Uppot

Introduction

Although multi-detector computed tomography (MDCT) is widely available, its use is curtailed in three groups of patients: pediatric patients, pregnant patients, and the morbidly obese.

Limitations on imaging pediatric and pregnant patients are self-imposed by radiologists to avoid radiation exposure to these patients. However, limitations for imaging morbidly obese patients are equipment-imposed, including the inability to accommodate the patient on imaging equipment or to obtain adequate-quality images [1, 2].

Thus, the use of MDCT to image the obese patient represents a dichotomy. If the patient fits on imaging equipment and the study is properly planned to take into account the large body habitus, MDCT can be the best and only available imaging tool for such patients. However, if the obese patient exceeds the table weight or gantry diameter limit, he or she cannot be imaged using MDCT and the remaining imaging options are few.

The purpose of this chapter is to discuss: (1) the clinical definition of obesity, its increasing incidence, and the factors that impact imaging; (2) the difficulties in CT imaging obese patients and considerations in acquiring images, including proper protocols, intravenous contrast, and radiation exposure; (3) positron emission tomography (PET) PET/CT, CT colonography, and CT-guided interventional procedures in the obese; and (4) pending technologies, such as dual-source CT, which could improve image quality when imaging obese patients.

Definition of Obesity

Clinically, obesity is defined by body mass index (BMI), defined as a person's weight in kilograms divided by his or her height in meters squared (kg/m^2). The definitions of overweight, obese, and morbidly obese are based on BMI (Table 1). The quantification of fat is important, because obesity is the cause of numerous associated health problems, including hypertension, type II diabetes, heart disease, and cancer (endometrial, breast, colon) [1]. Although BMI is used clinically to quantify fat, it is not useful for the purposes of acquiring diagnostic MDCT images. Instead, in MDCT imaging of obese patients, the body dimensions, i.e., body weight and body diameter, are more important.

Incidence of Obesity

The prevalence of obesity has progressively increased in the USA and throughout the world. Currently, in the USA, approximately 66% of the adult population is considered overweight, obese, or morbidly obese [1]. More than 60 million American adults (> 20 years old) have a BMI > 30 kg/m^2, with 6 million individuals in this group considered morbidly obese (BMI > 40 kg/m^2) [1]. Obesity trend maps from the Centers for Disease Control and Prevention (CDC) show a progressive increase in the prevalence of obesity from 1995 to 2006 in all 50 states [3] (Fig. 1). The incidence of obesity has also increased throughout the world. It is estimated that worldwide, approximately 1.7 billion people are considered overweight or obese [4].

Table 1. Clinical weight classification based on body mass index (BMI)

Weight classification	BMI
Underweight	<18.5 kg/m^2
Normal weight	18.5–24.9 kg/m^2
Overweight	25–29.9 kg/m^2
Obese	30–39.9 kg/m^2
Morbidly obese	> 40 kg/m^2

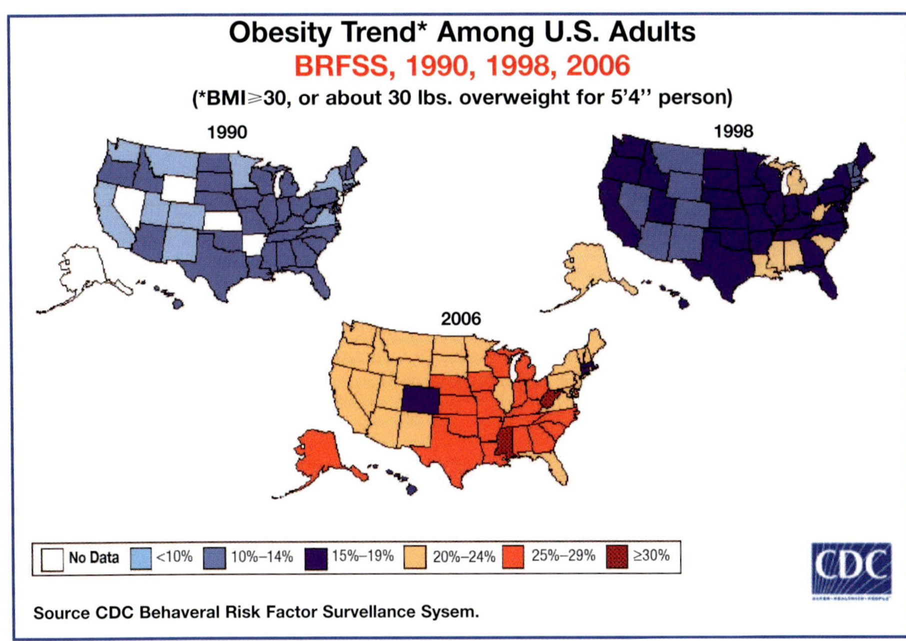

Fig. 1. Obesity trends among adults in the USA: 1990, 1998, 2006 for patients with BMI > 30 or 30 lbs overweight for 5'4" person. (From Centers for Disease Control and Prevention. Behavioral risk factor and surveillance. Available at:http://www.cdc.gov/nccdphp/dnpa/obesity/trend/maps. Accessed January 28, 2008)

Additionally, obese patients are entering health care facilities in increasing numbers due to the rise in popularity of gastric bypass or gastric banding surgery. In 2006, it is estimated that 170,000 gastric bypass procedures were performed in the USA [5]. Although not all patients who undergo laparascopic bariatric surgery require MDCT (they all need preoperative ultrasound and postoperative barium swallow), this imaging modality is valuable when the need arises to evaluate for potential postoperative complications. In addition, at many health centers, CT is used to determine total body and intraperitoneal fat. A single-slice CT image acquired at the level of the lumbar spine is used to quantify and monitor the amount of intraperitoneal fat [4].

Fitting Obese Patients on the MDCT Equipment

Factors that must be considered when a CT scan is acquired from an obese patient include table weight and gantry diameter limits, and the ability of the patient to remain in the prone position and motionless during image acquisition. However, compared with the design and function of other imaging modalities, such as ultrasound, fluoroscopy, and magnetic resonance imaging (MRI), CT offers a competitive option for imaging large patients (Table 2). In addition, "large-bore CT," which supports weight limits up to 390 kg (680 lbs) and accommodates gantry diameters up to 90 cm, is slowly becoming available for diagnostic imaging.

Weight Limits

The most important factor in the ability to acquire a CT scan is a patient's body weight. If a patient's weight exceeds the CT table weight limit, the patient cannot be placed on the CT scanner and images cannot be acquired.

Table-weight limits are defined by equipment manufacturers. The current industry standard table weight limit for CT is 205 kg (450 lbs). Although the

Table 2. Industry standard and industry maximum weight limits and aperture diameter limits for various imaging modalities

Modality	Standard weight limit	Standard aperture diameter	Industry maximum weight limit	Industry maximum aperture diameter
Ultrasound	None	None	None	None
Fluoroscopy	160 kg (350 lbs)	45 cm	318 kg (700 lbs)	47 inches
4- to 64-slice MDCT	204 kg (450 lbs)	70 cm	309 kg (680 lbs)	90 cm
Cylindrical-bore MRI 1.5–3.0 T	160 kg (350 lbs)	60 cm	250 kg (550 lbs)	70 cm
Vertical field MRI 0.3–1.0 T	250 kg (550 lbs)	55 cm	250 kg (550 lbs)	55 cm

MDCT multi-detector row computed tomography, *MRI* magnetic resonance imaging

CT table can physically sustain weights of more than 205 kg (450 lbs), the limitations are defined by how much weight the table motor can lift vertically and the accuracy with which the table can horizontally move the patient into the gantry. Industry standards require that the table be able to move into the gantry at a constant speed to an accuracy of 0.25 mm while supporting any weight load.

Knowing both the maximum allowable CT table weight limit and the patient's weight prior to scheduling CT examinations is important to avoid disruptions. If the patient's weight exceeds the table weight limit, the CT examination should not be scheduled and the radiologists must consult with the referring physician to assess possible alternatives, including standing plain radiographs, ultrasound (which will likely be very limited in image quality but not limited by weight), or MRI [which, for some models, can support weights up to 250 kg (550 lbs)].

Gantry Diameter Limit

A patient who meets the CT table weight limit must also meet the gantry diameter limit. The CT gantry diameter is defined by a fixed diameter. The current industry standard for diagnostic CT gantry diameter is 70 cm. This measurement is defined in the horizontal plane. The anteroposterior (AP) diameter of the gantry is approximately 12–15 cm less due to the table taking up space within the gantry (Fig. 2).

Prior to scheduling CT, if a patient's large weight suggests that his or her body diameter may approach the gantry limits, the patient's body diameter must be measured. One unique solution to determine body circumference is to use a hula hoop, with a circumference approximating the

gantry diameter [7]. The hula hoop can be taken to the patient's bedside by the technologists and fitted around the patient. If the patient can fit within the hula-hoop, the CT is scheduled. If the patient cannot fit within the hula hoop, the CT examination is canceled, and the disruption incurred by bringing the patient to the department and attempting to fit him or her through the gantry is avoided.

The ability to fit into the gantry is even more critical in CT-guided interventional procedures, in which both the patient and the instruments must fit through the gantry.

Ability to Remain in the Prone Position and Motionless

A third factor in the ability to acquire CT images or perform CT-guided interventional procedures in obese patients is the patient's ability to remain in the prone position and motionless.

Although CT technology has advanced to the stage at which an entire head-to-toe CT can be acquired in less than 30 s, the ability to remain prone and motionless during this brief time interval is important. A horizontal position may be a problem in obese patients, who often have associated sleep apnea, respiratory problems, or claustrophobia. Obese patients with respiratory problems, who typically lie inclined on their hospital beds may not tolerate lying flat on a CT table. In addition, obese patients whose body diameter approaches the gantry diameter and who are claustrophobic may not tolerate entering the gantry. One advantage of the CT gantry over closed-bore MRI is that the horizontal length of the CT gantry is typically shorter than that of the MRI bore. The short length of the CT gantry allows portions of the patient (such as the head) to be positioned outside the gantry while other parts of the body are imaged. Other solutions include using a pillow or wedge to allow the patient to be inclined, or to position the patient so that only the area to be imaged passes under the gantry (i.e., feet first to avoid putting the patient's head/chest through the gantry).

Acquiring Images

If the patient can be accommodated in the CT scanner then, of all the available imaging modalities, CT is an excellent modality to evaluate the obese patient. MDCT has a resolution as low as 0.625 cm and therefore can reliably detect small pathologies in a large patient. However, the quality of the CT can vary based on the distribution of fat within the obese patient's body, and equipment factors such as kilovolt peak (kVp), milliampere

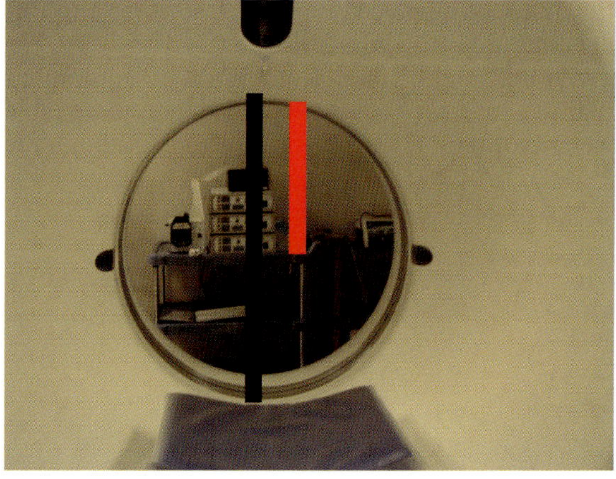

Fig. 2. Computed tomography (CT) gantry diameter is 70 cm (*black line*). Movement of the CT table into the gantry will decrease its vertical diameter to 55 cm (*red line*). Reprinted from [1], with permission from American Journal of Roentgenology

Table 3. Comparison of recommended computed tomography (CT) protocols for the 61-kg (135 lbs) vs. ≥ 91-kg (≥ 200 lbs) patient

CT parameters	61-kg patient (135 lbs)	≥ 91-kg patient (≥ 200 lbs)
Noise index	10	15
kilovolt peak (kVp)	120	140
milliampere-second (mAs)	Manual control	Automatic
Gantry rotation	1 rotation/ 0.5 s	1 rotation/1 s
Pitch	1.1	0.6

second (mAs), pitch, noise index, and field of view (FOV). Specific CT protocols for imaging obese patients are now available and can maximize image quality in these patients (Table 3). In addition, CT artifacts specific to obese patients must be recognized and corrected as necessary.

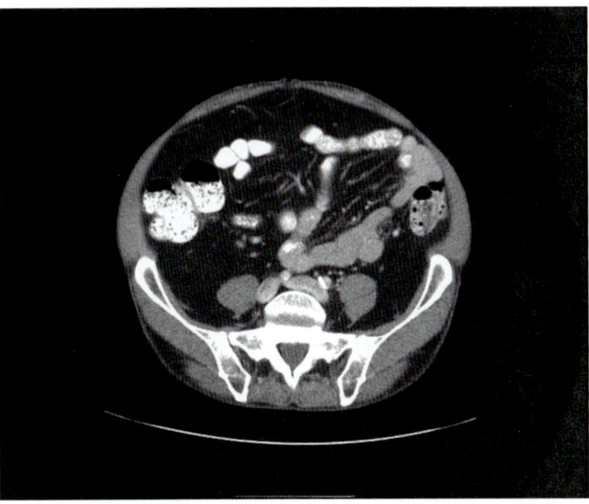

Fig. 3. Axial computed tomography (CT) in 56-year-old man with extensive intra-abdominal mesenteric fat shows separation of the small-bowel mesentery and internal organs, allowing for better visualization. Reprinted from [1], with permission from American Journal of Roentgenology

Fat Distribution

The distribution of fat, i.e., subcutaneous versus intraperitoneal, is important for image quality in CT. Good-quality images can be obtained from patients with an overabundance of intraperitoneal fat due to the wide separation of central bowel loops and intraperitoneal organs (Fig. 3), which allows for clear visualization of small structures. However, lower-quality images are obtained from patients with fat predominantly in a subcutaneous distribution; this is because not only is there less separation of the intraperitoneal organs, there is also increased attenuation of the penetrating X-ray beams as they pass through the thickness of the subcutaneous fat.

Noise Index/kVp/mAs

As with other imaging modalities, the limiting factor in obtaining diagnostic-quality images is poor penetration and increased image noise. Adjustments to the noise index, kVP, mAs, and pitch can be used to improve image quality in obese patients.

At our institution, one of the first adjustments for obese patients made on the CT scanner is the noise index. For patients weighing < 61 kg (135 lbs), the noise index is set at 10; for patients weighing 61–91 kg (135–200 lbs), it is set at 12.5; and for patients weighing > 91 kg (200 lbs) it is set at 15. The noise index determines the number of X-ray photons that will be used to create an image.

In addition, for obese patients, the standard kVp of 120 is increased to 140 kVp to penetrate through the adipose tissue. Studies using 45-cm water phantoms have shown that a kVp of at least 140 is mandatory for photons to be able to penetrate through a morbidly obese patient [8, 9]. Although increasing the kVp increases the overall radiation dose administered, it also has the inverse effect of decreasing the amount of skin dose absorbed, as the stronger photons penetrate through the subcutaneous tissue.

Another equipment adjustment to improve image quality in obese patients is an increase in the mAs. Most CT scanners have the option of delivering either a fixed mAs or an automatic mAs. In obese patients, the distribution of fat and soft tissues varies to a greater degree than in normal-sized individuals. In a head-to-toe scan, the least amount of fat is encountered in the head and chest; typically, there is more fat in the abdomen. If the CT is allowed to automatically regulate the amount of mA, the automatic mAs delivered per slice section results in an overall decrease in radiation dose to areas that do not require large mAs and allows for uniformity in the noise of the acquired image (Fig. 4).

Another option to increase the effective mAs is to decrease the gantry rotation speed. At the standard setting, images are acquired at one rotation in 0.5 s. In obese patients, slowing the gantry rotation to one rotation in 1 s has the same effect as doubling the effective mAs. Decreasing the pitch from 1.1 to 0.6 also has the effect of increasing the effective mAs.

Field of View

Standard CT equipment has an FOV of 50 cm; therefore, situations can arise in which patients are able to fit into a 70-cm gantry for imaging but still

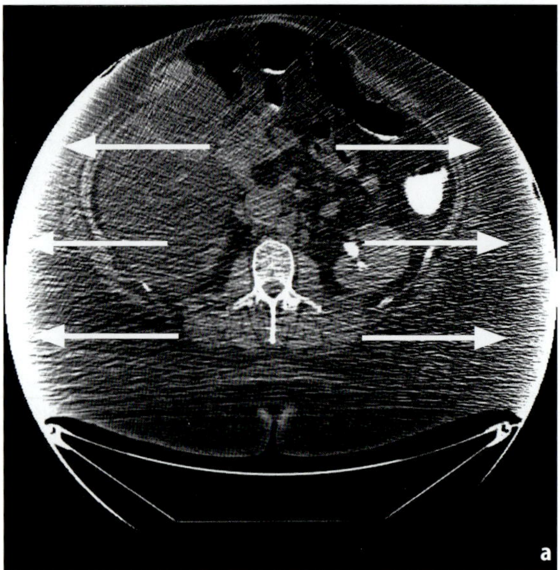
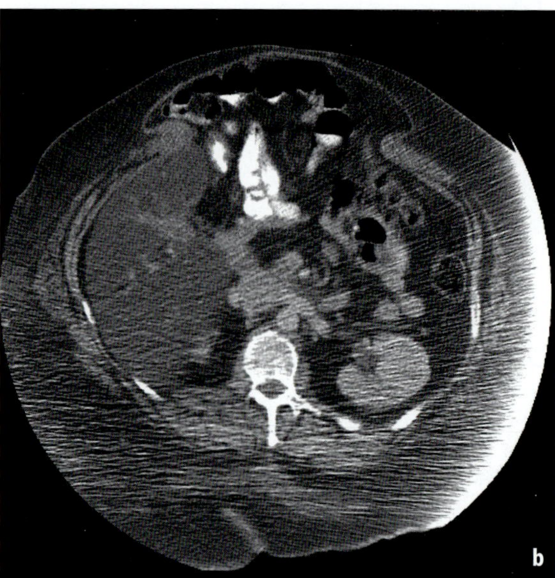

Fig. 4a, b. A 39-year-old 413-lb female patient. **a** Axial computed tomography (CT) of the abdomen with fixed milliampere-second (mAs), resulted in increased noise. Beam-hardening artifact is visualized where the patient's body exceeds the field of view (*arrows*). **b** Repeat axial CT of the abdomen with equipment setting switched to automatic mAs allows the CT to increase the mAs, thereby decreasing the noise. Reprinted from [1], with permission from American Journal of Roentgenology

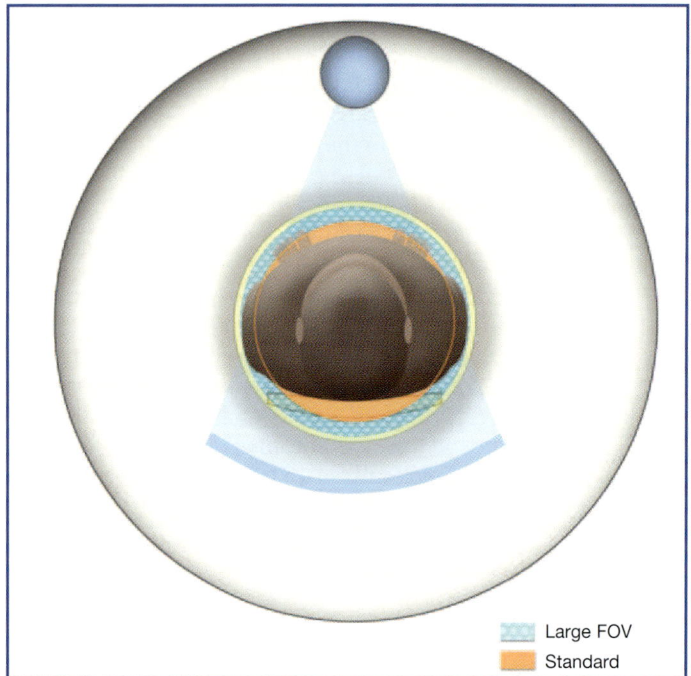

Fig. 5. Image showing gantry diameter, field of view (FOV) and extended field of view. *Thin yellow circle* represents standard computed tomography (CT) gantry diameter of 70 cm, which can accommodate a patient. However, the standard FOV of 50 cm (*orange circle*) may not cover the patient's periphery. Larger CTs with extended FOV of up to 70 cm may be able to cover the entire patient (*blue checkered area*)

exceed the 50-cm FOV. Typically, when this occurs, what is seen is similar to a beam-hardening artifact at the peripheral edge of the image. Body parts that lie beyond the 50-cm diameter FOV are not visualized, and the CT computers display them as hyperattenuating streaks, resembling beam-hardening artifacts. Solutions to this problem include adjusting the patient's body position so that the area of interest is re-imaged and placed within the 50-cm FOV. In addition, newer large-bore CTs have an increased FOV up to 70 cm (Fig. 5).

Artifacts

In addition to beam-hardening type artifacts, another image-quality issue that must be considered in obese patients occurs when images are cropped

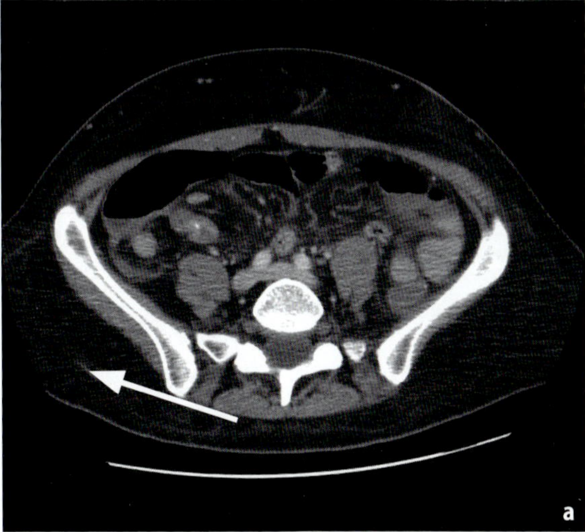

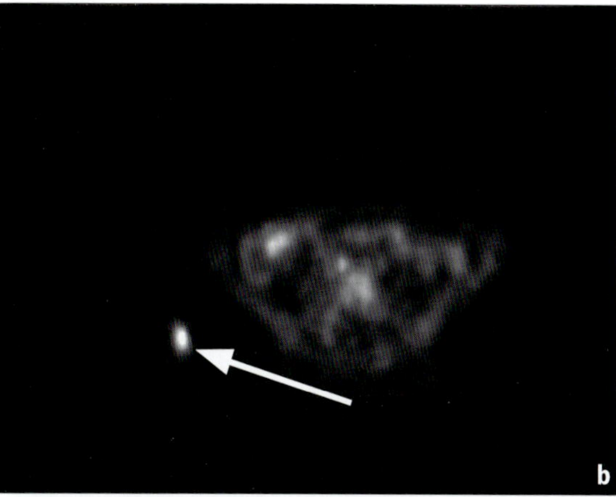

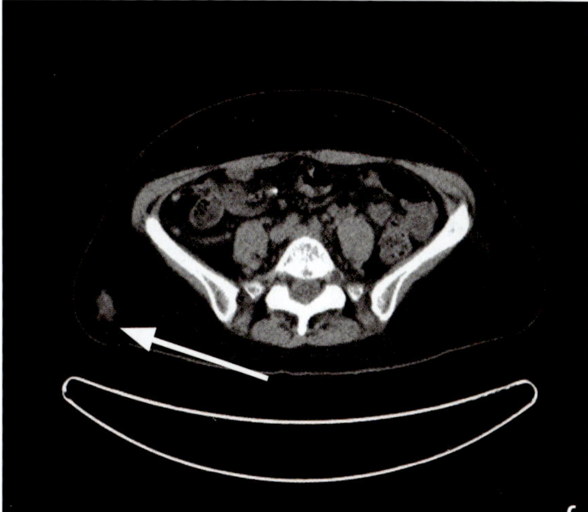

Fig. 6a-c. PET/CT in a 52-year-old, 177-lb female with history of carcinoid tumor. **a** Axial CT in a PET/CT study to look for metastasis. The CT image was cropped to focus on intra-abdominal structures. **b** PET portion of the study which was not cropped showed an area of FDG uptake (*arrow*). **c** Review of the un-cropped axial CT image showed a soft-tissue deposit (*arrow*) corresponding to the area of FDG uptake seen on PET. Reprinted from [1], with permission from American Journal of Roentgenology

by technologists to focus on internal organ structures. Such cropping in obese patients can result in the exclusion of large amounts of soft tissue and thus of pertinent information, particularly when metastatic or inflammatory processes are the focus of the evaluation (Fig. 6).

Intravenous Contrast

Obtaining intravenous access in obese patients can be challenging due to the excess subcutaneous tissues obscuring the deep superficial veins. Hospital inpatients will typically present with intravenous access; however, obese outpatients presenting for CT must be scheduled with sufficient time to allow adequate intravenous access to be established. Warm compresses, displacing the adipose tissues, guidance by anatomic landmarks, and the use of multiple tourniquets have been variously reported to aid in obtaining intravenous access in obese patients [10]. If peripheral intravenous access is not possible and intravenous contrast is needed, a cen-

tral access via a femoral or subclavian approach may be attempted by the radiologist.

The standard dose of contrast material administered in CT is weight-based (ml/kg), with the maximum dose typically being 120 ml of iodinated contrast. At our institution, the weight-based dose of Isovue 370 (370 mg iodine/ml; Bracco Diagnostics, Princeton, NJ, USA) is as follows: < 61 kg (135 lbs) = 80 ml, 61-91 kg (136-200 lbs) = 100 ml, and > 91 kg (200 lbs) = 120 ml. Obese patients (with no renal insufficiency) are typically administered the maximum 120 ml. This amount is not exceeded, as it is adequate for current scanners, which accommodate up to 205 kg (450 lbs). With the newer, larger gantry and table weight CTs, the need for increasing the weight-based contrast dose may need to be addressed.

Radiation

Increases in the kVp and, more importantly, the mAs can incrementally increase the radiation dose to the obese patients. The typical standard dose of 8 millisievert (mSv) for chest CT and 10 mSv for abdominal CT can be incrementally greater in obese patients. As noted above, increased kVp can actually decrease the skin dose absorbed as the stronger photons penetrate through the tissues.

In any CT examination, the risks of radiation must be balanced with the risks of not obtaining the CT examination. Ultrasound is likely not a viable option in obese patients due to the poor image quality obtained. There are 1.5-Tesla MRIs that can accommodate patients up to 250 kg (550 lbs).

PET/CT

Modifications to the design of PET/CT scanners to accommodate obese patients will probably only occur after the weight and gantry modifications of MDCT scanners are successfully marketed. Currently, most PET/CTs have a standard weight limit of 205 kg (250 lbs) and gantry-diameter limit of 70 cm. In addition, the co-morbidity of diabetes in obese patient must be taken into account. All diabetics require modifications to their medications prior to a PET/CT study.

CT Colonography

CT colonography provides an excellent alternative to standard optical colonoscopy in obese patients. Optical colonoscopy is typically performed under conscious sedation and requires passage of a 250-cm transrectally up to the cecum. The limitations in obese patients include the risk of conscious sedation in patients who may have a compromised airway and the possibility of encountering a lengthy tortuous colon that may not be reached with standard colonoscopy.

If an obese patient meets the weight- and gantry-limit criteria, CT colonography may be carried out with insufflation of gas via transrectal. Typically, images are acquired with the patient in the supine and prone positions; obese patients may not tolerate remaining prone, and a lateral decubitus position may be used instead.

CT-Guided Interventional Procedures

CT-guided interventional procedures are affected by the issues discussed above for diagnostic imaging in addition to other issues, including adequate positioning for the instruments to reach the target, adequate space for the instruments to clear the gantry, safe administration of conscious sedation, and the increased risk of post-procedure complications.

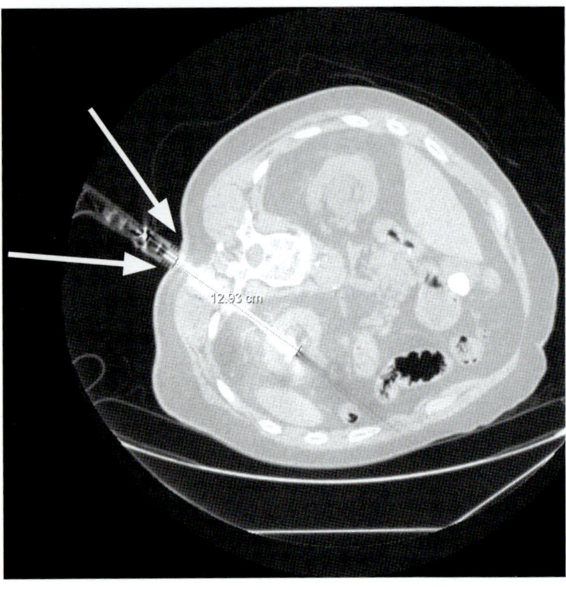

Fig. 7. Axial computed tomography (CT) in a radiofrequency ablation procedure shows pliability of the subcutaneous fat, which allows the probe to be pushed in further to gain a length advantage (*arrows*). Reprinted from [2], with permission from Elsevier

Adequate Positioning

Properly positioning the patient for CT-guided drainage or biopsy is important, as there are limitations in the length of the instruments used for these procedures (Table 3), and some instruments may be too short due the abundance of subcutaneous or intraperitoneal fat. Pre-planning the trajectory is important to find the shortest distance along the safest pathway. Properly positioning the patient can aid in decreasing the distance to the target. Occasionally, pushing the instrument in can help compress the subcutaneous fat and allow the instrument to reach its target (Fig. 7).

A second issue regarding positioning obese patients is the difficulty for one technologist alone to move the patient from the stretcher to the CT table and to safely position the patient. Several individuals may be needed to move the obese patient onto the CT table and various splints, pillows, and devices may be needed to position the patient.

Clearing the Gantry

Once the patient is properly positioned and before starting the procedure, it is necessary to determine whether portions of the instruments outside the patient are able to pass under the gantry for imaging. Positioning of an obese patient must account for the shortest distance to the target and for the ability of the instrument to pass under the gantry. Some equipment manufacturers have redesigned

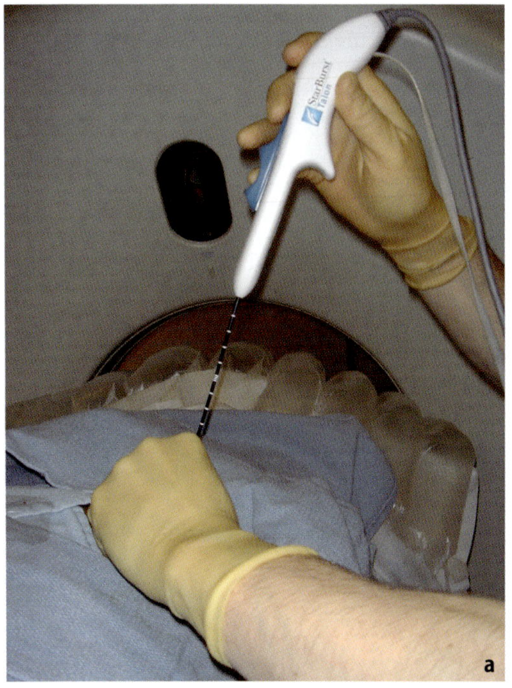 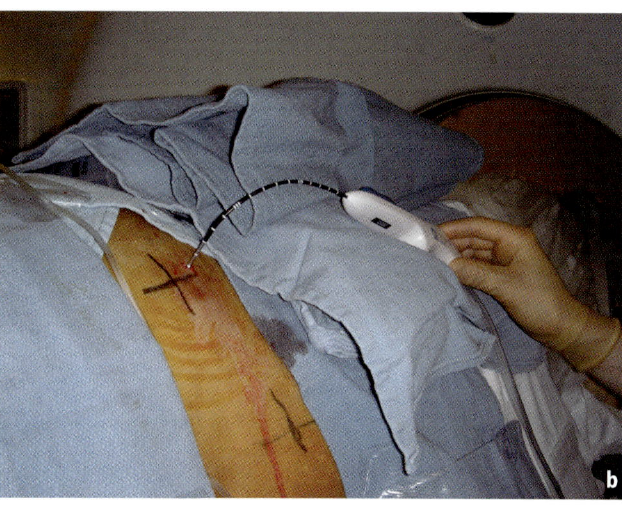

Fig. 8a, b. Radiofrequency ablation procedure. **a** Insertion of radiofrequency probe into the liver. Note minimal clearance space for the probe and the obese patient into the computed tomography (CT) gantry. **b** Radiofrequency probe is flexible and can bend, allowing the probe to clear the gantry for imaging. Reprinted from [2], with permission from Elsevier

their instruments to allow them to clear the gantry (Fig. 8).

Conscious Sedation

Administering conscious sedation to obese patients for a procedure may pose some difficulties, including adequate sedation and pain control and the risk of respiratory compromise.

Medications typically used in our institution for CT-guided procedures include lidocaine, midazolam hydrochloride, and fentanyl. Lidocaine administered locally has a maximum limit of 300 mg (30 ml of 1% lidocaine) and may not achieve adequate pain control in a 180-kg (400 lbs) patient. Intravenous medications are weight-based and do not have an absolute maximum limit. They can be administered as long as cardiac and respiratory functions are monitored. In obese patients, the dose of these weight-based drugs can be very large.

Post-procedure Complications

Obese patients have an increased risk of post-operative and post-procedure complications due to associated co-morbidities such as diabetes. In addition, the larger body mass can strain a healing wound.

New Developments

Dual-Source CT

The higher X-ray tube power of dual-source CT offers the potential for improved image quality in obese patients. Studies using water phantoms show that dual-source MDCT can provide more optimal image quality in large patients due to the higher power of the X-ray tube (160 kW; 80 kW from two sources) and data over-sampling from two detector arrays [11].

Conclusion

The increasing prevalence of obesity and the popularity of gastric bypass surgery will continue to challenge radiologists to provide diagnostic quality imaging in the subset of obese and morbidly obese patients. If a patient can be accommodated on a CT scanner, of all the imaging modalities currently available, MDCT remains the best tool for the diagnostic evaluation of obese patients. As large-bore CTs become increasingly available, the issue of accommodating obese patients on MDCT will improve. Properly designed protocols for MDCT studies and pre-planning of CT-guided interventional procedures will allow radiologists to address MDCT-related issues in obese patients.

References

1. Uppot RN, Sahani DV, Hahn PF et al (2007) Impact of obesity on Medical imaging and image-guided intervention. AJR Am J Roentgenol 188:433-440
2. Uppot RN (2007) Impact of obesity on radiology. Radiol Clin N Am 45:231-246
3. Centers for Disease Control and Prevention. Overweight and Obesity. Department of Health and Human Services Web site. http://www.cdc.gov/nccdphp/dnpa/obesity/trend/index.htm. Accessed January 28, 2008.
4. Deitel M (2003) Overweight and Obesity Worldwide Now Estimated to Involve 1.7 Billion People. Obes Surg 13(3):32-330
5. Trus TL, Pope GD, Finlayson SR (2005) National trends in utilization and outcomes of bariatric surgery. Surg Endosc 19(5):616-620
6. Zhao B, Colville J, Kalaigian J (2006) Automated quantification of body fat distribution on volumetric computed tomography. J Comput Assist Tomogr 30(5):777-783
7. Personal Communication Richard Benedikt
8. Vannier MW (2006) MDCT of massively obese patients. In: Stanford radiology 8th Annual International Symposium on Multidetector-Row CT. Stanford p 78-79
9. Vannier, MW, Johnson PJ, Dachman A et al (2005) Multidetector CT of massively obese patients. In: 2005 Radiological Society of North America Meeting (RSNA) Chicago 2005
10. Rosenthal K (2004) Selecting the best i.v. site for an obese patient. Nursing 34(11):14
11. Kalra M, Schmidt B, Suess C et al (2005) Comparison of single and dual source 64 channel MDCT scanner for evaluation of large patients: a phantom study. In: 2005 Radiological Society of North America Meeting (RSNA) Chicago, 2005

8

3-D Post-processing: Principles and Practical Applications

Unni K. Udayasankar, Zaheerabbas Momin, William C. Small

Introduction

Computed tomography (CT) has evolved considerably since its introduction more than three decades ago. In 1998, multi-detector row CT (MDCT) technology provided a key breakthrough in the field of radiology. Today, MDCT scanners enable the rapid acquisition of an exceptional number of thin sections during multiple phases of contrast enhancement. The increasing spatial and temporal resolutions have allowed major improvements to be made in differentiating and characterizing normal and abnormal structures and processes.

These technological advances present substantial new challenges, especially with respect to managing the immense amount of scan data acquired by the newer generation of MDCT scanners. One of the most important concerns is the vast quantity of images to be evaluated. The long-established technique of reviewing transverse images is giving way to nonaxial and volumetric techniques. Recent advances in MDCT technology and post-processing software have brought about excellent post-processing of axial images into superior-quality nonaxial images. Commonly performed post-processing techniques produce two-dimensional (2-D) images using multi-planar reformation (MPR) and maximum intensity projection (MIP), or three-dimensional (3-D) images using various types of volume rendering (VR) (Table 1) [1]. Older 3-D techniques, such as shaded-surface display (SSD), have fallen out of favor at most centers. Recent reports suggest significant benefits of MPR images combined with transverse images in the interpretation of diseases of various body systems [2–4]. The smaller anteroposterior and transverse compared with cranial-caudal dimensions of the body cavity generally translate into fewer total coronal and sagittal MPRs than is the case with axial images. This has the potential to result in decreased interpretation time, thus enabling prompt diagnosis in many clinical scenarios. Furthermore, the use of MPR images may improve communication with most referring physicians, who may be more familiar with anatomic relationships in the coronal and sagittal planes. Three-dimensional reformats have emerged as important diagnostic tools in noninvasive imaging of most body parts, as they allow visualization of CT images from any orientation. Furthermore, the images produced are closer to the anatomic appearance of the organ being examined. The increase in the number of thin sections generated by MDCT scanners and newer 3-D software provides enormous opportunities in 3-D post-processing and storage.

Table 1. Post-processing techniques in multi-detector row computed tomography (MDCT)

2-D techniques
Multi-planar reformation (MPR)
Coronal
Sagittal
Oblique
Curved-planar reformations (CPR)
Maximum intensity projections (MIP)
Minimum intensity projections (Min-IP)
Average intensity projections (AIP)
3-D techniques
Shaded surface display
Volume rendering
Virtual endoscopy
Virtual otoscopy
Virtual bronchoscopy
Virtual colonoscopy
Virtual cystoscopy
Virtual angiography/angioscopy

Isotropic Images

Understanding the principles of isotropic imaging is essential in formulating protocols to acquire im-

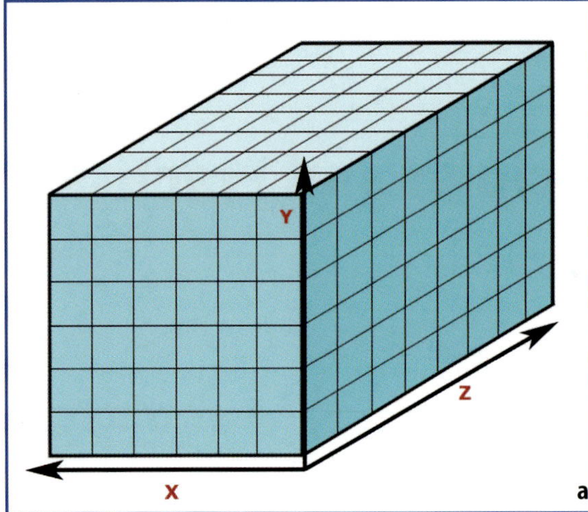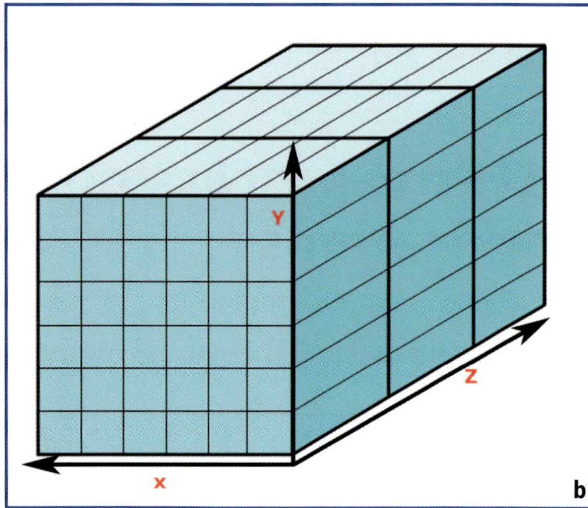

Fig. 1a, b. Geometrical representation of computed tomography (CT) data. Isotropic images (**a**) have equal dimensions in all three axes, whereas anisotropic images (**b**) have increased section thickness in z-axis compared with x- and y-axes

ages as well as to ultimately manipulate patient data using 3-D-CT protocols. The pixel sizes in axial images are determined by the field of view and the spatial resolution. The clarity of images obtained with any volumetric post-processing method relies on this spatial resolution of image data in the axial (x, y) plane as well as that acquired along the long axis of the patient (z-axis). If the reconstructed section thickness of CT images along the z-axis is equal to the pixel size within the x-y plane, the data are considered isotropic. Isotropic data have similar dimensions in all three axes, whereas anisotropic data typically have inferior spatial resolution in the longitudinal plane compared with the transverse plane (Fig. 1). Isotropic imaging directly correlates with section thickness; a section thickness of 0.5–0.8 mm is usually required to obtain the corresponding spatial resolutions in all three planes, resulting in truly isotropic images. This is achieved in present-day MDCT scanners by the narrow configuration of the detector arrays that expose the smallest detector. However, routine acquisition of isotropic data in MDCT imaging is not advocated by many investigators because of the higher patient radiation dose associated with thinner sections. As an acceptable alternative, recent generations of MDCT scanners have the ability to reconstruct thinner sections from the original data sets at need.

Post-processing Techniques in MDCT

2-D Techniques

Multiplanar reformation was one of the earliest and is still the most widely used of the 2-D post-

processing techniques. MPRs are generated from the volume of stacked axial images. Many departments routinely reformat axial data sets into coronal and/or sagittal images. A sagittal reformat is obtained from a stack of axial CT images by sampling in the y and z directions. Likewise, a coronal reformat is formed from a stack of axial images by sampling in the x and z directions. Many organs and systems in the human body cannot be accurately and completely visualized in routine coronal and axial reformats and are further benefited from oblique reformats (Fig. 2). Oblique reformats are constructed similarly to axial or coronal images, except for the orientation of the images. The axial stacks are sampled along an axis that is tilted

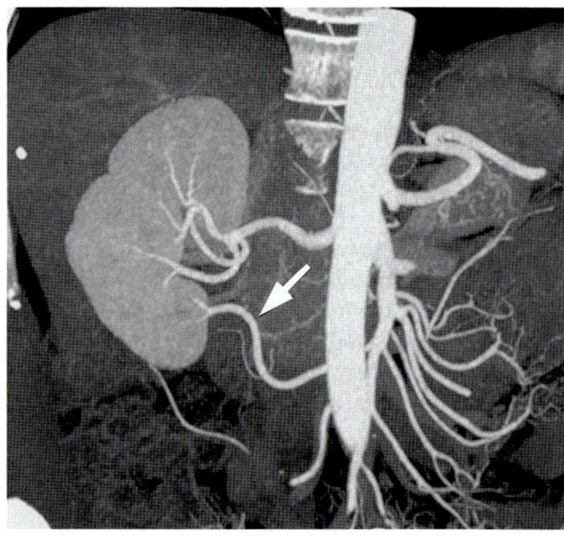

Fig. 2. Oblique MPR image shows the entire extent of the right kidney and accessory right renal artery (*arrow*)

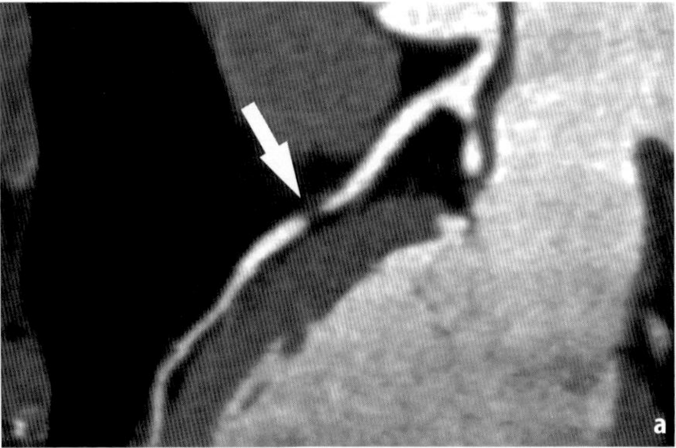
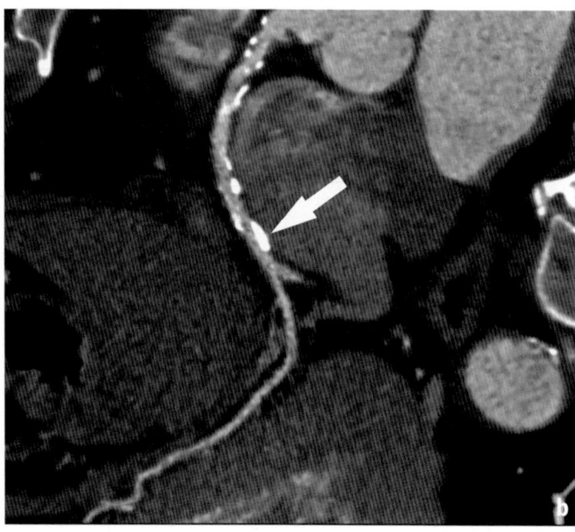

Fig. 3a, b. Curved reformat of the coronary arteries shows apparent straightening of the vessels. Note the presence of non-calcified (**a**) and calcified (**b**) plaque within the coronary arteries (*arrows*)

to the x or y axis to obtain images that may show the entire anatomic extent of the organ. Oblique reformats are particularly useful in cardiac, hepatic, and pancreatic imaging. MPRs are less intensive in terms of processing power requirements, and the modern workstations handle these reconstructions with ease.

Maximum intensity projection is similar to the MPR technique, but instead of averaging the density values in a selected slab, the MIP image displays the highest attenuation values detected when viewing rays are traced from the expected position of the operator through the object to the display screen. Unlike MPR images, this method tends to highlight bone and contrast-filled structures, and there is relative loss of low-density data in the final MIP image. MIP images are particularly useful in highlighting arterial calcium and high-density structures such as stents and prosthetic valves. They may facilitate interpretation of noisy images resulting from large body habitus or suboptimal bolus administration. Minimum intensity projection (Min-IP) is a similar technique that detects the minimum attenuation value along the ray paths. The plane selection using MIP and Min-Ip is similar to that of MPR.

Curved reformats are a variant of the multiplanar technique in which the plane of the image follows the organ and its course in its entirety. This technique is particularly useful when evaluating curved structures (mandible) or tortuous tubular structures (pancreatic or biliary ducts, blood vessels). The preferred curve is typically defined manually along the curve of the structure in question. The workstations from most vendors include automatic software that produces curved reformats of arteries by tracing the centerline for the vessel lumen and displaying the warped image around this axis. This results in a stretched out display of the

vessels. In some centers, curved reformats are the primary method of coronary artery evaluation (Fig. 3).

3-D Techniques

Surface rendering (SR), also known as shaded surface display, was the earliest 3-D rendering method developed for medical images. In surface rendering, the apparent surfaces of organs are determined within the volume of data, and an image representing the derived surfaces is displayed. Simple thresholding is a commonly used technique designed to segment structures of interest for surface rendering. In this technique, each voxel intensity within the data set is determined to be within some user-specified range of attenuation values. The volume data are converted into a list of polygons that represent the anatomic surface of interest, and the surfaces are modeled as overlapping polygons. Although surface rendering provides the clearest volume-depth cues of all 3-D images, its current use is limited to a very few specific indications. This is partly due to the development of better volume-rendering techniques, which, in addition to showing anatomic surfaces, produce excellent visualization of details beneath the surface. A common criticism of surface rendering is that it is not adequate for identifying structures that do not have naturally well-differentiated surfaces. Also, since the images are derived from only a small percentage of available data, they may fail to capture the entire extent of a particular pathology.

Volume rendering is a widely used 3-D technique in which pixels are shaded and colored depending on their attenuation values to generate a 3-D volume [5]. The CT numbers that make up the image are often allocated to be either visible or in-

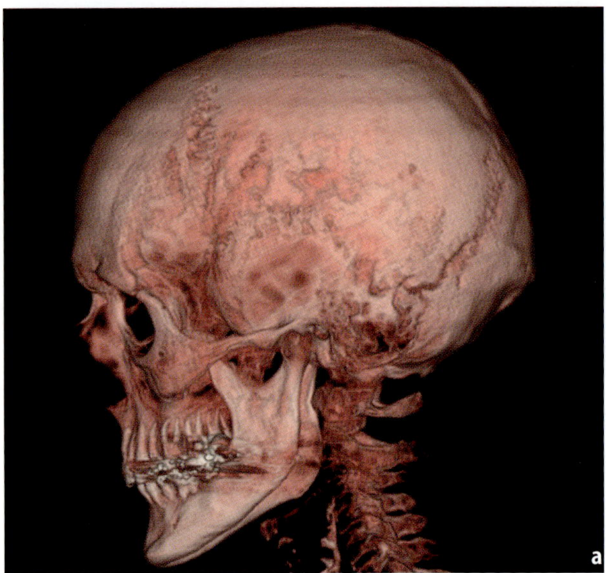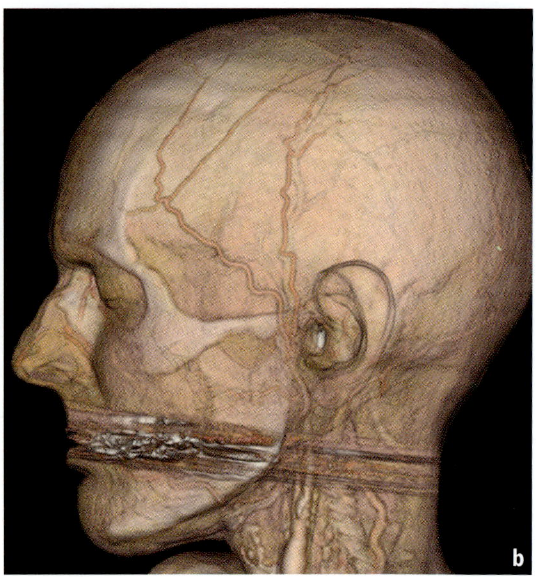

Fig. 4a, b. Effect of varying levels of transparency in 3-D VR images. Soft tissues are prominent in (**b**) compared with skeletal details in (**a**). Also note the increased circumferential artifacts from dental implants in (**b**)

visible, thus displaying the images with varying levels of transparency (Fig. 4). Different colors are assigned to ranges of attenuation values such as air, fat, soft tissue, and bone. VR not only gives surface information but also provides detail concerning interior structures, a differentiating feature from the previously used, now largely abandoned, SSD technique [6]. Adjustments of the coloring styles, opacities, and attenuation ranges highlight the structure of interest. The volume can be cut to expose the interior anatomy or to remove unwanted structures, thus resembling anatomic dissection.

The volume is automatically segmented to isolate the organ of interest, with the surrounding structures cut off, which makes the surface landmarks more prominent. Additionally, VR provides for a spherical clipping volume, which allows the operator to choose a boundary to demarcate the voxels that need to be visible from the voxels outside the sphere that remain invisible. This manual segmentation can be performed when automatic segmentation fails. VR techniques provide excellent views of the anatomic course and relationships of the vasculature, thus aiding in the diagnosis, classification, and surgical planning of many organ's systems. They are particularly useful in depicting complex anatomic relationships and vascular connections that are not well defined on traditional views. The images are excellent for conveying information to the referring physician and the patient. Impressive images can be generated with the VR technique for multimedia presentations and for teaching files.

Nonetheless, VR techniques are not without drawbacks. Accurate estimation of luminal stenosis cannot be made with VR images, and visualization of noncalcified plaque is difficult. Arterial calcium cannot be easily differentiated from the luminal contrast. Contrast-filled or high-density structures can sometimes obscure visualization of adjacent arterial branches, requiring manual removal of the impeding structure. Furthermore, the loss of additional diagnostic information contained in source axial images (for example, small metastatic foci within solid organs) compared with the information retained during volumetric reconstructions limits the routine use of VR methods.

Virtual endoscopy produces images similar to those obtained from standard invasive endoscopic procedures via post-processing of scan data sets obtained from MDCT scanners. High-quality VR or SSD endoscopic images are created from isotropic images acquired by present-day MDCT scanners to produce fly-through displays that allow the physician to navigate through the various hollow organs (Fig. 5). Virtual endoscopy images are used in the evaluation of the middle ear, trachea, esophagus, and colon. Many studies have shown that the images are comparable to standard endoscopies [7–12].

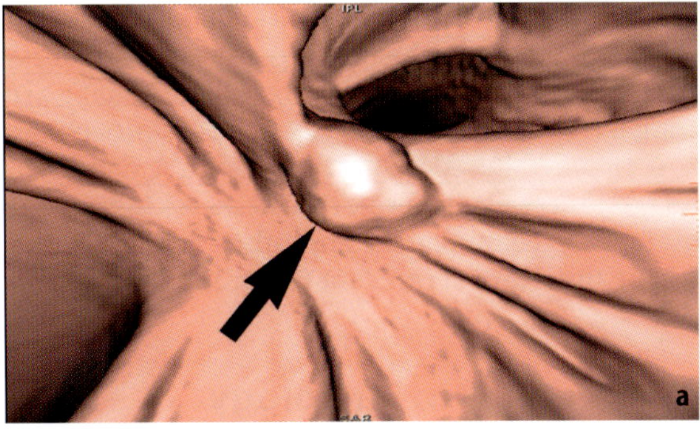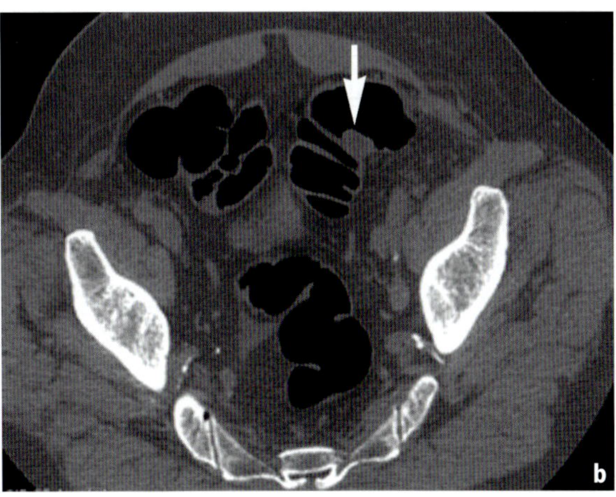

Fig. 5a, b. Virtual colonoscopy image (**a**) shows broad-based polyp (*arrow*) in the sigmoid colon. Note that the appearance closely matches that of conventional colonoscopy, although the polyp (*arrow*) is also seen in the axial image (**b**)

Implementation of 3-D Techniques

Scan Protocols

The newer helical CT scanners have the ability to acquire extremely thin-section images with isotropic resolution. Faster scanning technology allows for increased scan coverage within a single breath-hold. However, the major concern associated with reduced section thickness is the corresponding increase in radiation dose. Many new techniques have been introduced in MDCT imaging to minimize radiation exposure, including automatic tube current modulation (ATCM), bowtie filtering, re-sampling, and multi-phasic acquisition. ATCM attempts to maintain a constant image quality in the scanning plane (x-, y- or angular modulation), along the patient's long axis (z-axis modulation), or both (combined or xyz modulation) by adapting tube current to patient size and attenuation. Recent studies show significant dose savings with ATCM applied to various body parts [13–15] Re-sampling involves mapping of volumetric data into smaller volumes. Retrospective thin-section reconstructions obtained from newer helical CT scanners often produce high-quality MPRs and 3-D reformats. Individual scan protocols are chosen based on the body part to be analyzed and the specific pathology.

Scan Acquisition

Three-dimensional CT angiography (3-D-CTA) has become an important noninvasive clinical method for the evaluation of vascular structures. The degree of contrast enhancement is a crucial factor affecting the quality of 3-D-CTA, especially in systems with lower intrinsic amplitudes of contrast enhancement, including venous structures such as the portal system. Improvements in contrast enhancement result in better pre-operative planning of organ resection, transplantation, and vascular interventions such as those applied in the liver [16, 17]. The degree of enhancement is directly related to the concentration of the contrast agent, the injection rate, and the patient's body weight [18]. For a given patient weight and contrast volume, the two practical ways to increase intra-arterial enhancement at CT are: (a) increase the *injection rate*, and (b) increase the *iodine concentration*.

Although previous studies [19, 20] have shown that a higher degree of enhancement is obtained with a faster injection rate, many centers use an injection rate of 3–5 ml/s for 3-D-CTA. A recent report by Tanikake et al. [21] demonstrated that an injection rate of 5 ml/s was superior to 4 ml/s at both visual and quantitative evaluation of hepatic arterial enhancement for 3-D-CTA. An injection rate of 5 ml/s is recommended for sufficient visualization of peripheral branches of the hepatic artery on 3-D-CTA.

The concentration of intravenous iodinated contrast is also a crucial factor affecting the degree of contrast enhancement; for a given volume, contrast agents with higher iodine concentration result in increased contrast enhancement. A recent study showed greater enhancement and contrast-to-noise ratio of the cerebral vessels for a protocol based on 370 mg iodine/ml compared with one in which 300 mg iodine/ml was used. Interestingly, parenchymal enhancement was not significantly different [22]. In another study, a contrast-agent concentration of 400 mg/ml was shown to significantly improve contrast enhancement at 16-detector-row coronary CTA compared with 300 mg/ml, when injection rate was held constant (4 ml/s) [23].

Saline flush following contrast bolus has been advocated for reducing the extent of contrast material dilution [17]. By pushing the contrast, the saline flush results in reduced contrast mixing with the blood; it also prevents the retention of contrast material in the dead space between the peripheral and central veins. The contrast material otherwise retained in the dead space is thus effectively used for intravascular and organ enhancement and thus has the potential to reduce the overall contrast dose. Several studies have shown that use of the saline flush technique significantly reduces the amount of contrast material needed for vascular imaging of the thorax and abdomen [24, 25].

The synchronization of contrast-material administration with data acquisition (scan delay) is becoming increasingly important owing to the introduction of faster spiral CT scanners; however, controversies remain regarding the use of these techniques. Some studies that evaluated earlier-generation MDCT scanners reported consistently adequate study quality using *fixed delays*. For example, Macari et al. found uniform acceptability of enhancement during CTA in which there was a fixed 25-s delay during imaging of the abdominal aorta, with the intravenous administration of 150 ml of contrast material [26]. However, a standard delay time before initiation of scanning after the start of contrast administration overlooks the varying transit times of the contrast bolus among patients; this is especially true in patients with altered hemodynamic status. Such individual variation becomes increasingly important with the increased speed (and hence shorter scan duration) of the faster/newer-generation scanners and the gradual trend of using smaller volumes of higher-concentration contrast. Therefore, an *automatic bolus tracking* technique is followed in many centers, in which a region of interest (ROI) is placed on blood vessels and the contrast enhancement is measured. The initiation of scan acquisition is triggered when a pre-determined threshold is reached in the vessel [27, 28]. A study by Cademartiri et al. [29] compared the automatic bolus triggering technique with the test bolus method for coronary CTA. Their results showed that the bolus-tracking group had more homogeneous and steady enhancement than the test bolus group, with less pooling of contrast material in the pulmonary vessels and right side of the heart. With 16- or 64-detector-row scanners, optimal synchronization of contrast material passage and data acquisition is possible using the bolus-tracking technique, resulting in consistently high and homogeneous contrast enhancement [29].

Implementation of 3-D Techniques

A dedicated 3-D imaging laboratory and trained personnel substantially improve the overall workflow of modern radiology departments. The 3-D imaging laboratory at our institute takes care of all the 3-D reformats, which improves the turnaround time for interpretation. The axial scan data are transferred to the imaging lab and post-processing is performed based on clinical needs. A dedicated image-processing laboratory also serves to train radiologists, technologists, and other personnel and can be the site of significant research activity.

Applications in Radiology

Intracranial CTA

Although cerebral CTA has been increasingly used during the last decade for the early diagnosis of ruptured intracranial aneurysms, intra-arterial digital subtraction angiography (IA-DSA) is the accepted standard of reference for the detection and characterization of intracranial aneurysms as well as for pre-operative treatment planning of patients suffering from subarachnoid hemorrhage [30, 31] (Fig. 6). However, there are several disadvantages associated with DSA, including its invasive nature, need for greater operator skills, relatively higher cost, and a low but significant risk of neurological complications [32]. There has therefore been increasing interest in the use of noninvasive alternatives for accurate depiction of intracranial aneurysms. CTA is a noninvasive imaging technique that does not require arterial puncture or catheter manipulation. It can be easily performed immediately after the initial nonenhanced CT with a single bolus of intravenous contrast medium and allows for rapid diagnosis and treatment planning in the acute setting. Furthermore, CTA data can be viewed from almost unlimited projections, facilitating aneurysm detection and characterization [33].

Volume-rendered 3-D images are used for the detection of intradural aneurysm, characterization of arterial branching patterns at the neck, 3-D visualization of mural thrombi and calcification, depiction of the position and spatial orientation of the aneurysm neck and sac, and depiction of the relationship of the aneurysm to the local and regional bone anatomy [34]. Many previous studies with single-detector-row CT scanners showed limited diagnostic accuracy of this technique in identifying intracranial aneurysms < 3 mm in diameter [30, 31, 35, 36]. MDCT scanners have improved the accuracy of detection of smaller intracranial aneurysms. Recent studies showed that MDCTA with 3-D reformations using VR is an accurate imaging technique for the detection and characterization of intracranial aneurysms and has the potential to substitute for DSA in most cases [37, 38]. A recent study by Sakamoto et al. [39] showed that volume-subtracted 3-D-CTA is more effective than DSA for evaluating internal carotid artery aneurysms near the base

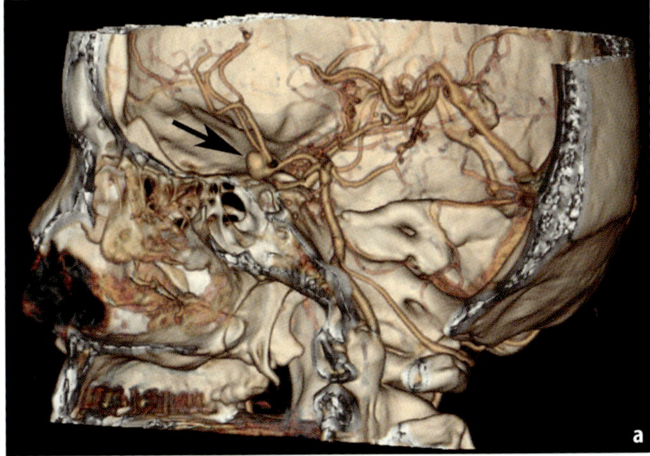
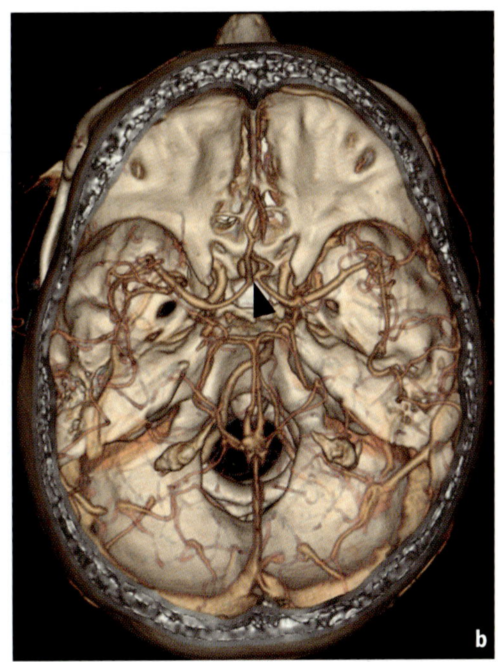

Fig. 6a, b. Anterior communicating artery aneurysm in a 56-year-old man. Although the aneurysm is noted in axial and MIP images, volume-rendered images (**a**, **b**) better depict 3-D information that helps in further characterizing the origin and extent of the aneurysm (*arrow*)

of the skull. The accuracy of 3-D-CTA was equal to that of DSA in the detection and characterization of these aneurysms, including further branching arteries at the aneurysm necks. Three-dimensional CTA with VR is also useful in the post-surgical evaluation of clipping surgery for intracranial aneurysms. VR 3-D CTA has been recommended as a noninvasive technique for routine post-operative evaluation. In fact, it has been suggested that intra-arterial DSA only be performed when 3-D-CTA is inconclusive [40].

Evaluation of Carotid Artery Stenosis

Carotid arteriography, color-Doppler ultrasonography, and magnetic resonance angiography (MRA) are currently used to evaluate carotid artery stenosis. CTA has also been shown to be highly accurate in diagnosing carotid artery stenosis. In a systematic review of CTA accuracy, the technique was found to accurately detect a 70–99% stenosis in the carotid artery and may be used as an alternative to arteriography and MRA. Carotid CTA with VR can be a valuable tool for grading carotid arterial stenosis because it provides excellent visualization of the lumen in calcified vessels as well as accurate assessment of circumferential high-density plaque [41].

Middle-ear Imaging

Two-dimensional images often fail to illustrate the detailed anatomy of the middle ear due to the

small size and complexity of this structure. A combination of 2-D, multi-planar, and 3-D rendering of the petrous bone provides an alternative approach-one that yields more reliable information relative to the middle-ear cavity and ossicles. Additionally, high-quality endoluminal views of the middle ear provide diagnostic information comparable with that obtained with transtympanic endoscopy. Virtual endoscopy has been shown to be especially useful when ossicular pathologic changes are present as well as for pre-operative and post-operative imaging of otologic procedures [10, 42]. However, according to a recent study, MPRs show anatomic features and pathologic conditions of the middle ear more precisely than axial images and virtual endoscopy in the majority of patients [43].

Maxillofacial Applications

Facial fractures are well-illustrated with SSD and VR techniques [26] (Fig. 7). There are controversial conclusions concerning the preferable algorithm. A study comparing various SR and VR protocols showed that SR images provide a sufficient and time-efficient means for 3-D visualization of facial fractures [44]. There was no diagnostic benefit of VR over SR according to that study. Three-dimensional-CT has emerged as the best imaging method for the diagnosis of Le Fort type fractures [45]. This approach provides valuable information concerning spatial relationships, which especially benefits the pre-surgical treatment planning of these fractures.

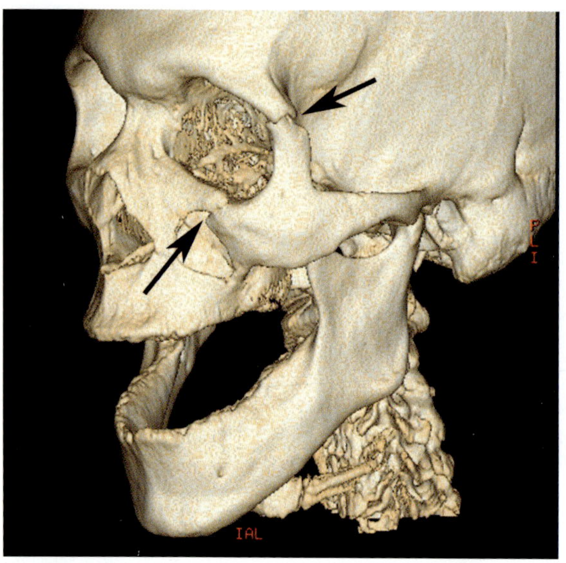

Fig. 7. Three-dimensional volume-rendered (3-D VR) images show the fractures involving the margins of the orbit (*arrows*) as well as the extent and direction of displacement

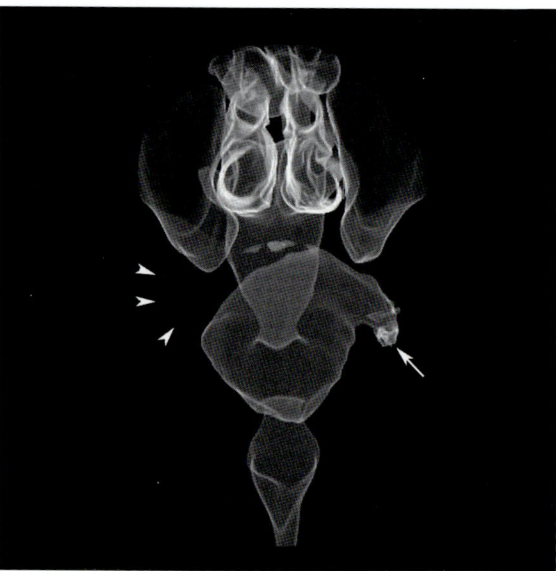

Fig. 8. Transparent 3-D reformatted image of the upper respiratory tracts demonstrate a filling defect involving the right vallecula (*arrowheads*). Note normal appearance of left vallecula (*arrow*)

Respiratory Tract

Thin-slab MIP technique facilitates detection of small parenchymal nodules and fine linear abnormalities. Peripheral perspective images of the lung give a visual impression of the extent of pleura surrounding the lung and thus help in the identification and surgical planning of peripherally placed masses and pleural pathologies. Endoluminal fly-through technique permits navigation of the interior of the tracheobronchial tree similar to tracheobronchoscopy. Virtual bronchoscopy has been found useful in guiding transbronchial biopsies, screening for endobronchial neoplasms, and guiding video-assisted thoracic surgery. Pre-operative simulation maps with 3-D-VR images enhance the surgeon's confidence, as they closely simulate the surgical field (Fig. 8) [46]. Visualization of bronchial segments distal to a severe narrowing and the relative hurdle in manipulating the bronchoscope through smaller airways, as in the pediatric population, are stumbling blocks in conventional bronchoscopy, both of which are overcome by 3-D-VR technique [47]. Additionally, VR allows better depiction of anomalous branching of the airways as well as the relationships of the airways with adjacent vascular structures, if CTA is performed concurrently [48]. Helical CT with 3-D reconstruction and virtual endoscopy has also been shown as a single noninvasive examination in support of endoscopy for tracheobronchial and esophageal stent planning [49].

Cardiovascular System

Axial, MPR, and curved reformat images are the cornerstones for diagnostic assessment of the coronary arteries in most cases. Three-dimensional techniques are usually supplemental but are useful for anatomic overview and patient communication (Fig. 9). The excellent temporal (165 ms) and spatial (0.4–0.6 mm) resolution of 64-slice MDCT scanners make them suitable for cardiac imaging [50, 51]. In contrast to catheter angiography, coronary CTA is noninvasive and depicts both the vessel wall and the lumen. It also gives functional information, such as ejection fraction (EF), left ventricular (LV) volumes, and wall motion abnormalities [52]. The coronary arteries have a complex, meandering course encompassing three dimensions; hence, their entire course cannot be evaluated in any single orthogonal or oblique plane. Estimation of luminal stenosis tends to be accurate because there is no distortion of data in MPR and because the entire range of density information is used to generate the image [53]. Curved reformats can be used to identify atheromatous disease and to grade stenosis. As noted earlier, in some centers, curved reformats are the primary method of coronary artery evaluation, although at most centers, they supplement MPR images. VR techniques provide excellent views of the anatomic course and relationship of the coronary vasculature, aiding in diagnosis, classification, and surgical planning aimed at the treatment of coronary anomalies [54,

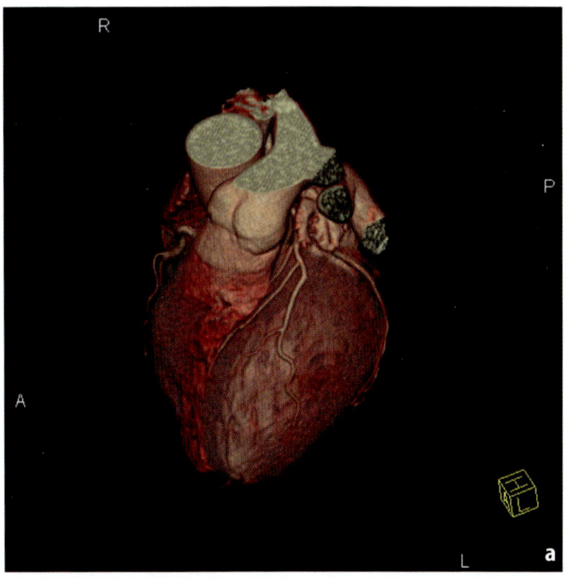
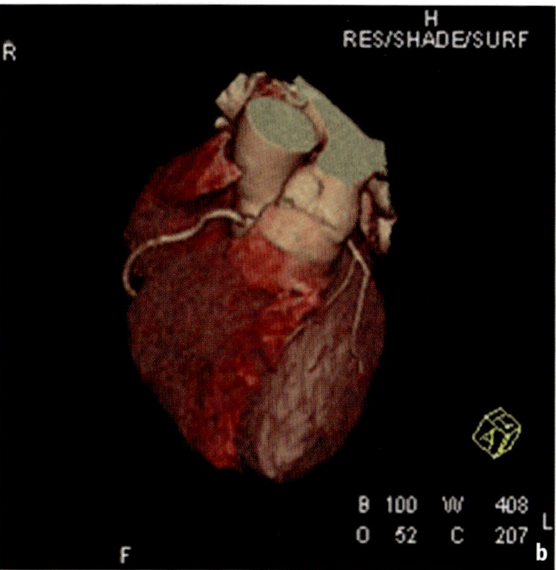

Fig. 9a, b. Three-dimensional volume-rendered (3-D VR) images showing excellent depiction of the cardiac surfaces and course of coronary arteries

55]. The VR technique is particularly useful in the evaluation of by-pass grafts because it depicts the sometimes complex anatomic relationships and vascular connections of the grafts, which may otherwise be confusing.

4-D techniques in Cardiac Imaging

The fourth dimension is the additional component of cardiac motion. This technique is used for assessment of LV function, wall motion, as well as native and prosthetic valves. The current generation of software allows for automatic segmentation of the LV cavity after the user identifies the mitral-valve plane and selects the end-systolic and end-diastolic phases. The software also allows running of a cine loop to simulate wall motion during the cardiac cycle, facilitating the identification of hypokinetic, akinetic, or dyskinetic segments.

Non-neurologic General Vascular Imaging

Three-dimensional VR techniques have gained widespread acceptance in the evaluation of vascular structures. VR images of the abdominal and thoracic aorta are extensively used to identify the extent of disease processes as well as in pre- and post-surgical evaluations (Fig. 10). Apart from detecting aneurysms along the entire extent of the aorta and in all three dimensions, VR images accurately assess branch-vessel involvement. Although axial and multi-planar views are usually adequate for identifying a vascular disorder, virtual angioscopic views better define its anatomic details [56].

Three-dimensional VR with CT virtual endoscopy of the intra-abdominal aorta has been shown to provide excellent post-grafting information on the 3-D relationship of intra-aortic stent struts to aortic branch ostia (in particular, the renal and superior mesenteric arteries) [11]. Virtual endoscopy findings aid clinicians in accurately assessing the effect of suprarenal intra-aortic stent-grafting on the renal arteries while MIP and VR images are excellent in demonstrating stenosis of these arteries.

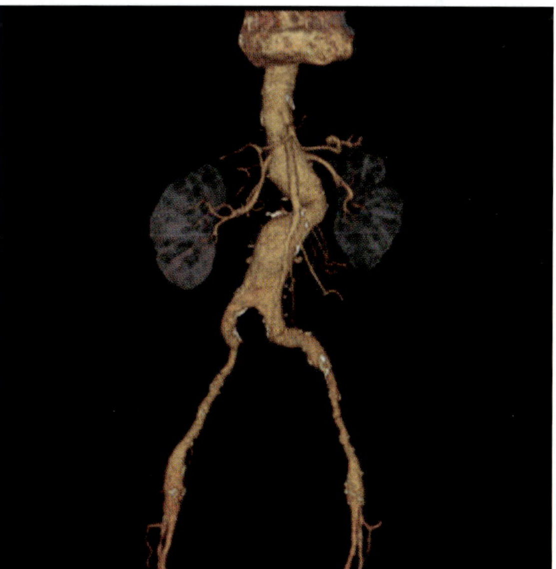

Fig. 10. Three-dimensional volume-rendered (3-D VR) image of the entire abdominal aorta and its branches demonstrates the extent of diffuse calcified atherosclerotic disease. There is aneurysmal dilatation of the abdominal aorta as well as ectasia of the superior mesenteric artery, left common iliac, and bilateral common femoral arteries

The accessory and main renal arteries are easily depicted, and stenosed segments are better demonstrated with 3-D techniques [57]. Three-dimensional-CTA with MDCT routinely replaces conventional invasive diagnostic angiography in patients with blunt or penetrating injuries of the extremities [58].

Accurate real-time interactive viewing of renal vascular anatomy in a format familiar to the surgeon can be achieved with 3-D-VR of MDCT data (Fig. 11). Noninvasive cross-sectional imaging combined with various image post-processing techniques has replaced conventional angiography for renal-donor evaluation in many centers. Normal and variant vascular anatomy can be viewed easily and accurately on videotape in a 3-D format by the surgeon. The vascular map provided by 3-D VR augments the technical performance of laparoscopic live-donor nephrectomy [59]. In addition, 3-D-VR has been used successfully in the pre-operative evaluation of patients undergoing partial nephrectomy or nephron-sparing surgery [60, 61].

Three-dimensional CT images are increasingly being used in the pre-operative evaluation of the hepatic vasculature in patients undergoing hepatectomy. This technique is useful for understanding the correlation between vessels and liver tumor and for pre-operative simulations–specifically, visualization of the peripheral branches of intrahepatic vessels [62]. Three-dimensional-CT clearly delineates portal and hepatic veins comparable to or better than the catheter angiogram and identifies the hepatic artery and its branches well enough to be considered as a replacement for angiography [63]. In patients evaluated for repeat hepatectomy, liver regeneration requires accurate pre-operative assessment of the involved segments. In these cases, 3-D-CT allows simultaneous demonstration of the hepatic veins, the portal vein, and the hepatic artery with their branches and elucidates the relationship of the tumor to these surrounding structures during either initial or repeat surgery.

In living-donor liver transplantation, VR images can be used in the pre-operative evaluation, as, together with CT hepatic venography, they clearly depict hepatic venous branches [64]. A better understanding of the branching patterns of the hepatic veins allows surgeons to plan the optimal hepatic resection technique and to chart suitable venous reconstruction [65]. All-inclusive, three-phase, dual-enhancement MDCT with 3-D reformatting was recently introduced, allowing delineation of the biliary, vascular, and parenchymal morphology [66]. As a single noninvasive imaging technique, this all-in-one approach provides adequate information for patient selection and surgical planning [67, 68].

The level of small-bowel obstruction can be identified with 3-D-CT imaging in addition to

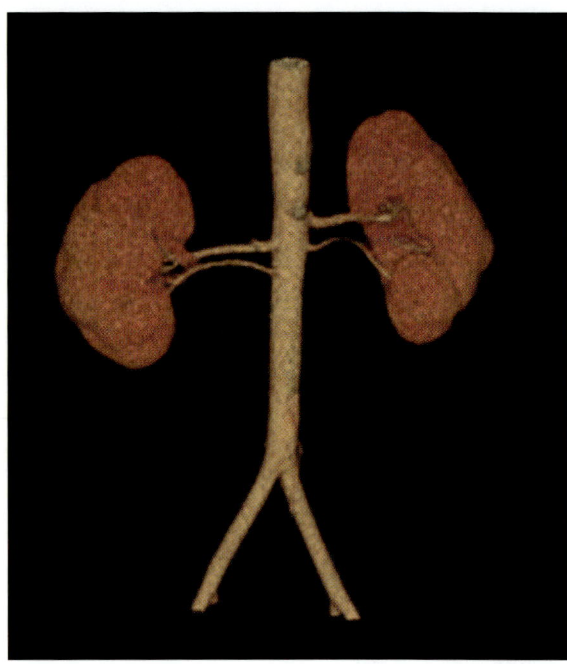

Fig. 11. Demonstration of renal vasculature using three-dimensional volume-rendered (3-D VR) technique. Note bilateral accessory renal arteries

evaluation of diseases of the stomach, pancreas, and adrenals. Several studies have reported varying levels of success in the 3-D-CT assessment of tumoral involvement of adjacent vascular and nonvascular structures [69–76].

Virtual Colonoscopy

The enormous amount of imaging data is a major limiting factor in routine CT colonography studies. Techniques such as 3-D fly-through and the newer VR applications have been shown to improve lesion detection, especially in small polyps located in colonic folds [77–79]. Virtual and conventional colonoscopy showed similar efficacy in the detection of polyps $\geq$ 6 mm in diameter in a recent study [8].

Urinary Tract

Three-dimensional reformatted images of the kidneys, ureters, and bladder in the coronal plane closely resemble images produced by excretory urography and demonstrate both upper and lower urothelial abnormalities (Fig. 12). Although none of the 3-D reconstruction algorithms evaluated (VR, MIP, or SSD) are known to significantly differ in terms of calyceal visualization and urinary-tract opacification from any of the other algorithms,

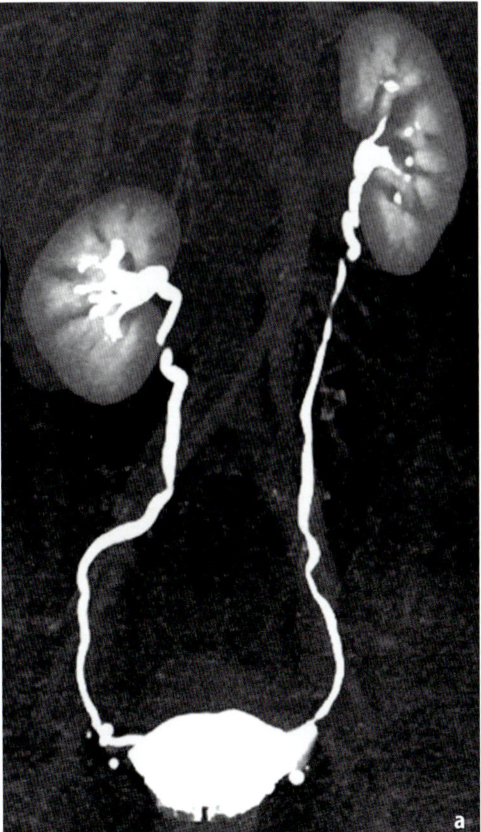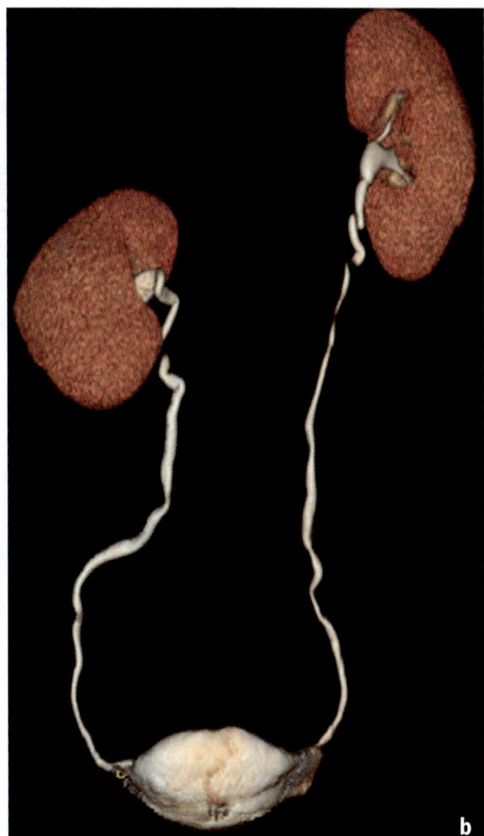

Fig. 12a, b. Three-dimensional volume-rendered (3-D VR) images (**a**, **b**) of the kidneys and urinary tract. Application of different color schemes allows adequate visualization of the collecting system and ureters along their entire extent

most centers rely on VR techniques because of their relative quick reformat time and less dependence on technical factors such as image acquisition timings. By excluding high-density skeletal structures anterior and posterior to the kidneys, excellent VR images can be obtained, all of which illustrate the urinary tract in its entirety [80]. Despite the ease and usefulness of 3-D reformatted images, according to the literature, axial CT images have significantly higher sensitivity in identifying urothelial neoplasms and therefore should be the primary set of images used in the interpretation of urinary-tract pathologies [81]. Endoluminal imaging of the bladder lumen using CT was introduced more than a decade ago and involves the differential attenuation of the lumen and bladder wall to increase bladder-tumor conspicuity. Either positive contrast media or low-density air can be used to distend the bladder prior to imaging. Studies show significant sensitivity and specificity for detection of bladder tumors measuring > 10 mm in diameter, with lower accuracy for smaller tumors [9, 81–83]. Virtual nephroureteroscopy has also been described as a potential technique to evaluate the upper urinary tract.

Skeletal Imaging

In the imaging of acute traumatic injuries to the spine and pelvis (Fig. 13), MDCT with MPR and 3-D reformations has replaced plain-film radiography. Three-dimensional reformats accurately delineate the extent of injury and yield a high degree of certainty in the diagnosis, with a higher level of reader confidence than is the case for plain films [4]. The one disadvantage often raised is the time delay in obtaining 3-D reformats; however, this can be overcome by the availability of post-processing software in those workstations where axial images are read. High-quality 3-D reformatted images aid in surgical planning for the correction of fracture and spinal deformities [84]. Computer-aided surgical techniques are also greatly facilitated by 3-D reformats [85].

Future Developments

Dynamic 3-D CTA is a promising new technique to demonstrate volumetric vascular hemodynamics [86]. This method allows the volumetric assess-

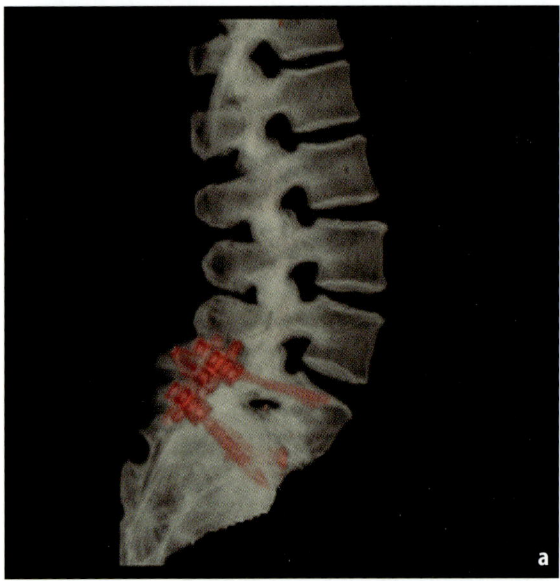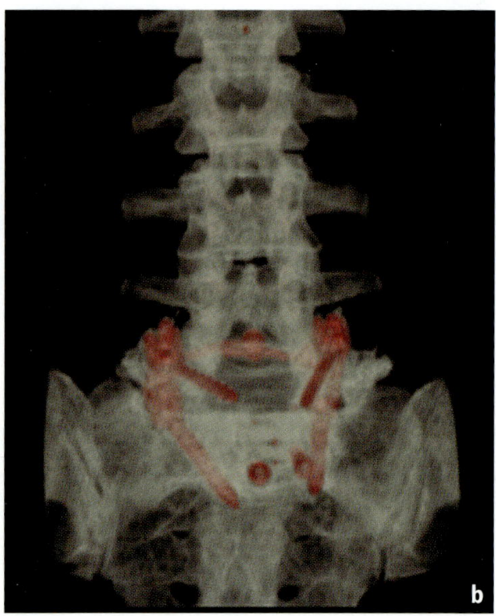

Fig. 13a, b. Assessment of metallic prosthesis using 3-D techniques. Differential color schemes again allow assessment of the position and depth of the metallic implants within the spine

ment of vascular anatomy and disease. Along with serial 3-D images of the dynamic blood flow, it allows simultaneous determination of cerebral perfusion in a single acquisition. However, increased radiation and contrast-agent dose are rate limiting factors in its broader application and acceptance.

Summary

Narrow collimation, multi-phasic imaging, and isotropic data sets provide the improved lesion detection, multi-planar capability, and ability to reformat high-quality 3-D images characteristic of modern-day MDCT scanners. However, the major concern associated with these protocols is the increased radiation dose. Narrow collimation results in increased radiation dose due to the increased number of rotations and the significant penumbra effect of the X-ray beam. An understanding of the technical parameters involved in MDCT protocols helps the radiologist to tailor MDCT protocols according to patient size and clinical question, so that diagnostically acceptable images are acquired with the lowest possible radiation dose. The process of 3-D reconstruction in general can be time consuming but continues to improve with software and workstation advances implemented by trained personnel.

References

1. Cuk V, Belina S, Fure R et al (2007) Virtual bronchoscopy and 3-D spiral CT reconstructions in the management of patient with bronchial cancer—our experience with Syngo 3-D postprocessing software. Coll Antropol 31:315-320
2. Jaffe TA, Nelson RC, Johnson GA et al (2006) Optimization of multiplanar reformations from isotropic data sets acquired with 16-detector row helical CT scanner. Radiology 238:292-299
3. Kozuka T, Tomiyama N, Johkoh T et al (2003) Coronal multiplanar reconstruction view from isotropic voxel data sets obtained with multidetector-row CT: assessment of detection and size of mediastinal and hilar lymph nodes. Radiat Med 21:23-27
4. Lucey BC, Stuhlfaut JW, Hochberg AR et al (2005) Evaluation of blunt abdominal trauma using PACS-based 2-D and 3-D MDCT reformations of the lumbar spine and pelvis. AJR Am J Roentgenol 185:1435-1440
5. van Ooijen PM, Ho KY, Dorgelo J, Oudkerk M (2003) Coronary artery imaging with multidetector CT: visualization issues. Radiographics 23:e16
6. Semba CP, Rubin GD, Dake MD (1994) Three-dimensional spiral CT angiography of the abdomen. Semin Ultrasound CT MR 15:133-138
7. Vining DJ (1996) Virtual endoscopy: is it reality? Radiology 200:30-31
8. Fenlon HM, Nunes DP, Schroy PC, 3rd et al (1999) A comparison of virtual and conventional colonoscopy for the detection of colorectal polyps. N Engl J Med 341:1496-1503
9. Bernhardt TM, Rapp-Bernhardt U (2001) Virtual cystoscopy of the bladder based on CT and MRI data. Abdom Imaging 26:325-332
10. Klingebiel R, Bauknecht HC, Kaschke O et al (2001) Virtual endoscopy of the tympanic cavity based on high-resolution multislice computed tomographic data. Otol Neurotol 22:803-807
11. Sun Z, Winder RJ, Kelly BE et al (2004) Diagnostic value of CT virtual intravascular endoscopy in aortic stent-grafting. J Endovasc Ther 11:13-25
12. De Wever W, Bogaert J, Verschakelen JA (2005) Virtual bronchoscopy: accuracy and usefulness—an overview. Semin Ultrasound CT MR 26:364-373
13. Kalra MK, Rizzo S, Maher MM et al (2005) Chest CT

performed with z-axis modulation: scanning protocol and radiation dose. Radiology 237:303-308

14. Namasivayam S, Kalra MK, Pottala KM et al (2006) Optimization of Z-axis automatic exposure control for multidetector row CT evaluation of neck and comparison with fixed tube current technique for image quality and radiation dose. AJNR Am J Neuroradiol 27:2221-2225

15. Kalra MK, Rizzo SM, Novelline RA (2005) Reducing radiation dose in emergency computed tomography with automatic exposure control techniques. Emerg Radiol 11:267-274

16. Uchida M, Ishibashi M, Abe T et al (1999) Three-dimensional imaging of liver tumors using helical CT during intravenous injection of contrast medium. J Comput Assist Tomogr 23:435-440

17. Matoba M, Kondou T, Yokota H et al (2005) Usefulness of a saline flush for intravenous 3-dimensional computed tomography portography using multidetector-row helical computed tomography. J Comput Assist Tomogr 29:780-785

18. Yamashita K, Mikami Y, Urakami A et al (2003) Three-dimensional images of pancreatic pseudocyst prior to percutaneous drainage. Am J Surg 185:219-220

19. Bae KT, Heiken JP, Brink JA (1998) Aortic and hepatic peak enhancement at CT: effect of contrast medium injection rate—pharmacokinetic analysis and experimental porcine model. Radiology 206:455-464

20. Kim T, Murakami T, Takahashi S et al (1998) Effects of injection rates of contrast material on arterial phase hepatic CT. AJR Am J Roentgenol 171:429-432

21. Tanikake M, Shimizu T, Narabayashi I et al (2003) Three-dimensional CT angiography of the hepatic artery: use of multi-detector row helical CT and a contrast agent. Radiology 227:883-889

22. Kloska SP, Fischer T, Nabavi DG et al (2007) Comparison of different iodine concentration contrast media in perfusion computed tomography of the brain: is high iodine concentration useful? Invest Radiol 42:564-568

23. Cademartiri F, Mollet NR, van der Lugt A et al (2005) Intravenous contrast material administration at helical 16-detector row CT coronary angiography: effect of iodine concentration on vascular attenuation. Radiology 236:661-665

24. Haage P, Schmitz-Rode T, Hubner D et al (2000) Reduction of contrast material dose and artifacts by a saline flush using a double power injector in helical CT of the thorax. AJR Am J Roentgenol 174:1049-1053

25. Schoellnast H, Tillich M, Deutschmann HA et al (2004) Improvement of parenchymal and vascular enhancement using saline flush and power injection for multiple-detector-row abdominal CT. Eur Radiol 14:659-664

26. Macari M, Israel GM, Berman P et al (2001) Infrarenal abdominal aortic aneurysms at multi-detector row CT angiography: intravascular enhancement without a timing acquisition. Radiology 220:519-523

27. Sandstede JJ, Tschammler A, Beer M et al (2001) Optimization of automatic bolus tracking for timing of the arterial phase of helical liver CT. Eur Radiol 11:1396-1400

28. Silverman PM, Roberts S, Tefft MC et al (1995) Helical CT of the liver: clinical application of an automated computer technique, SmartPrep, for obtaining images with optimal contrast enhancement. AJR Am J Roentgenol 165:73-78

29. Cademartiri F, Nieman K, van der Lugt A et al (2004) Intravenous contrast material administration at 16-detector row helical CT coronary angiography: test bolus versus bolus-tracking technique. Radiology 233:817-823

30. Velthuis BK, Rinkel GJ, Ramos LM et al (1998) Subarachnoid hemorrhage: aneurysm detection and preoperative evaluation with CT angiography. Radiology 208:423-430

31. Anderson GB, Steinke DE, Petruk KC et al (1999) Computed tomographic angiography versus digital subtraction angiography for the diagnosis and early treatment of ruptured intracranial aneurysms. Neurosurgery 45:1315-1320. Discussion 1320-1312

32. Cloft HJ, Joseph GJ, Dion JE (1999) Risk of cerebral angiography in patients with subarachnoid hemorrhage, cerebral aneurysm, and arteriovenous malformation: a meta-analysis. Stroke 30:317-320

33. Aoki S, Sasaki Y, Machida T et al (1992) Cerebral aneurysms: detection and delineation using 3-D-CT angiography. AJNR Am J Neuroradiol 13:1115-1120

34. Kangasniemi M, Makela T, Koskinen S et al (2004) Detection of intracranial aneurysms with two-dimensional and three-dimensional multislice helical computed tomographic angiography. Neurosurgery 54:336-340. Discussion 340-331

35. Korogi Y, Takahashi M, Katada K et al (1999) Intracranial aneurysms: detection with three-dimensional CT angiography with volume rendering-comparison with conventional angiographic and surgical findings. Radiology 211:497-506

36. Karamessini MT, Kagadis GC, Petsas T et al (2004) CT angiography with three-dimensional techniques for the early diagnosis of intracranial aneurysms. Comparison with intra-arterial DSA and the surgical findings. Eur J Radiol 49:212-223

37. Yoon DY, Lim KJ, Choi CS et al (2007) Detection and characterization of intracranial aneurysms with 16-channel multidetector row CT angiography: a prospective comparison of volume-rendered images and digital subtraction angiography. AJNR Am J Neuroradiol 28:60-67

38. Villablanca JP, Jahan R, Hooshi P et al (2002) Detection and characterization of very small cerebral aneurysms by using 2-D and 3-D helical CT angiography. AJNR Am J Neuroradiol 23:1187-1198

39. Sakamoto S, Kiura Y, Shibukawa M et al (2006) Subtracted 3-D CT angiography for evaluation of internal carotid artery aneurysms: comparison with conventional digital subtraction angiography. AJNR Am J Neuroradiol 27:1332-1337

40. Sakuma I, Tomura N, Kinouchi H et al (2006) Postoperative three-dimensional CT angiography after cerebral aneurysm clipping with titanium clips: detection with single detector CT. Comparison with intra-arterial digital subtraction angiography. Clin Radiol 61:505-512

41. Marcus CD, Ladam-Marcus VJ, Bigot JL et al (1999) Carotid arterial stenosis: evaluation at CT angiography with the volume-rendering technique. Radiology 211:775-780

42. Karhuketo TS, Dastidar PS, Ryymin PS et al (2002) Virtual endoscopy imaging of the middle ear cavity and ossicles. Eur Arch Otorhinolaryngol 259:77-83

43. Trojanowska A, Trojanowski P, Olszanski W et al (2007) How to reliably evaluate middle ear diseases? Comparison of different methods of post-processing based on multislice computed tomography examination. Acta Otolaryngol 127:258-264

44. Rodt T, Bartling SO, Zajaczek JE et al (2006) Evaluation of surface and volume rendering in 3-D-CT of facial fractures. Dentomaxillofac Radiol 35:227-231

45. Chen WJ, Yang YJ, Fang YM et al (2006) Identifica-

tion and classification in le fort type fractures by using 2-D and 3-D computed tomography. Chin J Traumatol 9:59-64

46. Ueno J, Murase T, Yoneda K et al (2004) Three-dimensional imaging of thoracic diseases with multidetector row CT. J Med Invest 51:163-170

47. Boiselle PM, Dippolito G, Copeland J et al (2003) Multiplanar and 3-D imaging of the central airways: comparison of image quality and radiation dose of single-detector row CT and multi-detector row CT at differing tube currents in dogs. Radiology 228:107-111

48. Lawler LP, Fishman EK (2001) Multi-detector row CT of thoracic disease with emphasis on 3-D volume rendering and CT angiography. Radiographics 21:1257-1273

49 Di Simone MP, Mattioli S, D'Ovidio F, Bassi F (2003) Three-dimensional CT imaging and virtual endoscopy for the placement of self-expandable stents in oesophageal and tracheobronchial neoplastic stenoses. Eur J Cardiothorac Surg 23:106-108

50. Klingenbeck-Regn K, Schaller S, Flohr T et al (1999) Subsecond multi-slice computed tomography: basics and applications. Eur J Radiol 31:110-124

51. Nikolaou K, Flohr T, Knez A et al (2004) Advances in cardiac CT imaging: 64-slice scanner. Int J Cardiovasc Imaging 20:535-540

52. van der Vleuten PA, Willems TP, Gotte MJ et al (2006) Quantification of global left ventricular function: comparison of multidetector computed tomography and magnetic resonance imaging. a meta-analysis and review of the current literature. Acta Radiol 47:1049-1057

53. Sirineni GK, Kalra MK, Pottala KM et al (2006) Visualization techniques in computed tomographic coronary angiography. Curr Probl Diagn Radiol 35:245-257

54. Datta J, White CS, Gilkeson RC et al (2005) Anomalous coronary arteries in adults: depiction at multidetector row CT angiography. Radiology 235:812-818

55. Shi H, Aschoff AJ, Brambs HJ, Hoffmann MH (2004) Multislice CT imaging of anomalous coronary arteries. Eur Radiol 14:2172-2181

56. Carrascosa P, Capunay C, Vembar M et al (2005) Multislice CT virtual angioscopy of the abdomen. Abdom Imaging 30:249-258

57. Tepe SM, Memisoglu E, Kural AR (2004) Three-dimensional noninvasive contrast-enhanced electron beam tomography angiography of the kidneys: adjunctive use in medical and surgical management. Clin Imaging 28:52-58

58. Fleiter TR, Mervis S (2007) The role of 3-D-CTA in the assessment of peripheral vascular lesions in trauma patients. Eur J Radiol 64:92-102

59. El Fettouh HA, Herts BR, Nimeh T et al (2003) Prospective comparison of 3-dimensional volume rendered computerized tomography and conventional renal arteriography for surgical planning in patients undergoing laparoscopic donor nephrectomy. J Urol 170:57-60

60. Coll DM, Uzzo RG, Herts BR et al (1999) 3-dimensional volume rendered computerized tomography for preoperative evaluation and intraoperative treatment of patients undergoing nephron sparing surgery. J Urol 161:1097-1102

61. Coll DM, Herts BR, Davros WJ et al (2000) Preoperative use of 3-D volume rendering to demonstrate renal tumors and renal anatomy. Radiographics 20:431-438

62. Yamazaki S, Takayama T, Watanabe Y et al (2007) Imaging modality of three-dimensional CT in caudate cholangioma: assessment for resectability. Hepatogastroenterology 54:397-399

63. Bogetti JD, Herts BR, Sands MJ et al (2001) Accuracy and utility of 3-dimensional computed tomography in evaluating donors for adult living related liver transplants. Liver Transpl 7:687-692

64. Onodera Y, Omatsu T, Nakayama J et al (2004) Peripheral anatomic evaluation using 3-D CT hepatic venography in donors: significance of peripheral venous visualization in living-donor liver transplantation. AJR Am J Roentgenol 183:1065-1070

65. Hiroshige S, Nishizaki T, Soejima Y et al (2001) Beneficial effects of 3-dimensional visualization on hepatic vein reconstruction in living donor liver transplantation using right lobe graft. Transplantation 72:1993-1996

66. Schroeder T, Radtke A, Kuehl H et al (2006) Evaluation of living liver donors with an all-inclusive 3-D multi-detector row CT protocol. Radiology 238:900-910

67. Smith PA, Klein AS, Heath DG et al (1998) Dual-phase spiral CT angiography with volumetric 3-D rendering for preoperative liver transplant evaluation: preliminary observations. J Comput Assist Tomogr 22:868-874

68. Schroeder T, Malago M, Debatin JF et al (2005) "All-in-one" imaging protocols for the evaluation of potential living liver donors: comparison of magnetic resonance imaging and multidetector computed tomography. Liver Transpl 11:776-787

69. Takeshita K, Furui S, Takada K (2002) Multidetector row helical CT of the pancreas: value of three-dimensional images, two-dimensional reformations, and contrast-enhanced multiphasic imaging. J Hepatobiliary Pancrat Surg 9:576-582

70. Matsuki M, Tanikake M, Kani H et al (2006) Dual-phase 3-D CT angiography during a single breath-hold using 16-MDCT: assessment of vascular anatomy before laparoscopic gastrectomy. AJR Am J Roentgenol 186:1079-1085

71. Matsuki M, Kanazawa S, Kanamoto T et al (2006) Virtual CT gastrectomy by three-dimensional imaging using multidetector-row CT for laparoscopic gastrectomy. Abdom Imaging 31:268-276

72. Kobayashi M, Morishita S, Okabayashi T et al (2006) Preoperative assessment of vascular anatomy of inferior mesenteric artery by volume-rendered 3-D-CT for laparoscopic lymph node dissection with left colic artery preservation in lower sigmoid and rectal cancer. World J Gastroenterol 12:553-555

73. Johnson PT, Heath DG, Hofmann LV et al (2003) Multidetector-row computed tomography with three-dimensional volume rendering of pancreatic cancer: a complete preoperative staging tool using computed tomography angiography and volume-rendered cholangiopancreatography. J Comput Assist Tomogr 27:347-353

74. Hurley ME, Herts BR, Remer EM et al (2003) Three-dimensional volume-rendered helical CT before laparoscopic adrenalectomy. Radiology 229:581-586

75. House MG, Yeo CJ, Cameron JL et al (2004) Predicting resectability of periampullary cancer with three-dimensional computed tomography. J Gastrointest Surg 8:280-288

76. Candocia FJ, Goldman I (2005) Three-dimensional computed tomography illustration of small bowel obstruction transition points in patients receiving oral contrast: report of 3 cases. J Comput Assist Tomogr 29:202-204

77. Yee J, Akerkar GA, Hung RK et al (2001) Colorectal neoplasia: performance characteristics of CT colonography for detection in 300 patients. Radiolo-

gy 219:685-692
78. Beaulieu CF, Jeffrey RB, Jr. et al (1999) Display modes for CT colonography. Part II. Blinded comparison of axial CT and virtual endoscopic and panoramic endoscopic volume-rendered studies. Radiology 212:203-212
79. McFarland EG, Brink JA, Pilgram TK et al (2001) Spiral CT colonography: reader agreement and diagnostic performance with two- and three-dimensional image-display techniques. Radiology 218:375-383
80. Noroozian M, Cohan RH, Caoili EM et al (2004) Multislice CT urography: state of the art. Br J Radiol 77 Spec No 1:S74-86
81. Chow LC, Sommer FG (2001) Multidetector CT urography with abdominal compression and three-dimensional reconstruction. AJR Am J Roentgenol 177:849-855
82. Kim JK, Ahn JH, Park T et al (2002) Virtual cystoscopy of the contrast material-filled bladder in patients with gross hematuria. AJR Am J Roentgenol 179:763-768
83. Song JH, Francis IR, Platt JF et al (2001) Bladder tumor detection at virtual cystoscopy. Radiology 218:95-100
84. Ohashi K , El-Khoury GY, Bennett DL et al (2005) Orthopedic hardware complications diagnosed with multi-detector row CT. Radiology 237(2):570-757
85. Holly LT (2006) Image-guided spinal surgery. Int J Med Robot 2(1):7-15
86. Matsumoto M, Kodama N, Endo Y et al (2007) Dynamic 3-D-CT angiography. AJNR Am J Neuroradiol 28:299-304

SECTION II

MDCT of the Abdomen

9

Dual-Phase Liver MDCT

Dushyant V. Sahani, Anandkumar H. Singh

Introduction

The advent of multidetector computed tomography (MDCT) scanners has provided an impetus for various changes in applications of computed tomography (CT) principles and their implementation in the design of CT protocols. The advanced MDCT scanners can produce isotropic voxel resolution, which can improve detection of subtle lesions in the organ. It thus remains the major imaging modality for detection of hepatic pathologies [1-4].

The main area of improvisation by MDCT for liver imaging appears to be in detection and characterization of small liver malignancies with better characterization of benign pathologies and vascular flow details [5]. Studies have shown that thinner images with MDCT provides some benefits, such as reduced volume-averaging artifacts, thereby improving diagnosis of focal hepatic lesions and hepatic vascular pathologies [6, 7]. Also, due to shorter hepatic arterial acquisition time and thin collimation with MDCT, multiplanar imaging and CT angiography are much better [8].

Basic Concepts for Liver Imaging

The enhancement pattern of the arterial phase is dependent on the contrast medium injection rate, injection duration, and the time of the scan performed relative to the contrast bolus. The arterial opacification can primarily be controlled by the iodine administration rate, which is further dependent on the flow rate and the concentration of medium administered. It is important that the injection duration be longer than the scanning time to ensure strong vascular enhancement by the recirculation of contrast.

On the other hand, the parenchymal enhancement is independent of the injection flow rate and depends on the total volume (dose) of contrast administered. Thus, to obtain optimal liver parenchymal enhancement, a sufficient volume of contrast medium is required (approximately 120–150 cc of 370 mgI contrast agent). The iodine dose is directly proportional to the contrast volume administered and/or the iodine concentration of the contrast medium. Thus, increasing either would lead to an increase in dose. For example, for vascular mapping of the liver [computed tomographic arteriography (CTA)], arterial phase imaging is of paramount importance, and administration of a smaller volume of high-concentration contrast medium at a higher rate would suffice.

Contrast material later enters the extracellular space by diffusion, and this reduces the conspicuity of the liver lesion and its contrast with the surrounding parenchyma, later causing obscuration of the lesion. This is called the equilibrium phase, and it is important that the scan be completed well before this stage sets in.

Dual-Phase Imaging

Normally, the liver derives only 25% of its blood supply from the hepatic arterial flow and the remaining 75% from the portal venous system [9]. After the administration of iodinated contrast medium, opacification of hepatic arteries is encountered first, usually at 15–25 s (arterial phase). Liver enhancement in the portal venous system usually occurs between 45 and 55 s, followed by hepatic venous opacification at 60–70 s after contrast injection (portal venous phase [PVP]). Based on the contrast circulation, the hepatic arterial phase (HAP) can be further divided into an early (true) arterial phase in which there is opacification of the hepatic arterial system without much parenchymal enhancement and a following late (dominant) arterial phase, which not only permits optimal opacification of the hepatic arteries but also higher parenchymal enhancement. This information is important in designing MDCT protocols, as hypervascular lesions are best visualized in the late arterial phase. In other words, better hepatic parenchymal contrast in the HAP is produced as a consequence of greater enhancement of hypervascular lesions and relatively less enhancement of the background liver parenchyma (Fig. 1). In the subsequent portal venous phase, these lesions are less conspicuous due to the higher enhancement of background liver parenchyma. Studies have demonstrated that HAP images reveal more numerous benign and malignant hypervascular liver lesions than PVP images [10], where most hypovascular lesions are evident (Table 1). Hence, dual-phase CT of the liver is performed in the late HAP and the PVP. Although initial reports supported the use of triple-phase scanning (early and late HAP and PVP) for evolution of hypervascular lesions, subsequent studies revealed no additional benefits of the early phase. Because of this and because of additional concerns relating to excess radiation dose, the early HAP is losing importance (Fig. 2) [11].

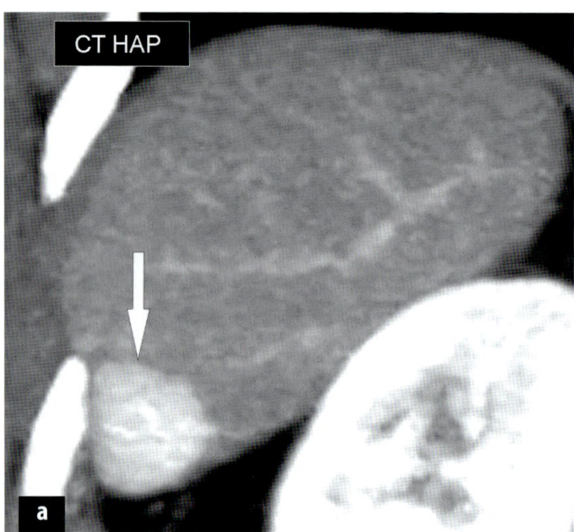

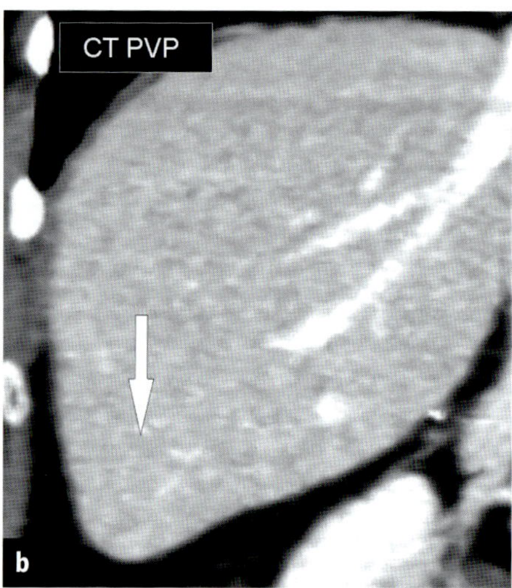

Fig. 1a, b. Hepatocellular carcinoma detection: coronal reformatted computed tomographic (CT) images of the liver in the arterial phase (**a**) showing intensely enhancing hepatocellular carcinoma (HCC) (*arrow*). Note better lesion-to-parenchymal contrast in the arterial-dominant phase in comparison with the portal venous phase image (**b**) where the lesion is not appreciated

Table 1. List of common hypervascular and hypovascular lesions encountered in the liver

Hypervascular lesions (arterial phase)	Hypovascular (PVP) lesions
Malignant	Metastases
• Primary malignancy	• Lung carcinoma
• Hepatocellular carcinoma	• Colon carcinoma
	• Breast carcinoma
Metastases	Benign
• Carcinoid	• Cysts
• Islet cell tumors	• Biliary hamartoma
• Renal cell carcinoma	
• Melanoma	
Benign	
• Hemangioma	
• Focal nodular hyperplasia	
• Hepatocellular adenoma	

PVP portal venous phase

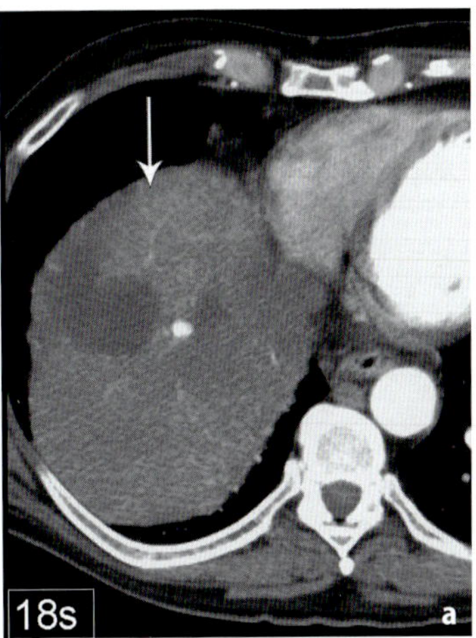

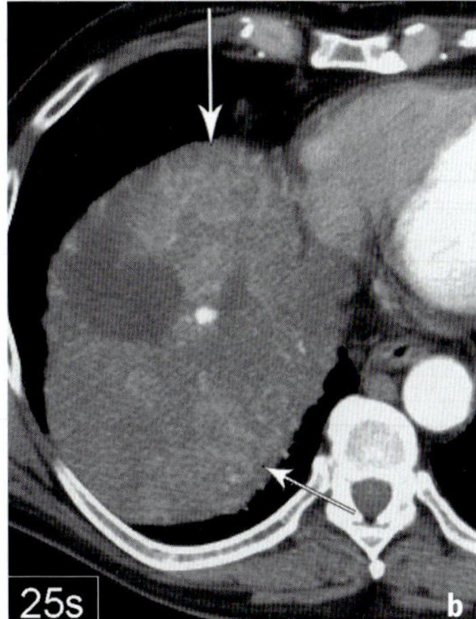

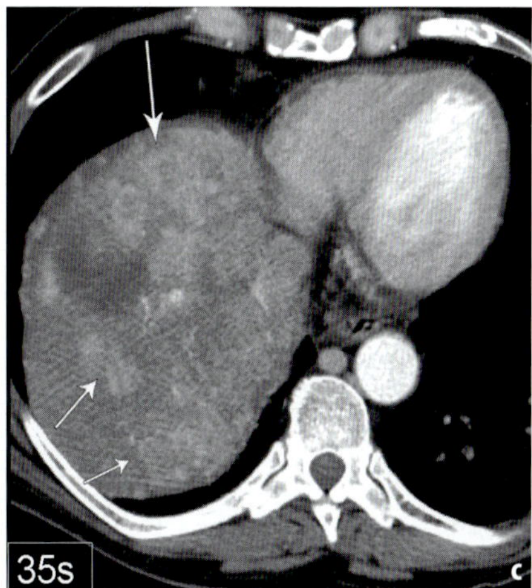

Fig. 2a-c. Improved detection of hepatocellular carcinoma (HCC) in the late arterial phase: serial images obtained at 18 s (**a**), 25 s (**b**), and 35 s (**c**) following initiation of contrast injection. Although arterially enhancing lesions are seen on images **a** and **b**, better enhancement and more lesions (*arrows*) are evident on the late arterial phase image (**c**)

Rationale for High-Concentration Contrast Medium

When a CT scan was performed with old scanners (conventional, helical, and dynamic), the liver was predominantly scanned during the preequilibrium phase due to slower scan speed and lengthened bolus time. With the evolution of MDCT, due to the reduction in scanning time, the scans can be performed during optimal phases with near perfection. One way of achieving this is by increasing the injection speed. The other way is to increase the concentration of the iodinated contrast medium.

There should be an optimal balance between iodine concentration in the contrast and the volume of material injected for the desired hepatic parenchymal enhancement. The use of high iodine concentration contrast medium has gained importance in patients with decreased cardiac output, obesity, in conditions such as cirrhosis of the liver or portal vein thrombosis, and other conditions where there is decreased liver perfusion. It has been observed that the maximum hepatic enhancement in obese patients is significantly lower than in those who are lighter in weight. This could be attributed to the decreased level of perfusion of the liver in obese patients [12]. Also, in cases of liver cirrhosis, due to decreased portal perfusion, the peak contrast enhancement in liver is late, and usually, the plateau of contrast enhancement occurs in the late portal phase. This is again secondary to decreased portal perfusion seen in these patients [13]. The injection of contrast medium with standard iodine concentration could increase the possibility of missing hypovascular metastases during the late phase in heavy patients or in patients with cirrhosis or chronic hepatitis.

The use of high-concentration contrast medium enables better visualization of the heterogeneous enhancement pattern in cirrhotic patients. The use of high-concentration contrast medium for MDCT enables greater enhancement of the aorta in the early and the late arterial phases [14, 15]. It also results in higher mean attenuation of the liver in the portal phase than would be achieved by use of contrast medium of lesser iodine concentration. Therefore, the lesion-to-liver contrast can be improved when high iodine concentration contrast medium is used (Fig. 3).

Other Technical Considerations for Liver Imaging

Appropriate selection of the delay for scan initiation is essential, along with modification of the contrast administration protocol. Various technical and physiological factors affect MDCT contrast enhancement of the liver [16, 17].

Scan Delay and Contrast Delivery

With increasing detector rows in CT scanners, scan delays and contrast delivery in liver protocols need to be altered accordingly. As discussed, if the volume of contrast to be administered is kept constant and the rate is increased, the delay for peak aortic enhancement decreases [16]. Also, in patients with decreased cardiac output or more body weight, a longer time is required for the contrast to demonstrate peak aortic enhancement and thereby liver parenchymal enhancement. Thus, optimal enhancement in larger patients can be achieved by

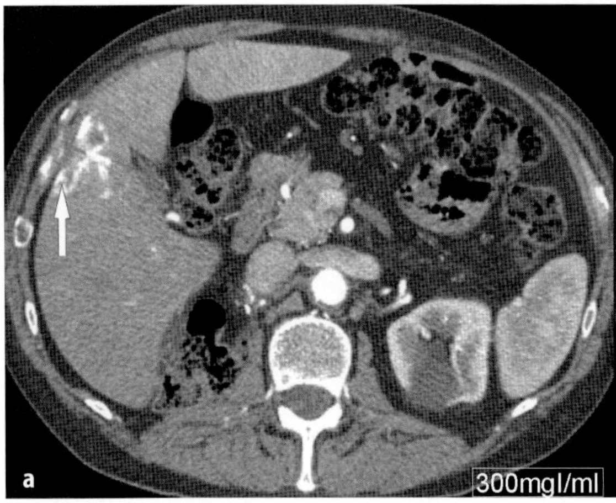

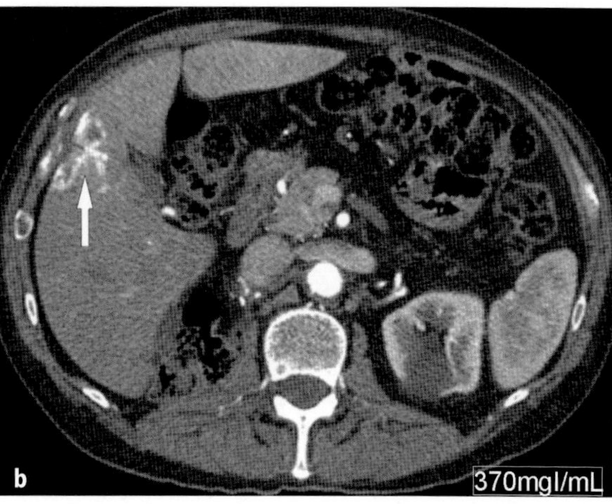

Fig. 3a, b. Comparison of low- and high-concentration contrast for characterization of a hemangioma: Arterial phase axial computed tomographic (CT) images of the liver performed with 300 mgI/ml (**a**) and 370 mgI/ml (**b**) concentration contrast media in a patient with a liver lesion. There is improved enhancement of the aorta and the liver hemangioma on the image obtained with the higher-concentration contrast medium

increasing the injection rate, and the time required for each of the phase acquisitions varies from patient to patient.

Techniques for Contrast Delivery Optimization

Timing of the hepatic arterial phase following contrast administration is of vital importance, and with the availability of computer-automated scanning technology (CAST), fixed time delays can be planned. However, fixed time delays do not take into account the patient-to-patient variability in cardiac output or the contrast circulation time.

Almost all recent scanners are now equipped with automated scanning trigger software wherein a threshold enhancement [Hounsfield units (HU)] in a vessel or an organ is preselected to initiate a scan after injection of contrast. A few initial images are obtained at a static table position, and after the contrast bolus arrives and the threshold of enhancement in the region of interest is reached, scans can be initiated either manually or automatically. Alternatively, a test bolus can be used wherein a small amount of contrast (10–15 ml at 3-4 cc/s) is injected and serial images are obtained through the upper aorta to judge its maximal opacification and determine the appropriate delay time for the patient. A test bolus is accurate but does entail additional contrast and time . With both the test bolus and automatic triggering techniques, the scan should be performed at the point of maximal opacification of the hepatic arterial system. This should enable creation of excellent images of the vascular anatomy of the liver.

However, for venous phase imaging, delays of 65–70 s, 60 s or less from the start of injection, are usually planned in 4-slice, 16-slice, and 64-slice scanners, respectively. This ensures optimal opacification of the portal vein and the hepatic veins.

Contrast Volume

Reduced volumes of contrast injection are not favored for liver imaging due to concerns about image quality. Unlike thoracic and vascular CT imaging, the authorities still recommend 120–150 ml of contrast medium of concentrations up to 300–370 mg of iodine [18]. However, in larger patients, an increased volume of up to 180 ml has been administered. In particular, patients with cirrhosis require a higher volume of contrast to achieve optimal parenchymal enhancement due to decreased liver perfusion.

Also, the volume of contrast to be injected varies depending on the iodine concentration in the contrast medium. Usually in cases of MDCT liver imaging, 120–150 cc of 300 mgI/ml of nonionic contrast is injected at a rate of 4 cc/s. On the other hand, if 370 mgI/ml is used, only 80–100 cc would be required, but this needs to be balanced with a slightly higher injection rate of 4–5 cc/s. Thus, with use of higher or lower iodine concentration contrast media, appropriate adjustments in injection rate and contrast volume are needed.

Pitch and Scan Collimation

The use of thinner collimations with increases in detector configuration of CT scanners has revolutionized the role of CT scans in imaging of liver pathologies. It has been shown that the use of 2.5 mm collimation markedly improves the detec-

Table 2. Multi-detector computed tomography (MDCT) liver protocols on different computed tomography (CT) scanners

Parameters	4 channel	16 channel	64 channel
DC (mm)	4 × 1.25	16 × 0.625	64 × 0.6
TS (mm/s)	15	18.75	38
Pitch 1.0–2.0	0.938	0.984	
Slice thickness (mm)			
Arterial phase (CTA)	1.25	1.0	1.0
Arterial phase (liver)	2.5–5.0	2.5	2.5
Venous phase (CTA)	2.5	2.0	2.0
Venous phase (liver)	5.0	5.0	5.0
Arterial delay (s)		Bolus tracking/automated trigger Empirical delay: 25–30 s	
Venous delay (s)	65–70 s	60 s	50–60 s

DC detector collimation, *TS* table speed, *CTA* computed tomographic arteriography

tion of liver lesions compared with imaging on scanners with higher collimation such as 10 mm, 7.5 mm, and 5 mm [6]. For hepatic parenchymal imaging, 2.5 mm collimation is typically selected with a 4-row MDCT, but with increasing detector rows, such as 16- and 64-slice CT, collimations as thin as 1.25 mm and 0.625 mm can be obtained.

One of the most important factors that determines the pitch is the table speed (Table 2). New-generation MDCT scanners provide better coverage using the maximum table speed, which is due to the presence of their respective detector configurations and more data elements (Table 2). However, it is possible that this may result in unacceptable noise in the images.

Reconstruction Interval

It was shown by Kawata et al. [19] that there is no significant difference in the images obtained by using intervals of 2.5 mm, 5 mm, and 7.5 mm for detection of hypervascular hepatocellular carcinomas. It is essential that overlap of reconstructions be at least 50% to obtain optimal image quality particularly for hepatic CT angiography. Although thinner slices are desirable, reconstruction intervals of less than 2 mm can add to the noise in the image and thus affect the rate of detection of liver lesions. However, retrospective reconstruction from thinner collimated images of isotropic voxel resolution promotes reduction of partial-volume artifacts.

Role of MDCT in Imaging of Liver Tumors

The advent of MDCT scanners has ensured the availability of fast data acquisition, thinner collimations, and near-isotropic voxel resolution, but along with this has come alterations in scan delay and rate of contrast administration as well as emphasis on the importance of contrast concentration.

The two most important factors that influence the detection of lesions is lesion size and its intrinsic vascularity. Lesions as small as 1 mm have been detected by MDCT. It is generally believed that a minimum of 10 HU difference between lesion and normal liver parenchyma is required for the lesion to be detected. Different tumors may enhance at different phases of the scans depending on tumor vascularity. It must be noted that most tumors derive their blood supply from the hepatic artery and its branches. However, some may be more vascular than others and thus show increased enhancement on the hepatic arterial phase of the scan. Such tumors are classified as hypervascular tumors. Examples are hepatocellular carcinomas, metastases from melanoma, breast cancer, carcinoid, thyroid medullary carcinoma, islet cell tumors, and renal cell carcinoma.

Certain benign lesions also show increased vascularity in the hepatic arterial phase of the scan, such as focal nodular hyperplasia (FNH) and hemangiomas less than 1 cm. This advantage of tiny lesion detection by MDCT scanners revealed that benign tumors in conditions such as cysts, focal nodular hyperplasia, hemangiomas, and adenomas occur in up to one third of the population without known malignancy [20]. In addition, MDCT detects tiny lesions, such as metastases in the liver, at an early stage, thereby ensuring early surgery, ablation therapy, or chemotherapy.

As we have moved to the era of 16- and 64-slice CT scanners, a study of the subtle enhancement pattern of tiny hypodense liver lesions in the hepatic arterial phase can be performed [21]. MDCT can detect the peripheral rim enhancement in hypovascular lesions and can very well depict involvement of the adjacent vasculature by the tu-

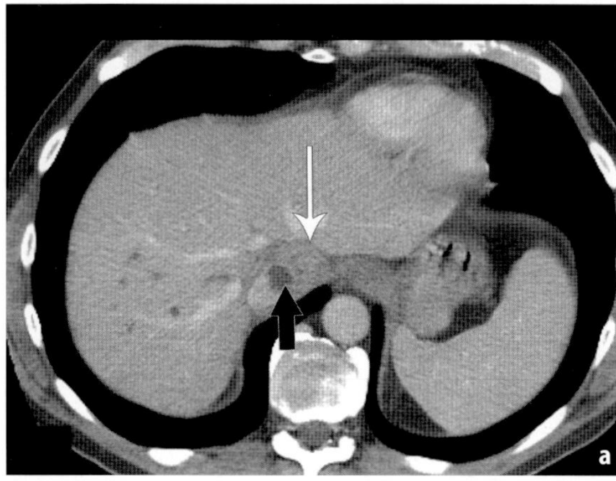
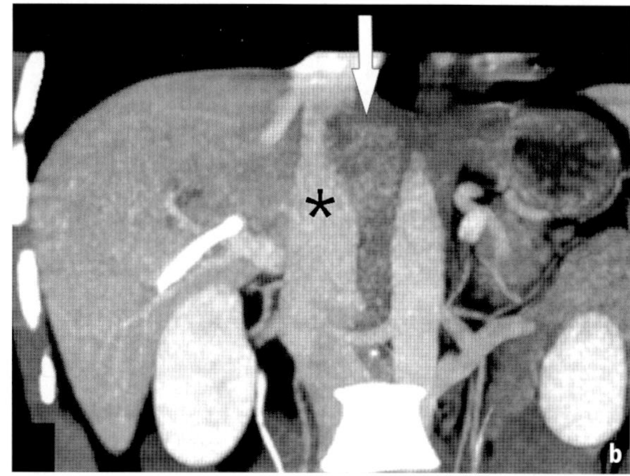

Fig. 4a, b. Preoperative planning of cholangiocarcinoma: contrast-enhanced axial image (**a**) shows an infiltrative mass in the dome of the liver with suspicion of inferior vena cava (IVC) invasion (*arrow*) seen as a filling defect. However, the corresponding coronal subvolume maximum intensity projection (MIP) image (**b**) confirmed only extrinsic compression and not invasion of the IVC (*asterisk*) by the tumor (*arrow*), and therefore surgery was feasible

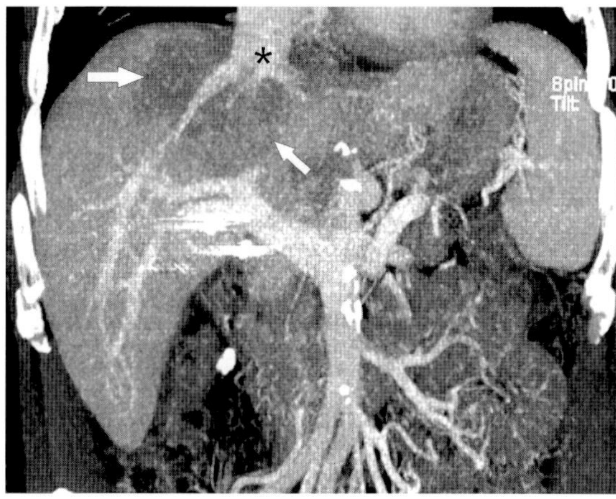

Fig. 5. Coronal reformat subvolume maximum intensity projection (MIP) image demonstrates an infiltrative cholangiocarcinoma (*arrows*) encasing the hepatic venous confluence and inferior vena cava (IVC) (*asterisk*) that makes the tumor unresectable

mor mass. It is also an important imaging modality for tumor staging (Figs. 4 and 5).

An important feature of the hepatic arterial phase for such lesions is the search for arterioportal shunting. Certain malignant lesions reveal the presence of arterioportal shunts (Fig. 6). This is due to the compression of portal or hepatic veins, which causes development of hepatic artery to portal venous collateral vessels. However, such shunts can also be visualized in the arterial phase in cases of abscess, small hemangiomas, and cirrhosis [22].

Importance of Early Tumor Detection by MDCT

Early detection of small hypervascular metastases and primary tumors by MDCT is important for early treatment planning. Due to the inherent capability of MDCT scanners to outline smaller and more subtle lesions much earlier in the disease process, routine screening for hepatitis B patients is performed to detect early development of neoplasia in the liver. In such patients, the ability of MDCT to pick up tiny lesions in different phases of the scan proves to be a crucial imaging modality. Patients with small tumors of less than 5-mm diameter may be candidates for liver transplantation. Studies have shown the importance of late arterial phase scans for detection of tiny liver tumors [23, 24]. But due to constraints posed by inaccurate bolus tracking methods, which may read to significant hepatic venous enhancement in the late arterial phase, the use of both phases is justified [25].

Hepatic artery catheter MDCT is an invasive procedure that involves injection of lipiodol into the hepatic artery. It can detect subtle intra-arterial enhancement, which may not be revealed on intravenous contrast injection. This procedure could thus have a significant impact on tumor treatment options.

Detection of Small Benign Lesions

The differentiation between tiny benign and malignant lesions poses a challenge for MDCT. The only factor that is of vital importance to consider is the pattern of enhancement following administration of contrast. Thinner collimation with MDCT helps in accurate detection of attenuation in tiny lesions such as simple cysts. MDCT also aids in better differentiation of hemangiomas from hypervascular metastasis. Attenuation of small hemangiomas is more or less like that of the aorta in

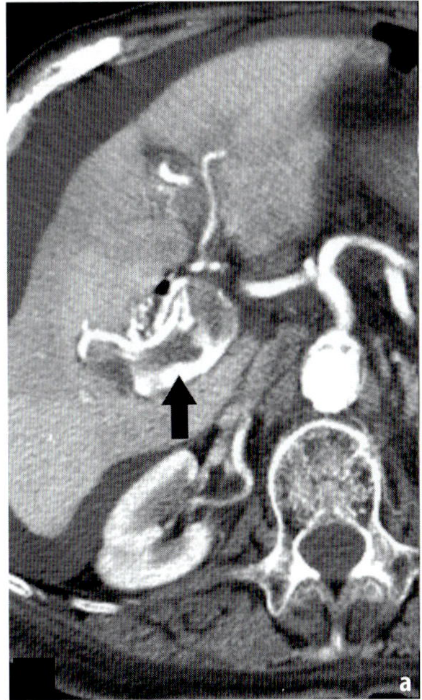
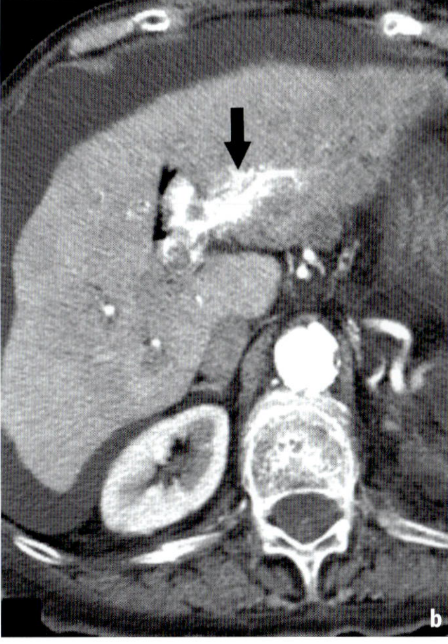

Fig. 6a, b. Tumor invasion in the portal vein from hepatocellular carcinoma (HCC). Two arterial phase axial images of the liver are shown. **a** Tumor thrombus is seen in the right portal vein (*arrow*). Also note the enhancement/contrast in the portal vein in the arterial phase. **b** Intensely enhancing arterioportal shunts from the tumor (*arrow*) around the left portal vein. Also seen is evidence of liver cirrhosis and ascites

MDCT in Liver Cirrhosis

With the availability of smart prep technology in the recent 16- and 64-slice scanners, the arterial and venous phases can be optimally timed, which is of paramount importance in cirrhotic patients who have decreased liver perfusion. In addition, the use of high-concentration contrast medium enables better visualization of the heterogeneous enhancement pattern in cirrhotics, which is mainly due to regenerative nodules, periportal fibrosis, and microcirculatory shunts between the portal venous and hepatic venous systems. Due to the thin slice collimation and accurate definition of the arterial and venous phase with MDCT scanners, better image quality and CTA reconstructions from data sets are possible. The collateral circulation in cases of portal hypertension is also seen more clearly and with prominent paraumbilical collaterals, esophageal varices, and periportal circulation.

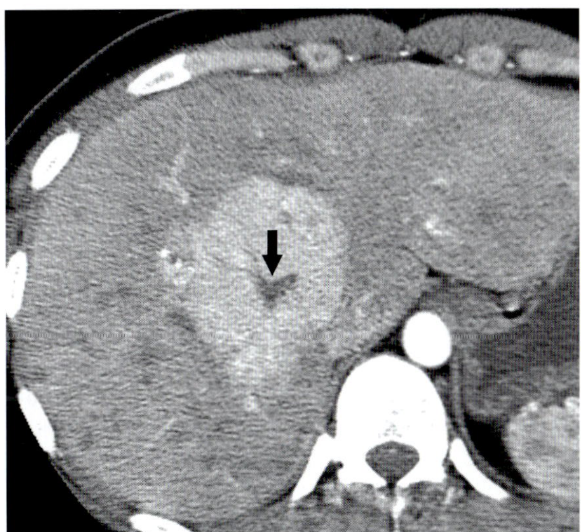

Fig. 7. Focal nodular hyperplasia: a dynamic late arterial phase axial image showing a well-defined, heterogeneously enhancing liver lesion with central scar (*arrow*), which appears as a hypoattenuating area

the arterial phases and similar to the hepatic veins in the venous phase. As MDCT can better define arterial and venous phases, detection of tiny hemangiomas is simplified to some extent.

Due to the capability of MDCT to highlight liver contrast in different phases of the scan, the detection of FNH is also simplified. The hallmark of FNH on dual-phase MDCT is its intense enhancement pattern, with or without a low attenuation central area, on arterial phase images and rapid wash out on venous phase images, in which it becomes more or less isoattenuating with the liver [26, 27] (Fig. 7).

MDCT for Preoperative Planning

Preoperative knowledge of the variations in vascular anatomy could help avoid complications such as inadvertent ligation or injury of various hepatic arteries, hepatic ischemia, and hemorrhage and biliary leak. Variations in the celiac axis anatomy are common, and preoperative knowledge is useful for surgery, especially in obese patients who have large amounts of lymphatic and fatty tissue in the duodenal hepatic ligament and the porta hepatis [28]. CT angiography images can provide excellent outlining of the vascular structures and demon-

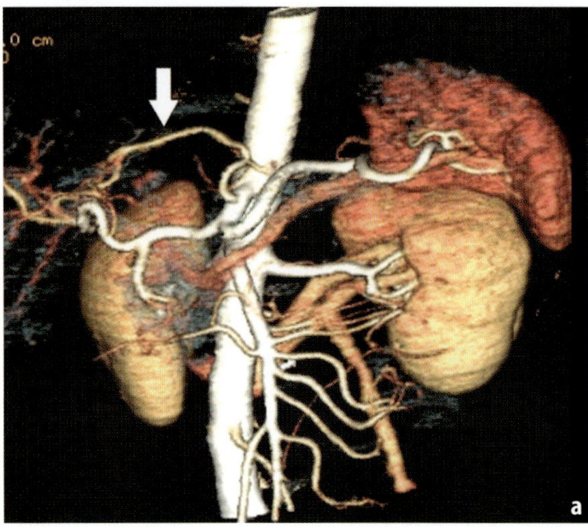

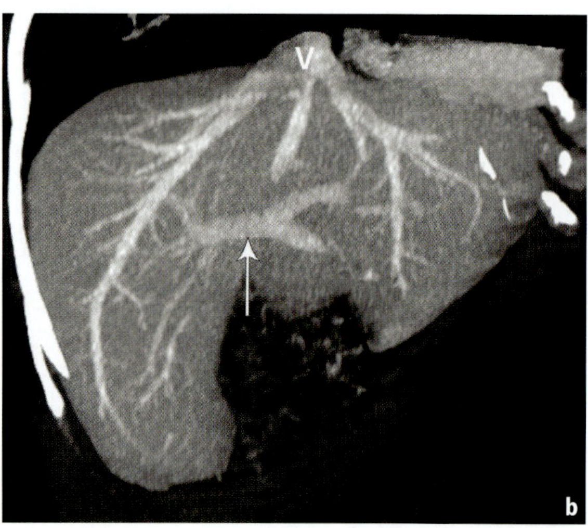

Fig. 8a, b. Preoperative planning for living-related liver transplantation: Color-coded volume-rendered computed tomographic arteriography (CTA) (**a**) demonstrates an anomalous origin of the left hepatic artery from the left gastric artery (*thick arrow*). A venous phase, subvolume maximum intensity projection (MIP) image in coronal oblique plane in venous phase (**b**) demonstrates normal portal and hepatic venous anatomy (*thin arrow*)

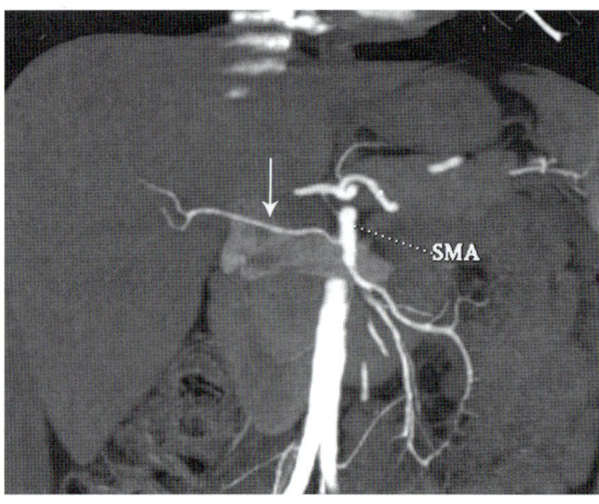

Fig. 9. Preoperative mapping of the arterial anatomy for intra-arterial chemotherapy pump placement. A coronal maximum intensity projection (MIP) computed tomographic arteriograph (CTA) displaying a replaced right hepatic artery (*arrow*) arising from the superior mesenteric artery (SMA)

strate the exact extent of involvement by lesions. CTA images are especially useful for understanding vascular variations prior to hepatic resection and the extent of vascular involvement by tumors before liver surgery (Fig. 8).

The newer MDCT scanners enable routine acquisition of submillimeter sections (up to 0.5 mm) with isotropic resolution [29, 30]. The quality of the three-dimensional (3-D) images is largely dependent on the source images for reconstruction. As with other forms of visualization, such as multiplanar reformation (MPR), volume rendering (VR), and maximum intensity projections (MIP), the source images should be of thin collimation,

have a greater longitudinal coverage with about 50 % overlap, and sufficient signal-to-noise ratio. These prerequisites are well provided by recent MDCT scanners [31].

The usual techniques for CT angiography of the liver are VR and MIP [32]. The MIP images provide no clue as to the depth of the structure but project the brightest structure, which in the hepatic arterial phase is the vascular detail (Fig. 9). Hence, optimal delay time, contrast medium concentration, and opacification are important. Due to the inherent capability of MDCT to provide desirable volumetric data and the required overlap, the reconstructed MIP images are of better quality than those obtained from older CT scanners. Some MDCT vendors allow users to save simplified scanning protocols on the user interface in the scanner so that exquisite MIP images can be obtained directly at the console.

Conclusion

MDCT offers several advantages, such as increased scanning speed and better definition of lesion conspicuity and characterization. However, to realize the maximum benefit, optimization of the acquisition parameters in different scanner types is important. Dual-phase imaging of the liver on MDCT is usually performed in the late arterial and portal venous phases, which not only enables better detection of small hypervascular lesions (in the arterial phase) at an early stage, but also plays an important role for early treatment planning. The availability of high-iodine concentration contrast medium ($\geq$370 mgI/ml) is an added benefit in such settings. These contrast media not only provide better opacification of vascular structures but also add to the quality of reconstruction images, especially for preoperative planning and placement of intra-arterial pumps [33-35]. To ensure better-quality images, technical details pertaining to planning scan delays and the right time of arterial contrast delivery are important.

References

1. Tsurusaki M, Sugimoto K, Fujii M, Sugimura K (2004) Multi-detector row helical CT of the liver: quantitative assessment of iodine concentration of intravenous contrast material on multiphasic CT–A prospective randomized study. Radiat Med 22(4): 239–245
2. Kanematsu M, Oliver JH 3rd, Carr B, Baron RL (1997) Hepatocellular carcinoma: the role of helical biphasic contrast-enhanced CT versus CT during arterial portography. Radiology 205(1):75–80
3. Hollett MD, Jeffrey RB Jr, Nino-Murcia M et al (1995) Dual-phase helical CT of the liver: value of arterial phase scans in the detection of small (< or = 1.5 cm) malignant hepatic neoplasms. AJR Am J Roentgenol 164(4):879–884
4. Abdelmoumene A, Chevallier P, Chalaron M et al (2005) Detection of liver metastases under 2 cm: comparison of different acquisition protocols in four row multidetector-CT (MDCT). Eur Radiol 15(9):1881–1887
5. Fishman EK, Jeffrey RB Jr (2004) Multidetector CT: Principles, techniques and clinical applications. Lippincott Williams & Wilkins, Philadelphia, p 85
6. Weg N, Scheer MR, Gabor MP (1998) Liver lesions: improved detection with dual-detector-array CT and routine 2.5-mm thin collimation. Radiology 209(2):417–426
7. Wang G, Vannier MW (1999) The effect of pitch in multislice spiral/helical CT. Med Phys 26(12): 2648–2653
8. Spielmann AL (2003) Liver imaging with MDCT and high concentration contrast media. Eur J Radiol 45 [Suppl 1]:50–52
9. Bader TR, Prokesch RW, Grabenwoger F (2000) Timing of the hepatic arterial phase during contrast-enhanced computed tomography of the liver: assessment of normal values in 25 volunteers. Invest Radiol 35(8):486–492
10. Hollett MD, Jeffrey RB Jr, Nino-Murcia M et al (1995) Dual-phase helical CT of the liver: value of arterial phase scans in the detection of small (< or = 1.5 cm) malignant hepatic neoplasms. AJR Am J Roentgenol 164(4):879–884
11. Ichikawa T, Kitamura T, Nakajima H et al (2002) Hyper vascular hepatocellular carcinoma: can double arterial phase imaging with multidetector CT improve tumor depiction in the cirrhotic liver? AJR Am J Roentgenol 179(3):751–758
12. Furuta A, Ito K, Fujita T et al (2004) Hepatic enhancement in multiphasic contrast-enhanced MDCT: Comparison of high- and low-iodine-concentration contrast medium in same patients with chronic liver disease. AJR Am J Roentgenol 183(1):157–162
13. Vignaux O, Legmann P, Coste J et al (1999) Cirrhotic liver enhancement on dual-phase helical CT: Comparison with non-cirrhotic livers in 146 patients. AJR Am J Roentgenol 173(5):1193–1197
14. Murakami T, Kim T, Takamura M et al (2001) Hyper vascular hepatocellular carcinoma: detection with double arterial phase multi-detector row helical CT. Radiology 218(3):763–767
15. Awai K, Takada K, Onishi H, Hori S (2002) Aortic and hepatic enhancement and tumor-to-liver contrast: Analysis of the effect of different concentrations of contrast material at multi-detector row helical CT. Radiology 224(3):757–763
16. Saini S (2004) Multi-detector row CT: principles and practice for abdominal applications. Radiology 233(2):323–327
17. Kalra MK, Maher MM, Toth TL et al (2004) Techniques and applications of automatic tube current modulation for CT. Radiology 233(3):649–657
18. Choi BI, Han JK, Cho JM et al (1995) Characterization of focal hepatic tumors. Value of two-phase scanning with spiral computed tomography. Cancer 76(12):2434–2442
19. Kawata S, Murakami T, Kim T et al (2002) Multidetector CT: diagnostic impact of slice thickness on detection of hypervascular hepatocellular carcinoma, AJR Am J Roentgenol 179(1):61–66
20. Jones EC, Chezmar JL, Nelson RC, Bernardino ME (1992) The frequency and significance of small (less than or equal to 15 mm) hepatic lesions detected by CT. AJR Am J Roentgenol 158(3):535–539
21. Schwartz LH, Gandras EJ, Colangelo SM et al (1999) Prevalence and importance of small hepatic lesions found at CT in patients with cancer. Radiology 210(1):71–74
22. Kim KW, Kim TK, Han JK et al (2001) Hepatic hemangiomas with arterioportal shunt: findings at two-phase CT. Radiology 219(3):707–711
23. Li L, Liu LZ, Xie ZM et al (2004) Multi-phasic CT arterial portography and CT hepatic arteriography improving the accuracy of liver cancer detection. World J Gastroenterol 10(21):3118–3121
24. Laghi A, Iannaccone R, Rossi P et al (2003) Hepatocellular carcinoma: detection with triple-phase multi-detector row helical CT in patients with chronic hepatitis. Radiology 226(2):543–549
25. Kim T, Murakami T, Hori M et al (2002) Small hyper vascular hepatocellular carcinoma revealed by double arterial phase CT performed with single breath-hold scanning and automatic bolus tracking. AJR Am J Roentgenol 178(4):899–904
26. Mortele KJ, Praet M, Van Vlierberghe H et al (2000) CT and MR imaging findings in focal nodular hyperplasia of the liver: Radiologic-pathologic correlation. AJR Am J Roentgenol 175(3):687–692
27. Carlson SK, Johnson CD, Bender CE, Welch TJ (200) CT of focal nodular hyperplasia of the liver. AJR Am J Roentgenol 174(3):705–712
28. Stemmler BJ, Paulson EK, Thornton FJ et al (2004) Dual-phase 3D MDCT angiography for evaluation of the liver before hepatic resection. AJR Am J Roentgenol 183(6):1551–1557
29. Hu H, He HD, Foley WD, Fox SH (2000) Four multidetector-row helical CT: image quality and volume coverage speed. Radiology 215(1):55–62
30. Flohr T, Prokop M, Becker C, Schoepf UJ et al (2002)

A retrospectively ECG-gated multislice spiral CT scan and reconstruction technique with suppression of heart pulsation artifacts for cardio-thoracic imaging with extended volume coverage. Eur Radiol 12(6):1497–1503

31. Kalender WA (1995) Thin-section three-dimensional spiral CT: is isotropic imaging possible? Radiology 197(3):578–580

32. Johnson PT, Halpern EJ, Kuszyk BS et al (1999) Renal artery stenosis: CT angiography comparison of real-time volume rendering and maximum intensity projection algorithms. Radiology 211(2):337–343

33. Takahashi S, Murakami T, Takamura M et al (2002) Multi-detector row helical CT angiography of hepatic vessels: depiction with dual-arterial phase acquisition during single breath hold. Radiology 222(1):81

34. Sahani D, Saini S, Pena C et al (2002) Using multidetector CT for preoperative vascular evaluation of liver neoplasms: Technique and results. AJR Am J Roentgenol 179(1):53–59

35. Sahani DV, Krishnamurthy SK, Kalva S et al (2004) Multidetector-row computed tomography angiography for planning intra-arterial chemotherapy pump placement in patients with colorectal metastases to the liver. J Comput Assist Tomogr 28(4): 478–484

10

Hepatobiliary Imaging by MDCT

Sebastian T. Schindera, Rendon C. Nelson

Introduction

Hepatobiliary imaging by computed tomography (CT) has advanced impressively since the introduction of multidetector CT (MDCT) scanners in the late 1990s. Over the last few years, the number of detector rows has increased progressively from four, to eight, to 16, and then up to 64. Two important advantages of MDCT are the routine use of thinner, submillimeter sections, which yield higher spatial resolution, along the Z-axis and decrease in gantry rotation time, which result in a significantly reduced scan time. Sixteen-, 32- and 64-slice scanners allow the acquisition of data sets with nearly isotropic voxels for multiplanar imaging (e.g., coronal and sagittal plane), which has similar spatial resolution compared with axial planes. These off-axis reformations are particularly helpful for evaluating the hepatic vascular anatomy, the biliary system, and the segmental distribution of hepatic lesions. Since thin-section collimation also reduces partial volume averaging, sensitivity and specificity for detecting and characterizing increases, especially for small focal hepatic lesions, whether benign or malignant. Furthermore, evaluation of the biliary tract improves, not only at the level of the porta hepatis and extrahepatic bile ducts, but all the way to the hepatic periphery.

Shorter scan durations make it possible to include the entire upper abdomen during a single, comfortable breath hold. This reduces motion artefacts, especially in critically ill patients. Another advantage of reduced scan duration is more precise timing of different hepatic enhancement phases following bolus administration of iodinated contrast material, thus improving depiction and differentiation of focal hepatic lesions.

The main indication for MDCT examination of the liver is the detection and characterization of hepatic lesions. The crucial part of a diagnostic workup of focal hepatic lesions is the differentiation between benign and malignant disease. Characterization of small incidental lesions still remains a challenging task for hepatic MDCT because of an overall lack of features. Schwartz et al. [1] have shown, however, that approximately 80% of small hepatic lesions (smaller than 1 cm) in patients with cancer diagnosed on MDCT are benign.

Urgent indications for MDCT scan of the liver include blunt and penetrating trauma, abscesses, and postoperative complications (e.g., bleeding, infection). Moreover, multiphasic MDCT plays an important role for pre- and postoperative evaluation of liver resection and transplant patients. MDCT is also highly useful for diagnosing hepatic parenchymal abnormalities (e.g., fatty infiltration, cirrhosis, iron deposition) and in some cases can provide quantitative information.

The gold standard for imaging the biliary tree is still endoscopic retrograde cholangiopancreatography (ERCP), even though this procedure is invasive, expensive, and physician intensive. In the last several years, magnetic resonance cholangiopancreatography (MRCP) has gained wide acceptance for noninvasive biliary imaging. In some practices and many academic centers, MRCP even functions as the first-choice technique for biliary tract imaging. Although spatial resolution of MDCT is superior to that of MRCP, MDCT, either with or without a cholangiographic agent, serves only as an alternative clinical tool for noninvasive evaluation of the biliary system.

In this chapter, we discuss technical principles and improvements of hepatobiliary MDCT. In addition, the principles of contrast media application and different phases of liver enhancement, including the typical enhancement pattern of various liver lesions, are reviewed.

Parameters and Technical Principles of Hepatobiliary MDCT

After introduction of the first 4-row MDCT scanner in 1998, the radiological community quickly accepted the new technology. With the development of 16-, 32-, and 64-slice scanners, data acquisition time has been further reduced. Coupling of wide collimation with large beam pitches and faster gantry rotation times has allowed for routine use of submillimeter collimation to acquire data sets with isotropic voxels. Rapid technological development, though, has increased the complexity of imaging options and scanning parameters. Radiologists using MDCT for hepatobiliary imaging should understand the imaging parameters and technical principles needed to acquire images with superior quality. The key parameters are:

- Acquisition parameters
- Reconstruction parameters
- Contrast media application
- Different phases of hepatic vascular and parenchymal enhancement

Acquisition Parameters

As the number of detector channels increases, application of thin collimation has become a routine part of MDCT. The minimum section collimation of 16-, 32-, and 64-slice scanners is 0.625 mm (GE, Philips), 0.60 mm (Siemens), or 0.50 mm (Toshiba). This submillimeter feature allows for isotropic data acquisition. An isotropic voxel is cubic, having equal dimensions in the X-, Y-, and Z-axis. Since the X- and Y-axes are determined by both field-of-view (FOV) and matrix size, isotropic voxels can be acquired only when slice thickness (Z-axis) measures 0.75 mm or less. The major advantage of these nearly isotropic data sets is the ability to reformat images in any desired plane, having similar spatial resolution to that of the axial plane. In recent studies, our group found multiplanar reformations particularly helpful for diagnosis of acute appendicitis and for evaluation of small-bowel obstruction [2, 3]. Further work is needed to evaluate the contribution of MDCT to hepatobiliary imaging.

Owing to increased spatial resolution and reduced partial volume averaging, thinner-slice collimation also results in an improved ability to detect small hepatic lesions. However, there is no consensus in the literature about the optimal collimation needed to detect small hepatic lesions [4–7]. The study performed by Haider et al. [7] using a 4-slice MDCT scanner did not find an improvement in the detection of hepatic metastases measuring 1.5 cm or smaller at collimation widths of less than 5 mm. Similar results were reported by Abdelmoumene et al. [5] when comparing four protocols with different slice collimations (5.0 and 2.5 mm) to detect small liver metastases (<2 cm). No improvement in lesion detection was found with a collimation width less than 2.5 mm. Furthermore, hepatic imaging with thinner sections caused an increase in image noise, with significantly lower performance in the detection of hepatic lesions [5]. To reduce noise associated with thinner sections, radiation dose to the patient should be increased. Typical scanning protocols for hepatobiliary imaging by MDCT are shown in Table 1. Section collimation should be tailored to the indication for hepatobiliary CT scan.

Reconstruction Parameters

With the development of 16-slice scanners, it became possible to scan the entire abdomen during a single, comfortable breath hold at a resolution of less than 1 mm in the X-, Y-, and Z-axes, resulting in a nearly isotropic data set. This three-dimen-

Table 1. Scan parameter for PVP and HAP using 4-, 16-, and 64- slice multidetector computed tomography (MDCT) (developed for GE scanners)

	4-slice MDCT		16-sclice MDCT		64-slice MDCT	
	HAP	*PVP*	*HAP*	*PVP*	*HAP*	*PVP*
Detector configuration (mm)	4 × 3.75	4 × 2.5	16 × 1.25	16 × 0.625	64 × 0.625	64 × 0.625
Pitch	1.5	1.5	1.38	1.75	1.38	1.38
Table speed (mm/rotation)	22.5	15	27.5	17.5	55.0	55.0
Rotation time (s)	0.8	0.8	0.6	0.5	0.5	0.5
kV	140	140	140	140	140	140
mA	220	220	300	380	450	450
Slice thickness (mm)	5.0	5.0	5.0	5.0	5.0	5.0
Axial slice thickness for MPR and 3-D- reconstruction (mm)	2.5	2.5	1.25	0.625	1.25	0.625

HAP hepatic arterial phase, *PVP* portal venous phase, *MPR* multiplanar reformation

sional (3-D) volume can be used for further two-dimensional (2-D) and 3-D postprocessing. The most important rendering techniques for hepatobiliary MDCT are straight or curved multiplanar reformation (MPR), maximum intensity projection (MIP), minimum intensity projection (minIP), and volume rendering (VR). The type of reconstruction primarily depends on the indication for the study.

MPR, representing a 2-D reformatted plane other than the axial plane, is mainly used as a tool to visualize complex hepatic anatomic and pathological findings. Using a 4-slice CT scanner, Hong et al. [8] evaluated image quality and diagnostic value of abdominal MPRs. There was superior visualization of liver segments and lesions with MPRs compared with axial images alone; however, no significant difference in liver lesion detection between axial and MPR images could be found. The key to optimizing image quality of MPRs is to increase the reconstruction thickness to several millimeters. Recently, our group demonstrated in a qualitative analysis that 2- and 3-mm-thick coronal reformations provide the best image quality [9]; 1-mm-thick sections were too noisy, whereas 4- to 5-mm slice thickness was too smooth, yielding little anatomical detail, especially for blood vessels and lymph nodes.

MIPs are routinely used to evaluate hepatic arteries and the portal veins, since these projections display the greatest attenuation difference between vessels and adjacent tissue. Another indication for MIP is CT cholangiography, which is well suited to visualization of the biliary tract anatomy and the presence of congenital anomalies [10–12]. In patients with bile duct obstruction, minIPs may be helpful for demonstrating the biliary tract when MDCT is performed without a cholangiographic agent [13–15]. To improve image quality of MIPs and minIPs, partial volume averaging effects can be reduced by choosing the volume of interest as small as possible.

The VR technique allows the user to view the entire volume data set in an appropriate 3-D context, including a range of different types of abdominal tissues (Fig. 1). Various opacity values can be applied to simultaneously display both the surface and the interior of the volume. These images are well appreciated by surgeons, since they offer a true 3-D view of the hepatic vascular anatomy. Other indications for VR are estimation of liver volume and virtual hepatectomy prior to living-related liver transplantation.

Contrast Media Application

Nonionic iodinated contrast agents are small molecular weight extracellular agents that are most

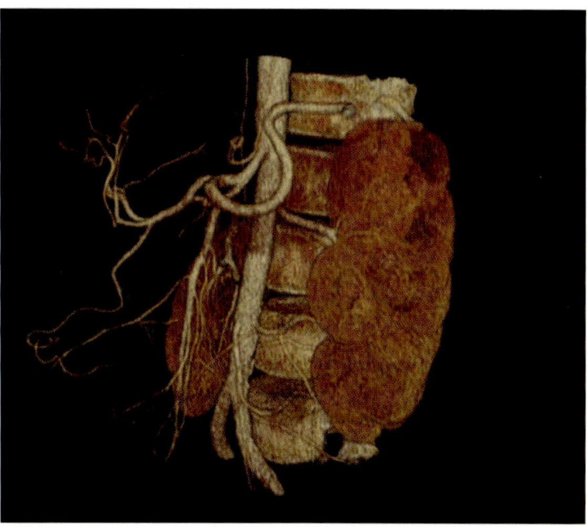

Fig. 1. Volume rendering technique of the hepatic arterial system. Note the anatomic variation of the celiac axis arising from the superior mesenteric artery (SMA)

commonly used with hepatobiliary MDCT to delineate blood vessels and hepatic parenchyma, as well as to detect and characterize focal and diffuse hepatic abnormalities. The degree of maximum enhancement of liver parenchyma during the portal venous phase (PVP) is directly proportional to the *total amount* of iodine administered. There is no difference between contrast material injection protocols specifying 100 ml of an agent with an iodine concentration of 370 mg/ml (37 g of iodine) and 125 ml of an agent with an iodine concentration of 300 mg/ml (37.5 g of iodine). Furthermore, the introduction of faster 16- and 64-slice CT scanners did not significantly reduce the necessary volume of injected contrast media for hepatobiliary imaging since the speed of the scanner did not improve enhancement during the venous phase. For most applications, 38–44 g of iodine is recommended, since 44 g has not been shown to statistically significantly improve hepatic enhancement [16]. Total iodine doses less than 30 g are also not recommended, as the duration and magnitude of hepatic enhancement will decrease, resulting in a lower detection rate of focal liver lesions.

Contrast materials with an iodine concentration up to 400 mg/ml are currently available. Most institutions administer a fixed amount of contrast agent (120–150 ml) when using iodine concentration of 300 mg/ml. However, previous studies have recommended tailoring the volume of contrast material to body weight [17–19]. Yamashita and coworkers achieved the best hepatic parenchymal enhancement with a dose of 2.0–2.5 ml/kg adjusted for body weight [18].

Opacification of the hepatic arterial system and detection of hypervascular hepatic lesions are improved primarily by the *rate* of iodine delivery and the *timing* of imaging relative to the contrast media bolus. Improved lesion-to-liver contrast can be attained either by an accelerated injection rate or by an increased iodine concentration. While the injection rate of contrast media (3–6 ml/s) may be physiologically limited, the use of contrast agents with higher iodine concentration (350–400 mgI/ml) is compelling. Regardless of iodine concentration, faster injection rates are superior in detection of hypervascular liver lesions. A recent study by Itoh et al. [20] reported improved arterial enhancement with contrast agents having high iodine concentration (350 mgI/ml) by shortening the injection duration. Awai et al. [21] found a significantly higher tumor-to-liver contrast with hepatocellular carcinoma (HCC) in the arterial phase after administration of contrast material with high iodine concentration (370 mgI/ml) compared with moderate iodine concentration (300 mgI/ml). However, there was no significant difference in hepatic enhancement during the PVP, since the same iodine load was administered to both groups. There may be a potential cost saving when using a contrast material with a higher iodine concentration, since the volume of contrast can be decreased to maintain the same number of grams of iodine per milliliter per second.

In the case of MDCT angiography, when only arterial enhancement is of interest, Ho et al. [19] reported a significant reduction of contrast material dose with the use of an interactive injection protocol that included an immediate interruption of the contrast injection after the aorta enhanced qualitatively. Contract media dose was reduced because of the increased speed of the MDCT scanner.

The recent development and introduction of double-syringe mechanical power injectors simplified the saline flush technique. Immediate injection of a saline bolus after contrast agent administration avoids accumulation of the contrast agent in the injection tubing and the venous system. The new injector results in superior contrast enhancement. Schoellnast et al. [22] noted a significantly higher parenchymal and vascular enhancement of the liver in a group of patients receiving a 20-ml saline flush with a double-syringe power injector compared with the same patient population using a single-syringe power injector without flush. The same contrast media protocol (100 ml of contrast agent with iodine concentration of 300 mgI/ml) was used in both groups. By using the saline flush technique, the same group showed a decrease in contrast media dose by 17% without a significant decrease in enhancement of hepatic parenchyma and vessels [23]. This injection technique may reduce total yearly amounts of contrast agent and individual patient doses, for example, for patients with renal insufficiency; however, the additional

costs of a second syringe must be taken into account.

To opacify the biliary tree for diagnostic imaging with MDCT (CT cholangiography), either oral or intravenous cholangiographic contrast agents can be administered. The intravenous cholangiographic contrast agent is infused over 30 min and is followed by a CT scan within 15–30 min. Most institutions administer intravenous diphenhydramine prior to infusion of cholangiographic contrast material to diminish the incidence of allergic reactions. For CT cholangiography with oral contrast medium, the patient has to ingest 6 g of iopanoic acid after a low-fat meal the night before. Several studies have shown that intravenous MDCT cholangiography is feasible for noninvasive evaluation of the biliary anatomy [11, 12, 24]. Nonetheless, intravenous cholangiography is rarely used in the United States, not only due to the high rate of allergic reactions and of renal and hepatic toxicity, but also due to the fact that there is suboptimal visualization of the biliary tract in up to 36% of patients [12, 25].

Different Phases of Hepatic Vascular and Parenchymal Enhancement

The increasing speed of MDCT scanners has improved the ability to perform multiphasic examinations of the liver. Most of the recently introduced 64-slice MDCT scanners image the whole liver in less than 2 s. Since acquisitions are becoming closer to a snapshot, timing of contrast-material bolus is even more important. Most of the recently introduced 64-slice MDCT scanners image the whole liver in less than 2 s, which may result in superior hepatic scans during multiple phases with more optimal enhancement. Table 2 demonstrates the indication for dynamic hepatobiliary MDCT imaging.

There are selected cases in which an unenhanced CT scan of the liver is helpful and recommended. Reasonable clinical indications for a noncontrast hepatic CT include:
- Depiction of acute hemorrhage of the liver
- Delineation of siderotic nodules
- Detection and characterization of hepatic calcification (e.g., calcified metastases, epithelioid hemangioendothelioma, hydatid cysts)
- Evaluation of parenchymal liver diseases (e.g., fatty infiltration, hepatic cirrhosis, hemochromatosis)
- Follow-up CT scan after embolization of hypervascular liver lesions.

Contrast-enhanced MDCT of the liver is complicated by the liver's dual blood supply (parenchyma receives 75% of its blood via the portal vein

Table 2. Indications for dynamic hepatobiliary multidetector computed tomography (MDCT) imaging

	Noncontrast	EAP	LAP	PVP	EQP
Hypovascular liver metastases				x	
Hypervascular liver metastases			x	x	
Hepatocellular carcinoma	x		x	x	x
Focal nodular hyperplasia			x	x	
Hepatocellular adenoma	x		x	x	
Evaluation of hepatic arterial system		x			
Cholangiocarcinoma				x	x
Primary sclerosing cholangitis				x	x
Cholecystitis				x	
Gallbladder carcinoma				x	x

EAP early arterial phase, *LAP* late arterial phase, *PVP* portal venous phase, *EQP* equilibrium phase

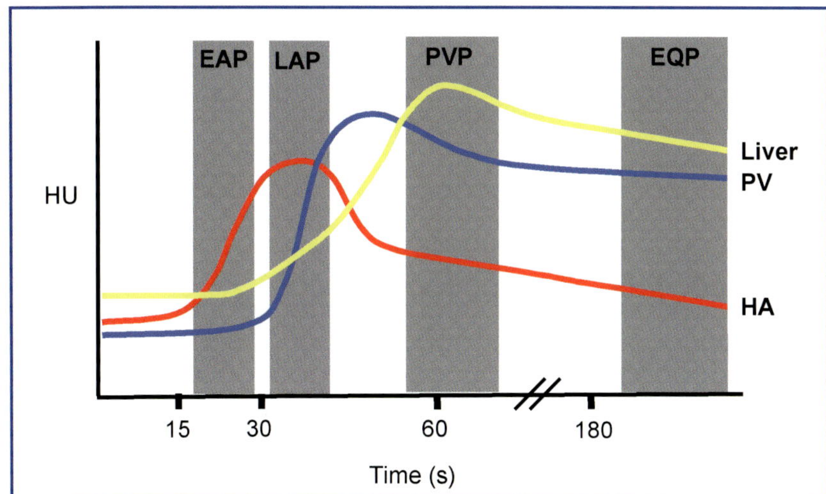

Fig. 2. Different phases of enhancement in dynamic hepatobiliary MDCT imaging. *EAP* early arterial phase, *LAP* late arterial phase, *PVP* portal venous phase, *EQP* equilibrium phase, *PV* portal vein, *HA* hepatic artery)

and 25% via the hepatic artery), resulting in various phases of enhancement. Figure 2 demonstrates the typical enhancement curves of the hepatic artery, the portal vein, and liver parenchyma. Following an intravenous bolus of contrast material, the hepatic artery enhances first at approximately 15 s and reaches peak attenuation at approximately 30 s. After the contrast medium returns from the splanchnic system, the portal vein starts to enhance at around 30 s. Enhancement of liver parenchyma begins later, reaching a plateau at 60–70 s. The plateau may last up to 20–30 s. Finally, there is the equilibrium phase (EQP) (3 min and later), which occurs when the amount of contrast material in the intra- and extravascular extracellular space is essentially the same. Arterial hepatic enhancement is regulated mainly by cardiovascular circulation time and iodine delivery rate, whereas parenchyma enhancement of the liver is related to total iodine dose administered. According to the different enhancement curves of the hepatic artery, portal vein, and hepatic parenchyma, four phases can be distinguished:

1. *Early arterial phase* (EAP) appears 20–25 s after administration of contrast material when there

is conspicuous enhancement in the hepatic arteries compared with almost no enhancement of liver parenchyma or hypervascular lesions. This phase typically provides the least information for imaging the liver, since the contrast media at that time has accumulated neither in hypervascular liver lesions nor in liver parenchyma. Nevertheless, this phase is well suited for CT angiography when used to evaluate the anatomical configuration of hepatic arteries prior to liver transplantation, hepatic tumor resection, or arterial chemoembolization.

To achieve optimum timing for EAP scanning for hepatic CT angiography, an automated triggering system may be used. This technique is superior to a fixed-delay or a test bolus. The scanner is typically set at the top of the liver with the trigger placed in the descending thoracic aorta. Following a 15-s delay after initiation of contrast material administration, a low-dose image is acquired every 3 s. When the trigger, which monitors the descending aorta, reaches a predefined attenuation (typically 90–100 HU), the scan begins for the EAP.

2. *Late arterial phase* (LAP) appears at about 30–35 s following initiation of contrast material administration. For optimum timing using the au-

tomated triggering technique, to avoid the EAP, an additional 8- to 10-s delay is required. The LAP is also referred to as the portal vein inflow phase, since the portal vein is already starting to enhance during this phase. The hepatic arterial systems as well as prominent neovasculature of hypervascular hepatic neoplasms continue to enhance during the LAP, while there is only minimal enhancement of hepatic parenchyma. At this point, there is a maximum attenuation difference between hypervascular liver lesions and the surrounding liver parenchyma (Fig. 3). Thus, LAP is the optimal phase for detecting hypervascular neoplasms of the liver. Foley et al. [26] were one of the first groups to propose three different hepatic circulatory phases using MDCT and showed that there was a significantly better delineation of hypervascular liver lesions during the LAP compared with the EAP. A few years later, Laghi et al. [27] investigated whether the use of the two arterial phases in combination improves the detection of hypervascular HCC with MDCT. Their data showed no significant difference between the late phase and the two combined arterial phases for depiction of HCC, so they concluded that acquisition of the LAP together with the PVP is considered sufficient for detection of HCC with MDCT.

3. *Portal venous phase* (PVP), or hepatic venous phase, appears at about 60–70 s following initiation of a contrast media bolus, when the enhancement of liver parenchyma reaches its peak and the portal vein and hepatic veins are well enhanced. For accurate timing of the PVP in a single-phase exam, we again recommend automated scanning technology instead of a fixed time delay. The trigger is placed in liver parenchyma to track the enhancement curve, and when attenuation reaches a predefined

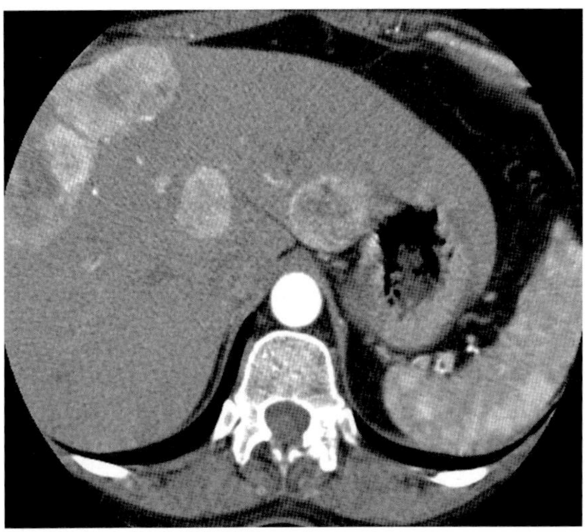

Fig. 3. Hyperenhancing or hypervascular liver metastases from a neuroendocrine tumor of pancreas during the late arterial phase (LAP)

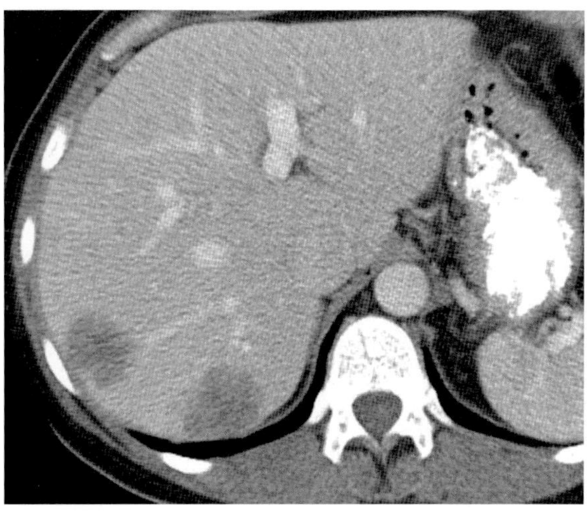

Fig. 4. Hypoenhancing or hypovascular liver metastases in the right hepatic lobe from a colon cancer detected during portal venous phase

threshold (e.g., 50–70 HU), the table is moved to the top of the liver and the diagnostic scan initiated. For a dual-phase exam, there is a fixed time delay of 40 s following the end of the LAP.

Hypovascular tumors are optimally detected during the PVP when enhancement of liver parenchyma is maximal and there is the greatest liver-to-lesion attenuation difference (Fig. 4). For detection of these tumors, a single scan during the PVP is sufficient, since there is no further advantage performing unenhanced or arterial-phase imaging. The PVP is also the appropriate phase for visualization and evaluation of intrahepatic bile ducts, when there is the greatest difference of attenuation between the maximally enhanced liver parenchyma and the hypoattenuating intraductal bile.

4. *Equilibrium phase* (EQP), or intersitial phase, appears at approximately 3 min postinjection, when there is an increased diffusion of contrast media into liver parenchyma and attenuation difference between parenchyma and vessels is minimal. Washout of the contrast material in different liver lesions may vary vastly depending on their histological nature. One clear indication for acquiring images during the EQP includes intrahepatic cholangiocarcinoma. This tumor when desmoplastic may accumulate the contrast agent and show a delayed washout compared with surrounding liver parenchyma. This delay causes hyperattenuating lesions (Fig. 5). In a study by Keogan et al. [28], 36% of proven cholangiocarcinomas on the EQP demonstrated as hyperattenuating lesions compared with the liver. By comparison, HCC may show a faster washout during the EQP relative to the surrounding liver parenchyma, representing a hypoattenuating mass (Fig. 6).

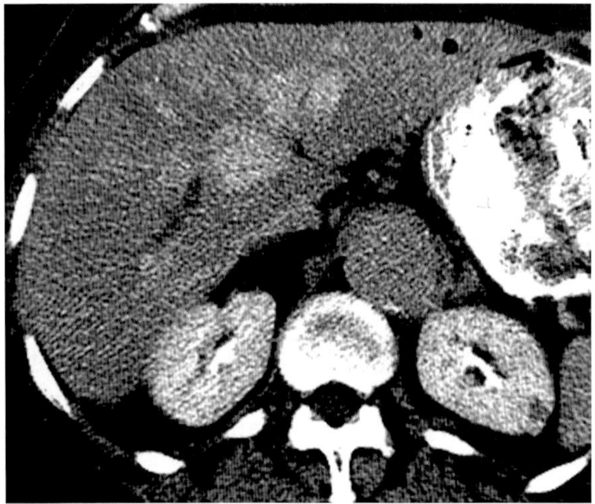

Fig. 5. Hyperattenuating lesion or delayed washout in the left hepatic lobe during the equilibrium phase (EQP) in a patient with cholangiocarcinoma

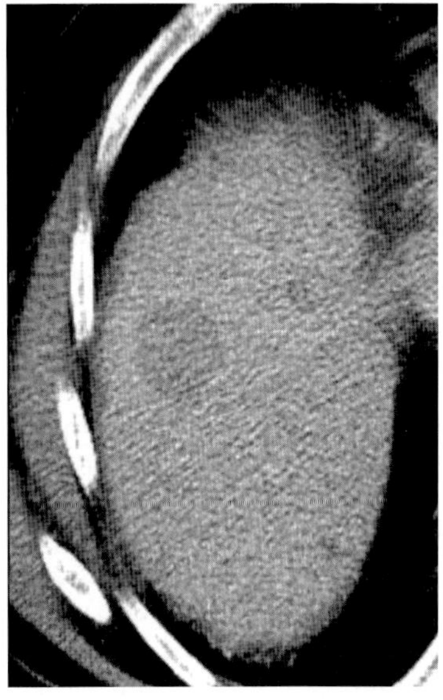

Fig. 6. Hypoattenuating mass representing faster washout of the hepatocellular carcinoma (HCC) during equilibrium phase (EQP)

Applications of Hepatobiliary MDCT

Liver

MDCT of the liver plays a crucial role in the detection of focal hepatic lesions as well as characterization of the mass as benign or malignant. Besides that, MDCT often functions as the technique of choice for tumor staging, monitoring response to treatment, diagnostic workup prior to hepatic resection or liver transplantation, or guidance of percutaneous biopsy and ablation. Superior detection of liver lesions with 16-slice or 64-slice MDCT scanners is a result of their increased speed, which

allows routine use of thinner collimation to increase spatial resolution and decrease acquisition time. The diagnostic impact of the technical advances of MDCT will be discussed for different hepatic tumors.

Liver Metastases
One of the major indications for hepatic MDCT is the detection of metastatic liver disease, which is by far the most common malignant hepatic tumor in patients without cirrhosis. The CT image appearance of liver metastases may vary widely depending on the histologic nature of the lesion and its vascularity. The type of MDCT protocol for depiction of liver metastases mainly depends on the degree of primary tumor vascularization.

Hypovascular Metastases
Most hepatic metastases are hypovascular and arise from primary tumors of the gastrointestinal tract (e.g., colon, rectum, stomach), pancreas, urothelium, lung, and head and neck, as well as from gynecologic tumors. During the PVP, these lesions are typically hypoattenuating owing to superior enhancement of adjacent liver parenchyma. In the periphery of these metastases, there may be increased enhancement during either the arterial phase or the PVP, represented by a hypervascular rim or halo. Most authorities recommend a single-phase CT during the PVP for evaluation of hypovascular metastases. Several studies have shown that the additional use of unenhanced or hepatic arterial-phase images does not detect more lesions [29–31]. However, the adjunct use of arterial-phase images may be valuable in the depiction of hypovascular metastases with a hypervascular rim, for example, colon cancer. A recent study, which investigated the enhancement pattern of focal liver lesions during the arterial phase, reported a complete ring enhancement in about 85% of hypovascular metastases [32]. Although dual-phase MDCT may be beneficial for special cases, for routine imaging of hypovascular liver metastases, arterial-phase imaging is not necessary. The reported detection rate of hypovascular liver metastases for MDCT during the PVP is between 85% and 91% [29, 33]. In a study performed by Soyer et al. [29], CT depicted all hypovascular metastases with a diameter greater than 1 cm during the PVP but only two out of six metastases (33%) with a diameter smaller than 0.5 cm. None of these small metastases could be detected on the unenhanced images or during the hepatic arterial phase.

Hypervascular Metastases
Primary tumors that tend to be associated with hypervascular liver metastases include neuroendocrine tumors (e.g., islet cell carcinoma, carcinoid tumor), renal cell carcinoma, thyroid carci-

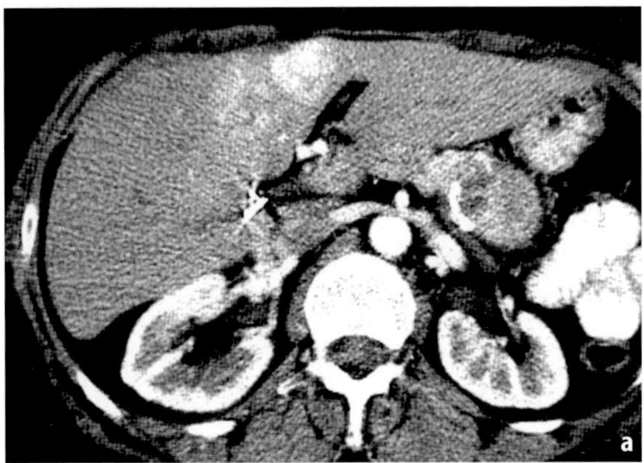

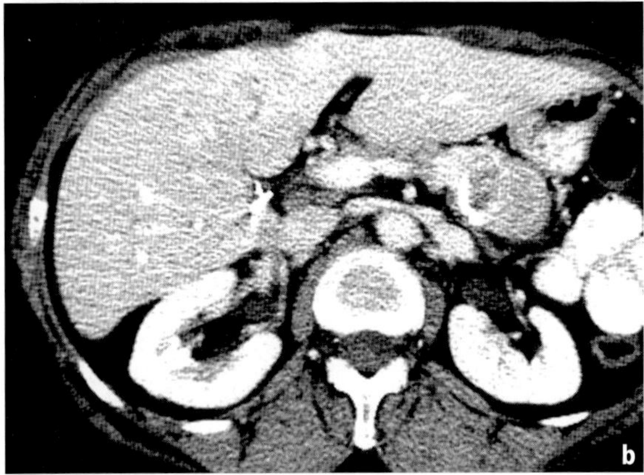

Fig. 7a, b. Hypervascular metastases from a neuroendocrine tumor of the pancreas during the late arterial phase (LAP) (**a**) and the portal venous phase (PVP) (**b**). Note that the tumors are much less apparent during the PVP

noma, melanoma, and occasionally breast cancer. The imaging protocol for hypervascular metastases is significantly different from hypovascular metastases. Hypervascular lesions are typically hyperattenuating during the late hepatic arterial phase due to an earlier and increased contrast media uptake compared with adjacent hepatic parenchyma. Blake et al. [34] investigated the sensitivity of different multiphasic contrast-enhanced CT protocols for the detection of liver metastases from melanoma. The study reported that the detection rate decreased by 14% when using only the PVP instead of obtaining an additional arterial phase. The MDCT protocol of choice for the detection of hypervascular metastases currently includes the LAP and PVP (Fig. 7a, b) [26, 27]. Other techniques that help improve the detectability of focal hypervascular liver lesions during biphasic MDCT are a contrast medium with a higher iodine concentration and a higher injection rate [20, 35]. At our institution, we evaluate hypervascular liver metastasis with a flow rate of 3.5 ml/s and contrast medium with an iodine concentration of 370 mgI/ml. The reported sensitivity of dual-phase CT for hypervascular liver metastases ranges between 78% and 96% [34, 36].

Hepatocellular Carcinoma

HCC is by far the most common primary malignant hepatic neoplasm as well as one of the most prevalent malignancies worldwide. The main predisposing factor in the Western Hemisphere is cirrhosis due to alcohol abuse, whereas in Africa and Asia, the most common underlying causes are hepatitis B and C infections and exposure to aflatoxin A. While surgical resection and liver transplantation provide the best long-term outcome and are the treatments of choice for HCC, most patients are not candidates for surgical therapy [37, 38]. Before considering these treatment options, early diagnosis of HCC in a more curable stage as well as detection of the precise number of nodules must be determined.

Multiphasic MDCT plays a central role in HCC screening of high-risk cirrhotic patients. The CT appearance of HCC is extremely variable and depends on the neoplasm's growth pattern (solitary mass, multifocal masses, or diffusely infiltrating neoplasm), size, histological nature, and vascularity. Up to 36% of HCCs are associated with fatty change, which may aid detection on unenhanced images [39]. The majority of HCCs are hypoattenuating on precontrast images; however, some tend to be isoattenuating compared with adjacent liver parenchyma (Fig. 8a-d). Many HCCs are hypervascular neoplasms, which enhance significantly during the LAP because of increased blood supply from the hepatic artery (Fig. 8b). Small HCCs (<3 cm) generally demonstrate a more homogenous enhancement during the arterial phase, whereas larger tumors show a heterogeneous enhancement pattern due to necrosis or hemorrhage. During the PVP, HCC usually becomes iso- to hypoattenuating to liver parenchyma depending on the extent of washout of the mass (Fig. 8c). During the EQP, the tumors themselves wash out more rapidly than hepatic parenchyma (Fig. 8d), but a tumor capsule and fibrous septation, if present, may be hyperattenuating due to delayed washout of the contrast material.

Detection of HCCs within cirrhotic liver parenchyma is challenging because of large amounts of fibrosis, distorted anatomy, and atrophy of various portions of the liver. Peterson et al. [40] investigated the sensitivity of preoperative helical CT for detecting HCC in cirrhotic patients undergoing liver transplantation [41]. In 320 patients with advanced cirrhosis, only 59% of the lesions confirmed by surgical pathology were detected on helical triphasic CT scans. In pretransplantation patients with cirrhosis, Valls et al. [41] reported a sensitivity of 94% for the detection of HCC (larger than 2 cm) with biphasic helical CT. However, the detection rate of HCC less than 2 cm was just 61%. Hence, the detection of HCCs in the setting of cirrhosis seems to depend largely on the

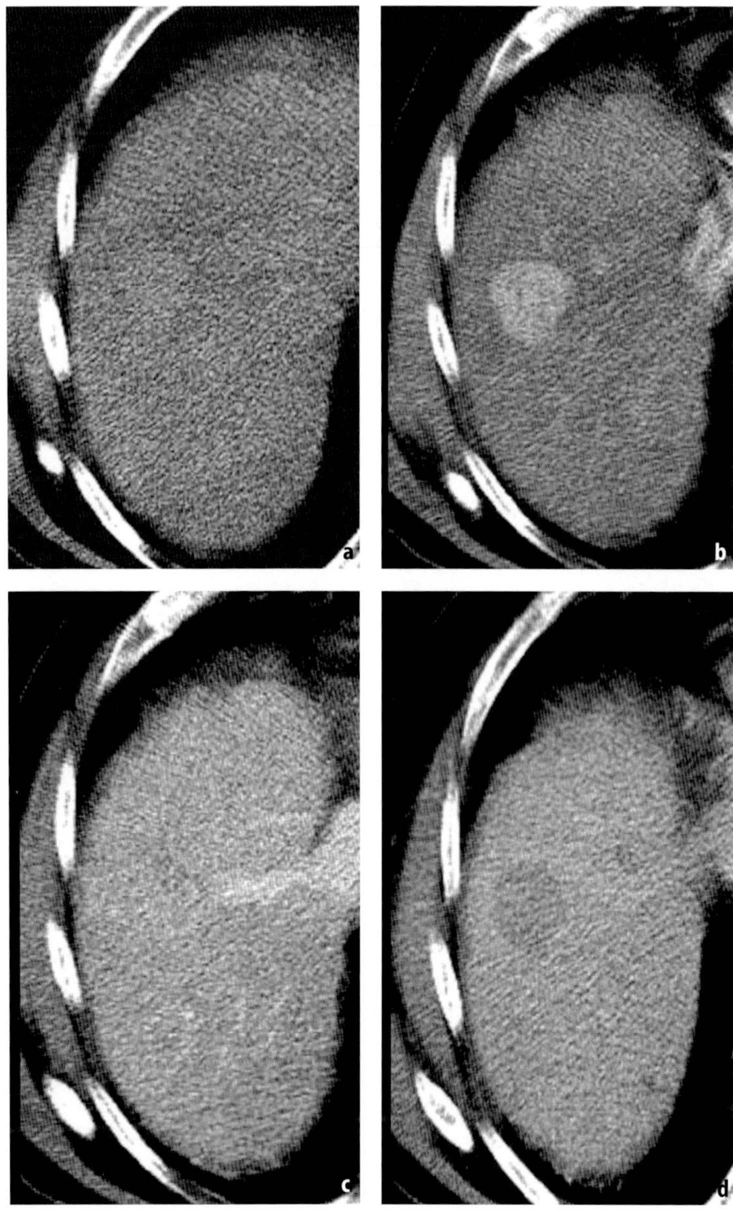

Fig. 8a-d. HCC in a cirrhotic patient during the unenhanced state (**a**), late arterial phase (LAP) (**b**), portal venous phase (PVP) (**c**) and equilibrium phase (EQP) (**d**). Note that the tumor is most conspicuous during the LAP and EQP

size of the neoplasm.

In the last few years, several investigators have demonstrated that the use of a biphasic MDCT protocol, a LAP followed by a PVP, significantly improves the depiction of HCC [26, 27, 42]. Additional EAP images in conjunction with bi- or triplephasic MDCT protocol did not improve detection of HCC [27, 42]. Furthermore, the role of unenhanced and delayed phase images for detection of HCC with MDCT remains controversial. A recent investigation reported a significant increase in HCC detection in cirrhotic patients, with the addition of a delayed or EQP (180 s postinjection) acquisition in conjunction with a biphasic MDCT protocol [43]. Moreover, 10% of detected HCCs showed a tumor capsule, which again could only be visualized on the EQP images. Regarding the use of

unenhanced images, the study did not present any significant advantages for depiction of HCC; however, the authors believe that unenhanced images are particularly helpful in the differentiation of hyperattenuating siderotic nodules from hyperenhancing HCC nodules. At our institution, the CT protocol for detection of HCC includes all four phases: unenhanced, LAP, PVP, and EQP.

Several studies have indicated that the administration of higher-concentration contrast material (370–400 mgI/ml) significantly increases liver-to-lesion contrast during the arterial phase. This method may improve depiction of HCC [21, 44, 45]. However, it is noteworthy that a study performed by Marchiano et al. [45] did not observe a significant increase in the overall number of HCCs detected after the injection of a high concentration

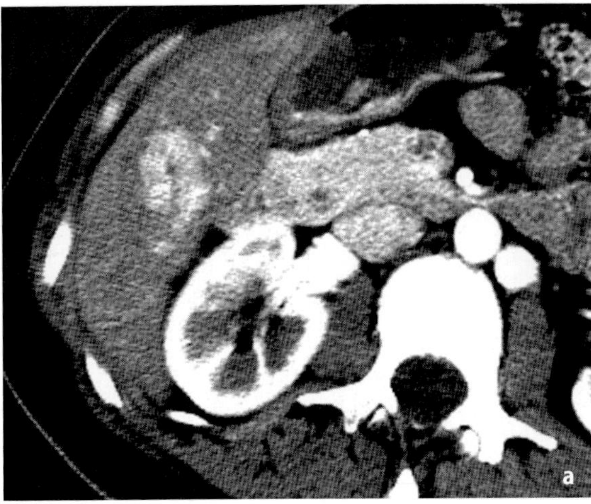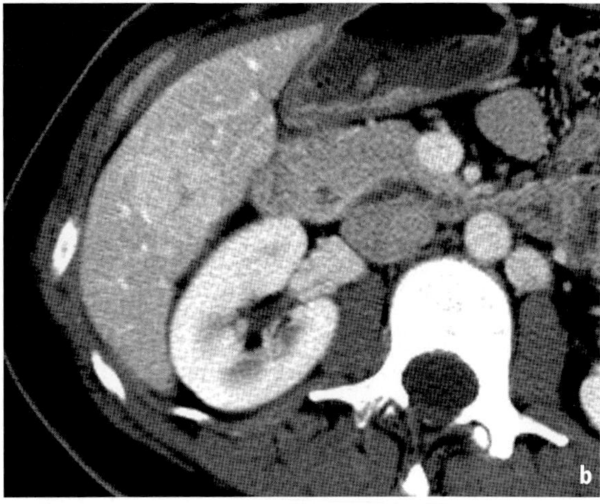

Fig. 9a, b. Focal nodular hyperplasia with a central scar during the late arterial phase (LAP) (**a**) and portal venous phase (PVP) (**b**). Note that the central scar enhances slowly

of iodinated contrast material. There is also a clear trend toward the use of faster injection rates (4–5 ml/s), which may improve conspicuity of HCCs due to superior liver-to-lesion contrast in the arterial phase [20, 46]. Oliver et al. [47] reported about a 74% detection rate for HCC with a flow rate of 4–5 ml/s during the hepatic arterial phase compared with a 58% detection rate with a flow rate of 3 ml/s. While only 19% of the detected lesions in this study showed an increase in enhancement with a flow rate of 3 ml/s, up to 83% of HCCs demonstrated as hyperattenuating on arterial-phase images using the higher flow rate.

Focal Nodular Hyperplasia
Focal nodular hyperplasia (FNH) is the second most common benign neoplasm of the liver after hemangioma. FNH arises predominately in women. The tumors are usually solitary, in a subcapsular location and, are often discovered incidentally during radiological imaging. The pathogenesis of FNH is believed to be a congenital vascular malformation having an increased arterial blood flow. A recent study by Mathieu et al. [48] suggested that FNH is not associated with the use of oral contraceptives. The neoplasm often contains a stellate central scar surrounded by small nodules of proliferating hepatocytes, bile ducts, and malformed vessels of different caliber [49, 50]. Recently, a significantly higher prevalence of hemangiomas in patients with FNH was reported by Vilgrain et al. [51], perhaps because both neoplasms are vascular malformations. The differential diagnosis of FNH includes other hypervascular liver lesions, such as hepatocellular adenoma, HCC, and hypervascular metastases. Therefore, distinction between FNH and other hypervascular liver tumors is crucial to ensure proper therapy.

Multiphasic MDCT is an excellent imaging technique for the accurate diagnosis of FNH [50, 52]. On unenhanced CT, FNH is typically either hypoattenuating or isoattenuating to surrounding liver parenchyma. During the LAP, FNH becomes homogenously hyperattenuating with the exception of the central scar (Fig. 9a). This is felt to be the most reliable CT sign. During the portal venous and equilibrium phases, the neoplasm usually becomes isoattenuating relative to hepatic parenchyma (Fig. 9b). On EQP images, the central scar may demonstrate delayed washout. This characteristic dynamic enhancement pattern is mainly due to a prominent arterial supply of the tumor and its large draining veins. On the basis of this enhancement pattern, most authorities recommend multiphasic MDCT, including LAP and PVP images [50, 52].

Hepatocellular Adenoma
Hepatocellular adenoma is a rare benign neoplasm that is usually detected incidentally in women of childbearing age who have taken oral contraceptives for a long period. Other risk factors for hepatocellular adenoma include type 1 glycogen storage disease and, in men, the ingestion of anabolic steroids. Most hepatic adenomas are solitary; however, it is not unusual to detect two or three adenomas in one patient, particularly in patients with glycogen storage disease [53, 54]. The histological features of hepatocellular adenomas are sheets of proliferated hepatocytes surrounded by numerous dilated sinusoids with poor connective tissue support. The tumor tissue may contain a few Kupffer cells but usually lacks bile ducts. Deposition of lipid and glycogen in hepatic adenomas is not uncommon and may be valuable in diagnosing these neoplasms. Hepatocellular adenomas have a tendency to spontaneously hemorrhage, which can be fatal. Since these lesions may also undergo malig-

nant transformation to an HCC, they are considered surgical [53, 54].

Because of different therapeutic management, accurate differentiation of FNH and HCC is crucial. Unfortunately, the appearance on CT is variable and not specific. On unenhanced CT images, hepatocellular adenomas demonstrate either a hypoattenuating mass because of lipid and glycogen accumulation in the tumor or a hyperattenuating mass due to fresh hemorrhage (Fig. 10a). During the LAP, hepatocellular adenomas enhance rapidly and are hyperattenuating relative to the normal liver (Fig. 10b). Small lesions tend to demonstrate a more homogenous enhancement, whereas larger lesions tend to enhance heterogenously [53]. During portal-venous- and equilibrium-phase imaging, most adenomas are nearly isoattenuating compared with surrounding liver parenchyma (Fig. 10c). Due to the variable CT appearances of hepatocellular adenoma, a triphasic MDCT protocol, including unenhanced, LAP, and PVP images, has been recommended for detection and characterization [54, 55].

The Biliary System

Although MDCT is not generally considered to be a first-line imaging technique for patients with suspected biliary pathology, advances in MDCT scanners have resulted in an increased capability to detect and characterize various biliary diseases. The advantages of MDCT of the biliary tract are increased speed and reduction of acquisition time and respiratory motion artefacts. Furthermore, the thinner slices of MDCT result in reconstructed data sets with isotropic voxels for MPR and 3-D displays. Straight and curved MPR are especially valuable for visualization and evaluation of the biliary tree, which is typically oriented either perpendicular or tangential to the axial plane.

The intrahepatic bile ducts, which are linear structures accompanying the portal vein and hepatic arterial branches, can be best visualized during the PVP when there is an optimal attenuation difference between hypodense bile ducts and the adjacent enhanced vessels and parenchyma. Using thin collimation, normal intrahepatic bile ducts with a diameter of up to 2 mm can be visualized routinely, even out to the periphery of the liver. On unenhanced images, the diameter of the intrahepatic bile ducts must measure at least 2 mm to be distinguished from adjacent vascular structures and liver parenchyma. The low-attenuation extrahepatic bile ducts (common hepatic duct and common bile duct), which measure between 3 mm and 6 mm, are routinely visualized on thin-section MDCT images. Their thin walls (1 mm) usually enhance after administration of contrast media,

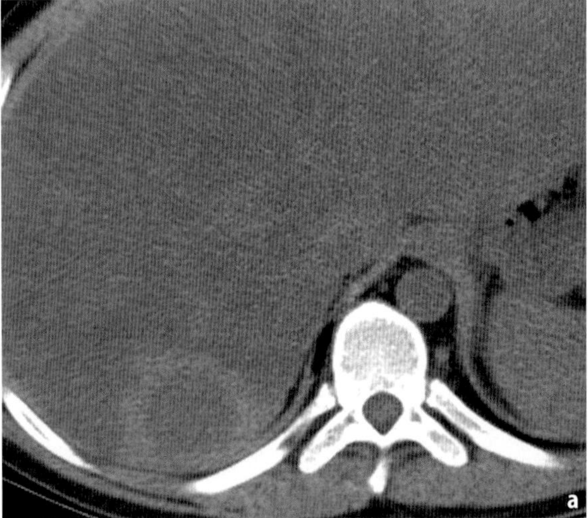

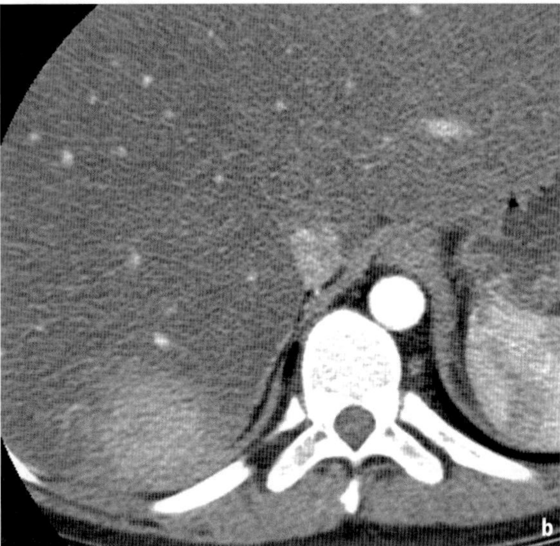

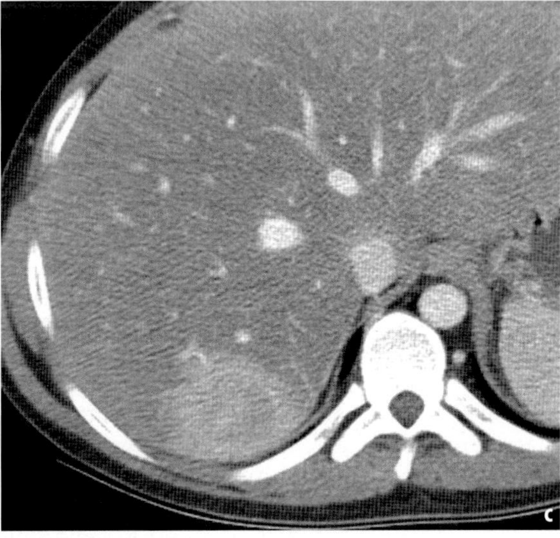

Fig. 10a-c. Hepatocellular adenoma in a patient with glycogen storage disease type 1A (von Gierke's disease) during the unenhanced state (**a**), late arterial phase (LAP) (**b**) and portal venous phase (PVP) (**c**). The liver is enlarged, and there is diffuse fatty infiltration. While this particular tumor has no internal hemorrhage, there is a thin fibrous capsule

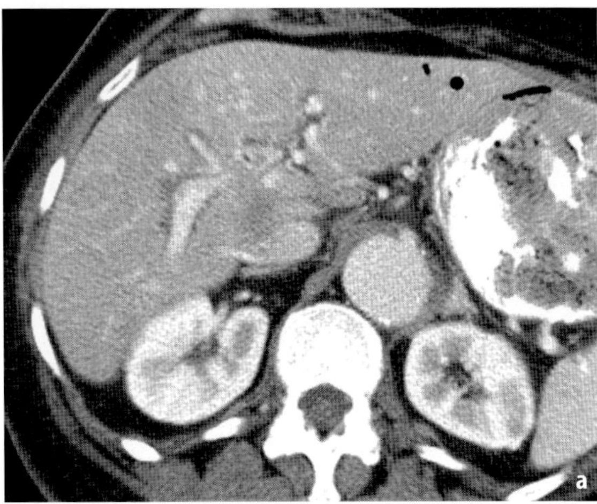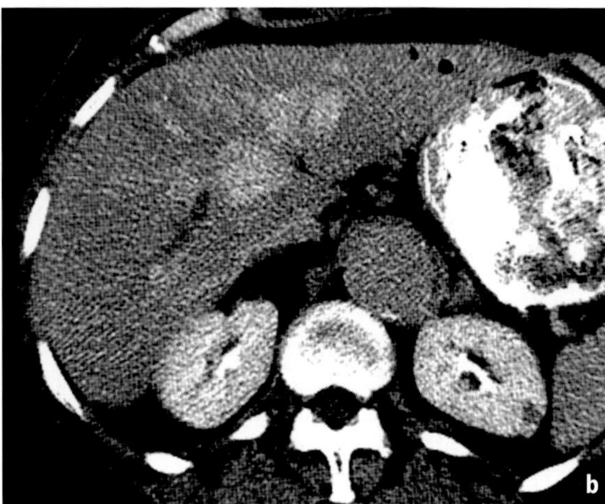

Fig. 11a, b. Hilar cholangiocarcinoma during portal venous phase (PVP) (**a**) and equilibrium phase (EQP) (**b**). Delayed washout in the tumor during the EQP is apparent and indicates a high fibrous content

which helps to differentiate them from the adjacent vessels. The normal gallbladder wall, which is 1- to 3-mm thick, also enhances postcontrast. The enhancement and thickness of the gallbladder wall may vary depending on luminal distension and on pathologic conditions (e.g., inflammation, tumor). There are several pathological situations in which density of bile in the gallbladder increases significantly. Examples include deposition of sludge and milk of calcium. The role of MDCT in the evaluation of different biliary pathologies and their characteristic imaging findings are discussed below.

Cholangiocarcinoma

Cholangiocarcinoma is the most common primary malignancy of the intra- and extrahepatic biliary tract. Patients usually present with painless jaundice due to biliary obstruction. The majority of cholangiocarcinomas, adenocarcinomas, are found in the extrahepatic ducts. A tumor originating at the confluence of the left and right hepatic duct is referred to as a Klatskin tumor. Predisposing factors for cholangiocarcinoma include ulcerative colitis, sclerosing cholangitis, and congenital biliary anomalies (choledochal cyst and Caroli's disease). MDCT imaging of cholangiocarcinoma is usually employed to evaluate the extent of the neoplasm and its resectability, since radical surgical tumor removal with negative histologic margins is the only curative option.

The CT appearance of cholangiocarcinoma varies depending on the site of origin – peripheral intrahepatic, hilar, or extrahepatic. Peripheral cholangiocarcinoma appears as either a well-defined or an irregular mass along the course of dilated intrahepatic ducts. On MDCT, during both the LAP and PVP, intrahepatic cholangiocarcinoma usually demonstrates as a hypoattenuating mass with incomplete peripheral enhancement (Fig. 11a) [56, 57]. The central portion of the tumor may show prolonged enhancement and be hyperattenuating on EQP images (10–15 min postinjection) due to slow washout of the contrast material by the abundant fibrous tissue in the tumor (Fig. 11b). Up to 36% of cholangiocarcinomas demonstrate hyperattenuation during the EQP [28]. A time delay of 10–20 min after contrast media administration is optimal for EQP images [28]. With infiltrating hilar cholangiocarcinoma – the most common type of hilar cholangiocarcinoma – contrast-enhanced CT images may detect focal duct wall thickening, which appears hyperattenuating relative to liver parenchyma during the PVP [58]. A supplementary CT finding of hilar cholangiocarcinomas includes lobar atrophy due to either severe, long-standing ductal obstruction or portal venous encasement and obstruction [59, 60]. Contrast-enhanced CT appearances of infiltrating extrahepatic cholangiocarcinoma are hyperenhancing thickened walls in the common bile duct or a small hyperattenuating intraluminal mass at the point of abrupt termination of bile duct dilatation. Unfortunately, all the above CT findings may also occur with benign diseases that cause bile duct strictures. The CT protocol for diagnosing suspected cholangiocarcinoma should contain at least two enhancement phases (PVP and EQP) acquired with thin collimation to obtain multiplanar reconstructions [61].

Primary Sclerosing Cholangitis

Primary sclerosing cholangitis (PSC) is a rare

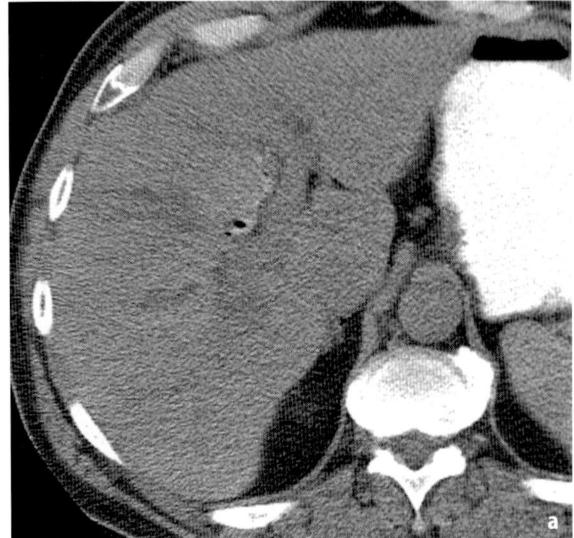

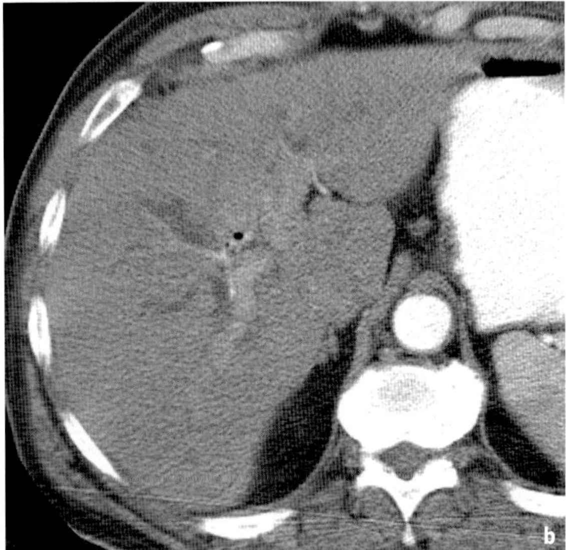

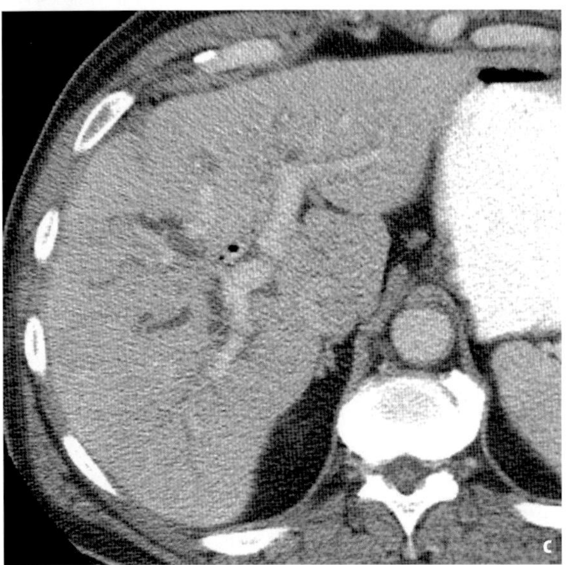

Fig. 12a-c. Early primary sclerosing cholangitis during the unenhanced state (**a**), LAP (**b**), PVP (**c**). Note the scattered intrahepatic ductal dilatation

chronic inflammatory condition of the intra- and extrahepatic bile ducts. It is associated with ulcerative colitis, Sjögren's syndrome, Riedel's thyroiditis, retroperitoneal fibrosis, and, occasionally, Crohn's disease. The etiology of PSC is unknown, although it is probably autoimmune. PSC occurs predominantly in men during the third to fifth decade of life. The typical presentation is intermittent jaundice and recurrent episodes of cholangitis.

CT findings in PSC usually reflect pathological changes, such as ductal and periductal fibrosis, that result in segmental stricturing and dilatation of the bile ducts. In the majority of cases, both the intra- and extrahepatic bile ducts are involved. Long-standing biliary obstruction may lead to cirrhosis. Morphological changes of PSC-induced cirrhosis include fibrosis, regenerative nodules, parenchymal atrophy, and marked hypertrophy of the caudate lobe.

MDCT in patients with PSC may demonstrate closely alternating dilatation and strictures of the intrahepatic bile ducts, thereby giving them a beaded appearance (Fig. 12a-c). Other characteristic CT findings of PSC include skip dilatation, a solitary dilatation of a peripheral duct, and pruning of the bile ducts representing dilated segmental duct without any dilatation of the side branches. According to Teefey et al. [62], none of these CT findings are specific to PSC except skip dilatations.

Since ERCP and biopsy are still the gold standard for diagnosing PCS, MDCT plays a central role in the evaluation of the extent of cirrhosis, portal hypertension, and cholangiocarcinoma and their complications. In a study by MacCarty et al. [63], 13% of 104 patients with PCS developed a cholangiocarcinoma, proven either by biopsy or autopsy. In a more recent investigation, Campbell et al. [64] demonstrated that CT provides higher sensitivity than cholangiography in detecting cholangiocarcinoma complicated by PCS.

Acute and Chronic Cholecystitis

Acute cholecystitis is mainly caused by an impacted stone in the cystic duct, resulting in bile stasis and gallbladder distension. Ultrasound is the diagnostic method of choice for the initial workup of suspected gallbladder pathologies. Since the clinical symptoms of acute cholecystitis are usually nonspecific, MDCT often serves as the initial imaging modality for evaluation of the acute abdomen. MDCT is also the preferred technique for diagnosing acute cholecystitis complications. The most common features on CT in acute cholecystitis include gallstones, thickening of the gallbladder wall (>3 mm), gallbladder distension or hydrops (>5 cm), hyperattenuating bile, and pericholecystic fluid and stranding (Fig. 13) [65]. Fur-

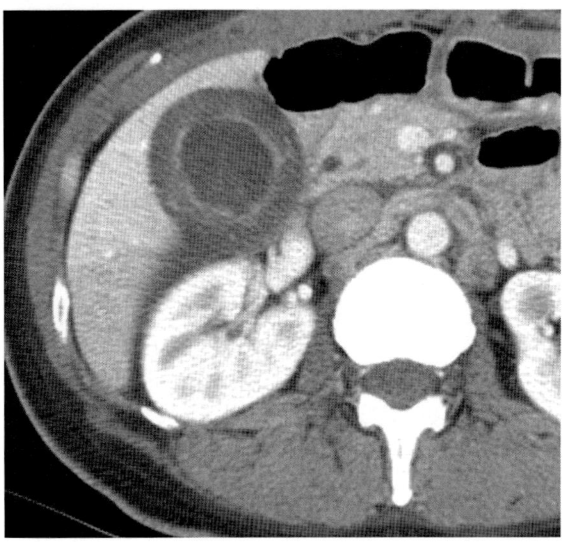

Fig. 13. Multidetector computed tomography (MDCT) image of the gallbladder in a patient with acute cholecystitis. Note the hyperenhancement of adjacent liver parenchyma

thermore, contrast-enhanced MDCT may reveal increased enhancement of the gallbladder wall, though this is a nonspecific finding. Yamashita et al. reported hyperenhancement in liver parenchyma adjacent to the gallbladder, likely due to hyperemia and to early venous drainage (Fig. 13) [66]. Common complications of acute cholecystitis include emphysematous cholecystitis, gangrene, and perforation of the gallbladder. In emphysematous cholecystitis, which occurs more commonly in elderly and diabetic patients, intramural gas secondary to gas-producing bacteria such as *Clostridium perfringens* can be detected on CT. No intravenous contrast material is required for a CT scan, which is the most accurate imaging technique to depict gas within the gallbladder wall [67].

Chronic cholecystitis may demonstrate many of the same findings on CT as acute cholecystitis. However, patients with chronic cholecystitis do not tend to have significant pericholecystic inflammation or fluid. The most common findings include calculi and mild to moderate thickening of the gallbladder wall. Since gallbladder carcinoma may show radiological features similar to chronic cholecystitis, to ensure adequate therapeutic management, it is important to differentiate between neoplasia and a chronic inflammatory process. Yun et al. [68] evaluated enhancement of the gallbladder wall during arterial and PVP CT images in patients with chronic cholecystitis and gallbladder carcinoma. With inflammation, the inner layer of the gallbladder wall was isoattenuating during the arterial phase and PVP. With neoplasia, the inner

layer of the gallbladder wall was hyperattenuating during both phases. Furthermore, the gallbladder wall tends to be thicker and more irregular in patients with carcinoma.

Gallbladder Carcinoma
Gallbladder carcinoma is the most common biliary tract neoplasm, being the fifth most common malignancy of the gastrointestinal (GI) tract, and it occurs predominantly in elderly women. Adenocarcinoma is the main histological type, accounting for up to 90% of cases. Predisposing factors for gallbladder carcinoma include chronic cholecystitis, inflammatory bowel disease, familial adenomatous polyposis, and porcelain gallbladder. The reported incidence of gallbladder carcinoma found in patients with calcified or porcelain gallbladders ranges from 12% to 61% [69]. However, a more recent study demonstrated a lower incidence of 5%, and another group found no association between gallbladder carcinoma and porcelain gallbladder [69, 70]. Both clinical symptoms and CT appearances of gallbladder carcinoma are nonspecific, and as a result, most tumors are detected at an unresectable stage.

There are three different morphological types of gallbladder carcinoma: (1) a mass replacing the gallbladder, (2) an intraluminal mass, and (3) thickening of the gallbladder wall [71]. The mass in the gallbladder bed, the most common type, appears on unenhanced scans as a nodular hypoattenuating mass, which often infiltrates adjacent liver parenchyma (Fig. 14a). After administration of intravenous contrast material, the tumor demonstrates variable but heterogeneous enhancement (Figs. 14b, c). The soft tissue mass may also show enclosed gallstones and central necrosis. The intraluminal mass type, which is less invasive, usually presents as a polypoid mass, which must be differentiated from a benign polyp. Polyp size is an indicator of malignancy, since benign lesions are usually smaller than 1 cm [72]. CT diagnosis of the least common type of gallbladder carcinoma, thickening of the gallbladder wall, is challenging due to this carcinoma's similar CT appearance to cholecystitis [73]. Additional CT findings of gallbladder carcinoma include biliary obstruction, direct invasion into adjacent liver parenchyma, liver metastases, lymphadenopathy, and peritoneal carcinomatosis.

Several investigators have recently demonstrated that CT is a very useful tool in preoperative evaluation of the resectability of gallbladder carcinoma [74, 75]. The accuracy for staging ranges from 83% to 93%. Detection of gallbladder carcinoma in the early stage, however, remains a challenge [74, 75].

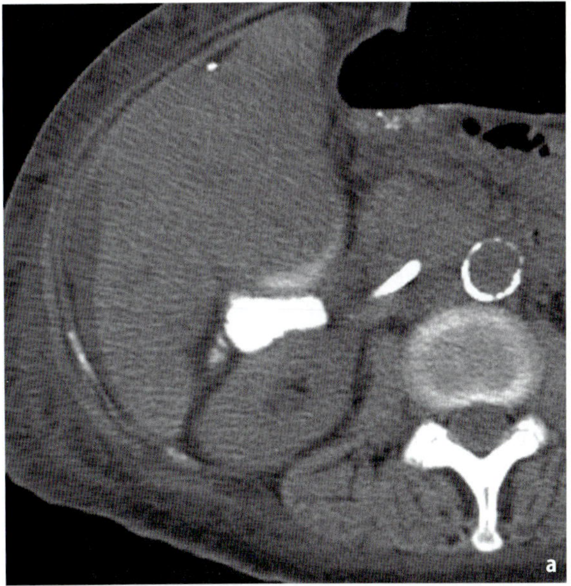
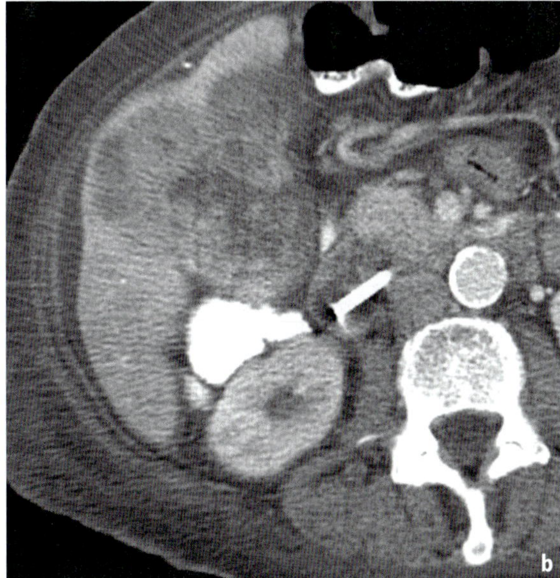
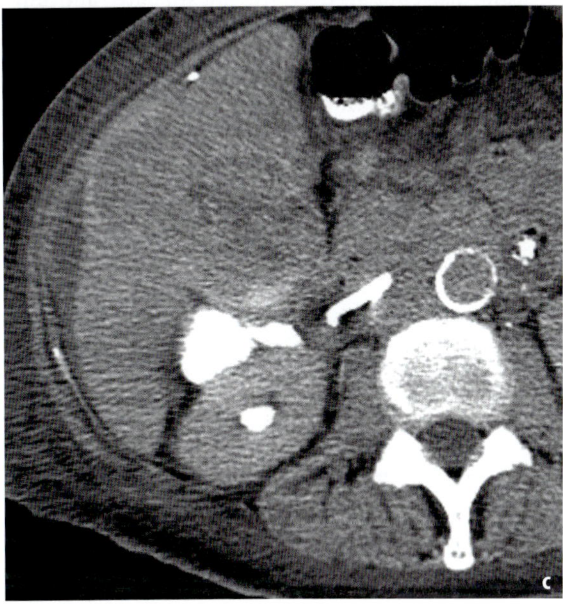

Fig. 14a-c. Gallbladder carcinoma during unenhanced state (**a**), portal venous phase (PVP) (**b**), and equilibrium phase (EQP) (**c**). Note that the tumor has invaded adjacent liver parenchyma, seen best during the PVP

References

1. Schwartz LH, Gandras EJ, Colangelo SM et al (1999) Prevalence and importance of small hepatic lesions found at CT in patients with cancer. Radiology 210:71–74
2. Paulson EK, Harris JP, Jaffe TA et al (2005) Acute appendicitis: added diagnostic value of coronal reformations from isotropic voxels at multi-detector row CT. Radiology 235:879–885
3. Caoili EM, Paulson EK (2000) CT of small-bowel obstruction: another perspective using multiplanar reformations. AJR Am J Roentgenol 174:993–998
4. Kawata S, Murakami T, Kim T et al (2002) Multidetector CT: diagnostic impact of slice thickness on detection of hypervascular hepatocellular carcinoma. AJR Am J Roentgenol 179:61–66
5. Abdelmoumene A, Chevallier P, Chalaron M et al (2005) Detection of liver metastases under 2 cm: comparison of different acquisition protocols in four row multidetector-CT (MDCT). Eur Radiol 15:1881–1887
6. Weg N, Scheer MR, Gabor MP (1998) Liver lesions: improved detection with dual-detector-array CT and routine 2.5-mm thin collimation. Radiology 209:417–426
7. Haider MA, Amitai MM, Rappaport DC et al (2002) Multi-detector row helical CT in preoperative assessment of small (< or = 1.5 cm) liver metastases: is thinner collimation better? Radiology 225:137–142
8. Hong C, Bruening R, Schoepf UJ et al (2003) Multiplanar reformat display technique in abdominal multidetector row CT imaging. Clin Imaging 27:119–123

9. Jaffe TA, Nelson RC, Johnson GA et al (2006) Optimization of multiplanar reformations from isotropic datasets acquired on a 16-element multidetector helical CT scanner. Radiology (*in press*)
10. Stabile Ianora AA, Memeo M, Scardapane A et al (2003) Oral contrast-enhanced three-dimensional helical-CT cholangiography: clinical applications. Eur Radiol 13:867–873
11. Wang ZJ, Yeh BM, Roberts JP et al (2005) Living donor candidates for right hepatic lobe transplantation: evaluation at CT cholangiography – initial experience. Radiology 235:899–904
12. Caoili EM, Paulson EK, Heyneman LE et al (2000) Helical CT cholangiography with three-dimensional volume rendering using an oral biliary contrast agent: feasibility of a novel technique. AJR Am J Roentgenol 174:487–492
13. Zandrino F, Benzi L, Ferretti ML et al (2002) Multislice CT cholangiography without biliary contrast agent: technique and initial clinical results in the assessment of patients with biliary obstruction. Eur Radiol 12:1155–1161
14. Kim HC, Park SJ, Park SI et al (2005) Multislice CT cholangiography using thin-slab minimum intensity projection and multiplanar reformation in the evaluation of patients with suspected biliary obstruction: preliminary experience. Clin Imaging 29:46–54
15. Rao ND, Gulati MS, Paul SB et al (2005) Three-dimensional helical computed tomography cholangiography with minimum intensity projection in gallbladder carcinoma patients with obstructive jaundice: comparison with magnetic resonance cholangiography and percutaneous transhepatic cholangiography. J Gastroenterol Hepatol 20:304–308
16. Brink JA, Heiken JP, Forman HP et al (1995) Hepatic spiral CT: reduction of dose of intravenous contrast material. Radiology 197:83–88
17. Heiken JP, Brink JA, McClennan BL et al (1995) Dynamic incremental CT: effect of volume and concentration of contrast material and patient weight on hepatic enhancement. Radiology 195:353–357
18. Yamashita Y, Komohara Y, Takahashi M et al (2000) Abdominal helical CT: evaluation of optimal doses of intravenous contrast material – a prospective randomized study. Radiology 216:718–723
19. Ho LM, Nelson RC, Thomas J et al (2004) Abdominal aortic aneurysms at multi-detector row helical CT: optimization with interactive determination of scanning delay and contrast medium dose. Radiology 232:854–859
20. Itoh S, Ikeda M, Achiwa M et al (2005) Multiphase contrast-enhanced CT of the liver with a multislice CT scanner: effects of iodine concentration and delivery rate. Radiat Med 23:61–69
21. Awai K, Takada K, Onishi H, Hori S (2002) Aortic and hepatic enhancement and tumor-to-liver contrast: analysis of the effect of different concentrations of contrast material at multi-detector row helical CT. Radiology 224:757–763
22. Schoellnast H, Tillich M, Deutschmann HA et al (2004) Improvement of parenchymal and vascular enhancement using saline flush and power injection for multiple-detector-row abdominal CT. Eur Radiol 14:659–664
23. Schoellnast H, Tillich M, Deutschmann HA et al (2003) Abdominal multidetector row computed tomography: reduction of cost and contrast material dose using saline flush. J Comput Assist Tomogr 27:847–853
24. Chopra S, Chintapalli KN, Ramakrishna K et al (2000) Helical CT cholangiography with oral cholecystographic contrast material. Radiology 214:596–601
25. Ott DJ, Gelfand DW (1981) Complications of gastrointestinal radiologic procedures: II. Complications related to biliary tract studies. Gastrointest Radiol 6:47–56
26. Foley WD, Mallisee TA, Hohenwalter MD et al (2000) Multiphase hepatic CT with a multirow detector CT scanner. AJR Am J Roentgenol 175:679–685
27. Laghi A, Iannaccone R, Rossi P et al (2003) Hepatocellular carcinoma: detection with triple-phase multi-detector row helical CT in patients with chronic hepatitis. Radiology 226:543–549
28. Keogan MT, Seabourn JT, Paulson EK et al (1997) Contrast-enhanced CT of intrahepatic and hilar cholangiocarcinoma: delay time for optimal imaging. AJR Am J Roentgenol 169:1493–1499
29. Soyer P, Poccard M, Boudiaf M et al (2004) Detection of hypovascular hepatic metastases at triple-phase helical CT: sensitivity of phases and comparison with surgical and histopathologic findings. Radiology 231:413–420
30. Miller FH, Butler RS, Hoff FL et al (1998) Using triphasic helical CT to detect focal hepatic lesions in patients with neoplasms. AJR Am J Roentgenol 171:643–649
31. Ch'en IY, Katz DS, Jeffrey RB Jr et al (1997) Do arterial phase helical CT images improve detection or characterization of colorectal liver metastases? J Comput Assist Tomogr 21:391–397
32. Nino-Murcia M, Olcott EW, Jeffrey RB Jr et al (2000) Focal liver lesions: pattern-based classification scheme for enhancement at arterial phase CT. Radiology 215:746–751
33. Valls C, Andia E, Sanchez A et al (2001) Hepatic metastases from colorectal cancer: preoperative detection and assessment of resectability with helical CT. Radiology 218:55–60
34. Blake SP, Weisinger K, Atkins MB, Raptopoulos V (1999) Liver metastases from melanoma: detection with multiphasic contrast-enhanced CT. Radiology 213:92–96
35. Furuta A, Ito K, Fujita T et al (2004) Hepatic enhancement in multiphasic contrast-enhanced MDCT: comparison of high- and low-iodine-concentration contrast medium in same patients with chronic liver disease. AJR Am J Roentgenol 183:157–162
36. Oliver JH 3rd, Baron RL, Federle MP et al (1997) Hypervascular liver metastases: do unenhanced and hepatic arterial phase CT images affect tumor detection? Radiology 205:709–715
37. Figueras J, Jaurrieta E, Valls C et al (2000) Resection or transplantation for hepatocellular carcinoma in cirrhotic patients: outcomes based on indicated treatment strategy. J Am Coll Surg 190:580–587
38. Island ER, Pomposelli J, Pomfret EA (2005) Twenty-year experience with liver transplantation for hepatocellular carcinoma. Arch Surg 140:353–358

39. Kutami R, Nakashima Y, Nakashima O (2000) Pathomorphologic study on the mechanism of fatty change in small hepatocellular carcinoma of humans. J Hepatol 33:282–289

40. Peterson MS, Baron RL, Marsh JW Jr (2000) Pretransplantation surveillance for possible hepatocellular carcinoma in patients with cirrhosis: epidemiology and CT-based tumor detection rate in 430 cases with surgical pathologic correlation. Radiology 217:743–749

41. Valls C, Cos M, Figueras J et al (2004) Pretransplantation diagnosis and staging of hepatocellular carcinoma in patients with cirrhosis: value of dual-phase helical CT. AJR Am J Roentgenol 182:1011–1017

42. Kim SK, Lim JH, Lee WJ et al (2002) Detection of hepatocellular carcinoma: comparison of dynamic three-phase computed tomography images and four-phase computed tomography images using multidetector row helical computed tomography. J Comput Assist Tomogr 26:691–698

43. Iannaccone R, Laghi A, Catalano C et al (2005) Hepatocellular carcinoma: role of unenhanced and delayed phase multi-detector row helical CT in patients with cirrhosis. Radiology 234:460–467

44. Sultana S, Morishita S, Awai K et al (2003) Evaluation of hypervascular hepatocellular carcinoma in cirrhotic liver by means of helical CT: comparison of different contrast medium concentrations within the same patient. Radiat Med 21:239–245

45. Marchiano A, Spreafico C, Lanocita R et al (2005) Does iodine concentration affect the diagnostic efficacy of biphasic spiral CT in patients with hepatocellular carcinoma? Abdom Imaging 30:274–280

46. Kim T, Murakami T, Takahashi S et al (1998) Effects of injection rates of contrast material on arterial phase hepatic CT. AJR Am J Roentgenol 171:429–432

47. Oliver JH, Baron RL (1999) High flow injection rates versus low flow injection rates: does increasing the injection rate result in greater detection of enhancement of hepatocellular carcinoma during hepatic arterial phase CT? 213:92–96

48. Mathieu D, Kobeiter H, Maison P et al (2000) Oral contraceptive use and focal nodular hyperplasia of the liver. Gastroenterology 118:560–564

49. Hussain SM, Terkivatan T, Zondervan PE et al (2004) Focal nodular hyperplasia: findings at state-of-the-art MR imaging, US, CT, and pathologic analysis. Radiographics 24:3–19

50. Brancatelli G, Federle MP, Grazioli L (2001) Focal nodular hyperplasia: CT findings with emphasis on multiphasic helical CT in 78 patients. Radiology 219:61–68

51. Vilgrain V, Uzan F, Brancatelli G (2003) Prevalence of hepatic hemangioma in patients with focal nodular hyperplasia: MR imaging analysis. Radiology 229:75–79

52. Carlson SK, Johnson CD, Bender CE, Welch TJ (2000) CT of focal nodular hyperplasia of the liver. AJR Am J Roentgenol 174:705–712

53. Grazioli L, Federle MP, Brancatelli G et al (2001) Hepatic adenomas: imaging and pathologic findings. Radiographics 21:877–892

54. Ichikawa T, Federle MP, Grazioli L, Nalesnik M (2000) Hepatocellular adenoma: multiphasic CT and histopathologic findings in 25 patients. Radiology 214:861–868

55. Ruppert-Kohlmayr AJ, Uggowitzer MM, Kugler C et al (2001) Focal nodular hyperplasia and hepatocellular adenoma of the liver: differentiation with multiphasic helical CT. AJR Am J Roentgenol 176:1493–1498

56. Kim TK, Choi BI, Han JK et al (1997) Peripheral cholangiocarcinoma of the liver: two-phase spiral CT findings. Radiology 204:539–543

57. Valls C, Guma A, Puig I et al (2000) Intrahepatic peripheral cholangiocarcinoma: CT evaluation. Abdom Imaging 25:490–496

58. Han JK, Choi BI, Kim AY et al (2002) Cholangiocarcinoma: pictorial essay of CT and cholangiographic findings. Radiographics 22:173–187

59. Vazquez JL, Thorsen MK, Dodds WJ et al (1985) Atrophy of the left hepatic lobe caused by a cholangiocarcinoma. AJR Am J Roentgenol 144:547–548

60. Jarnagin WR, Fong Y, DeMatteo RP et al (2001) Staging, resectability, and outcome in 225 patients with hilar cholangiocarcinoma. Ann Surg 234:507–517

61. Zech CJ, Schoenberg SO, Reiser M, Helmberger T (2004) Cross-sectional imaging of biliary tumors: current clinical status and future developments. Eur Radiol 14:1174–1187

62. Teefey SA, Baron RL, Schulte SJ et al (1992) Patterns of intrahepatic bile duct dilatation at CT: correlation with obstructive disease processes. Radiology 182:139–142

63. MacCarty RL, LaRusso NF, May GR et al (1985) Cholangiocarcinoma complicating primary sclerosing cholangitis: cholangiographic appearances. Radiology 156:43–46

64. Campbell WL, Peterson MS, Federle MP et al (2001) Using CT and cholangiography to diagnose biliary tract carcinoma complicating primary sclerosing cholangitis. AJR Am J Roentgenol 177:1095–1100

65. Grand D, Horton KM, Fishman EK (2004) CT of the gallbladder: spectrum of disease. AJR Am J Roentgenol 183:163–170

66. Yamashita K, Jin MJ, Hirose Y et al (1995) CT finding of transient focal increased attenuation of the liver adjacent to the gallbladder in acute cholecystitis. AJR Am J Roentgenol 164:343–346

67. Grayson DE, Abbott RM, Levy AD, Sherman PM (2002) Emphysematous infections of the abdomen and pelvis: a pictorial review. Radiographics 22:543–561

68. Yun EJ, Cho SG, Park S et al (2004) Gallbladder carcinoma and chronic cholecystitis: differentiation with two-phase spiral CT. Abdom Imaging 29:102–108

69. Stephen AE, Berger DL (2001) Carcinoma in the porcelain gallbladder: a relationship revisited. Surgery 129:699–703

70. Towfigh S, McFadden DW, Cortina GR et al (2001) Porcelain gallbladder is not associated with gallbladder carcinoma. Am Surg 67:7–10

71. Itai Y, Araki T, Yoshikawa K et al (1980) Computed tomography of gallbladder carcinoma. Radiology 137:713–718

72. Koga A, Watanabe K, Fukuyama T et al (1988) Diagnosis and operative indications for polypoid lesions of the gallbladder. Arch Surg 123:26–29

73. Kim BS, Ha HK, Lee IJ et al (2002) Accuracy of CT in

local staging of gallbladder carcinoma. Acta Radiol 43:71–76

74. Kumaran V, Gulati S, Paul B et al (2002) The role of dual-phase helical CT in assessing resectability of carcinoma of the gallbladder. Eur Radiol 12:1993–1999

75. Yoshimitsu K, Honda H, Shinozaki K et al (2002) Helical CT of the local spread of carcinoma of the gallbladder: evaluation according to the TNM system in patients who underwent surgical resection. AJR Am J Roentgenol 179:423–428

11

Soft Organ MDCT Imaging: Pancreas and Spleen

Dushyant V. Sahani, Zarine K. Shah

Introduction

Imaging is now integral for diagnosing pancreatic disease and neoplasms. The use of multidetector computed tomography (MDCT) scanners has dramatically reduced scan acquisition time, with resultant improvement in patient compliance and image quality. Fast scanning time enables the acquisition of multiple phases of enhancement, which is of paramount importance in imaging the pancreas. The improved Z-axis resolution permits excellent image reconstructions, which play a critical role in diagnosis and staging of pancreatic neoplasms due to the anatomic layout of the pancreas and its vasculature. The cross-sectional imaging of splenic pathology has also improved due to the improvement in MDCT technology. MDCT can rapidly image the spleen and is valuable in the diagnosis of a variety of congenital, neoplastic, inflammatory, and traumatic lesions of the spleen.

Concepts in Pancreatic Imaging

Detection of lesions within the pancreas on CT depends largely on the enhancement pattern of the lesion and the alteration in contour of the normal pancreas. Before initiation of contrast-enhanced MDCT of the pancreas, administration of negative oral contrast medium is performed to distend the stomach and duodenum, which facilitates detection of abnormalities in the pancreatic bed. The use of negative oral contrast medium has an added advantage in that it does not mask radiopaque stones in the common bile duct, and it may aid in the evaluation of gastric and duodenal wall lesions [1].

Enhancement of the pancreatic parenchyma and lesions is influenced by volume, iodine concentration, and injection rate of the contrast medium. Contrast-enhanced imaging of the pancreas can be performed in three distinct phases [2]. The early arterial phase, which is seen at approximately 20 s after contrast administration, demonstrates contrast uptake preferentially within the arterial tree with almost no enhancement of the pancreatic parenchyma. The next phase is the delayed arterial phase or the pancreatic phase, which is acquired at about 35–40 s following contrast administration. In this phase, there is optimal enhancement of the pancreatic parenchyma and excellent delineation of the arterial vascular system [2]. The third phase is the portal venous phase, which is usually acquired at 65–70 s after contrast administration. This phase offers the highest contrast uptake by the portal venous vessels, with good enhancement of the liver parenchyma. The exact timing of scan delay is variable based on the individual patient and can be optimized using bolus tracking techniques, where the initiation of the scan is based on the time when arterial enhancement peaks to a predetermined Hounsfield unit (HU) value. The Smart Prep technique used at our institute involves placing the region of interest (ROI) in the aorta just above the level of the pancreas and setting an HU value between 120 and 130 as the trigger. Scanning for the pancreatic phase starts 15 s after this threshold is reached.

Rationale for High-Concentration Contrast Media

An important determinant of image quality is contrast medium dynamics. The use of intravenous iodinated contrast media is routine with MDCT, and the dose and rate of contrast injection must be adapted to the higher scanning speeds of multidetector systems. The recommended maximum amount of iodine is 35–45 g, which should not change based on the concentration of the contrast medium used [3].

Higher concentrations of contrast in the ROI can be achieved by either an increase in injection rate or increase in the iodine concentration of the contrast medium. Since the contrast injection rate is limited by IV access and vessel diameter, the concentration of iodine (total iodine dose being kept constant) becomes an important factor. For a description of contrast enhancement of organs, a computer-generated, two-compartment model was used [4]. According to this model, organ enhancement is a result of enhancement of intravascular and extracellular–extravascular spaces. Contrast enhancement of the extracellular–extravascular space depends on the concentration gradient between intravascular and extracellular–extravascular spaces, the volume of the extracellular–extravascular space, the permeability of organ microvasculature and cellular interfaces, and surface area and time. A high concentration gradient between intravascular and extracellular–extravascular spaces allows a high influx of contrast material into the extracellular–extravascular space and contributes to high organ enhancement.

In a study by Fenchel et al. [5], the use of 400 mgI/ml of contrast medium concentration (Iomeprol 400) led to a significantly higher arterial and portal venous phase enhancement as compared with 300 mgI/ml concentration, the rate of contrast injection and the total dose of iodine being kept constant. It is likely that the use of high concentrations of contrast medium would improve conspicuity of hypovascular and hypervascular lesions in the pancreas.

Scanning Technique

A noncontrast CT of the upper abdomen is performed using 10-mm slice collimation to cover the pancreas. Depending on the scanner type, a pancreatic phase is performed using 1- to 2-mm slice collimation. Acquisition of the pancreatic phase is usually at a delay of 35–40 s following a bolus of 125–150 cc of iodinated contrast medium injected at a rate of 4–5ml/s. The scanned area extends from the diaphragm to below the transverse duodenum in a single breath hold [6]. A weight-based approach to IV contrast medium administration is now considered more appropriate in order to optimize the iodine dose for a study. An iodine dose of 550 mg/kg body weight can be used for both pancreatic and vascular enhancement that translates into 1.8–2.0 cc/kg body weight.

For the next phase, the patient is instructed to breathe deeply following the pancreatic phase acquisition, and a second spiral acquisition is performed at a 70–80 s scan delay. This is the portal venous phase, which covers the entire upper abdomen using 2.5- to 5-mm slice collimation, depending on the patient's body habitus (Table 1). This phase is critical for the detection of small hypodense liver metastases and in the diagnosis of venous encasement by a tumor. Early arterial phase scans can be performed if a CT angiogram is desired.

Dual-Phase Imaging for the Pancreas

Dual-phase MDCT of the pancreas is typically undertaken in the late arterial (pancreatic) phase and the portal venous phase and is considered optimal for assessment of pancreatic adenocarcinoma [2]. The gland enhances avidly during the pancreatic phase, thus, most pancreatic adenocarcinomas appear as low-density lesions compared with the normal enhancing pancreatic parenchyma, making tumor conspicuity maximal during this phase [7, 8] (Figs. 1a, b and 2a, b) The pancreatic phase also facilitates visualization of major arterial structures and permits staging the tumor and determining resectability based on vascular involvement (Fig. 3a, b). The criteria of unresectability of pancreatic adenocarcinoma now includes extrapancreatic invasion of major vessels (defined as

Table 1. Multidetector computed tomography (MDCT) parameters for the pancreas: Protocols for GE Scanners at our institute

Parameters	4 channel	16 channel	64 channel
DC (mm)	1.25	0.625	0.6
TS (mm/s)	15	18.75	38
		Beam Pitch 1.0–2.0	
Slice thickness (mm)			
Arterial (CTA)	1.25	1.0	1.0
Arterial (liver)	2.5–5.0	2.5	2.5
Venous (CTA)	2.5	2.0	2.0
Venous (liver)	5.0	5.0	5.0
		Delay arterial bolus tracking empirical delay 25–30 s	
Venous delay (s)	65–70	65–70	65–70

DC detector collimation, *TS* table speed, *CTA* computed tomographic arteriography

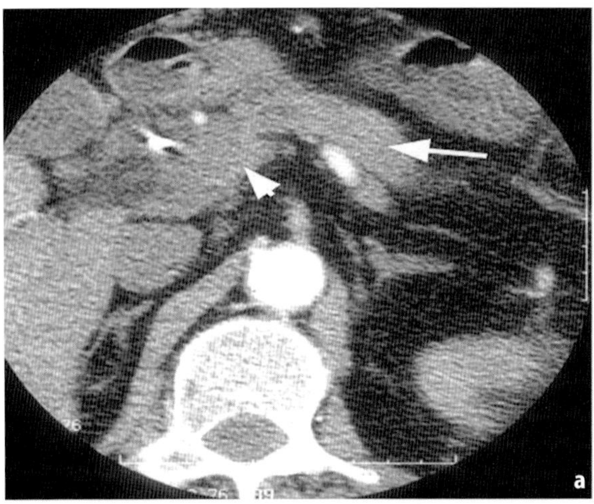
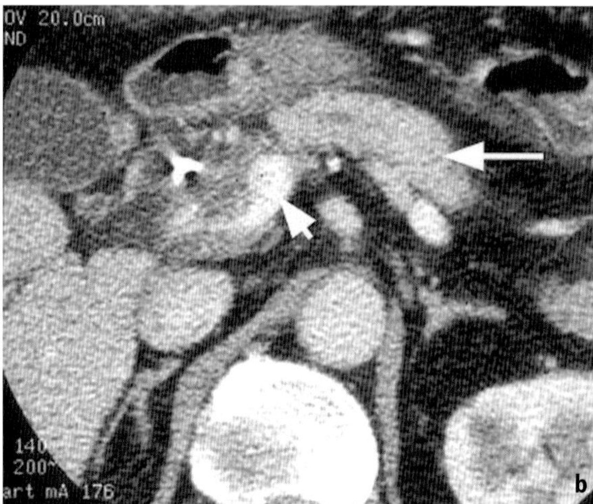

Fig. 1a, b. Importance of optimal phase imaging: **a** Early arterial phase axial multidetector computed tomography (MDCT) image in a patient with adenocarcinoma of the pancreatic head. Suboptimal enhancement of the normal pancreas (*long white arrow*) and portal vein (*short white arrow*). **b** Pancreatic phase helical computed tomography (CT) in the same patient, demonstrating optimized parenchymal (*long white arrow*) and vascular enhancement. Furthermore, the tumor is clearly identified and encases the portal vein (*short white arrow*)

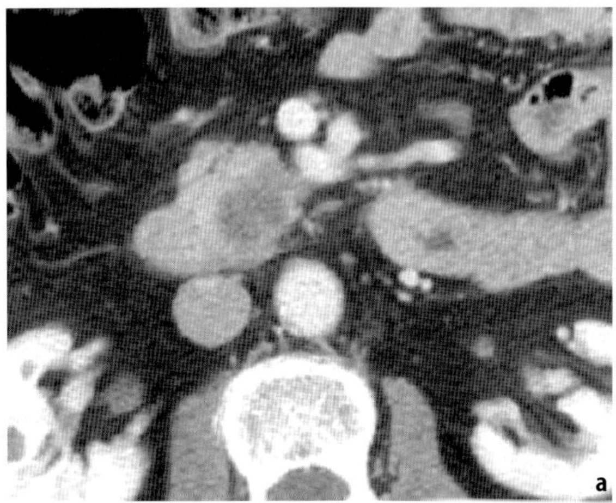
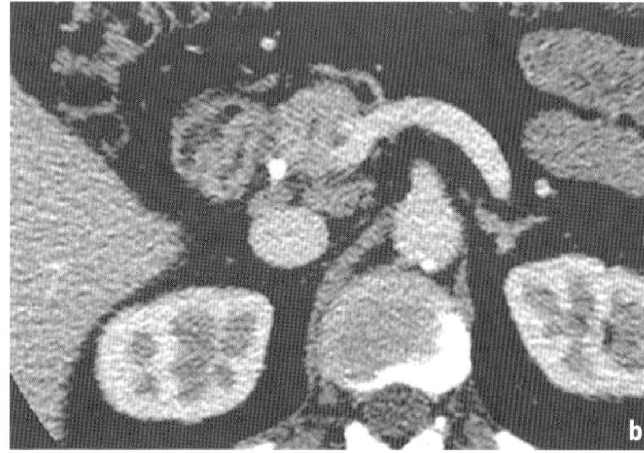

Fig. 2a, b. Importance of optimal "pancreatic phase" imaging: **a** Image acquired in the pancreatic phase clearly reveals the relatively hypodense mass in the pancreatic head. **b** Axial multidetector computed tomography (MDCT) image in a different patient taken later than the pancreatic phase shows a soft tissue invading into the superior mesenteric vein (SMV); however, the mass is not conspicuous on this phase due to equal enhancement of the mass and the normal pancreatic parenchyma

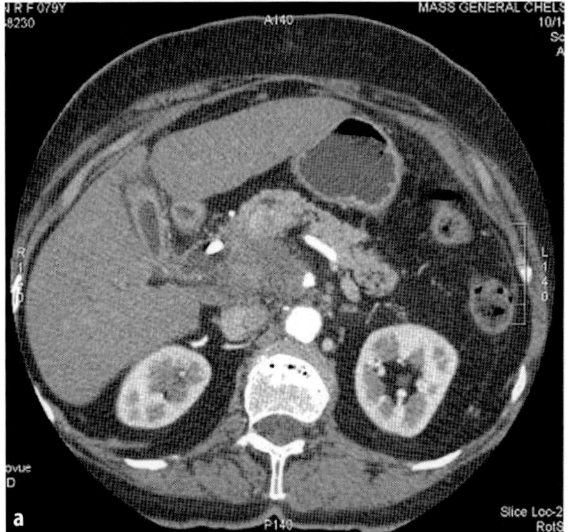
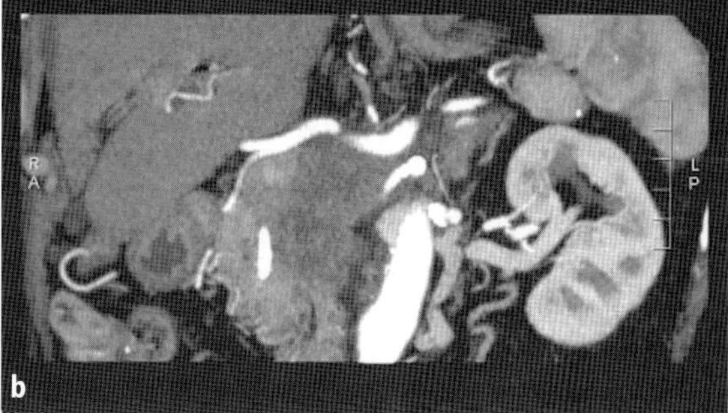

Fig. 3a, b. Axial contrast-enhanced 16-channel multidetector computed tomography (MDCT) image in a 79-year-old woman demonstrates an infiltrating mass involving the head and uncinate process of the pancreas, which encases the origin of the celiac axis, superior mesenteric artery (SMA), and invades into the inferior vena cava (IVC). **a** Coronal reformatted image in the same patient gives a better idea of the true extent of the tumor in the vertical dimension **b**

Table 2. Comparative results for detection and resectability of pancreatic adenocarcinoma

Image mode	Sensitivity	Specificity	Accuracy
Single-slice CT	81–89%	81–89%	69–87%
	Nishiharu T et al. [11]	Nishiharu T et al. [11]	Trede M et al. [12]
MDCT	96%	77%	85–90%
	Ellsmere J [13]	Grenacher L [14]	Kulig J et al. [15]
EUS	89–100%	100%	69–87%
	DeWitt J et al. [16]	Wiersema MJ [17]	Trede M et al. [12]

CT computed tomography, *MDCT* multi-detector computed tomography, *EUS* endovascular ultrasound

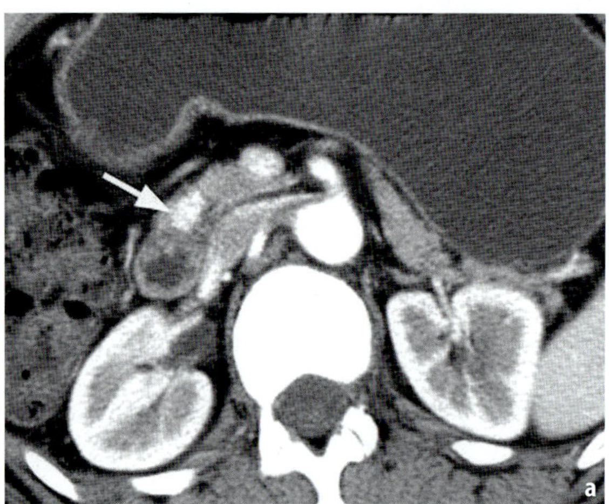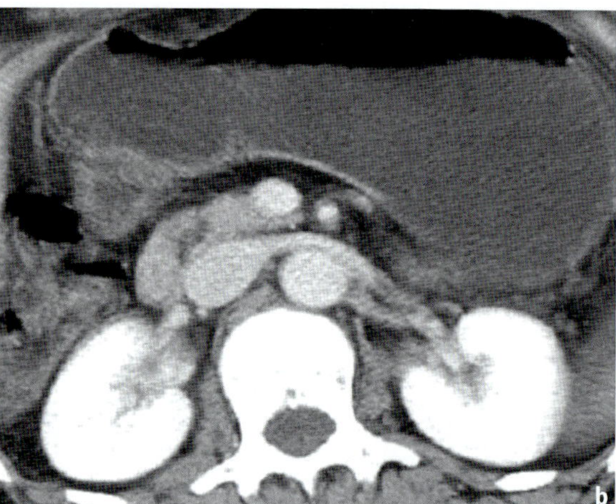

Fig. 4a, b. Pancreatic arterial phase helical computed tomography (CT) demonstrating a hypervascular tumor (*white arrow*) in the head of the pancreas. **a** Portal venous phase image reveals a hypodensity in the region of the tumor. It is imperative to perform an arterial phase CT in a patient with suspected endocrine tumor to allow adequate characterization of the mass, which is well demonstrated in this case (**b**)

tumor-to-vessel contiguity >50%) such as celiac artery, hepatic artery, portal vein, superior mesenteric artery or superior mesenteric vein, or massive venous invasion with thrombosis (Fig. 3a, b). Likewise, the presence of distant metastasis to the liver, regional lymph nodes, or omentum is a contraindication for surgical resection. However, partial venous invasion (tumor-to-vessel contiguity <50%) without thrombosis or obliteration of the venous lumen can still be classified as resectable adenocarcinoma [9, 10]. (Table 2).

Functioning or hormone-producing neuroendocrine tumors are typically hypervascular, and they enhance in the early arterial phase (20–25 s). Therefore, the scanning protocol for these tumors should be optimized to include arterial phase imaging. Neuroendocrine tumors are often seen as homogenously enhancing discrete lesions in the arterial phase [18] (Fig. 4a, b). Gouya et al., in their study comparing endovascular ultrasound (EUS) and CT, observed that MDCT alone has 94.4% diagnostic sensitivity for detecting insulinomas using the multiphasic protocol. EUS had a sensitivity

of 93.8% and a combination of MDCT and EUS a sensitivity of 100% [19]. Although other modalities such as gadolinium-enhanced magnetic resonance imaging (MRI), somatostatin-receptor imaging, and EUS have emerged as possible diagnostic modalities for pancreatic endocrine neoplasm, multiphasic MDCT is far superior in both detection and staging of pancreatic islet-cell tumors [20]. The presence of hypervascular metastatic deposits to the pancreas can be detected in the arterial phase (Fig. 5). Arterial-enhancing liver metastasis from neuroendocrine tumors is also well seen during this phase.

Cystic Lesion Detection and Characterization

Cystic lesions in the pancreas are now frequently diagnosed due to the increased utilization of CT. These lesions encompass true neoplasms as well as inflammatory lesions. The accurate characterization of a cystic lesion is critical to triage a treat-

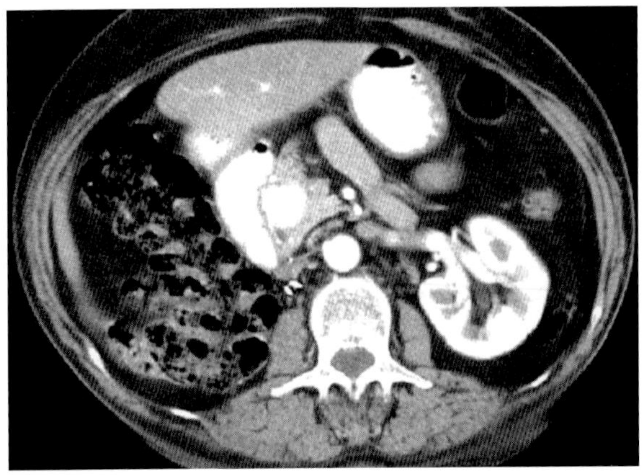

Fig. 5. Axial contrast-enhanced 16-channel multidetector computed tomography (MDCT) image reveals a hypervascular lesion in the head of pancreas. This patient is status postright nephrectomy for a renal call carcinoma. The lesion in the pancreas is an enhancing metastatic deposit from the renal cell carcinoma

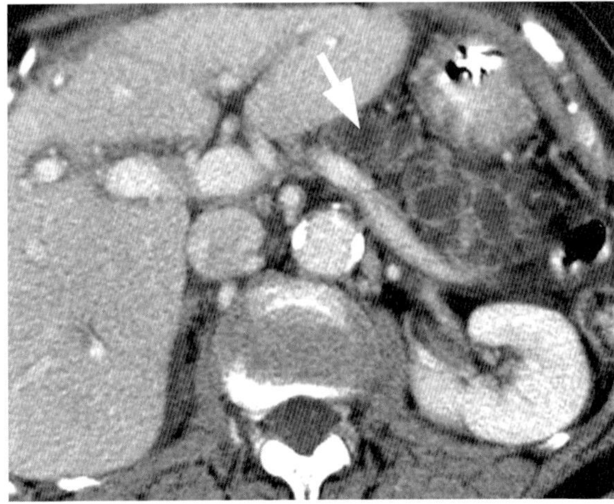

Fig. 6. Portal venous phase helical computed tomography (CT) in a 77-year-old man with chronic abdominal pain, demonstrating diffuse dilatation of the pancreatic duct (*white arrow*) with numerous side-branch cysts, consistent with a diagnosis of combined main duct and side branch intrapancreatic mucinous neoplasm (IPMN)

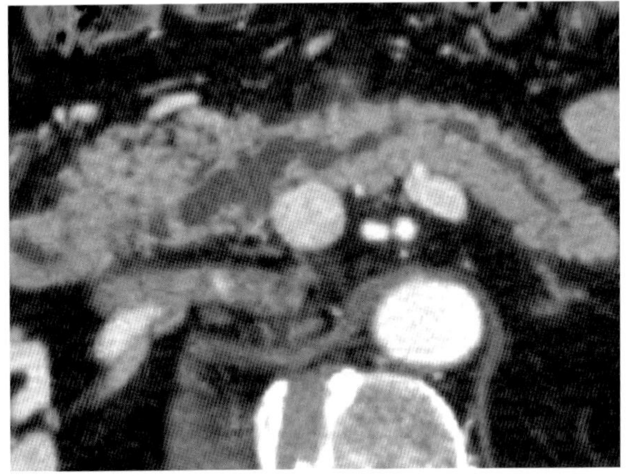

Fig. 7. Curved reformatted image in a middle-aged woman reveals segmental dilatation of the pancreatic duct without transition. These findings are consistent with main duct intrapancreatic mucinous neoplasm (IPMN)

ment decision in these patients. Serous cystadenoma is seen as a solid lesion, with a "honeycomb" appearance due to presence of microcysts [21]. The previously described appearance of a large mass with a central scar and "sunburst" calcification is uncommonly seen, as these lesions are being detected at early stages. Central scar when present is considered characteristic for serous cystadenoma. Mucinous neoplasms, on the other hand, are macrocystic, with few discrete compartments [22]. The classical septal or peripheral eggshell calcification, which is diagnostic of mucinous cysts, is an uncommon feature [23, 24]. Intrapancreatic mucinous neoplasms (IPMN) arise from the epithelium of the main pancreatic duct

and its side branch and may be benign or malignant. Demonstration of communication between the ductal system and the cystic neoplasm is diagnostic of IPMNs [25] (Fig. 6). MDCT with postprocessing is now considered excellent for the comprehensive evaluation of cystic lesions. Pancreatic ductal anatomy and pathology, including cyst communications, can be reliably detected with CT (Fig. 7).

Inflammatory Pathologies of the Pancreas

Although inflammatory pathologies in the pancreas are primarily diagnosed from clinical and laboratory findings, such as serum amylase, lipase, etc., CT is often used to confirm the diagnosis, determine the severity, and evaluate for any associated complication. There have been some minor changes in the protocol for imaging patients suspected of having pancreatitis with the use of MDCT. The use of positive oral contrast is no longer required to distinguish collections from hollow viscus since the high resolution of the MDCT scanners and the availability of reformatted images allow easy differentiation of the two. Intravenous contrast-enhanced multiphasic MDCT can detect all but the mildest forms of pancreatitis. The subtle findings of relatively poor enhancement of the pancreatic parenchyma, either diffusely or focally, and the loss of normal parenchymal lobulations can be a clue to the diagnosis of this condition (Fig. 8). Dual phase imaging for pancreatitis can be beneficial if a vascular complication, such as a pseudoaneurysm, is suspected clinically.

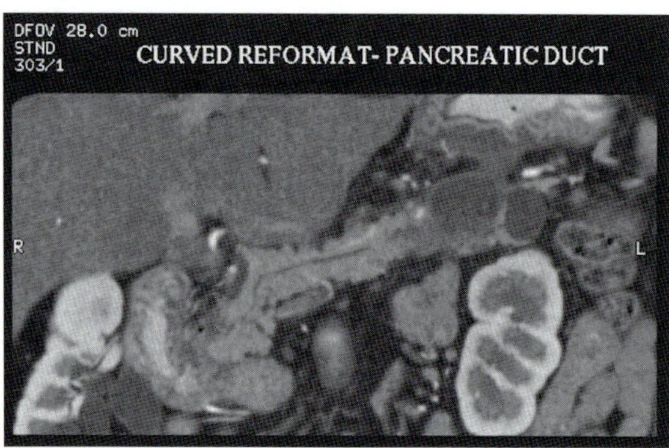

Fig. 8. Curved reformatted image along the pancreatic duct in a patient who presented with abdominal pain reveals an area of poor enhancement of the pancreatic parenchyma at the body due to parenchymal edema and presence of two pseudocysts in the tail of the pancreas. These features are typical of pancreatitis. The excellent resolution of 16-channel multidetector computed tomography (MDCT) permits accurate diagnosis of even subtle pancreatic inflammatory processes

Autoimmune pancreatitis is a rare form of diffuse or focal enlargement of the pancreas. Diffuse "sausage-shaped" enlargement of the pancreas with a rim or "halo" around it is considered a characteristic finding for this entity. Also, lack of vascular encasement may aid in distinguishing the focal form of autoimmune pancreatitis or focal chronic pancreatitis from adenocarcinoma of the pancreas [26].

Chronic pancreatitis, on the other hand, occurs due to repeated episodes of inflammation, which can lead to glandular atrophy and subsequent glandular scarring and fibrosis. The presence of calcifications within part or all of the gland or intraductal calculi may be associated with these features. These findings may occur alone or with pancreatic ductal dilatation.

Image Processing and Display

Various types of image postprocessing can be used for the evaluation of tumor resectability. The advantage of MDCT is the ability to obtain a volumetric data set with near-isotropic voxels. This improves the quality of two-dimensional (2-D) and three-dimensional (3-D) reformations. The evaluation of peripancreatic vasculature is of paramount importance in the diagnosis of locally advanced pancreatic adenocarcinoma. The addition of 2-D and 3-D reformatted images provides information regarding tumor extent, which may be difficult to evaluate on axial images alone. The presence of reconstructed images allows rapid identification of salient features by surgeons and gastroenterologists [27].

It is important to perform overlapping reconstructions at one half the slice thickness of the scan acquisition so as to ensure optimal spatial resolution [6]. A variety of image processing options are available, such as curved reformatted images, minimum-intensity projections, volume-rendered images, standard coronal and sagittal plane reformations, and coronal oblique reformations. Curved reformations are easily understood by surgeons and gastroenterologists. These are routinely obtained in two orthogonal planes. Curved-transverse and curved-coronal reformations are both useful. Since soft tissues are displayed with the ductal and vascular structures, curved reformations are important in determining vascular involvement and ductal abnormalities [28].

Minimum-intensity projections are used to visualize low-attenuation structures, such as pancreatic and common bile ducts [29]. Maximum-intensity projections evaluate high attenuation structures, such as peripancreatic vasculature. Volume-rendered images aid in peripancreatic vessel and tumor encasement.

MDCT Imaging of the Spleen

Evaluation of the spleen is most often done in conjunction with the liver and pancreas. Focal lesions in the spleen are encountered in patients with or without a risk of malignancy. There exists a significant overlap in the imaging features of these lesions, and thus accurate characterization of a lesion into benign or malignant histopathologic subtypes is often difficult.

When MDCT is performed specifically for imaging the spleen, images are obtained at 50–70 s after contrast injection, which is the phase of homogenous parenchymal enhancement of the spleen. When the splenic parenchyma is imaged in the arterial phase, a typical inhomogeneous "tigroid" enhancement pattern is noted due to differential enhancement of the white and red pulp [3] (Fig. 9a, b). At least 50% of normal spleens demonstrate heterogeneous enhancement on dynamic CT, which is more pronounced on MDCT due to high levels of bolus contrast opacification [30]. Ideally, thin-detector collimation (2.5 mm) is preferred for evaluation. Image reconstructions are performed at 1–2 mm, which improves the quality of the 3-D images. Three-dimensional and multiplanar reconstructions are very helpful in detecting splenic and perisplenic processes.

Splenomegaly can be due to a variety of conditions. MDCT can determine whether the spleen is enlarged and the degree of enlargement. Infiltrating conditions, such as malignancy, lymphoma (Fig. 10), and leukemia; and infectious processes,

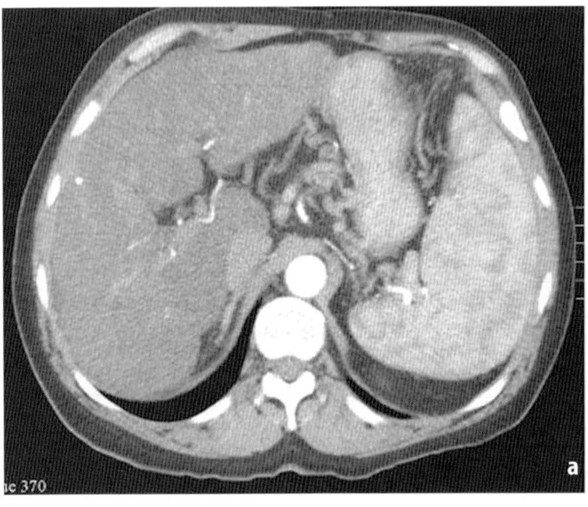
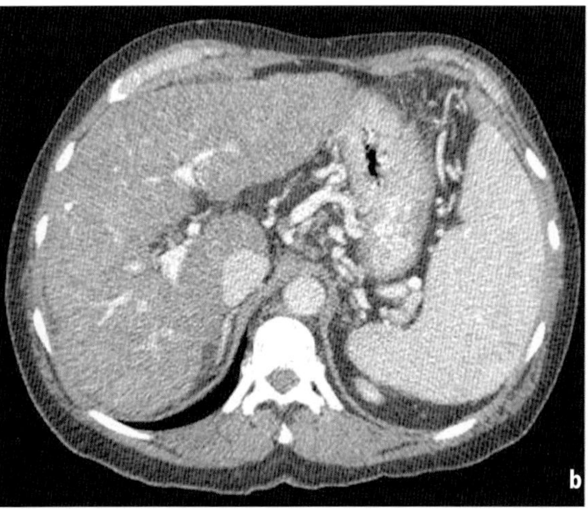

Fig. 9a, b. Arterial phase multidetector computed tomography (MDCT) of the abdomen shows the typical heterogenous enhancement pattern of the spleen sometimes called "tigroid" enhancement. **a** Equilibrium (venous) phase confirms the absence of pathology in the splenic parenchyma with homogenous enhancement of the spleen (**b**)

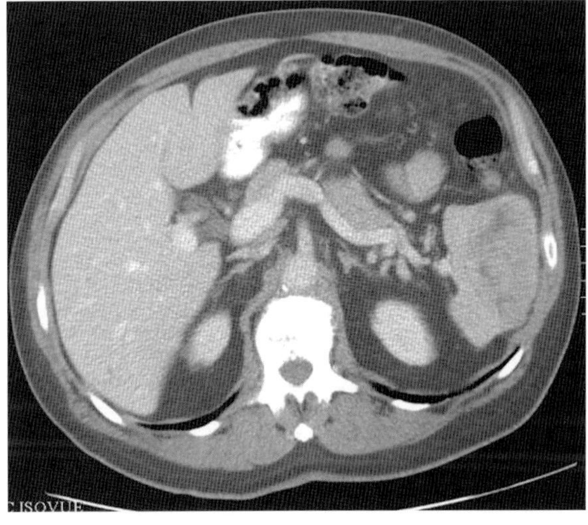

Fig. 10. Axial multidetector computed tomography (MDCT) image of the abdomen demonstrates an exophytic heterogeneously enhancing mass within the spleen. Abnormal periportal and portocaval lymphadenopathy is also visualized. These findings were suspicious of lymphoma on MDCT scan. Pathology examination proved this to be a non-Hodgkin's lymphoma

such as infective endocarditis and mononucleosis, can result in splenomegaly. Systemic processes, such as Gaucher's disease and sarcoidosis, can present with splenomegaly with or without focal masses. Angiosarcoma is the most common malignant primary nonlymphoid tumor of the spleen [31]. It has an aggressive growth pattern on CT, with cystic and necrotic areas seen within the tumor.

Splenic cysts may be congenital-epithelial true cysts, acquired posttraumatic pseudocysts, or parasitic cysts (echinococcal cysts). True epithelial-lined cysts are relatively uncommon (20%) [32]. Congenital cysts are well-defined, low-density lesions with sharply defined borders and no enhancement following contrast administration.

Splenic hemangiomas are often cavernous lesions, which may be from a few millimeters to several centimeters in size. Central punctate calcifications in the solid component and curvilinear peripheral calcifications may be seen. MDCT can identify these lesions as low density with enhancing periphery due to the vascular nature of the pathology. Lymphangiomas may be single or multiple and filled with proteinaceous material. Cystic variants may contain thin-walled, septated cysts, which do not enhance on contrast administration.

Splenic metastases on MDCT are usually low attenuation single or multiple foci. Distinction of cystic splenic metastasis from benign cysts is often difficult. MDCT may detect an enhancing component within the lesion, which favors malignancy (Fig. 11a, b). Splenic abscesses are typically focal and hypodense with a thick enhancing capsule. Presence of gas is a critical feature in making the diagnosis, and MDCT with multiplanar reconstruction is useful in detection of gas when present [33]. Splenic infarcts occur due to embolic occlusion of the splenic artery. A focal wedge-shaped area of decreased attenuation is the typical CT finding of splenic infarct (Fig. 12). Traumatic involvement of the spleen results in lacerations, subcapsular hematomas, or frank splenic rupture. These conditions can be diagnosed using MDCT.

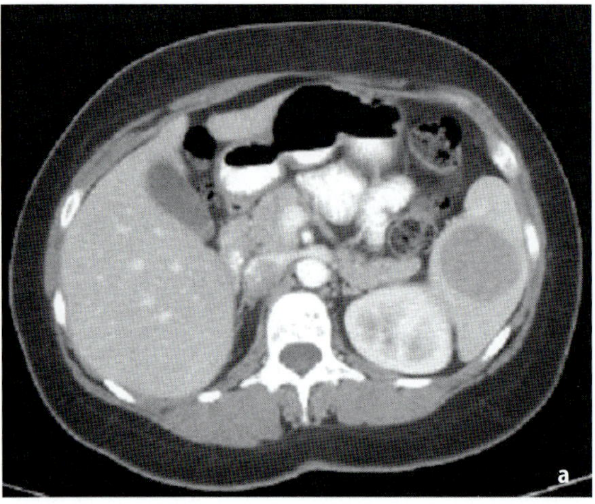

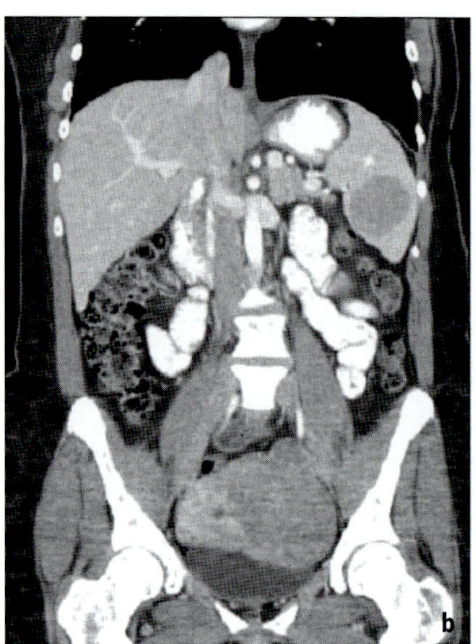

Fig. 11a, b. Axial contrast-enhanced 16-channel multidetector computed tomography (MDCT) in a 39-year-old woman with breast carcinoma reveals a predominantly hypodense mass lesion within the spleen, which has increased in size since the previous study. The presence of some enhancement within the lesion points toward a metastatic pathology as the likely cause. **a** Coronal reformatted image of the same patient shows the entire extent of the lesion (**b**)

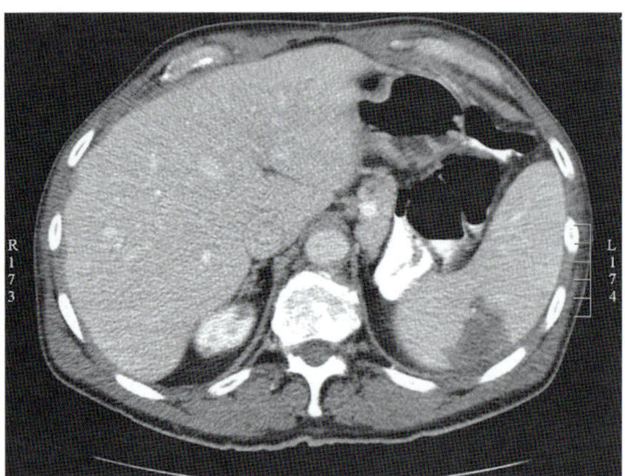

Fig. 12. Axial contrast-enhanced multidetector computed tomography (MDCT) image of the abdomen in the portal venous phase (PVP) shows a wedge-shaped hypodensity in the spleen typical for a splenic infarct

Conclusion

The availability of MDCT scanners has added new dimensions to spatial and temporal resolutions in CT imaging. The use of appropriately designed scanning protocols is the key issue for obtaining optimal quality studies. Availability of thinner-slice collimations leads to almost isotropic voxels and permits high-quality 2-D and 3-D reconstructions. Multiphasic imaging is especially important in the pancreas, where conspicuity of a tumor may change dramatically in the optimal phase. For pancreatic cancer detection, a pancreatic phase is con-

sidered optimal whereas for hypervascular lesion detection, early arterial phase scanning is required. Three-dimensional imaging with MDCT is now an integral part of preoperative staging and surgical planning. The use of high-concentration contrast media may further improve contrast enhancement in the tissue and vasculature.

MDCT has improved the diagnostic confidence for splenic lesions as well. Since there is considerable overlap between benign and malignant pathologies affecting the spleen, it is often difficult to accurately classify a lesion into a histopathological subtype. However, the use of multiphasic imaging and postprocessing techniques has considerably improved the scope for diagnosis of splenic pathology.

References

1. Tunaci M (2004) Multidetector row CT of the pancreas. Eur J Radiol 52:18–30
2. McNulty NJ, Francis IR, Platt JF et al (2001) Multidetector row helical CT of the pancreas: effect of contrast enhanced multiphasic imaging on enhancement of the pancreas, peripancreatic vasculature, and pancreatic adenocarcinoma. Radiol 220:97–102
3. Fenchel S, Boll DT, Fleiter TR (2003) Multislice helical CT of the pancreas and spleen. Eur J Radiol 45:S59–S72
4. Bae KT, Heiken JP, Brink JA (1998) Aortic and hepatic contrast medium enhancement at CT. Part I. Prediction with a computer model. Radiology 207:647–655
5. Fenchel S, Fleiter TR, Aschoff AJ et al (2004) Effect

of iodine concentration of contrast media on contrast enhancement in multislice CT of the pancreas. Br J Radiol 77:821–830

6. Elliot K Fishman, Jeffrey RB Jr (2004) Multidetector CT: Principles, techniques and clinical applications. Lippincott Williams & Wilkins, Philadelphia, pp 85

7. Boland GW, O'Malley ME, Saez M et al (1999) Pancreatic-phase versus portal vein-phase helical CT of the pancreas: optimal temporal window for evaluation of pancreatic adenocarcinoma. AJR Am J Roentgenol 172:605–608

8. Lu DSK, Vedantham S, Krasny RM et al (1996) Two-phase helical CT for pancreatic tumors: pancreatic versus hepatic phase enhancement of tumor, pancreas and vascular structures. Radiology 199: 697–701

9. Warshaw AL, Fernandez-del-Castillo C (1992) Pancreatic carcinoma. N Engl J Med 326:455–465

10. LU DS, Reber HA, Krasny RM et al (1997) Local Staging of pancreatic cancer: criteria for unrectability of major vessels as revealed by pancreatic phase, thin-section helical CT. AJR Am J Roentgenol 168:1439–1443

11. Nishiharu T, Yamashita Y, Abe Y et al (1999) Local extension of pancreatic carcinoma: assessment with thin-section helical CT versus with breath-hold fast MR imaging – ROC analysis. Radiology 212:445–452

12. Trede M, Rumstadt B, Wendl K et al (1997) Ultrafast magnetic resonance imaging improves the staging of pancreatic tumors. Ann Surg 226:393–405

13. Ellsmere J, Mortele K, Sahani D et al (2005) Does multidetector-row CT eliminate the role of diagnostic laparoscopy in assessing the resectability of pancreatic head adenocarcinoma? Surg Endosc 19:369–373

14. Grenacher L, Klaus M, Dukic L et al (2004) Diagnosis and staging of pancreatic carcinoma: MRI versus multislice CT – a prospective study. Rofo 176: 1624–1633

15. Kulig J, Popiela T, Zajac A et al (2005) The value of imaging techniques in the staging of pancreatic cancer. Surg Endosc 19:361–365

16. DeWitt J, Devereaux B, Chriswell M et al (2004) Comparison of endoscopic ultrasonography and multidetector computed tomography for detecting and staging pancreatic cancer. Ann Int Med 141(10):753–763

17. Wiersema MJ (2001) Accuracy of endoscopic ultrasound in diagnosing and staging pancreatic carcinoma. Pancreatology 1:625–632

18. Sheth S, Hruban R, Fishman E (2002) Helical CT of islet cell tumors of the pancreas: typical and atypical manifestations. AJR Am J Roentgenol 179:725–730

19. Gouya H, Vignaux O, Augui J et al (2003) CT, endoscopic sonography, and a combined protocol for preoperative evaluation of pancreatic insulinomas. AJR Am J Roentgenol 181:987–992

20. Ichikawa T, Peterson M, Federle M et al (2000) Islet cell tumor of pancreas: Biphasic CT versus MR imaging in tumor detection. Radiology 216:163–171

21. Procacci C, Graziani R, Bicego E et al (1997) Serous cystadenoma of the pancreas: report of 30 cases with emphasis on the imaging findings. J Comput Assist Tomogr 21:373–382

22. Grogan JR, Saeian K, Taylor AJ et al (2001) Making sense of mucin-producing pancreatic tumors. AJM Am J Roentgenol 176:921–929

23. Curry C, John Eng, Karen M et al (2000) CT of primary cystic pancreatic neoplasms: Can CT be used for patient triage and treatment? AJM Am J Roentgenol 175:99–103

24. Wilentz RE, Albores-Saavendra J, Zahurak M et al (1999) Pathologic examination accurately predicts prognosis in mucinous cystic neoplasms of the pancreas. Am J Surg Pathol 23:132–137

25. Sugiyama M, Atomi Y (1998) Intraductal papillary mucinous tumors of the pancreas: imaging studies and treatment strategies. Ann Surg 228:685–691

26. Sahani D, Kalva SP, Farrell J et al (2004) Autoimmune Pancreatitis: Imaging Features. Radiology 233:345–352

27. Rubin GD (2000) Data explosion: the challenge of multidetector row CT. Eur J Radiol 36:74–80

28. Nono-Murcia M, Jeffrey RB Jr, Beaulieu CF et al (2001) Multidetecotr CT of the pancreas and bile duct system: value of curved planar reformations. AJR Am J Roentgenol 176:689–693

29. Raptopoulos V, Prassopoulos P, Chuttani R et al (1998) Multiplanar CT pancreatography and distal cholangiography with minimum intensity projections. Radiology 207:317–324

30. Donnelly LF, Foss JN, Frush DP et al (1999) Heterogenous splenic enhancements patterns on spiral CT images in children: minimizing misinterpretation. Radiology 210:493–497

31. Smith VC, Eisenberg Bl, McDonald EC (1985) Primary splenic angiosarcoma. Case report and literature review. Cancer 55:1625–1627

32. Warshauer DM, Koehler RE (1998) Spleen. In: Lee JKT, Sagel SS, Stanley Rj, Heiken JP (eds) Computed body tomography with MRI correlation, 3rd ed. Lippincott–Raven,1New York, pp 845–872

33. Urrutia M, Mergo PJ, Ros LH et al (1996) Cystic masses of the spleen: radiologic-pathologic correlation. Radiographics 16:107–129

Mesenteric and Renal CT Angiography

Lisa L. Wang, Christine O. Menias, Kyongtae T. Bae

Introduction

Multidetector-row computed tomography (MDCT) is changing the spectrum of vascular imaging as a result of its fast image acquisition speed and spatial resolution. When coupled with high-quality three-dimensional (3-D) image representations, MDCT angiography effectively permits the evaluation of the abdominal visceral vasculature and is preferred to conventional angiography because of its noninvasiveness.

Abdominal applications of CT angiography (CTA) are growing. This chapter focuses on CTA evaluation of the mesenteric and renal vessels. Common indications include staging and surgical planning of tumors, evaluation for renal donor transplantation, workup of renovascular hypertension, and assessment of mesenteric ischemia and inflammatory bowel disease.

General Contrast Medium Principles

For CTA, contrast administration technique should be optimized to best delineate the vascular structure. Positive oral contrast is not administered because the anatomical separation of the intravenously enhanced vascular structures from the opacified gastrointestinal (GI) tract is difficult and can be problematic when displaying vasculature in 3-D. Prior to imaging, patients can drink approximately 1 l of water to distend the proximal GI tract. Optimal CTA contrast enhancement requires accurate timing of data acquisition with rapid and precise intravenous delivery of contrast medium. The amount of contrast medium required to achieve a desirable enhancement in CTA may be reduced because of a faster acquisition time with MDCT. An increased injection rate and high contrast medium concentration can compensate for the somewhat decreased magnitude of aortic enhancement achieved with the smaller contrast medium volume [1–3]. Contrast medium volumes ranging from 90 to 120 ml with 350–400 mgI/ml concentration are injected intravenously at rates of 4–5 ml/s. Given high injection rates, an intravenous access of at least 20 gauge or larger in the antecubital fossa should be used. In order to maintain an equivalent degree of contrast enhancement, larger patients require a larger iodine dose while smaller patients require smaller iodine dose. A saline flush improves the efficiency of contrast medium use and reduces artifact [4] and is particularly beneficial when a small total amount of contrast medium is used.

Precise arterial timing is critical to the CTA technique. Either a test bolus or bolus-tracking technique is used to determine the contrast bolus arrival time ($Tarr$). The $Tarr$ is derived by placing the region of interest within the reference vessel of interest. To ensure adequate vascular opacification, the scan delay is determined with an additional delay of 5–15 s plus the $Tarr$, as described in Section II [4, 5].

3-D CTA Postprocessing

CTA protocols generate a large amount of data. Interactive 3-D workstations are becoming more efficient in both managing the large data set and generating 3-D angiographic presentations [6]. Initially, reviewing axial images can be performed expeditiously by scrolling. Multiple planes can be selected on the interactive dedicated 3-D workstation to evaluate the vessel of interest. Volumetric data, reconstructed at 0.7–1.0 mm, can be reviewed using several available 3-D display techniques: maximum intensity projection (MIP), multiplanar reformatting (MPR), curve planar reformatting (CP), and volume rendering (VR).

The MIP technique displays only the maximum

intensity voxel values along a viewer projection in a given volume of 3-D data. Thus, additional image processing steps are often required to remove bones and other hyperdense structures that are of high CT attenuation value and superimpose over and obscure the vascular structure of interest. MPR illustrates all structures within a particular plane. Thus, to circumvent this restriction in evaluating a vessel, curved planar reformatting, which can be also time consuming, is utilized. VR is an easily adaptable technique, as it requires minimal data editing by the operator and can dexterously display complex anatomy [7–11]. As VR preserves spatial depth and relationships, it has been proven to be better than MIP in evaluating the peripancreatic and renal vessels [9, 12, 13]. Nonetheless, MIP images readily simulate conventional angiographic images and are effective in evaluating atherosclerotic burden in the vessels. The workstation should be user friendly and flexible for radiologists to switch rapidly from one display mode to another to depict anatomy and pathology in the most informative manner.

Mesenteric Vascular Imaging

CTA of the mesenteric vasculature includes the superior mesenteric artery (SMA) (Fig. 1), the inferior mesenteric artery (IMA) (Fig. 1), the superior mesenteric vein (SMV), and the inferior mesenteric vein (IMV) (Fig. 2). MDCT can be used to delineate involvement of the mesenteric vessels from disease processes such as neoplasm, mesenteric ischemia, and inflammatory bowel disease [12].

Imaging Techniques

For any type of CTA, attention to patient preparation, intravenous contrast medium administration, scanner features, data quality, and postprocessing

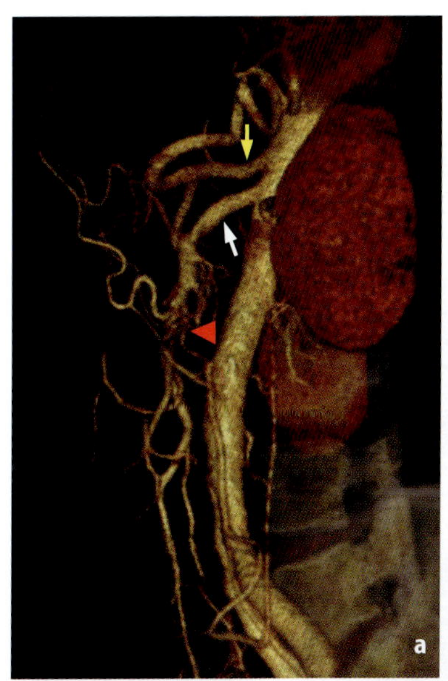
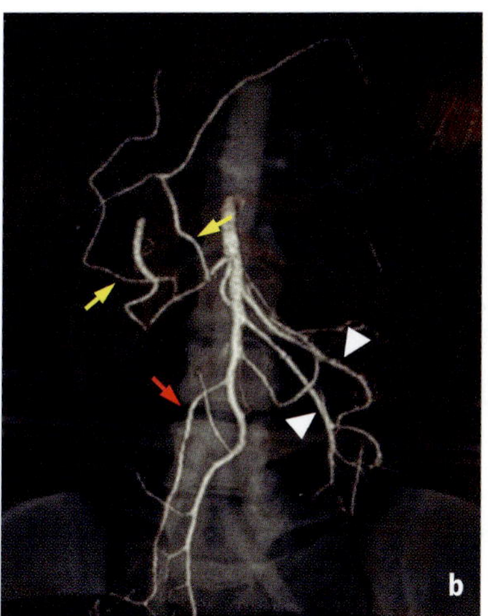
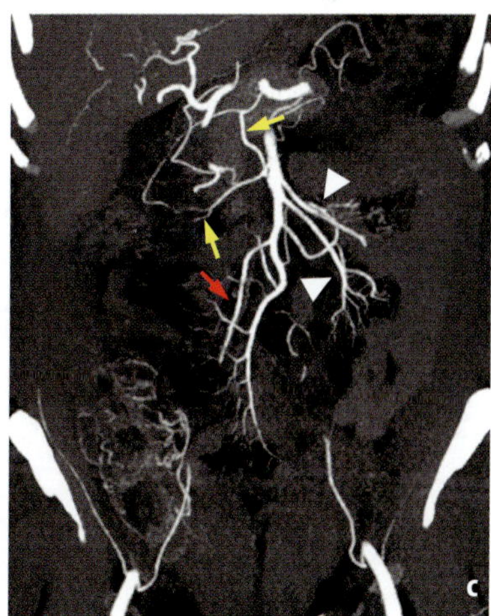
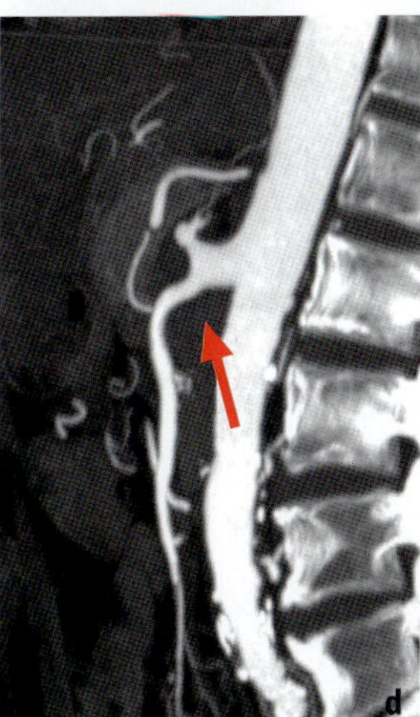
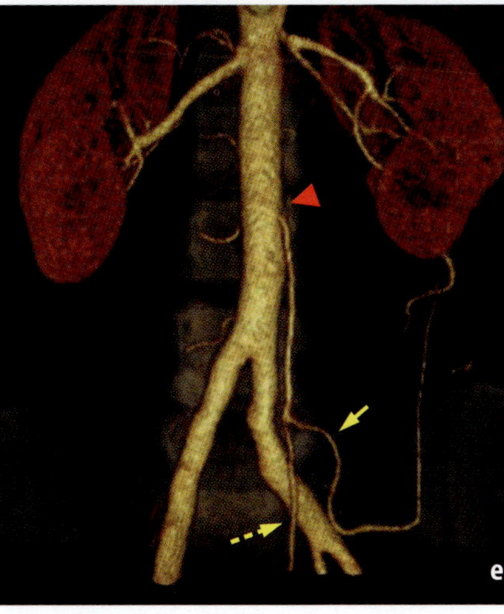

Fig. 1a-e. Normal superior and inferior mesenteric arteries. **a** Sagittal three-dimensional (3-D) volume rendering (VR) demonstrates the normal anatomy of the superior mesenteric artery (SMA) (*white arrow*) arising from near the L2 body approximately 1 cm caudal to the celiac axis (*yellow arrow*). Inferior mesenteric artery (IMA) (*red arrowhead*) arises approximately 7 cm caudal to the SMA. **b** Coronal VR and **c** coronal maximum intensity projection (MIP) demonstrating SMA branches: intestinal branches (*white arrowheads*), ileocolic artery (*red arrow*), middle colic artery (*short thick yellow arrow*), and right colic artery (*long thin yellow arrow*). **d** Uncommon variant of celiacomesenteric trunk (1%) (*red arrow*), which gives rise to the celiac axis and SMA in a different patient. **e** Coronal three-dimensional (3-D) VR of IMA (*red arrowhead*) with left colic artery (*short yellow arrow*) and superior rectal artery (*dashed yellow arrow*) [33]

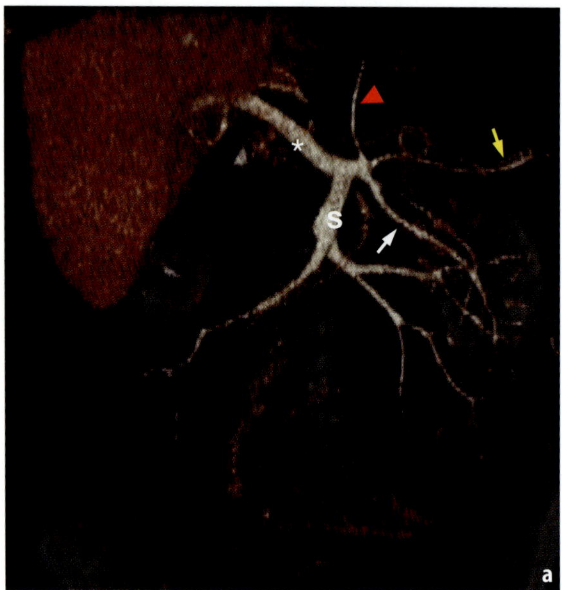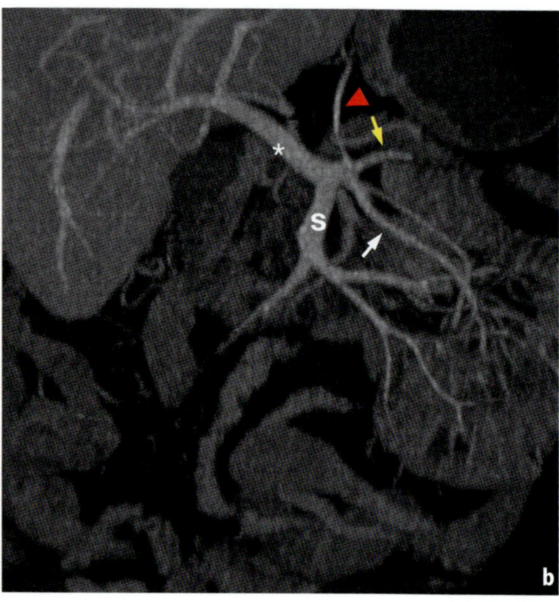

Fig. 2a, b. Normal portal venous system. Coronal volume rendering (VR) showing main portal vein (*), splenic vein (*yellow arrow*), and superior mesenteric vein (SMV) (*S*) joining at the portal confluence. The inferior mesenteric vein (IMV) (*white arrow*) and the gastroepiploic vein (*red arrowhead*) can drain into the splenic vein

Table 1. Mesenteric computed tomography angiography (CTA) parameters for 64-slice multidetector-row computed tomography (MDCT)[a]

Phase	Noncontrast	Arterial	Portal venous
kVp/effective mAs/rotation time (s)	120/240/0.5	120/240/0.5	120/240/0.5
Detector collimation (mm)	0.6	0.6	0.6
Slice thickness (mm)	5	1	2
Beam pitch	1:1	1:1	1:1
Recon increment (mm)	5	0.7	2
Scan delay		Bolus tracking	60 s

[a] Scan parameters from Siemens Sensation 64

Table 2. Mesenteric computed tomography angiography (CTA) parameters for 16-slice multidetector-row computed tomography (MDCT)[a]

Phase	Noncontrast	Arterial	Portal venous
kVp/effective mAs/rotation time (s)	120/160/0.5	120/180/0.5	120/180/0.5
Detector collimation (mm)	1.5	0.75	1.5
Slice thickness (mm)	5	1	2
Feed/rotation (mm)	24	12	24
Recon increments (mm)	5	0.8	2
Scan delay		Bolus tracking	60 s

[a] Scan parameters from Siemens Sensation 16

Table 3. Mesenteric computed tomography angiography (CTA) parameters for 4-slice multidetector-row computed tomography (MDCT)[a]

Phase	Noncontrast	Arterial	Portal venous
kVp/effective mAs/rotation time (s)	120/180/0.5	120/180/0.5	120/180/0.5
Detector collimation (mm)	2.5	1.25	2.5
Slice thickness (mm)	5	1.25	3
Feed/rotation (mm)	10	4	10
Recon increment (mm)	5	1	2
Scan delay		Bolus tracking	60 s

[a] Scan parameters from Siemens VolumeZoom

techniques is crucial. The mesenteric CTA protocol depends on the scanner type available. These protocols are summarized in Tables 1–3. Negative oral contrast such as water allows simultaneous detailed characterization of bowel-wall enhancement and 3-D vascular reconstruction without interference from bowel content [14]. The noncontrast phase is used to delineate bowel hemorrhage and vascular calcifications, the arterial phase is used for arterial vascular mapping and treatment planning, and the portal venous phase is used for portal-venous vascular mapping and visceral evaluation [15].

Applications

Neoplasms

Among numerous neoplastic processes, pancreatic cancer most commonly involves the mesenteric vessels. SMA invasion (Fig. 3) precludes surgery for pancreatic cancer [16, 17]. Limited involvement of the portal vein or confluence may not be an absolute contraindication for surgical resection. When a vessel is either narrowed or occluded by an adjacent soft tissue mass, vascular involvement is suspected (Fig. 4). Also, collateral vessels can be an ancillary sign of vascular involvement [12].

Other conditions such as carcinoid tumor, lymphoma (Fig. 5), or sclerosing mesenteritis (Fig. 6), can present as masses that infiltrate and encase the mesenteric vessels. The masses enveloping the mesenteric vessels are readily delineated on CTA but not on conventional digital subtraction angiography (DSA). For this reason, 3-D CTA is highly beneficial for planning surgery or biopsy.

Mesenteric Ischemia

Compromise (occlusion, thrombosis, or poor perfusion) of the major mesenteric vessels (SMV or SMA) (Figs. 7 and 8) can lead to bowel ischemia or

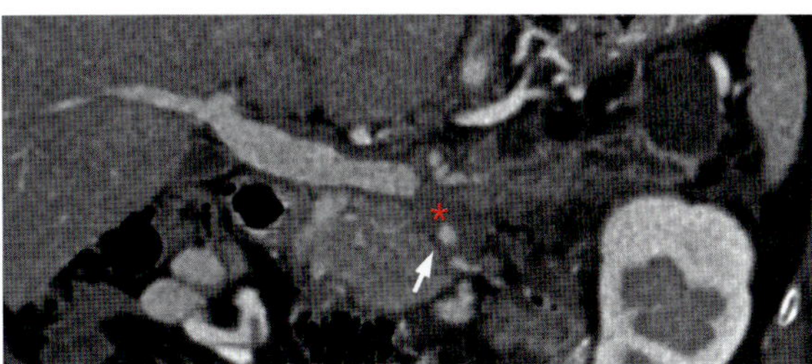

Fig. 3. Curved planar multiplanar reformat (MPR) reveals that the pancreatic adenocarcinoma (*) has totally encased the superior mesenteric artery (SMA) (*white arrow*). This finding is a contraindication for surgical treatment. Note the atrophy of the pancreatic body and tail to the *left* of the mass

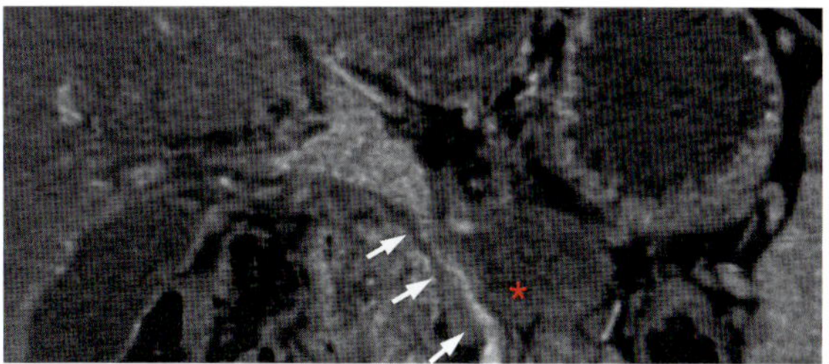

Fig. 4. Curved planar multiplanar reformat (MPR) demonstrating the pancreatic adenocarcinoma (*) severely narrowing the portal venous system at the portal confluence (*white arrows*)

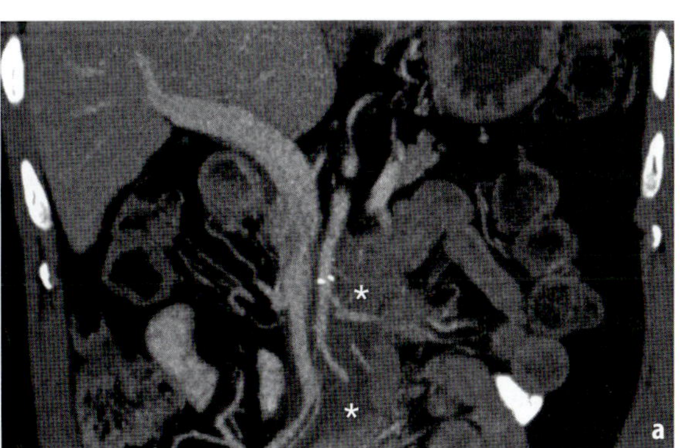

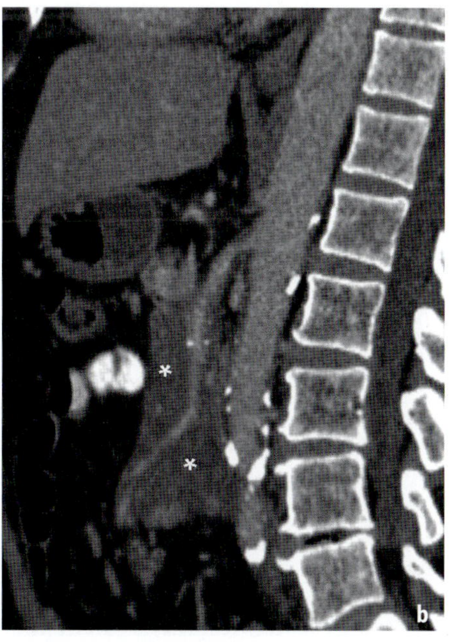

Fig. 5a, b. Lymphoma (*) encasing the superior mesenteric artery (SMA) and superior mesenteric vein (SMV) seen on **a** coronal and **b** sagittal multiplanar reformatting (MPR) views

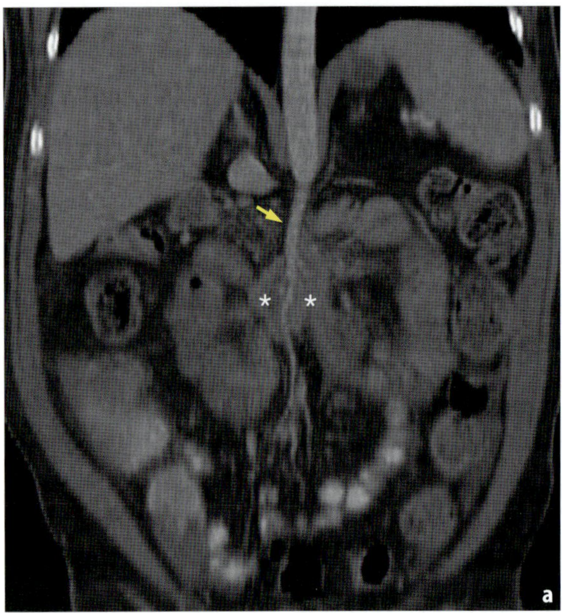

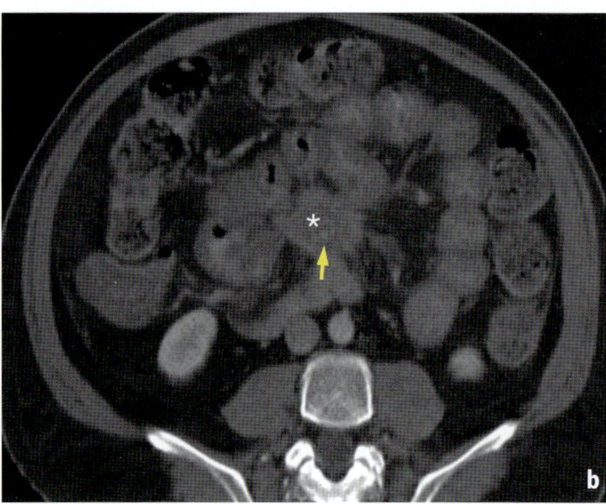

Fig. 6a, b. a Thick-section coronal and **b** axial multiplanar reformat (MPR) images demonstrate a soft tissue mass (*) encasing the superior mesenteric artery (SMA) (*yellow arrow*) with mesenteric tethering. Open surgical biopsy revealed the mass to be sclerosing mesenteritis

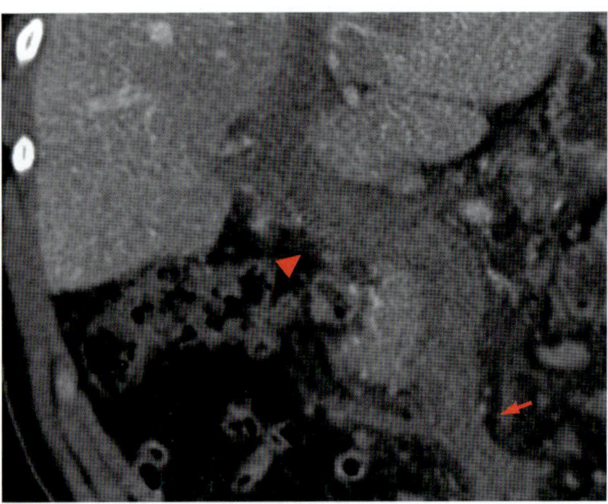

Fig. 7. Coronal multiplanar reformat (MPR) revealing acutely thrombosed portal venous system (*red arrows*). This patient, who had distal pancreatectomy and splenectomy for intraductal papillary mucinous neoplasm and subsequently developed acute pancreatitis of the remaining pancreas, now presents with thrombosed portal venous system

thickened bowel loops with either intramural low attenuation suggesting edema or high attenuation representing submucosal/intramural hemorrhage (Fig. 8g). Bowel caliber can increase, and bowel-wall enhancement can be decreased due to compromised blood supply or be increased due to hyperemia. Pneumatosis suggests irreversible infarction, but this is not specific, as it can be seen in mucosal ischemia (Fig. 8h) [14, 18–20].

Inflammatory Disease

Three-dimensional MDCTA may be helpful in assessing changes of active inflammation in patients with inflammatory bowel disease or vasculitis such as systemic lupus erythematosus (Fig. 11) and cystic medial necrosis (Fig. 12). Enlargement of the mesenteric vessels feeding the affected intestine may indicate hyperemia [12, 21].

Gastrointestinal Bleed

Oftentimes, when a patient presents with GI bleed, the source of the bleed is very difficult to find. CTA may be helpful in depicting the region or source and planning treatment of the patient's underlying disease condition (Fig. 13). Mesenteric vessel aneurysms or pseudoaneurysms (PSA) are accurately depicted with CTA (Fig. 14). CTA is particularly efficient in acquiring diagnostic information quickly for a patient in trauma in order for surgeons and interventional radiologists to plan and expedite an appropriate treatment (Fig. 15).

infarction. Thrombosis of the main mesenteric vessels can be seen on the axial images (Fig. 8c, d), and, if chronic, occlusions can present with collaterals (Figs. 9 and 10). Narrowing or occlusion of the origins of the major mesenteric vessels from atherosclerotic disease may be best seen on 3-D CTA (Figs. 9 and 10). Evaluation of the distal branches may also be improved with 3-D reformatted images.

Acute mesenteric ischemia can present with a variety of appearances. Manifestations can include

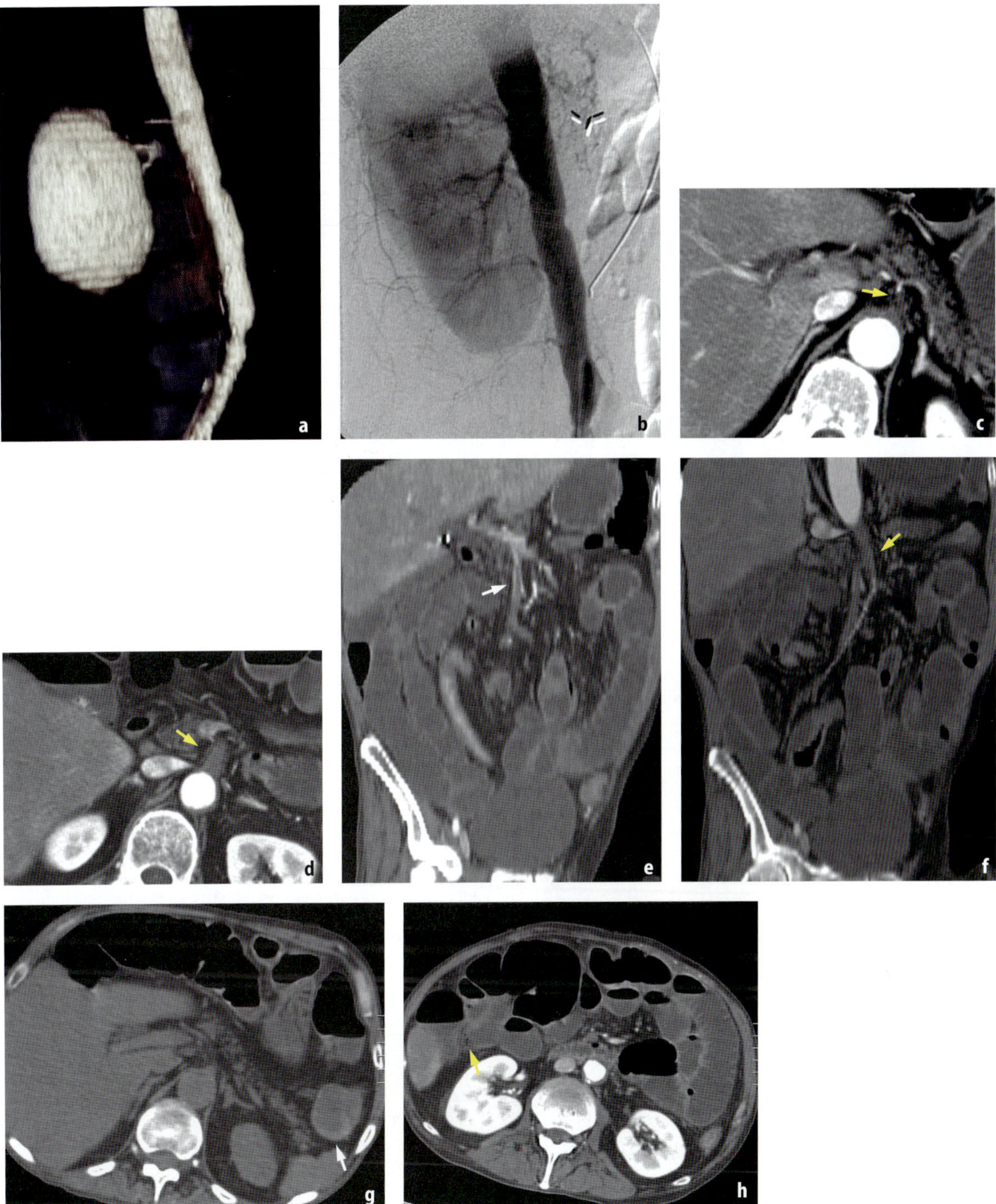

Fig. 8a-h. With history of worsening chronic abdominal pain and weight loss, this 59-year-old man was found to have ischemic bowel. All his major mesenteric vessels were occluded, as shown on **a** three-dimensional (3-D) volume rendered (VR) computed tomography angiography (CTA) and **b** conventional angiography, which demonstrate no major mesenteric vessel opacification. **c** Thrombosis of the celiac axis and **d** superior mesenteric artery (SMA) can be seen on axial plane. **e** Thick-section curved planar image demonstrates thrombus in the SMV. **f** Curve planar reformat reveals the SMA thrombosis. **g** Noncontrast axial image revealing submucosal hemorrhage (*arrow*). **h** Pneumatosis (*arrow*) in this case represents necrotic bowel

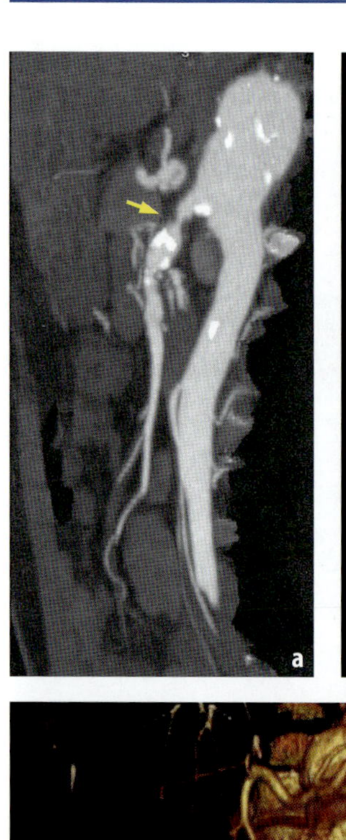
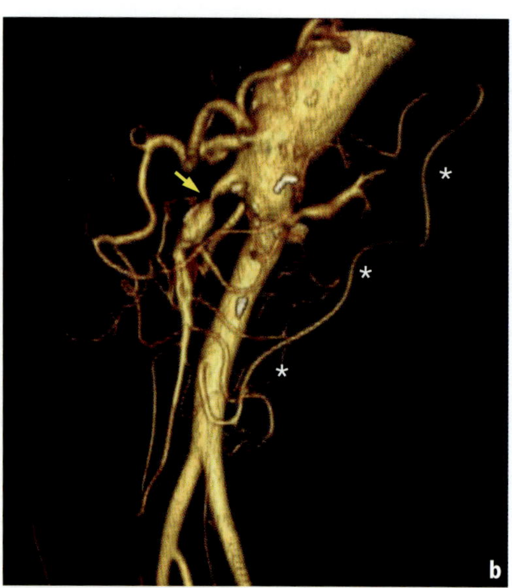
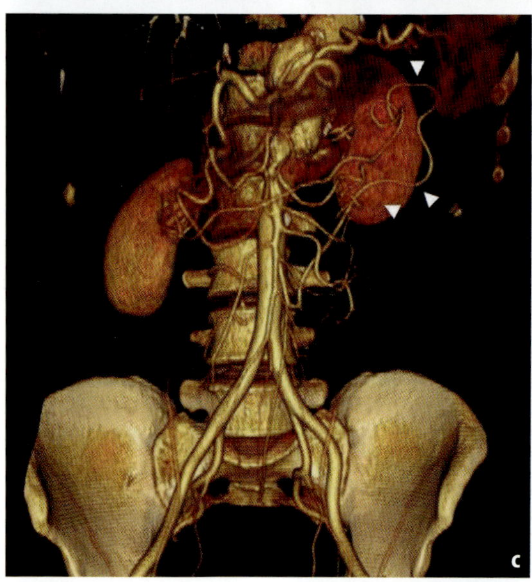

Fig. 9a-c. A 43-year-old man with thoracic and suprarenal abdominal aneurysm with an atherosclerotic superior mesenteric artery (SMA) stenosis just distal to its origin. **a** Thick-section multiplanar reformatting (MPR) and **b** and **c** three-dimensional (3-D) volume rendering (VR) reveal atherosclerotic plaque narrowing the SMA (*arrow*) with poststenotic aneurysmal dilatation. Collaterals between the inferior mesenteric artery (IMA) and the SMA (*white arrowhead*) are formed via the arc of Riolan [33]

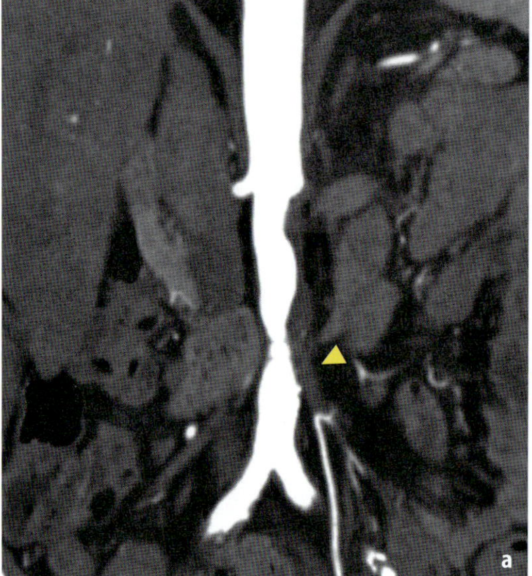
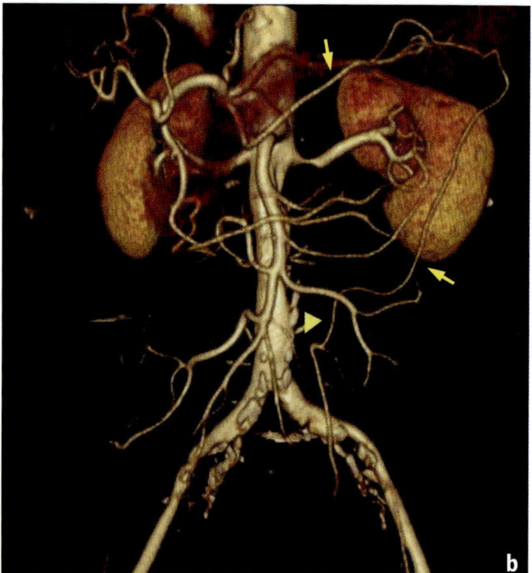

Fig. 10a, b. a Coronal multiplanar reformat (MPR) demonstrating the occluded proximal inferior mesenteric artery (IMA) (*arrowhead*) from atherosclerotic mural thrombus in a 69-year-old man with peripheral vascular disease. **b** Volume rendered (VR) image demonstrates the arc of Riolan (*yellow arrows*) that provides collateral to the IMA distal to the site of occlusion [33]

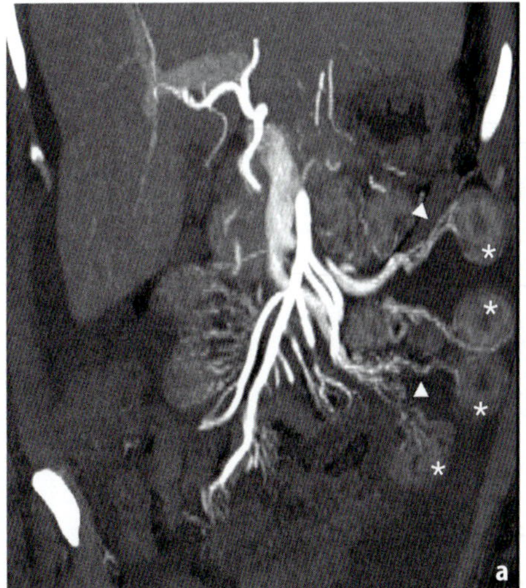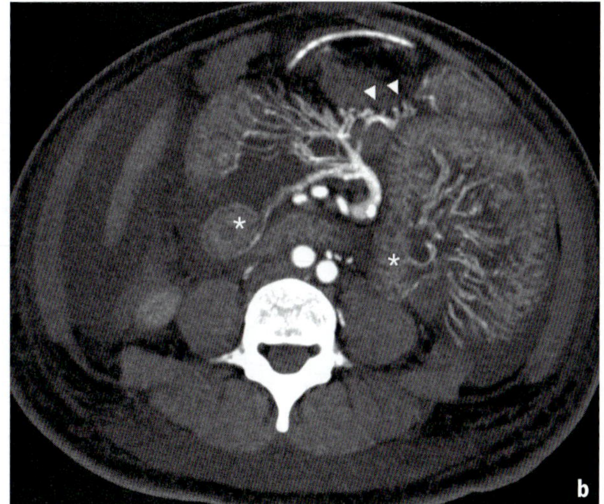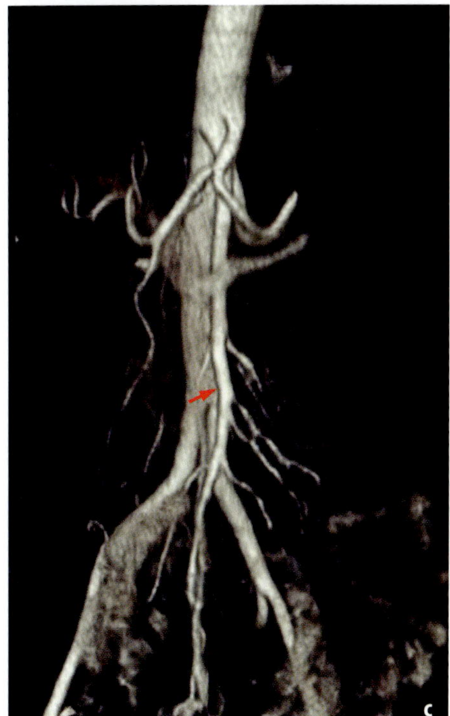

Fig. 11a-c. Thick-section multiplanar reformat (MPR) images demonstrating diffuse wall thickening (*) of the small bowel and small vessel collateralizations (corkscrew collaterals) of the jejunal branches of the superior mesenteric arteries (SMA) (*white arrowhead*) (**a, b**). Volume rendering (VR) image demonstrating the SMA (*red arrow*) (**c**) and its collateral vessels affected with vasculitis resulting in ischemia [34]. This patient is a 37-year-old woman with history of systemic lupus erythematosus who presented post-partum with several days of bloody stool. Similar arteriographic findings of corkscrew collaterals can be seen in patients with scleroderma, CREST syndrome, Buerger's disease, rheumatoid vasculitis, mixed connective-tissue disease, antiphospholipid-antibody syndrome, diabetes mellitus [35]

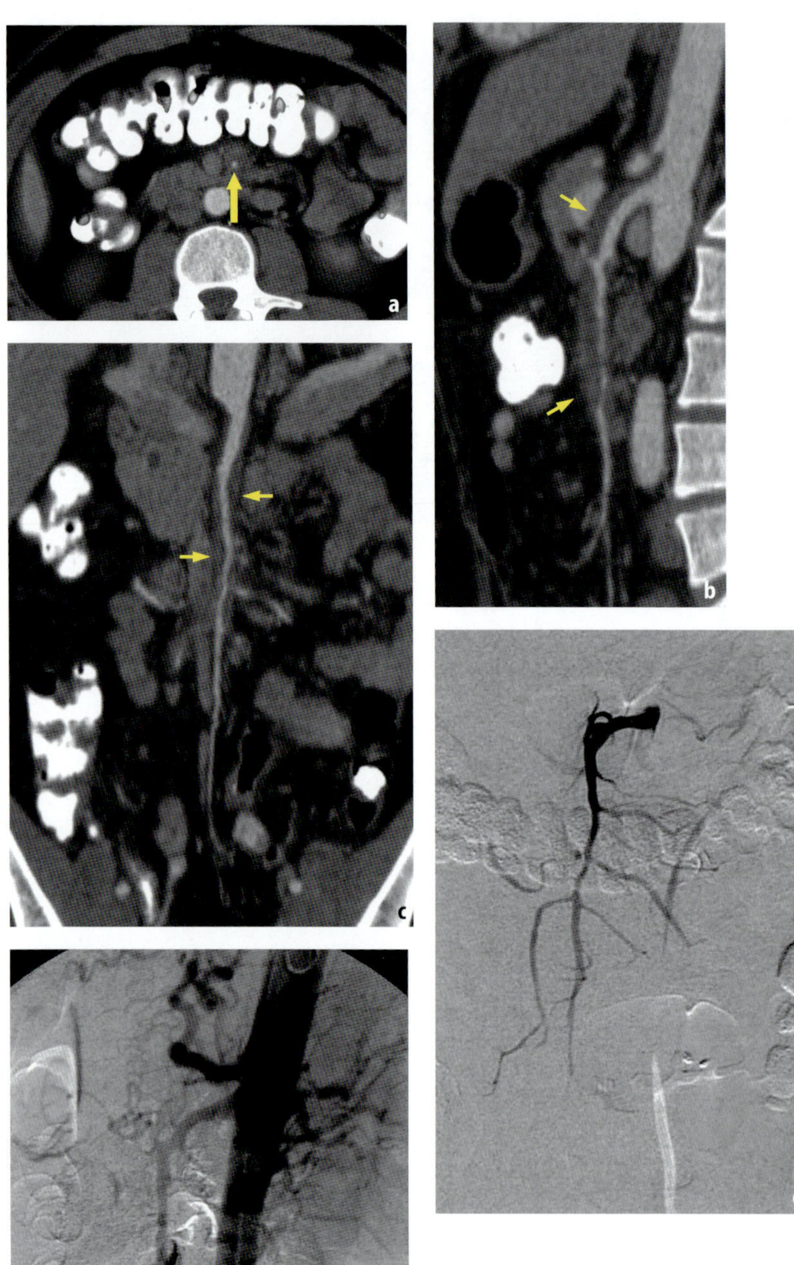

Fig. 12a-e. Multiplanar reformat (MPR) images (**a-c**) demonstrating a dissection with intramural hematoma in the superior mesenteric artery (SMA) (*yellow arrows*) in a 40-year-old man with a 6-month history of abdominal pain and a recent onset of diarrhea. **d, e** This abnormality of the SMA is not appreciated with the conventional angiogram because only opacified lumen is visualized. Surgical pathology demonstrates cystic medial necrosis as the etiology. Isolated SMA dissection is uncommon, and when it is seen, the reported causes include trauma, cystic medial necrosis, fibromuscular dysplasia, and hypertension [36]

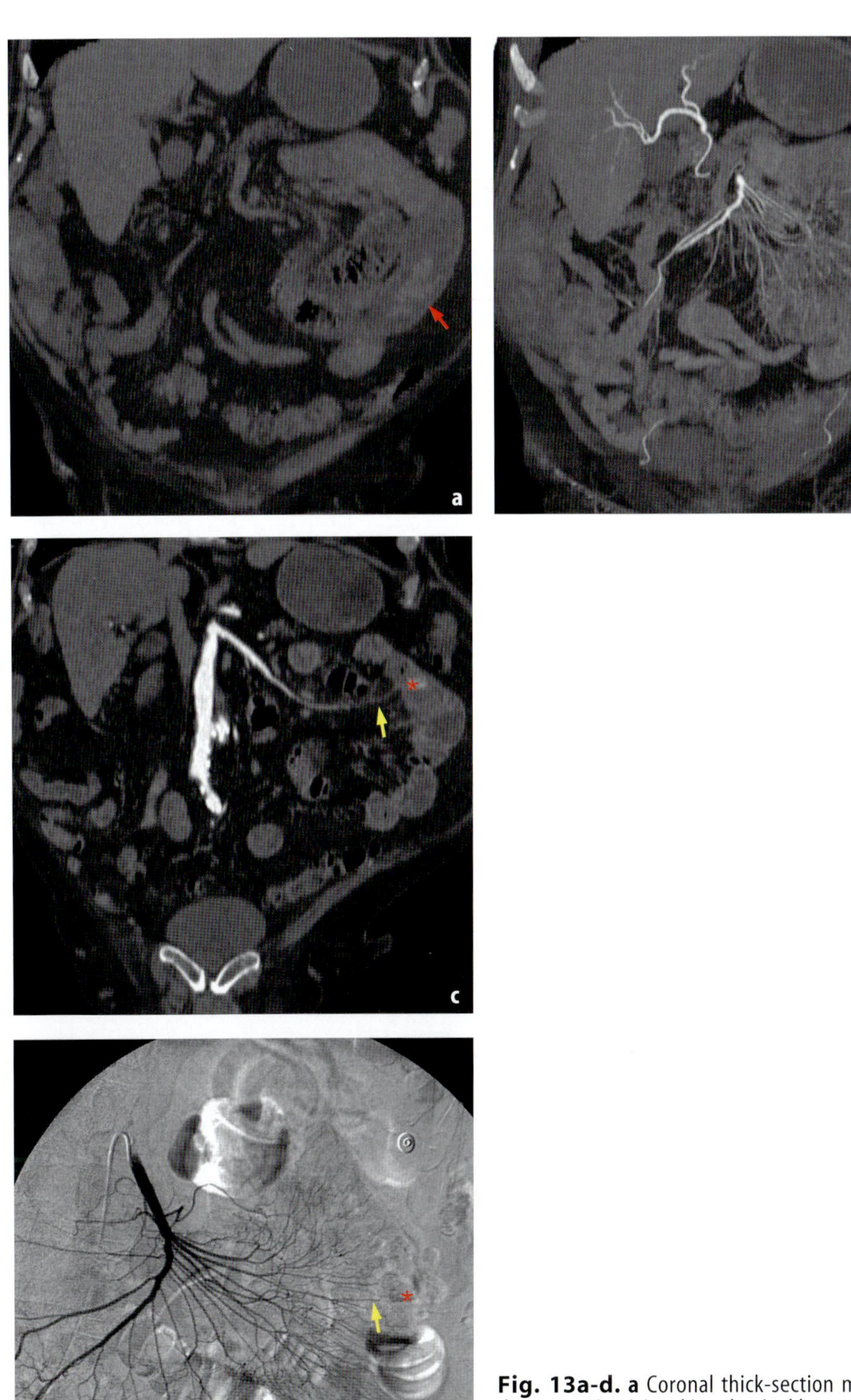

Fig. 13a-d. a Coronal thick-section multiplanar reformat (MPR) images demonstrating jejunal intraluminal hematoma (*red arrow*) on the unenhanced exam. **b, c** Active intravenous contrast extravasation (*) in a jejunal arterial branch (*yellow arrow*) on the enhanced images in a 76-year-old man with gastrointestinal (GI) bleed. **d** The leak is not as well seen on the conventional angiography

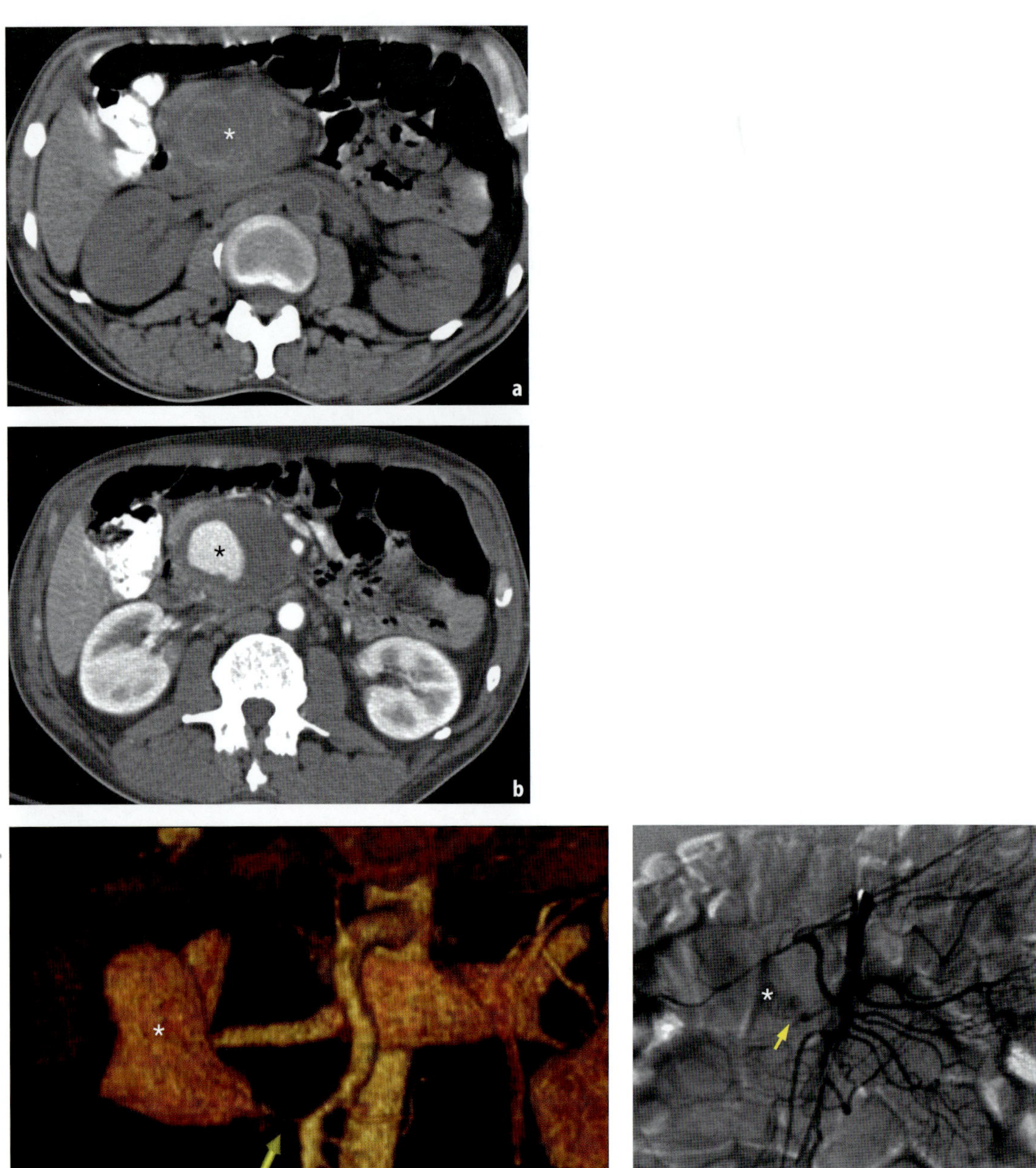

Fig. 14a-d. a A reported pancreatic "mass" (*) seen on unenhanced computed tomography (CT); **b** corresponds to a gastroduodenal artery pseudoaneurysm (*) apparent on the enhanced CT. This is a 53-year-old man with a history of alcohol-induced pancreatitis who presented with a diagnosis of a pancreatic mass. **c** Feeding vessel (*arrow*) from the superior mesenteric artery (SMA) was identified on the volume rendering (VR) image, **d** subsequently confirmed on the conventional preembolization angiogram

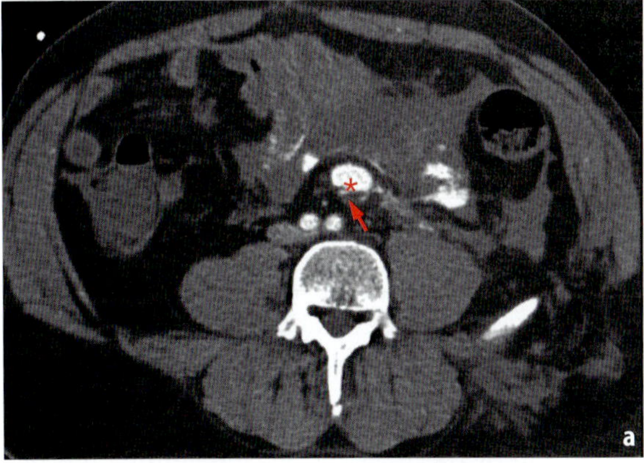

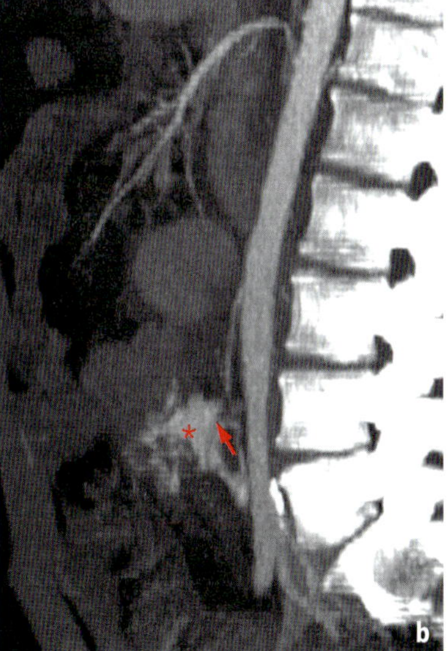

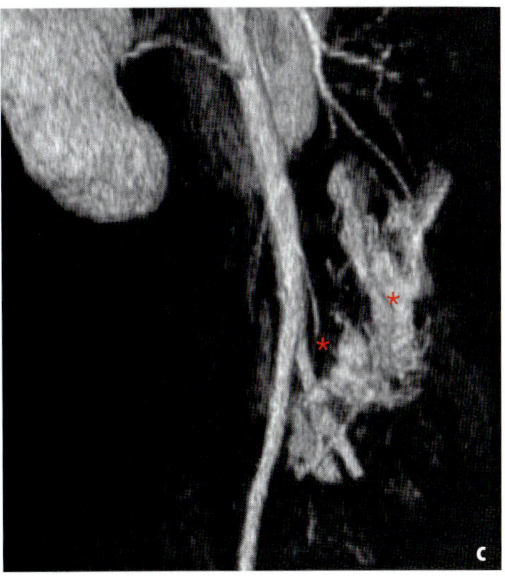

Fig. 15a-c. Active extravasation (*) from the inferior mesenteric artery (IMA) (*arrow*) depicted on the **a** axial computed tomography (CT), **b** sagittal maximum intensity projection (MIP), **c** and volume rendering (VR) images from a 44-year-old man who became hypotensive and unresponsive after suffering a motor vehicle collision

Renal Vascular Imaging

CTA is replacing conventional angiography in evaluation of renal vascular anatomy and pathology. Indications for renal CTA include renal donor transplant evaluation, renovascular hypertension workup and posttreatment assessment, oncologic perioperative staging, planning, and surveillance, and renal anomaly/variant workup. Advancement in technology, optimization of CTA protocols, and improvement of contrast application have allowed reliable and accurate depiction of renal vascular pathology [7–11, 22–24].

Imaging Techniques

After drinking approximately 1 liter of water for enteric contrast, patients should have an intravenous line at least 20 gauge or larger placed in the antecubital fossa. The patient lies supine, head first, on the CT table. Scanning is performed with the patient holding his or her breath at end inspiration. For concomitant assessment of the kidneys,

including calcification and hemorrhage, unenhanced CT images are obtained. For assessment of renal artery anatomy for surgical planning and renovascular disease, MDCT with 16 detector rows or more should be used to acquire thin-section (<1-mm) arterial images. Nephrographic-phase renal imaging is critical for evaluation of the renal parenchyma and mass. Scanning protocols for 16- and 64-slice MDCT are shown in Tables.

Applications

Living Renal Donor Evaluation and Renal Mass Surgical Planning

Renal CTA is extremely accurate in delineating the renal artery and vein anatomy [25] (Fig. 16). As laparoscopic surgery for renal harvesting is common, to prevent an undesirable or possibly life-threatening outcome, accurate preoperative knowledge of the presence of renal arterial and venous location and variant is essential for planning [26]. Almost 30% of patients may have variant renal vascular anatomy [7] (Fig. 17). Renal MDCTA has a mean accuracy of 94% in detecting accessory arteries, 95% in depicting early branching (Fig. 17c), and 98% in demonstrating renal-vein anomalies [27, 28]. Atypical location and diameter of adjacent vessels, such as lumbar, adrenal, and gonadal veins, must be identified to prevent or minimize complications during surgery [27]. Imaging is also crucial to define vascular anatomy in patients with renal anomalies for treatment planning (Fig. 18).

Renal Artery Pathology

Renovascular Hypertension (RVH) Assessment

Given its low prevalence of approximately 1%, RVH is usually screened with a minimally inva-sive or noninvasive imaging technique for high-risk patients [29]. Renovascular hypertension re-sults from decreases renal perfusion secondary to a severe renal arterial lesion; the most common cause is atherosclerotic renal artery stenosis (RAS) near the origin (Fig. 19). Fibromuscular dysplasia (FMD) (Fig. 20) is the second most com-mon cause, with the most prevalent type being medial fibroplasia, which presents with the "string-of-beads" appearance [11]. CTA is highly sensitive in the diagnosis of FMD [30]. As RVH is potentially treatable, its diagnosis is important. Because the renal arteries have a circuitous path, evaluation of these vessels is challenging and ne-cessitates the use of a 3-D image display worksta-tion. The caliber of the renal artery is evaluated more accurately with MPR than MIP reconstruc-

Table 4. Renal computed tomography angiography (CTA) parameters for 64-slice multi-detector row computed tomography (MDCT)[a]

Phase	Noncontrast	Arterial/corticomedullary	Nephrographic
kVp/effective mAs/rotation time (s)	120/240/0.5	120/240/0.5	120/240/0.5
Detector collimation (mm)	0.6	0.6	0.6
Slice thickness (mm)	3	1	2
Beam pitch	1	1	1
Recon increment (mm)	3	0.7	1
Scan delay		Bolus tracking	90 s

[a] Scan parameters from Siemens Sensation 64

Table 5. Renal computed tomography angiography (CTA) parameters for 16-slice multidetector-row computed tomography (MDCT)[a]

Phase	Noncontrast	Arterial/corticomedullary	Nephrographic
kVp/effective mAs/rotation time (s)	120/240/0.5	120/240/0.5	120/240/0.5
Detector collimation (mm)	1.5	0.75	1.5
Slice thickness (mm)	3	1	2
Feed/rotation (mm)	24	10	24
Recon increment (mm)	3	0.7	1
Scan delay		Bolus tracking	90 s

[a] Scan parameters from Siemens Sensation 16

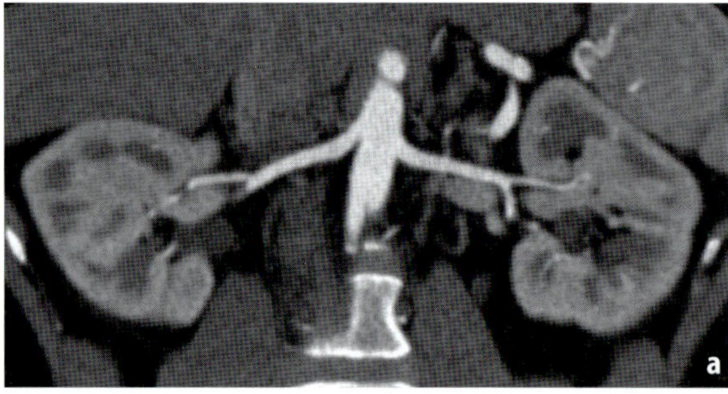
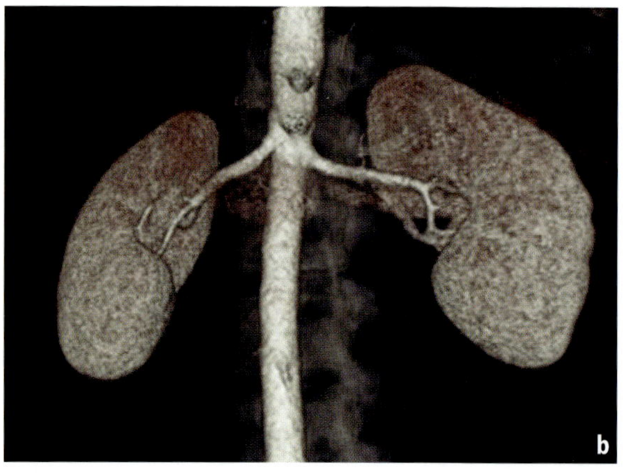

Fig. 16a, b. Single bilateral normal renal arteries seen on the **a** multiplanar reformatting (MPR) and **b** volume rendering (VR) im-age in a 32-year-old woman being evaluated for a potential renal donor

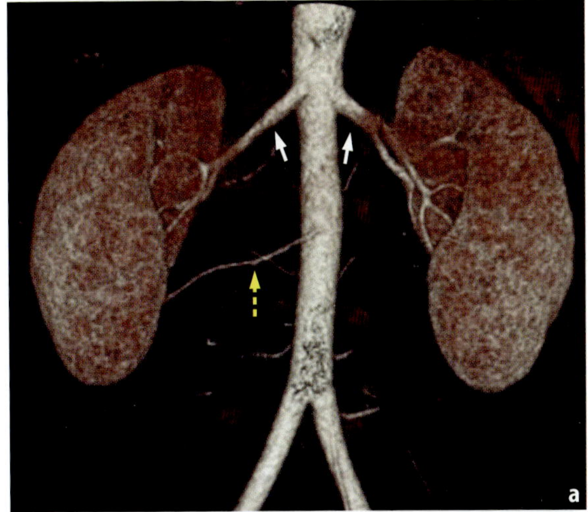
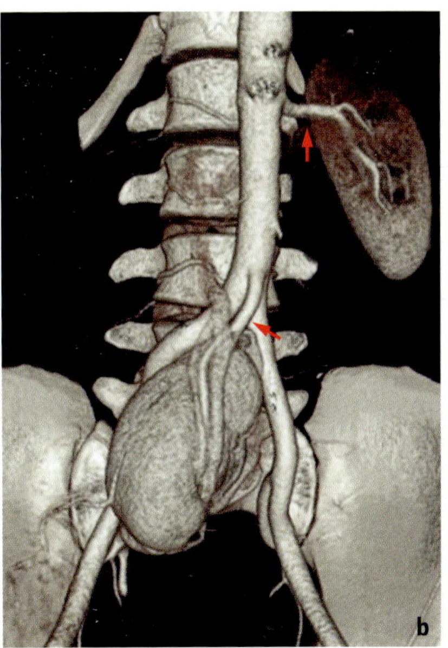
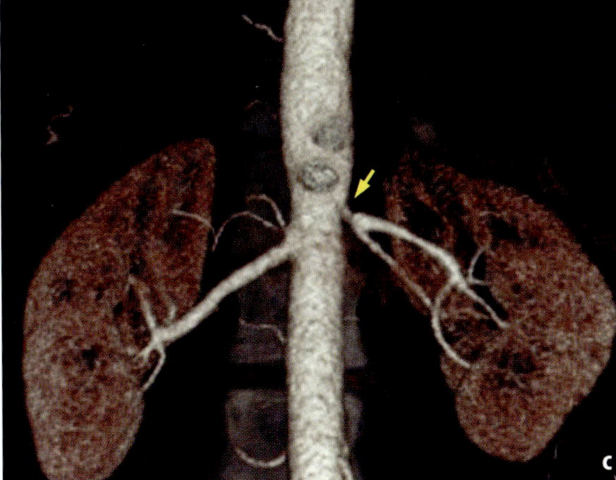

Fig. 17a, b. Volume rendering (VR) images of the renal arteries from three different patients being evaluated for potential renal donors. **a** Right-sided accessory renal artery (*dashed yellow arrow*), **b** right-sided pelvic kidney (*red arrow*), and **c** left-sided early bifurcating renal artery with incidentally discovered renal artery stenosis (*yellow arrow*) at the origin

tion [31]. VR technique is reported to have a higher specificity (99%) than MIP (87%) for demonstrating RAS [9]. Indirect findings of RAS include a smooth but atrophic kidney, poststenotic dilatation, delayed and prolonged nephrogram, and thinned renal cortex [7] (Fig. 21). After revascularization of RAS, CTA can be used to evaluate renal stent patency [32].

Renal Artery Aneurysms

Renal artery aneurysms (RAA) can be readily depicted with MIP and VR images. RAA is mainly due to atherosclerosis but can be seen with pregnancy, FMD, and neurofibromatosis. Pseudoaneurysms may be seen secondary to trauma, inflammation, and surgical complications (Fig. 22) [7].

Renal Venous Disorder

Renal vein thrombosis can be readily assessed with MDCTA. The etiology of renal vein thrombosis includes renal or adrenal malignancies, glomerulonephritis, collagen vascular disease, sepsis, diabetes, and severe dehydration. The renal venous enhancement typically peaks during the corticomedullary phase [7], unless the scan delay used for the corticomedullary phase is too early to allow a complete drain of the renal vein.

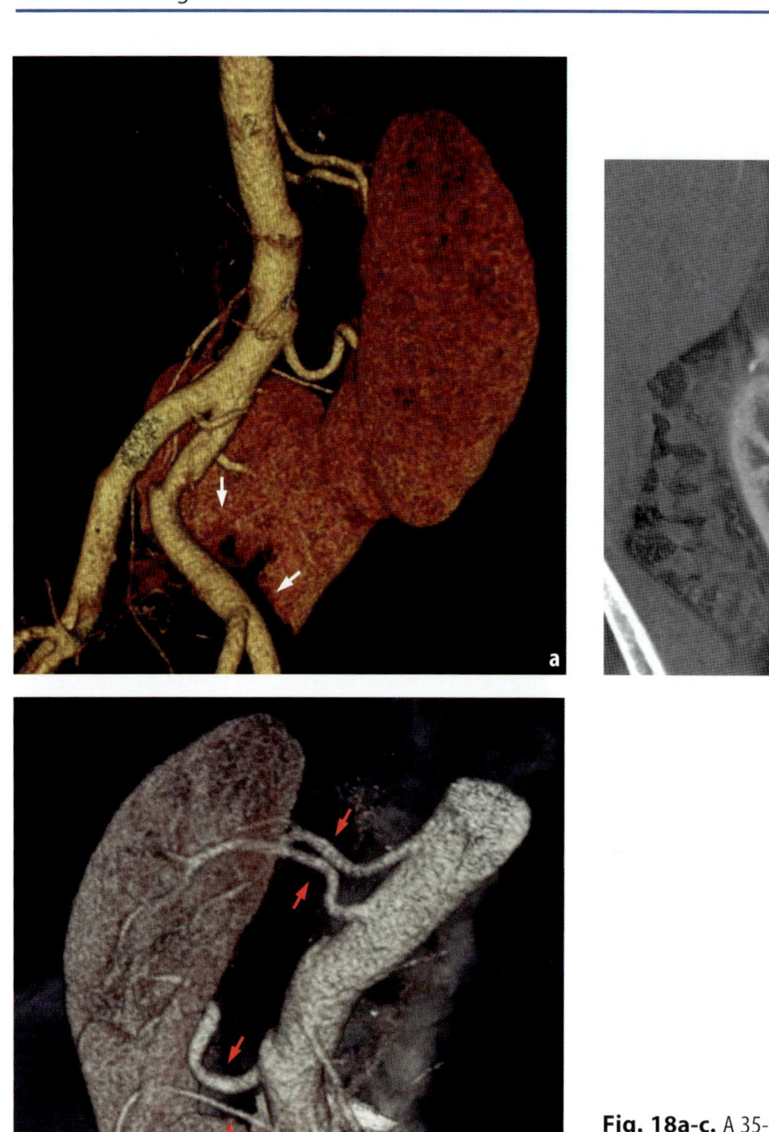

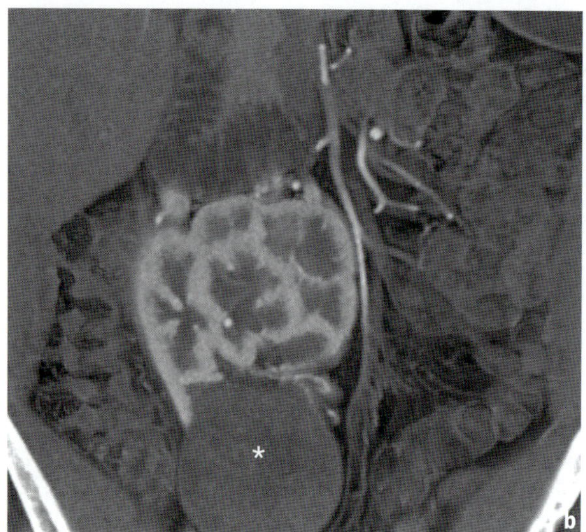

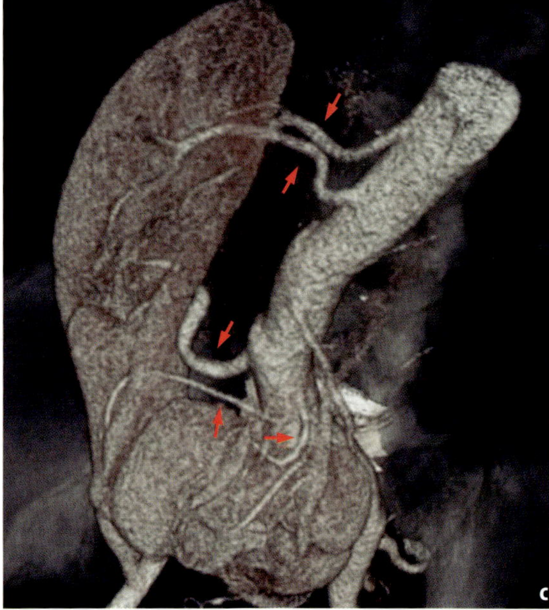

Fig. 18a-c. A 35-year-old man with crossed fused renal ectopia who was diagnosed with a renal mass suspected to be renal cell carcinoma underwent renal computed tomography angiography (CTA) to delineate the vascular anatomy for surgical planning. **a** Volume rendering (VR) in the prone projection reveals a mass (*arrows*) in the inferior aspect of the anomalous kidney. **b** On the coronal multiplanar reformatting (MPR) image, the hypovascular mass (*) is depicted. **c** Five renal arteries (*red arrows*) are identified on the oblique VR projection

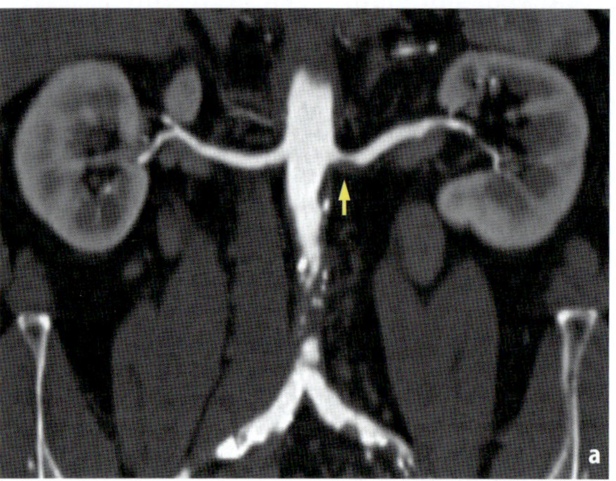

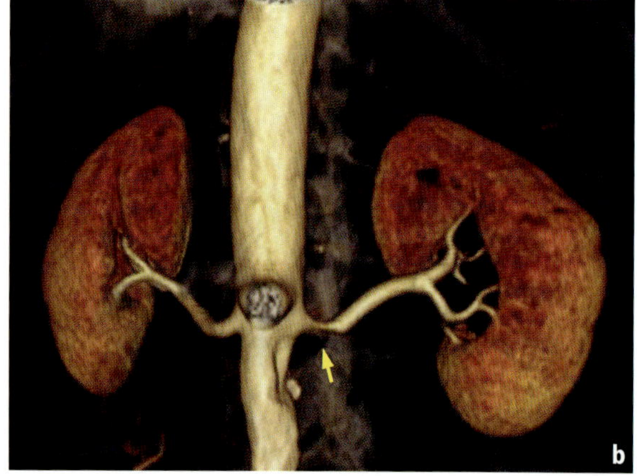

Fig. 19a, b. A significant left-sided renal artery stenosis (*arrow*) near the ostium from atherosclerotic mural plaque is seen on the **a** curved planar reformatting (CP) and **b** volume rendering (VR) images in a 68-year-old man with hypertension and peripheral vascular disease

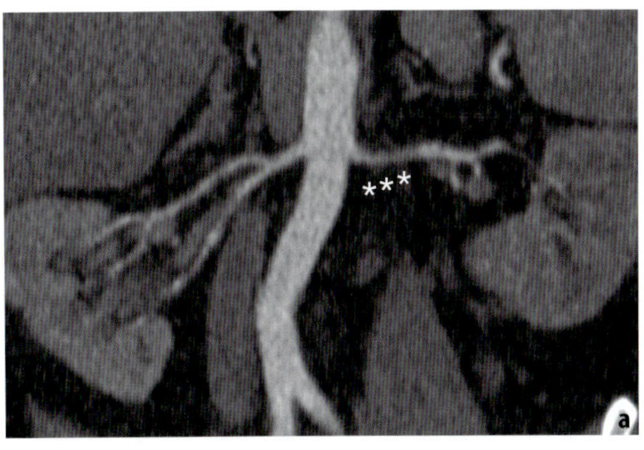

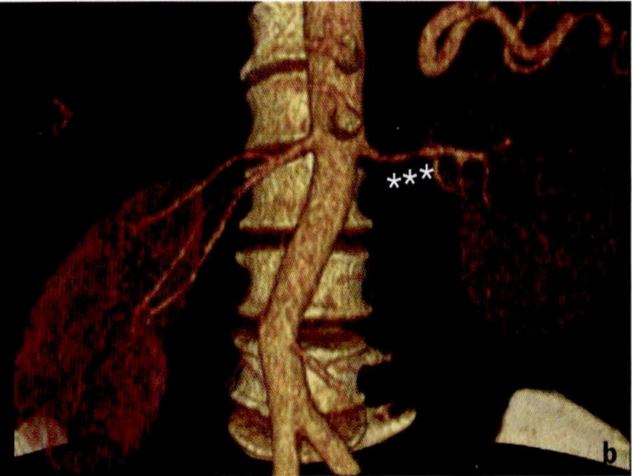

Fig. 20a,b. Irregularly beaded left renal artery (*arrows*) consistent with fibromuscular dysplasia seen on the **a** coronal curved planar reformatting (CP) and **b** volume rendering (VR) images in a 40-year-old man with refractory hypertension

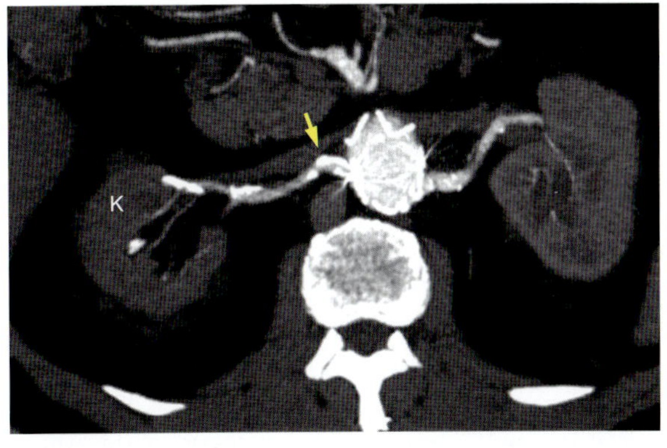

Fig. 21. Right renal artery stenosis from calcified atherosclerotic plaques (*arrow*) near the ostium as shown on this axial thick-section maximum intensity projection (MIP) with right renal atrophy and delayed perfusion

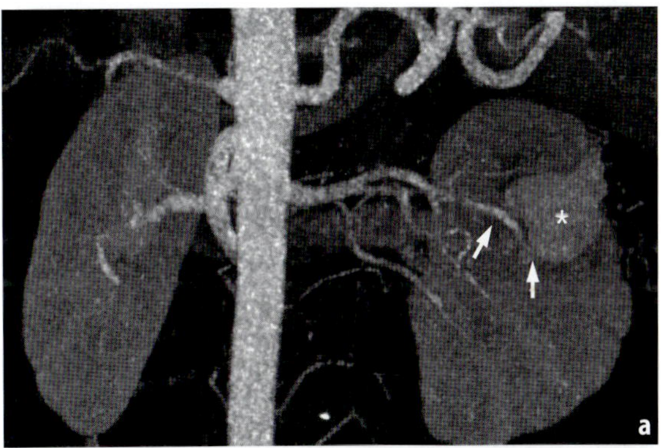

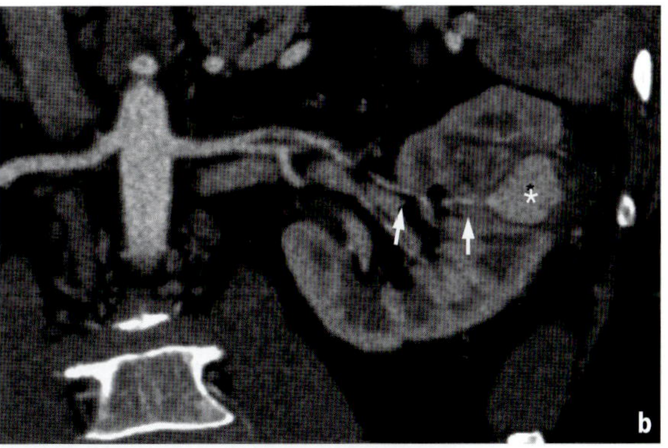

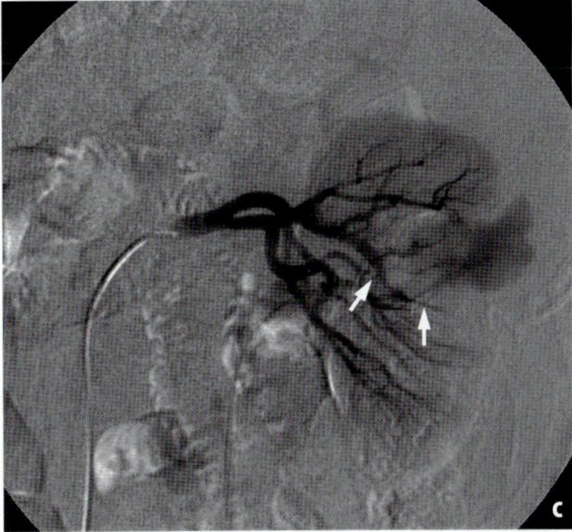

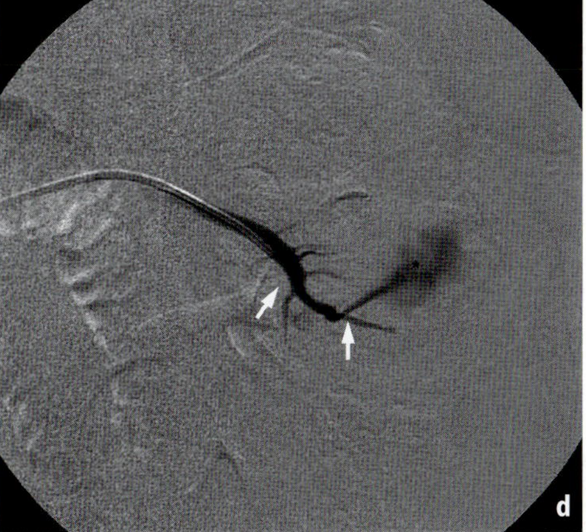

Fig. 22a-d. Pseudoaneurysm (*) with a feeding renal artery (*arrows*) in the left kidney near the postsurgical bed seen on **a** maximum intensity projection (MIP) and **b** curved planar reformatting (CP) images. This is a 47-year-old man status post a partial nephrectomy of the left kidney for renal cell carcinoma. **c, d** Computed tomography angiography (CTA) findings are confirmed on the conventional renal angiogram

Conclusion

Because of its minimal invasiveness and depiction of 3-D cross-sectional anatomy, CTA is supplanting conventional angiography for many diagnostic applications. The use of CTA to delineate the anatomy and to detect pathology of the mesenteric and renal vessels is growing. CT scanning and contrast administration protocols are rapidly evolving, as with the advance of MDCT technology. CT radiation dosage to the patient should be minimized and limited by diligently customizing the scanning protocols to adapt to each patient's clinical question. Magnetic resonance angiography can be used when radiation exposure is a concern or when iodinated contrast medium is contraindicated. The storing of immense image data sets can be a challenge. Advancing technology has kept abreast of this issue. The evaluation of 3-D vascular anatomy often involves a review of numerous images and detail anatomy and thus may take longer than the evaluation with conventional angiography. Furthermore, one must also pay attention to the extravascular findings, as alternative or additional pathology may be detected from the CT images.

References

1. Bae KT, Heiken JP, Brink JA (1998) Aortic and hepatic contrast medium at CT part I. Prediction with a computer model. Radiology 207:647–655
2. Bae KT, Heiken JP, Brink JA (1998) Aortic and hepatic contrast medium at CT part II. Effect of reduced cardiac output in a porcine model. Radiology 207:657–662
3. Fleischmann D (2002) Present and future trends in multiple detector-row CT applications: CT angiography. Eur Radiol 12[Suppl 2]:S11–S16
4. Haage P, Schmitz-Rode T, Hubner D et al (2000) Reduction of contrast material dose and artifacts by a saline flush using a double power injector in helical CT of the thorax. AJR Am J Roentgenol 174:1049–1053
5. Van Hoe L, Marchal G, Baert AL et al (1995) Determination of scan delay-time in spiral CT-angiography: Utility of a test bolus injection. J Comput Assist Tomogr 19:216–220
6. Rubin GD (2003) 3-D imaging with multidetector CT. Eur J Radiol 45[Suppl 1]:S37–S41
7. Sheth S, Fishman E (2004) Multi-detector row CT of the kidneys and urinary tract: Techniques and applications in the diagnosis of benign disease. Radiographics 24:e20 http://radiographics.rsnajnls.org/cgi/content/full/e20v1. Cited 30 Jan 2006
8. Kuszyk BS, Heath DG, Ney DR et al (1995) CT angiography with volume rendering: imaging findings. AJR Am J Roentgenol 165:445–448
9. Johnson PT, Halpern EJ, Kuszyk BS et al (1999) Renal artery stenosis: CT angiography – comparison of real-time volume rendering and maximum intensity projection algorithms. Radiology 211:337–343
10. Kattee R, Beek F, de Lange E et al (1997) Renal artery stenosis: detection and quantification with spiral CT angiography and optimized digital subtraction angiography. Radiology 205:121–127
11. Urban BA, Ratner LE, Fishman EK (2001) Three-dimensional volume rendered CT angiography of the renal arteries and veins: Normal anatomy, variants, and clinical applications. Radiographics 21:373–386
12. Horton KM, Fishman EK (2002) Volume-rendered 3D CT of the mesenteric vasculature: normal anatomy, anatomic variants, and pathologic conditions. Radiographics 22:161–172
13. Hong KC, Freeny PC (1999) Pancreaticoduodenal arcades and dorsal pancreatic artery: comparison of CT angiography with three dimensional volume rendering, maximum intensity projection, and shaded-surface display. AJR Am J Roentgenol 172:925–931
14. Horton KM and Fishman EK (2001) Multi-detector row CT of the mesenteric ischemia: Can it be done? Radiographics 21:1463–1473
15. Foley WD (2002) Multidetector CT: abdominal visceral imaging. Radiographics 22:701–719
16. Lu DS, Reber HA, Krasny RM et al (1997) Local staging of pancreatic cancer: criteria for unresectability of major vessels as revealed by pancreatic phase, thin section helical CT. AJR Am J Roentgenol 168:1439–1443
17. Raptopoulos V, Steer ML, Sheiman RG et al (1997) The use of helical CT and CT angiography to predict vascular involvement from pancreatic cancer: correlation with findings at surgery. AJR Am J Roentgenol 168:971–977
18. Taourel PG, Deneuville M, Pradel JA et al (1996) Acute mesenteric ischemia: diagnosis with contrast enhanced CT. Radiology 199:632–636
19. James S, Balfe DM, Lee JKT et al (1987) Small bowel disease, categorization by CT examination. AJR Am J Roentgenol 148:863–868
20. Bartnicke BJ, Balfe DM (1994) CT appearance of intestinal ischemia and intramural hemorrhage. Radiol Clin North Am 32:845–860
21. Fishman EK (2001) CT Angiography: Clinical applications in the abdomen. Radiographics 21:S3–S16
22. Platt JF, Ellis JH, Korobkin M, Reige K (1997) Helical CT evaluation of potential kidney donors: findings in 154 subjects. AJR Am J Roentgenol 169:1325–1330
23. Smith PA, Ratner LE, Lynch FC et al (1998) Role of CT angiography in the preoperative evaluation for laparoscopic nephrectomy. Radiographics 18:589–601
24. Rubin GD, Alfrey EJ, Dake MD et al (1995) Assessment of living renal donors with spiral CT. Radiology 195:457–462
25. Rankin SC, Jan W, Koffman CG (2001) Noninvasive imaging of living related kidney donors: evaluation with CT angiography and gadolinium enhanced MR angiography. AJR AM J Roentgenol 177:349–355
26. Rydberg J, Kopecky KK, Tann M et al (2001) Evaluation of prospective living renal donors for laparoscopic nephrectomy with multisection CT: the marriage of minimally invasive imaging with minimally invasive surgery. Radiographics 21:S223–S236
27. Kawamoto S, Montgomery RA, Lawler LP et al

(2003) Multidetector CT angiography for preoperative evaluation of living laparoscopic kidney donors. AJR Am J Roentgenol 180:1633–1638

28. Sahani DV, Rastogi N, Greenfield AC et al (2005) Multi-detector row CT in evaluation of 94 living renal donors by readers with varied experience. Radiology 235:905–910

29. Grenier N, Trillaud H (2000) Comparison of imaging methods for renal artery stenosis. BJU International 86[Suppl 1]: 84–94

30. Beregi JP, Louvegny S, Gautier C et al (1999) Fibromuscular dysplasia of the renal arteries: comparison of helical CT angiography and arteriography. AJR Am J Roentgenol 172:27–34

31. Galanski M, Prokop M, Chavam A et al (1993) Renal artery stenoses: spiral CT angiography. Radiology 189:185–192

32. Behar JV, Nelson RC, Zidar JP et al (2002) Thin-section multidetector CT angiography of renal artery stents. AJR Am J Roentgenol 178:1155–1159

33. Lin PH, Chaikof EL (2000) Embryology, anatomy, and surgical exposure of the great abdominal vessels. Surg Clin North Am 80(1):417–433

34. Lalani TA, Kanne JP, Hatfield GA et al (2004) Imaging findings in systemic lupus erythematosus. Radiographics 24: 1069–1086

35. Olin JW (2000) Thromboangiitis obliterans (Buerger's disease). NEJM 343:864–869

36. Nakamura K, Nozue M, Sakakibara Y et al (1997) Natural history of a spontaneous dissecting aneurysm of the proximal superior mesenteric artery: Report of a case. Surg Today 27:272–274

13

Multi-detector Computed Tomography in the Gastrointestinal System

Avinash R. Kambadakone, Dushyant V. Sahani

Introduction

The advent of multi-detector computed tomography (MDCT) has opened new paradigms in the imaging of the abdomen and pelvis, particularly in the evaluation of the gastrointestinal tract (GIT). The use of MDCT scanners that acquire isotropic volume data and the advances in imaging workstations that allow multi-planar and three-dimensional (3-D) evaluation of these isotropic data sets have allowed accurate depiction and characterization of bowel pathology. Substantial information regarding the GIT can now be obtained due to recent technological advances and accumulated experience in image interpretation [1].

The benefits of MDCT over single-detector CT include increased temporal resolution, improved spatial resolution, increased concentration of intravascular contrast material, decreased image noise, efficient X-ray tube use, and longer anatomic coverage, which increases the diagnostic accuracy of the examination [2]. Better z-axis resolution and larger scan volumes also result in improved multiplanar reconstruction in the coronal and sagittal planes. The reduced scanning time achieved by MDCT also reduce respiratory and motion artifacts. The diagnostic capabilities of MDCT examinations of the GIT have been enhanced by the ability of these scanners to visualize the bowel wall and to distend the lumen with the use of neutral luminal oral contrast materials (OCMs) [3].

An emerging and nearly well-established application of MDCT in the GIT is virtual endoscopy, which involves perspective volume rendering of the isotropic data. Virtual techniques (virtual gastroscopy, virtual enteroscopy, and virtual colonoscopy) not only provide endoscope-like views of the bowel, but they also depict extra-luminal pathology. Here we discuss the key concepts in MDCT evaluation of the GIT, with emphasis on the practical aspects. A brief review of the clinical applications of MDCT in the various bowel pathologies then follows.

Protocol Design

The key determinants for optimal evaluation of the GIT on MDCT examination are adequate bowel distension, intravenous contrast administration, volume acquisition, and post-processing. In addition, good contrast between the bowel lumen and the bowel wall is an indispensable component of GIT evaluation.

Bowel Distension and Oral Contrast

Adequate distension of the bowel wall is obligatory for the evaluation of wall thickness, since collapsed loops of bowel can falsely show bowel wall thickening. The normal thickness of the gastric wall is ≤ 5 mm at CT, whereas a thickness of > 1 cm can be caused by any abnormality, benign or malignant [4, 5]. The thickness of the normal small-bowel wall depends on the degree of luminal distension and is between 1 and 2 mm when the lumen is well-distended [1]. A measurement of < 3 mm is used as the upper limit of normal thickness [6]. The normal colonic wall is often imperceptible but is usually < 3 mm in thickness when well distended [7, 8]. The colon normally contains fecal contents and fluid, which can sometimes make the assessment of true thickness difficult.

Bowel distension and optimal contrast between the bowel wall and lumen are achieved by the administration of intraluminal (oral/rectal) contrast agents. The intraluminal oral contrast media used can be positive or negative/neutral; either works well in delineating the bowel. The degree of distension achieved by these contrast agents is proportional to the amount of contrast material ad-

Table 1. Positive oral contrast agents: salient features

- Oral contrast of choice for demonstration of hollow viscus perforation/contrast media extravasation
- Preferred agent for the demonstration of fistulas/sinus tracts
- Preferred agent in routine scans of abdomen and pelvis
- Other indications: pelvic peritoneal metastases, post-operative cases, intra-abdominal abscess, acute appendicitis, tube pre-check procedure, ascites, and extra-intestinal masses

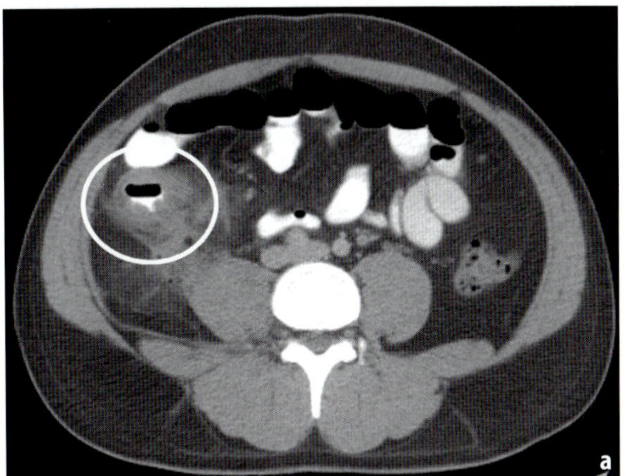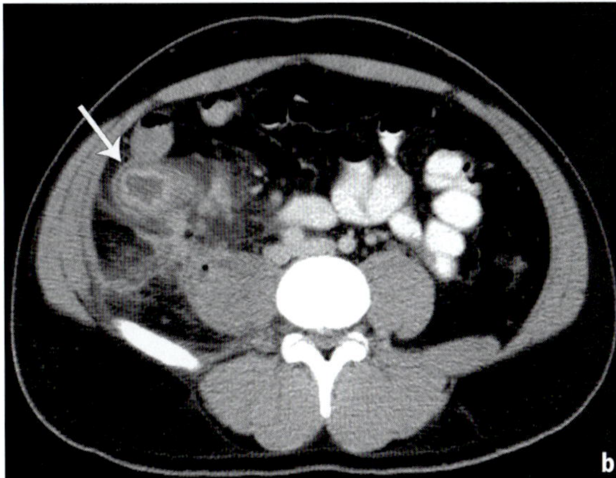

Fig. 1a, b. A 22-year-old man with known Crohn's disease who had two multi-detector computed tomography (MDCT) exams within a short interval. The gastrointestinal tract was labeled with positive and neutral oral contrast medium (OCM). **a** Representative axial image of contrast-enhanced CT exam with positive oral contrast shows mural thickening and regional stranding in the terminal ileum (*circle*). **b** On the corresponding axial CT image with neutral OCM, the changes in bowel inflammation, mainly mural and mucosal enhancement (*arrow*), are better appreciated

ministered, the rate at which it is administered, the bowel transit time, and the time delay of the examination itself [9].

The positive oral contrast materials (POCM) used include dilute barium (2–5%) and diluted water-soluble iodinated contrast medium. Because of the vast experience with positive contrast materials and unequivocal identification of the opacified bowel loop, they have been routinely used as oral contrast agents in GIT studies (Table 1). Positive oral contrast materials rely on structural changes in the bowel to demonstrate pathological lesions. These compounds have been found to be particularly well suited in evaluating thin patients without a lot of intraperitoneal fat, and oncology patients, in whom implants and lymph nodes will stand out from the small bowel [9]. The distinct advantage of positive OCMs includes their ability to demonstrate extravasations in the event of hollow viscus perforation. However, their potential limitation in evaluation of the bowel is the problem of obscuration of the mucosal enhancement by luminal contrast material [9] (Fig. 1). Positive OCMs can thus mask subtle pathological lesions in the gut wall, making evaluation of the pattern of enhancement difficult. Poor mixing of these contrast agents can also mimic pseudo-lesions on CT examinations.

Neutral oral contrast materials (NOCM) refers to agents that have an attenuation value similar to that of water (10–30 HU) (Table 2). Due to their

Table 2. Negative/neutral oral contrast agents: salient features

Negative oral contrast agent
- Negative contrast agents (air) are used for virtual endoscopic studies (virtual gastroscopy/virtual colonoscopy)

Neutral oral contrast agent
- Neutral contrast agents are contrast agents of choice for CT enterography
- Recommended for identifying mucosal enhancement and subtle mucosal abnormalities
- Do not interfere with data manipulation during 3-D imaging (CT angiography)
- Preferred agents for non-GIT indications: liver/pancreatic/renal mass, and CT urography
- Recommended for PET/CT examinations since they eliminate correction artifacts
- Indications: inflammatory bowel disease, GIT polyps and tumors, GIT bleeding, and mesenteric ischemia

CT computed tomography, *GIT* gastrointestinal tract

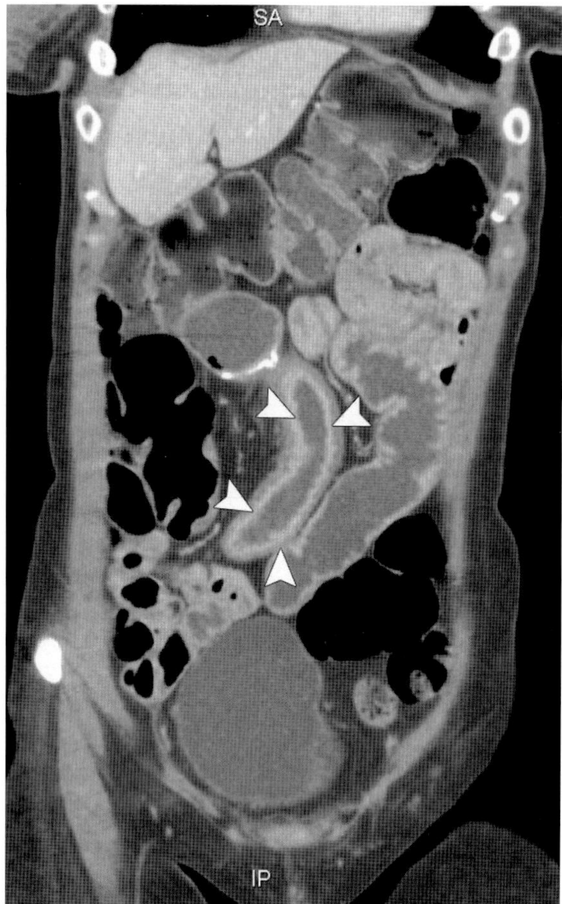

Fig. 2. Contrast-enhanced coronal reformatted computed tomography (CT) enterography image from a patient with Crohn's relapse. The presence of mural enhancement (*arrowheads*) after intravenous administration of contrast medium is an indicator of active disease. These changes are more conspicuous due to neutral oral contrast material (OCM), which provides the appropriate background

low attenuation, these agents allow complete visualization of the bowel wall and help in analysis of the degree and pattern of bowel-wall enhancement [10] (Figs. 1, 2). Low-attenuation neutral OCMs are preferred over positive agents when a mucosal abnormality is suspected [11]. Neutral OCMs are extremely comfortable to work with in angiographic studies, since they do not interfere with data manipulation during 3-D imaging. For neutral contrast agents to be effective, they must be used with intravenous contrast media and bowel distension must be optimal. Several neutral contrast agents have been evaluated, including water, water in combination with methylcellulose or locust bean gum, polyethylene glycol solutions, and a commercially available low-density barium solution (VoLumen) [3, 10, 12]. Water, although freely available and more acceptable, is rapidly absorbed across the small-intestinal mucosa, resulting in suboptimal distension of the distal bowel. VoLumen and polyethylene glycol solutions are

less rapidly absorbed and have been found to be superior to both water and methylcellulose in achieving bowel distension. VoLumen consists of gum system, sorbitol, and barium (0.1%, w/v). It has an attenuation value of 15–30 HU and has a berry taste because of the small amount of grape Kool-Aid added to it. A pitfall of the neutral contrast agents is their inability to identify extravasations. A practical outline of the oral contrast protocol is discussed below.

Inhibition of Bowel Peristalsis
Intramuscular or intravenous scopolamine butylbromide 20 mg (Buscopan, Boehringer International, Ingelheim, Germany) can be administered 10–15 min before the study to relax the bowel wall and reduce peristaltic bowel movement [13]. This is particularly helpful in virtual endoscopic procedures, such as CT gastrography and CT colonography, to achieve adequate distension of the bowel and to prevent spasm.

Stomach and Duodenum
Prior to the CT examination, the patient should be prepared by fasting overnight or at least for 5 h so that the stomach is devoid of food residue. A water-filling technique in which 600–1000 ml of tap water is ingested is frequently used for optimal distension of the stomach [14, 15]. For oral contrast agents, around 900–1000 ml of neutral contrast agent yields optimal distension and allows evaluation of various gastroduodenal lesions (Fig. 3). For CT gastrography/virtual gastroscopy, 8 g of effervescent granules taken with 10 ml tap water results in adequate gaseous distension of the stomach and duodenum through the release of bicarbonate granules [13, 16, 17]. Although desirable, positioning the patient in the right and left posterior oblique positions [11, 18] to maximize opacification of the duodenum is not usually performed due to workflow constraints.

Small Intestine
Depending on the clinical indication, the small intestine is evaluated by routine abdominopelvic CT scan or CT enterography. The protocol for the administration of positive oral contrast agents for visualization of the small intestine is discussed in Table 3.

CT enterography is performed for the focused evaluation of the small bowel with neutral oral contrast agents (Fig. 4). The use of thin sections and of large volumes of enteric contrast material in CT enterography accounts for the superior display of the small-bowel lumen and wall compared with routine abdominopelvic CT [12]. CT enterography helps in the excellent assessment of hypervascular lesions and hyperenhancing segments through the use of neutral OCMs and intravenous

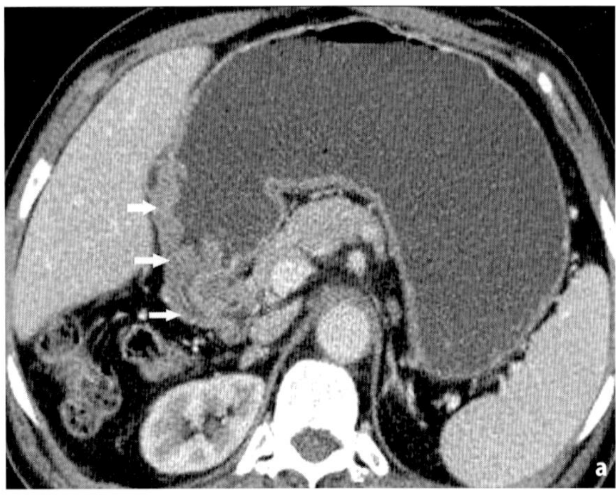
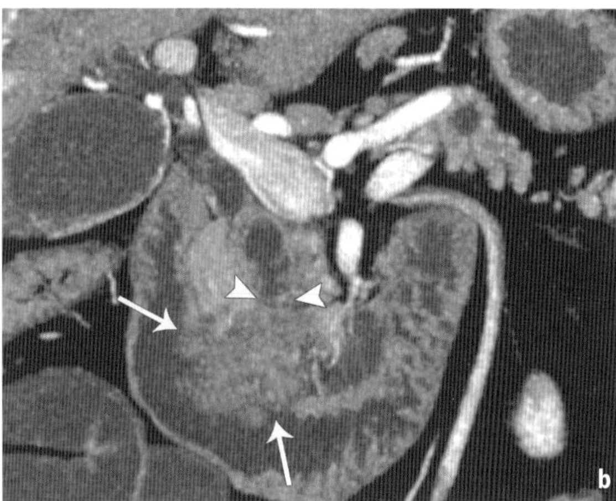

Fig. 3a, b. Post-contrast multi-detector row computed tomography (MDCT) images from two different patients studied with neutral oral contrast material (OCM). **a** Axial image in a patient with gastric carcinoma shows distended stomach and nodular wall thickening (*small arrows*) in the antrum. **b** Coronal reformatted image in another patient with peri-ampullary carcinoma demonstrates a well-distended duodenum with a polypoidal ampullary tumor extending into the lumen (*large arrows*) and causing distal obstruction of the common bile duct (*arrowheads*). Note that distension of the duodenal lumen with neutral contrast agent improves the accuracy of diagnosing the luminal component

Table 3. Positive oral contrast protocol for MDCT of small intestine

Barium 2% (Readicat 2) protocol
- Total volume: 900 ml (2 bottles of 450 ml each)
- 1st drink given over 40 min
- 2nd drink given over 20 min
  Scan to be done within 60 min of the 1st drink

Gastrografin protocol
- Dilute 7.5 ml of Gastrografin in 10 ounces (300 ml) of liquid (one drink)
- Three drinks given over 60 min prior to the scan
  1st drink given over 20 min
  2nd drink given over 20 min
  3rd drink given over 20 min

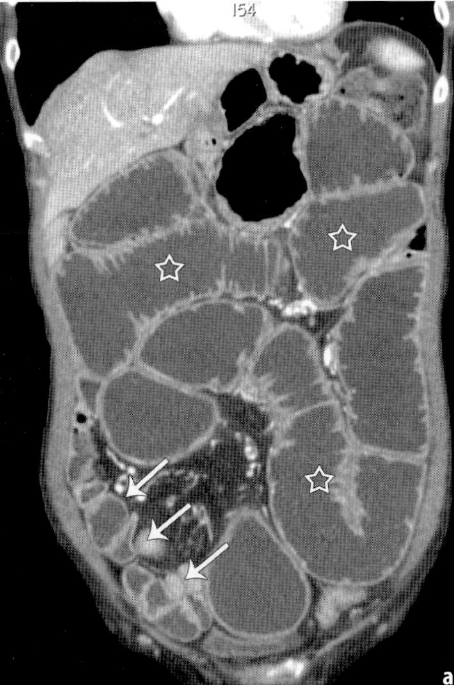

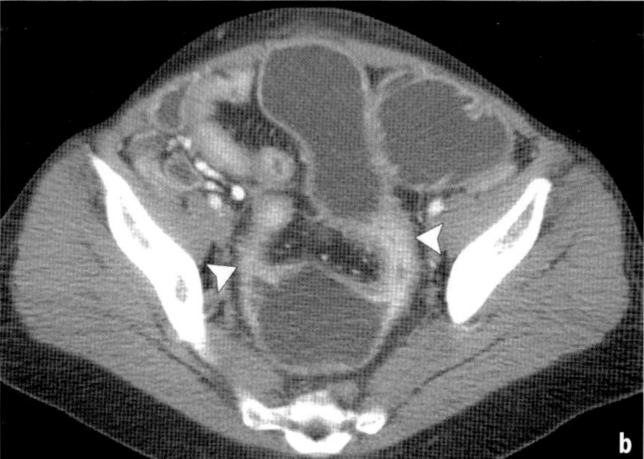

Fig. 4a, b. Computed tomography (CT) enterography images from a 30-year-old man presenting with small-bowel obstruction. **a** Contrast-enhanced coronal reformatted image shows multiple dilated jejunal loops (*stars*) with collapsed distal bowel segments (*white arrows*). **b** On the representative axial image, two strictures (*arrowheads*) with associated mural enhancement and wall thickening are evident. Diagnosis of Crohn's disease was established on histopathology

Table 4. Computed tomography (CT) enterography: oral contrast protocol for small bowel

- Total oral contrast volume: 1,800 ml (1,350 ml of VoLumen + 450 ml of water)
- Started 60 min prior to CT scan:
  - 450 ml of VoLumen over 20 min (total 3 bottles: 1,350 ml)
  - One glass of water (450 ml) on scanner table 5–10 min prior to scanning

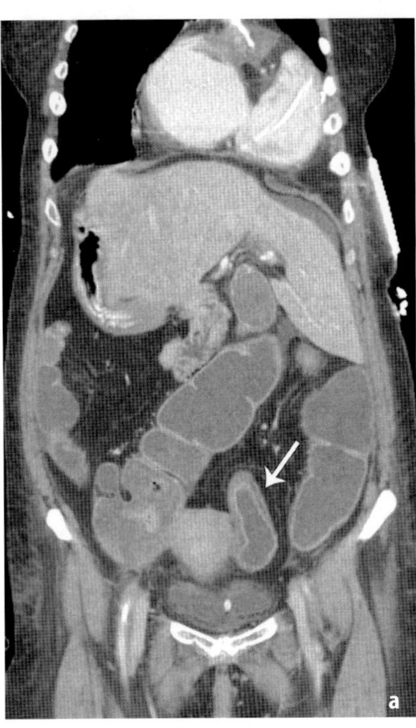
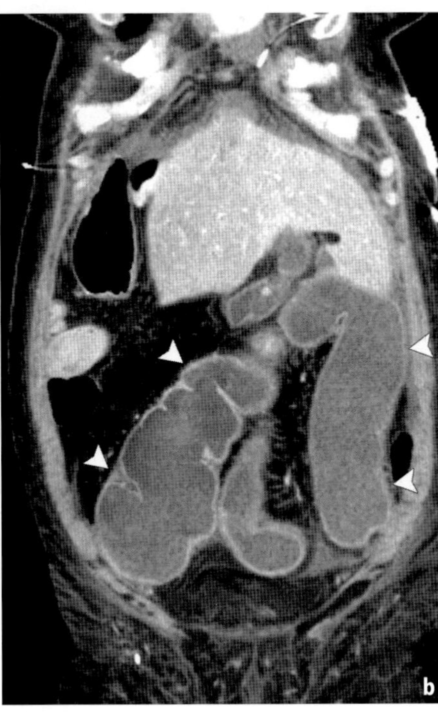

Fig. 5. Coronal reformatted multi-detector computed tomography (MDCT) enterography images obtained with neutral oral contrast material (OCM) in a 24-year-old man with ulcerative colitis. The extent of diffuse changes (*arrowheads*) of mucosal enhancement and mural thickening (*arrow*) typical to inflammatory bowel disease are eloquently displayed on the coronal images in the background of neutral OCM

contrast [12]. The ability of this technique to display the entire thickness of the intestinal wall, its surrounding mesentery, and peri-enteric fat and to allow examination of the deep ileal loops in the pelvis without superimposition makes it the preferred approach compared with traditional small-bowel follow-through examinations [12]. It also helps in the assessment of the solid organs and thus provides a global overview of the abdomen [12]. CT enterography is a useful and well-tolerated study for the evaluation of diseases affecting the mucosa and bowel wall, since it obviates the need for naso-enteric intubation and attains satisfactory luminal distension by oral hyperhydration [12].

The neutral contrast agent VoLumen is the oral contrast used for CT enterography in our department. A total volume of 1,350 ml VoLumen is administered over a period of 60 min prior to the CT examination (Table 4). Patients ingest three 450-ml bottles of VoLumen, the first one 60 min before the CT, the second one 40 min before, and the third one 20 min before the procedure. The patient consumes a glass of water on the scanner table 5–10 min prior to scanning. The role of water as a final contrast agent is intended primarily for the distension of the stomach and duodenum [9].

When water is used as a contrast agent for abdominal exams, two glasses of water are to be ingested: the first glass in the waiting room over 20 min and the second glass 20 min later, when the patient is on the table. For CT examinations of the abdomen and pelvis, three glasses of water are used: the first at 40 min before CT, the second 20 min later, and the third when the patient is on the table.

The oral contrast protocol needs to be modified according to the clinical situation. For patients with bowel obstruction, either positive or neutral oral contrast can be used. In patients in whom mesenteric ischemia is suspected, the administration of oral contrast depends upon the patient's clinical condition (Table 2).

Colon

Comprehensive assessment of the colon requires the administration of both oral and rectal contrast agents. In the evaluation of inflammatory colonic diseases, a combination of oral, rectal, and intravenous contrast is recommended to accurately demonstrate the inflammatory changes in the colonic wall and to assess the extent of the disease [19] (Fig. 5). A delay of 1–1.5 h is recommended following the administration of oral contrast for adequate opacification of the colon (Table 5).

More often, it is the radiologist who decides

Table 5. Oral contrast protocol for colon

Positive contrast (Readicat 2) protocol
- 1st drink given over 40 min
- 2nd drink given over 30 min
- 3rd drink given over 20 min
  Scan to be done within 90-120 min of the 1st drink

VoLumen protocol
- Total oral contrast volume: 1800 ml (1350 ml of VoLumen + 450 ml of water)
- Started 60-90 min prior to CT
  - 450 ml of VoLumen to be taken over 30 min (total: 3 bottles)
  - 1 glass of water with patient on scanner table 5–10 min prior to scanning

whether or not rectal contrast material is required. The administration of rectal contrast has been suggested to achieve adequate distension of the rectum and colon and hence prevent confusion between collapsed bowel wall and mural thickening due to inflammation [19]. As an alternative approach, positive oral contrast can be given the night before the examination [19]. The rectal contrast material can be either positive or neutral. If an enterovesical or rectovaginal fistula is suspected, an unenhanced scan is obtained combined with the use of positive oral and rectal contrast material in order to show the contrast in the bladder or vagina [19]. In a similar fashion, positive contrast material can easily be detected in an enterocutaneous or peri-anal fistulous tract [19].

Enhancement/Intravenous Contrast

The enhancement characteristics of the gut wall form an essential part of bowel evaluation, particularly in the assessment of inflammatory and vascular disorders. The normal bowel wall enhances after an adequate bolus of intravenous contrast material. The presence of low-attenuation contrast agents within the lumen facilitates identification of the enhancing wall, with enhancement greater on the mucosal aspect [1] (Fig. 2). Intravenous contrast material enables differentiation between lymphadenopathies and masses, with fine visualization of the parietal features, and therefore optimizes lesion characterization [20-23].

The portovenous phase (60-s delay) is suitable for optimal visualization of the different layers of the parietal wall [23]. For CT enterography at the start of the procedure, 80-150 ml of nonionic, high-concentration, iodinated (350–370 mg I/ml) contrast material is injected intravenously through a 20-gauge cannula at a rate of 3–4 ml/s using a power injector. After a delay of 50–70 s from the start of contrast material administration; the GIT tract is scanned in the portovenous phase (using the Smart Prep protocol, a liver enhancement threshold of 50 HU is followed).

In patients with mesenteric ischemia, a dual-phase protocol is followed: 130 ml of nonionic, high-concentration iodinated contrast media is injected at a rate of 5 ml/s. The arterial phase is either started at 40 s (extending from the celiacs up to the iliac crest) or bolus tracking is used at the level of the diaphragm, which starts scanning at 120 HU. The latter technique is especially helpful in elderly patients or in patients with impaired cardiac output. A venous phase is acquired at 70 s for adequate bowel-wall enhancement. For other indications such as bowel obstruction, uniphasic scans can be performed in which the intravenous contrast agent is administered in a volume of 100-120 ml at a rate of 3 ml/s with a scanning delay of 50–70 s.

In the evaluation of gastric cancer for improved differentiation of tumor tissue from normal mucosa, the injection of intravenous contrast material injection must be optimized [24]. Incremental dynamic MDCT has been used for the evaluation of gastric cancer, with lesion detection in the arterial phase, differentiation of the stomach from adjacent organs and lymph-node evaluation in the portovenous phase, and the depth of gastric-wall invasion in the delayed phase [25-27].

Volume Acquisition and Post-processing

Various post-processing techniques are routinely used in the evaluation of the GIT. These include standard reformatting, curved reformatting, maximum intensity projection (MIP), and volume-rendering (VR) techniques. Multi-planar and 3-D reconstruction techniques are reserved for problem solving in gastrointestinal pathologies [28]. Multi-planar reformations (MPRs, coronal, sagittal, and oblique) aid in identifying the precise anatomic location of gastric, small-intestinal, and colonic lesions [28] (Table 6). The ability to visualize an abnormality in multiple planes raises diagnostic confidence and aids in better depiction of the morphologic features of the lesion [29].

MPRs are crucial in the evaluation of bowel obstruction, as the reformatted images in different

Table 6. Applications of multi-planar reformations and 3-D imaging in the gastrointestinal tract

- Increases confidence and helps better characterize the morphologic features of the lesion
- Identification of the transition zone in bowel obstruction when not seen on axial scans
- Excellent depiction of the anatomy in closed-loop obstruction and volvulus
- Assessment of surrounding peritoneum, mesentery, and mesenteric vasculature
- Evaluation of the extent of involvement in inflammatory bowel disease
- Accurate demonstration of strictures and fistulas

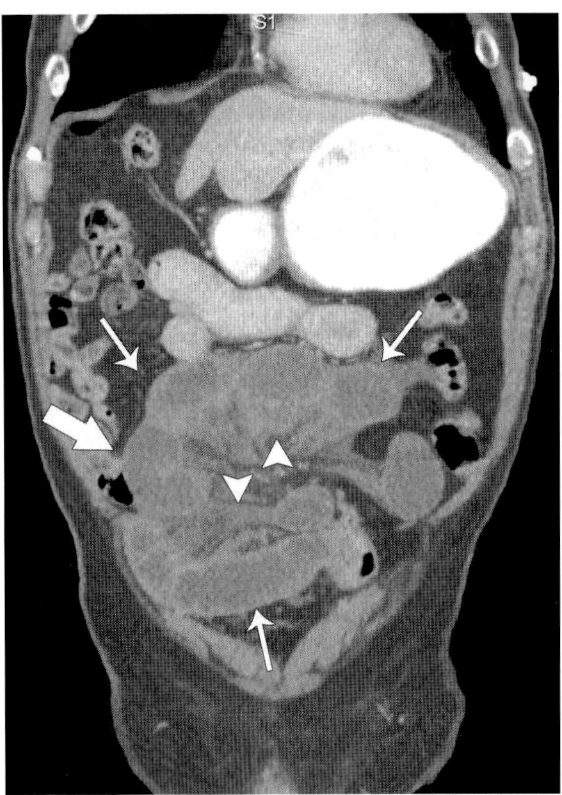

Fig. 6. Coronal multi-planar reformatted image from a patient with closed-loop obstruction displays the radial array of dilated bowel loops (*arrows*) and mesenteric vessels converging to a central point. Patchy areas of enhancement (*thick white arrow*) of small-bowel wall and mesenteric edema (*arrowheads*) are indicative of bowel ischemia complicating closed-loop obstruction

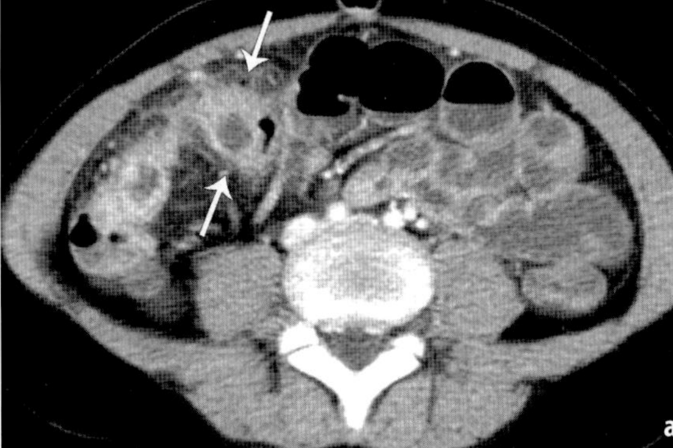

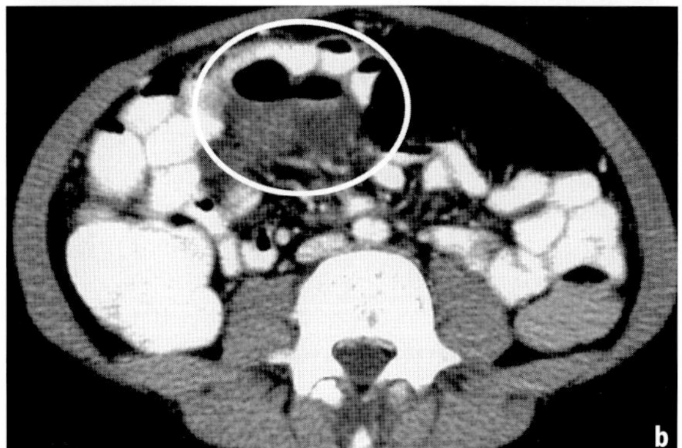

Fig. 7a, b. Two multi-detector computer tomography (MDCT) studies performed 2 weeks apart in a 16-year-old patient with known active Crohn's disease. These images highlight the advantages and limitation of neutral oral contrast material (OCM) for evaluating inflammatory bowel disease. **a** Post-contrast axial CT image from the initial CT enterography using neutral OCM reveals mural stratification and mucosal enhancement with regional mesenteric fat stranding, an indicator of active disease. A low-attenuation lesion (*arrows*) with a faint enhancing rim adjacent to the inflamed bowel segment was mistaken as a bowel loop. **b** However, on the exam repeated after 2 weeks but with positive OCM, there is an obvious enlarging extra-luminal abscess (*circle*) in the same location

planes help to locate the site of obstruction and to identify the transition between normal and abnormal loops. In cases of volvulus or closed-loop obstruction, post-processing yields excellent depiction of the abnormal bowel anatomy (Fig. 6). MPR not only allows evaluation of the bowel loop but also assessment of the surrounding structures, including peritoneum, mesentery, and mesenteric vasculature (Fig. 7). In inflammatory bowel diseases, MPRs demonstrate the extent of disease and provide detailed information on extra-intestinal

complications [19]. Coronal and sagittal reformatted images demonstrate fistulas better than on axial scans. Oblique coronal reformations along the axis of the bowel loops are particularly valuable in picking up subtle fistulous communications.

The main benefits of 3-D VR over two-dimensional (2-D) MPR are added perspective and enhanced depth perception, which allow visualization of a complex lesion in its entirety with better determination of its relationship to adjacent structures [29].

Scanning Technique

Initially, unenhanced scanning is done from the diaphragmatic dome to the iliac crest during a single breath-hold. Patients are instructed to suspend respiration during scanning. Contrast-enhanced CT scanning is then performed after intravenous injection of contrast. Imaging in the supine and prone positions helps to shift fluid that may obscure underlying lesions and to distend collapsed segments that are dependent on the other positioned images. Delayed scans clarify subtle bowel findings, such as colonic leak or perforation, pneumatosis, fistulas, and sinus tracts [19].

The scanning parameters for CT enterography on a 16- to 64-slice scanner include a detector configuration of 0.625–1.25 mm, axial reconstruction at a 2.5- to 5-mm interval, with retro-reconstruction at 1.25/0.625 mm (Table 7). Reconstruction of raw data obtained from the CT scanning should be controlled according to the method of imaging analysis. Usually, we reconstruct raw data sets with a standard-body reconstruction algorithm, available on the CT scanner and routinely used for abdominal CT scanning. The 2.5- to 5-mm axial slices are used for global interpretation. Post-processing is performed with 2-D in the form of coronal thin MIPs at a thickness of 2.5–3 mm. Three-dimensional post-processing with stack mode/cine displays are superior to tile mode for detecting transition zones.

Clinical Indications

Stomach and Duodenum

Among the gastroduodenal lesions, MDCT has made significant impact in the imaging of gastric cancer. To achieve precise diagnosis and tumor staging, accurate lesion depiction at CT is a prerequisite in the evaluation of this disease [13]. The common imaging manifestations of gastric carcinomas on CT include a focal area of mural thickening with or without ulceration, polypoidal lesions, generalized mural thickening, or the linitis plastica pattern (diffuse thickening of the gastric wall with obliteration of the gastric folds) [24].

The greatest benefits of MDCT in the evaluation of gastric cancer have been in the detection of early gastric cancer. Knowledge of the normal anatomy of the gastric wall on MDCT is therefore essential to diagnose early lesions. The normal gastric wall on MDCT is a three-layered structure composed of an inner layer of high attenuation, a middle layer of low attenuation, and an outer layer of intermediate attenuation between the inner and middle layers [14]. When the gastric wall shows focal thickening of ≥6 mm or focal enhancement and irregularity, it is considered to be abnormal [4] (Fig. 3a). Kim et al. [13] classified the depth of tumor invasion on CT as follows: T1, gastric-wall thickening with or without enhancement of the inner surface but with preservation of the low-attenuation stripe, corresponding submucosal layer, at the base of the lesion; T2, thickened gastric wall with loss or disruption of low-attenuation stripe but with a clear and smooth outer gastric surface around the lesion and a clear perigastric fat plane; T3, nodular or irregular outer border of the thickened gastric wall or perigastric fat infiltration; and T4, direct extension and invasion of tumor into a contiguous organ or structure.

Chen et al. noted that the use of MPR images allow the radiologist to choose the optimal imaging plane to accurately evaluate the depth of tumor invasion of the gastric wall and perigastric fat plane infiltration [26]. The use of MPR images also allows the identification of a thin fat plane between the tumor and adjacent organs, as well as the avoidance of partial volume averaging effects [26]. MPR images provide a good preoperative prediction of stage T1–T4 lesions [26].

Volumetric CT imaging has improved the detec-

Table 7. Scanning parameters for computed tomography (CT) enterography using 16- and 64-slice multi-detector computed tomography (MDCT)

	16-slice MDCT	64-slice MDCT
Phase	Hepatic (portal venous)	Hepatic (portal venous)
Detector configuration (mm)	16 × 0.625	64 × 0.625
Pitch	1.375	1-1.375
Table speed (mm/rotation)	13.75	40
Rotation time (s)	0.5	0.5
kilovolt peak (kVp)	120 – 140 (dependent on body habitus)	
milliampere (mA)	Noise index- 10-15	Noise index- 10-15
Reconstruction algorithm	Standard	Standard
Prospective slice thickness (mm)	2.5	2.5-5
Reconstruction interval (mm)	2.5	2.5
Coronal reconstruction (mm)	2.5-3	2.5-3

tion rate for early gastric cancers [16, 30]. In particular, the depiction of early gastric cancer (T1) on volumetric CT imaging is markedly improved compared with transverse imaging alone (96% vs. 69% of early gastric cancers) [13]. Small T1 cancers have a very low rate of nodal involvement; hence, if detected on MDCT, they are candidates for endoscopic or laparoscopic resection [13]. Kim et al. [13] found that the accuracy of tumor staging with volumetric CT imaging was superior to that with transverse CT imaging (overall accuracy, 84% vs. 77%). The superiority of volumetric CT imaging was more evident in pathologic staging of T1 and T3 cancers. These authors also noted that differences in the staging of lymph nodes and metastases between transverse CT imaging and volumetric CT imaging however were not significant [13].

MDCT can improve the overall accuracy of detection of perigastric invasion and peritoneal metastases because of good spatial resolution, an optimal imaging plane, and decreased partial-volume-averaging effects. It can correctly detect metastatic lesions smaller than those identified by previous-generation CT imaging [26]. Early detection of liver, peritoneal cavity, and retroperitoneal metastases, especially prior to surgery, is extremely important for patient survival because it enables the planning of combined treatment of primary and secondary disease.

MDCT can be used to more accurately define the group of patients for whom primary surgical therapy will be curable vs. those for whom it is unsuitable [24]. Ba-Ssalamah et al. [24] noted that if CT shows definitive transmural extension with peritoneal tumor spread, presurgical chemotherapy is used to downstage the tumor after which the tumor is restaged; this approach can lead to curative surgical therapy if there is a positive response. The authors concluded that pre-operative staging of gastric cancer is by far the main clinical indication of MDCT [24]. MDCT also plays a major role in the evaluation of postoperative complications and the detection of tumor recurrence following partial gastrectomy [24].

There are certain limitations of MDCT in the evaluation of gastric cancer. These include the inability to detect flat type of early gastric cancer, even in combination with virtual gastroscopy and MPR images [31, 32], overstaging in T2 cancers with perigastric inflammation or vascular or lymphatic engorgement, and understaging in T3 cancers with penetration of the serosal layer by a microscopic infiltration of cancer cells [33]. Tiny peritoneal metastases or ovarian metastases without associated ascites may lead to understaging [15]. MDCT is also still relatively insensitive in the detection of nodal metastases, as it cannot detect microscopic nodal invasion [34].

In patients with suspected gastric lymphoma, MDCT not only allows depiction of the gastric lesion but is also used for staging of generalized lymphoma in the abdomen and chest [24]. In addition, MDCT aids in the early diagnosis of disease progression in patients treated and followed-up for low-grade mucosa-associated lymphoid tissue (MALT) lymphoma, which may progress to high-grade B-cell lymphoma [24].

MDCT enhances the diagnostic accuracy of evaluating duodenal tumors and peri-ampullary carcinomas. This advantage is principally due to the excellent duodenal distension achieved by neutral contrast agents and to multi-planar capabilities, allowing better assessment of adjacent organ and vascular invasion (Fig. 3b). The assessment of vascular invasion is enhanced by using image planes that correspond to the oblique orientation of the pancreas within the retroperitoneum [35]. Three-dimensional CT is an accurate predictor of resectability for peri-ampullary neoplasms and for patients who will eventually undergo a margin-negative resection and thus derive a significant survival benefit [36].

Disorders of the Small Bowel

Patients with small-intestinal disorders are best examined by CT enterography. Certain criteria have been used to aid in the evaluation of abnormal small bowel: the pattern of enhancement, the length of involvement, the degree and symmetry of wall thickening, the precise location of the lesion along the course of the small bowel (proximal or distal) and in the wall (mucosal, submucosal, or serosal), and associated abnormalities in the mesentery and vessels [9]. Our emphasis in this section is on the MDCT features of the most common small-bowel disorders, i.e., bowel obstruction, inflammatory bowel disorders, and mesenteric ischemia.

Bowel Obstruction

The diagnosis of bowel obstruction is made on MDCT by the demonstration of dilated proximal bowel and collapsed distal bowel as well as the presence of a transition zone [37] (Fig. 4, Table 8). Identification of a transition zone is a key point in the diagnosis of obstruction, unlike the degree of dilatation, which is not a reliable criterion for differentiating bowel obstruction from ileus [37]. Coronal and sagittal reformatting are helpful in identifying the transition zone when it is not clearly shown on axial slices [37]. A small-bowel diameter of > 2.5 cm, "small-bowel feces sign," and air fluid levels are other CT signs of obstruction [38-40].

While MDCT also identifies the cause and severity of the small-bowel obstruction, its most crucial role is in the identification of signs of bow-

Table 8. Multi-detector row computed tomography (MDCT) in small bowel obstruction

- Confirm the presence or absence of obstruction and identify the site and level of transition zone
- Identify the cause and severity of obstruction
- Identify indeterminate cases on axial scans: volvulus, internal hernias
- Look for signs of closed-loop obstruction and strangulation: thickening and increased attenuation of the bowel wall, serrated beak-like narrowing at the site of obstruction, target or halo sign, pneumatosis intestinalis, and gas in the portal vein

el strangulation. The exact point of obstruction may not be visualized in the presence of adhesions, which are the most common cause of small-bowel obstruction [41]. In such situations, the diagnosis is made by visualizing the proximal dilated and distal collapsed bowel loops and an inability to establish a cause of obstruction [41]. Reformatting views may highlight a beak-like narrowing at the obstruction site and, although the actual adhesion may not be seen, the absence of any focal intestinal or adjacent lesion at that point is confirmed by MDCT, thus increasing diagnostic confidence [37]. MPR produces planes that highlight the relationship between normal and pathologic bowel wall in the characterization of intrinsic intestinal lesions such as neoplasms, inflammatory lesions, vascular lesions, and hematomas, as well as in the staging of these lesions [37]. In addition, reformatting can be used to analyze internal or external hernias in that it provides a better view of the location of the bowel loops [37].

MDCT evaluates the risk and severity of obstruction by looking for signs of closed-loop obstruction, volvulus, and of bowel ischemia [37] (Fig. 6). Closed-loop obstruction may be seen on CT as a C-shaped, U shaped or "coffee bean" configuration of the bowel loops, more often better appreciated on reformatted or 3-D VR images [37, 42]. However, the most specific sign is when two segments of bowel converging toward the same point are identified with a beak-like narrowing of these segments at this point. Anatomic views of this are obtained on oblique or curved reformatting [37]. "Whirl sign", a key feature of volvulus, may not be very apparent on axial CT if the axis of rotation is not perpendicular to the imaging plane [37]. Aufort et al. highlighted the benefit of coronal and sagittal reformatting when the axis of rotation of the twisted mesentery is in the axial plane. They also noted the use of 3-D VR CT angiography in illustrating the abnormal whirling course of the mesenteric vessels [37].

Bowel ischemia complicating bowel obstruction is diagnosed by identifying abnormalities of the bowel wall and of the mesentery attached to the ischemic bowel loops [37]. The best sign of ischemia is a lack of enhancement of the bowel wall; however, post-processing does not improve upon the findings on axial slices [37, 43]. Findings of haziness or obliteration of the mesenteric vessels, localized mesenteric fluid, and hemorrhage are seen in the mesentery attached to the ischemic bowel loops (Fig. 6).

Aufort et al. concluded that, although axial slices enable accurate diagnosis of bowel obstruction, post-processing enhances detection of the site of obstruction, the diagnosis of adhesions, and an analysis of the relationship between pathologic and normal bowel wall [37]. There are certain limitations in the use of MDCT for the diagnosis of small-bowel obstruction, such as false-positive diagnosis of the obstruction site caused by incomplete luminal distension owing to overly rapid passage of contrast material, or transient luminal narrowing caused by peristaltic movement [44].

Inflammatory Diseases of the GIT

Conventional CT has traditionally been used to guide the management of extra-intestinal complications of inflammatory bowel diseases but it has had a limited role in the identification of the small-bowel disease per se [12]. CT has also been preferred for evaluation of the transmural extent of disease suggested by the degree of wall thickening and to look for skip lesions beyond severe luminal stenoses [45] (Fig. 4). However, CT enterography is fast becoming the first-line modality in the evaluation of suspected inflammatory bowel disease due to its ability to demonstrate the activity of the inflammatory process (Fig. 2, Table 9). The higher spatial resolution, together with the use of neutral contrast agents, enables CT enterography to exquisitely demonstrate active Crohn's disease and its complications, such as small-bowel strictures [12, 46, 47].

The CT enterographic findings of active Crohn's disease correlate well with active mucosal and mural inflammation [48-51] (Table 9). Mural hyperenhancement on CT enterography refers to segmental mural hyperenhancement of distended small-bowel loops relative to normal-appearing loops, which correlates with histological findings of Crohn's disease [12, 52]. As jejunum enhances to a greater degree than ileum when scanning is done in the enteric phase of enhancement (40–60 s after the injection of contrast material), and since collapsed bowel loops have higher attenuation than distended ones, it is important to examine the

Table 9. Computed tomography (CT) enterographic features of active Crohn's disease [12]

* Mural hyperenhancement and stratification
* Bowel-wall thickening (asymmetric and along the mesenteric border)
* Soft-tissue stranding in the peri-enteric mesenteric fat and engorged vasa recta

Table 10. Multi-detector row computed tomography (MDCT) in mesenteric ischemia

* Circumferential bowel wall thickening
* Low attenuation or increased attenuation of the bowel wall
* Absent enhancement of the bowel wall or, occasionally, hyperenhancement
* Intramural gas, portal venous gas, and multi-organ infarctions
* CT angiography to assess the mesenteric vasculature: arterial stenosis/occlusion, venous thrombosis, and collaterals in chronic ischemia

enhancement patterns in segments that are properly distended [12, 53]. In nondistended bowel loops, active inflammation can be diagnosed based on secondary signs of small-bowel inflammation, such as mural stratification, engorged vasa recta, or stranding in the peri-enteric fat [12].

Mural stratification refers to visualization of layers of the intestinal wall at contrast-enhanced CT and is due to the avid enhancement of the mucosa and serosa [12]. Depending on the pathologic process involved, the intervening bowel wall may show intramural fat, indicating past or chronic inflammation, or intramural edema (water attenuation), indicating active inflammation [12]. The "comb sign" created by the engorged vasa recta vessels penetrating the bowel wall perpendicular to the lumen is an indication of active inflammation and has been associated with elevated C-reactive protein levels and longer hospital stays in patients with severe Crohn's disease [12, 54].

CT enterography is also superior to conventional CT in the detection of extra-intestinal complications such as fistulas, abscesses, and phlegmon. Fistulas usually appear as fluid- or air-filled tracts with an enhancing rim originating from actively inflamed bowel loops, except for peri-anal fistulas which are often isoattenuating relative to anorectum [12]. Coronal and/or oblique reformations are helpful in outlining these hyperenhancing tracts. Abscesses complicating Crohn's disease are often seen either within the leaves of the mesentery or in a retroperitoneal location (Fig. 7). MDCT often demonstrates the sinus tract connecting it to an inflamed bowel [12].

Mesenteric Ischemia

The vital role of MDCT in mesenteric ischemia is not only to detect the ischemic changes in the affected bowel loops but also to determine the cause of ischemia [44]. The specific findings that suggest acute mesenteric ischemia include demonstration of mesenteric vascular occlusion, intramural gas, absent intestinal-wall enhancement, and multi-organ infarctions [44] (Table 10, Fig. 8). However, more common but nonspecific findings seen on CT are luminal dilatation, circumferential bowel-wall thickening, mesenteric stranding, and ascites [44].

The ischemic bowel wall may demonstrate low or high attenuation depending on the pathological process involved. Low attenuation reflects submucosal edema and inflammation, while increased attenuation is due to the submucosal hemorrhage that is often seen in ischemia [55, 56]. After intravenous contrast administration, the affected loops may demonstrate either absent or decreased enhancement due to compromised blood flow or increased enhancement due to hyperemia [57-59].

In addition to detecting changes in the small bowel, MDCT with 3-D reformatting can help to evaluate the mesenteric vessels in patients with acute mesenteric ischemia. Mesenteric emboli and focal infarction of the affected bowel loops can be directly shown on an MDCT scan. Mesenteric venous thrombosis, an uncommon but potentially lethal cause of bowel ischemia, is well-demonstrated on MDCT, with 3-D reconstructions showing the entire mesenteric venous anatomy. Nonocclusive mesenteric ischemia shows changes in the bowel similar to those of occlusive mesenteric ischemia; however, the abrupt arterial occlusion is not seen in these patients [44]. MDCT provides a rapid definite diagnosis in nonocclusive mesenteric ischemia, with 3-D images that provide vascular information comparable to that obtained during angiography [60].

MDCT is extremely useful to demonstrate atherosclerotic changes, including calcified plaque in the aorta and mesenteric arteries in patients with chronic mesenteric ischemia. Mesenteric collateral vessels, which are formed in chronic mesenteric ischemia to preserve the blood flow to the intestines, are also identified at MDCT with 3-D reformatting (Fig. 8).

Hong et al. described certain limitations of us-

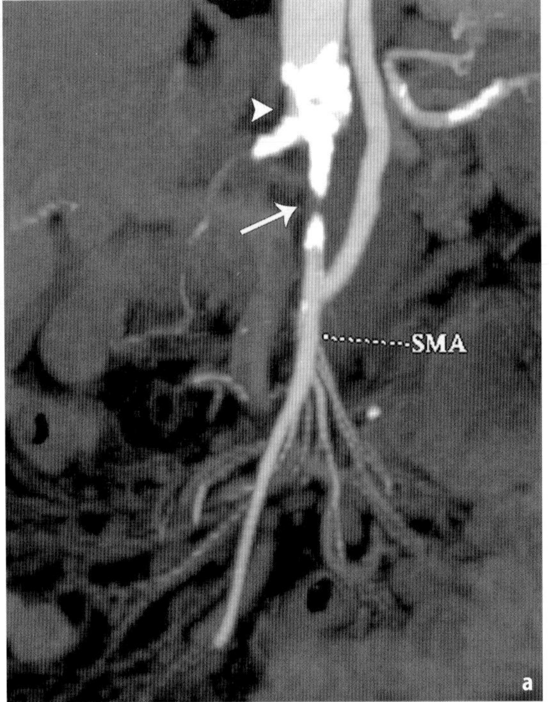
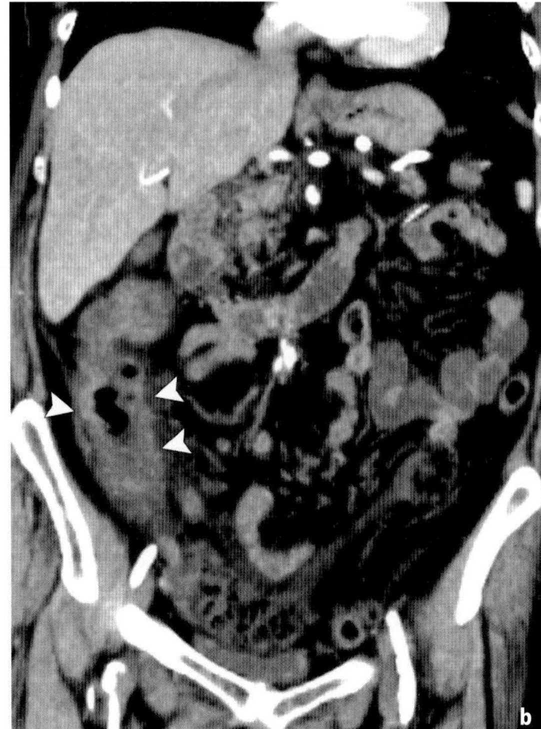
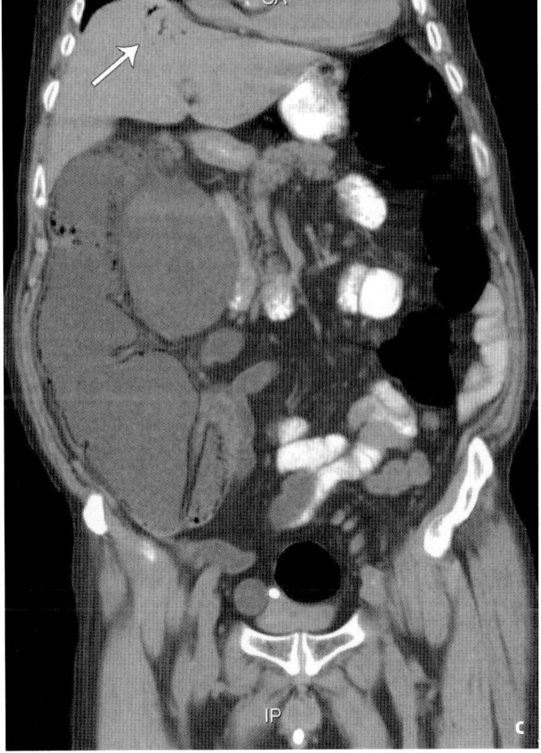

Fig. 8a-c. Multi-detector row computed tomography (MDCT) images of mesenteric ischemia in two different patients who presented with a history of bloody diarrhea. **a** In the first patient, there is severe stenosis of the superior mesenteric artery (*arrow*) just distal to the origin, with extensive calcific atherosclerotic changes (*arrowhead*) and distal reformation by collaterals seen on the thick section multi-planar reformatted image. **b** Coronal reformatted image in the same patient shows mural thickening and surrounding fat stranding, which suggests bowel insult from ischemia (*arrowheads*). **c** Coronal reformatted image from another patient shows more advanced changes of bowel ischemia evident as intramural gas in the ascending colon and intrahepatic portal venous gas (*arrow*). SMA superior mesenteric artery

ing MDCT to diagnose mesenteric ischemia [44]. The main limitation is the possibility of a false-positive diagnosis due to hypovolemia or spasm, which causes inadequate or nonopacified blood in the mesenteric vessels [44]. The other limitation is the frequent lack of association between the demonstration of calcified plaque in vessels and the presence of clinical symptoms. Calcified atherosclerotic plaque often can be observed at the origin of the mesenteric arteries in older individuals lacking clinical symptoms, whereas the small intestine can appear normal in patients with chronic mesenteric ischemia [44]. This necessitates careful correlation of the clinical picture with the CT findings in the evaluation of patients with suspected mesenteric ischemia [44].

Small-bowel Masses

Small-bowel neoplasms appear at CT enterography as focal intraluminal masses, focal areas of bowel-wall thickening, or areas of increased mural enhancement [12] (Fig. 9). Certain appearances may be present in particular tumors, e.g., a predominantly exoenteric mass in a gastrointestinal stromal tumor, adjacent lymphadenopathy in lymphoma, and avidly enhancing polyps or carpet lesions in carcinoid tumors [12]. MDCT and 3-D im-

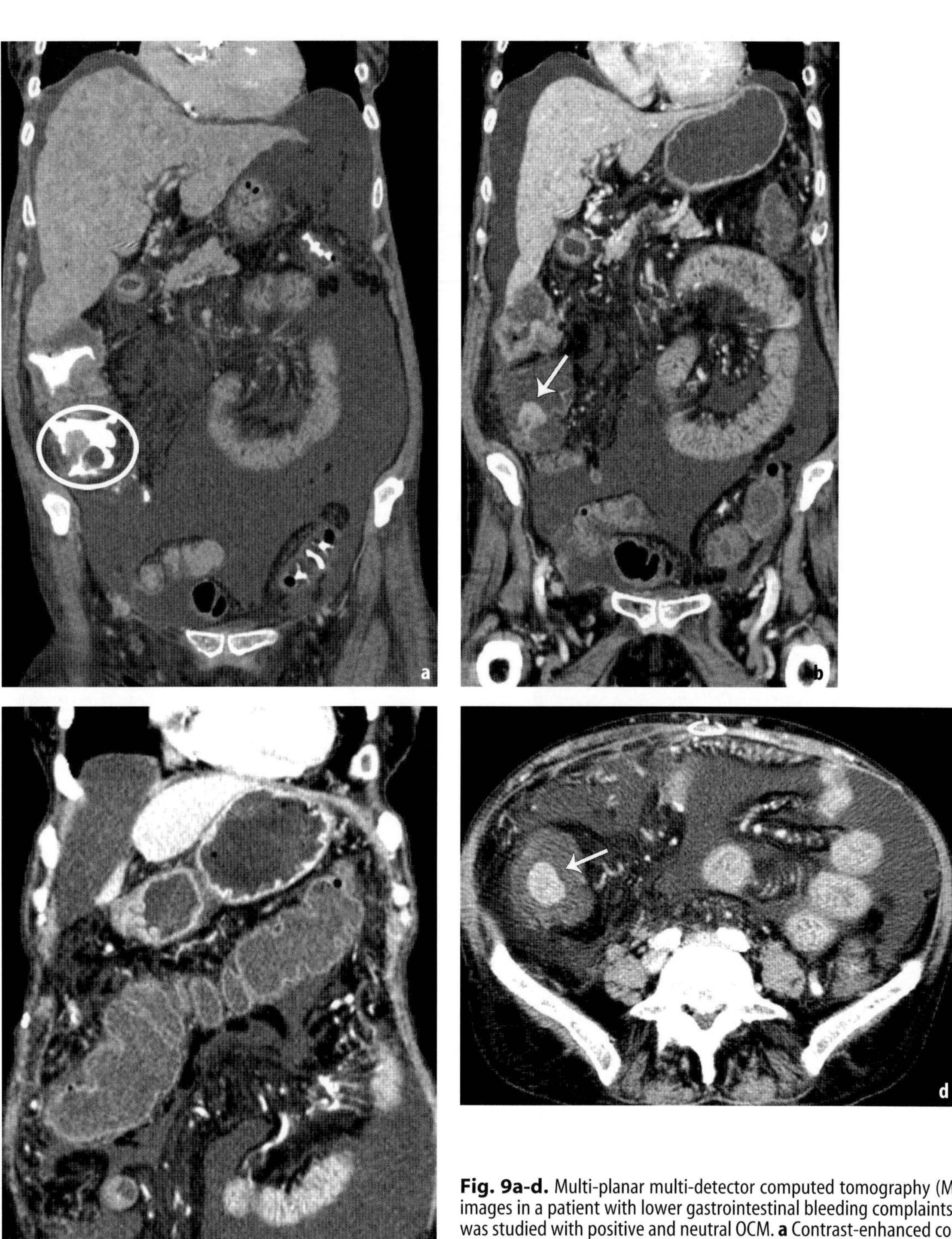

Fig. 9a-d. Multi-planar multi-detector computed tomography (MDCT) images in a patient with lower gastrointestinal bleeding complaints who was studied with positive and neutral OCM. **a** Contrast-enhanced coronal CT image with positive oral contrast material (OCM) shows ascites and a suspicious polypoidal lesion in the cecum (*circle*), which was interpreted as fecal residue. **b, d** Axial and coronal reformatted post-contrast CT images obtained after labeling the gastrointestinal tract with a neutral OCM demonstrates an avidly enhancing polypoid mass (*arrows*) that was the source of gastrointestinal (GI) bleeding. **c** Note the presence of colitis in the transverse colon. Diagnostic colonoscopy confirmed these findings

age processing play an important role in the diagnosis and staging of small-bowel neoplasms. The surgeon can make use of 3-D imaging in planning a resection based on better definition of the site of origin of these neoplasms [44]. In addition, MDCT angiography provides valuable information regarding the vascular supply of these tumors and the extent of their vascular invasion. Neutral OCMs are preferred in the evaluation of small-bowel neoplasms because they preserve the vascular information regarding the tumor, the affected bowel segment, and related vascular structures. Neutral contrast agents also help the clinician to better appreciate the intraluminal component of the enhancing polypoidal masses (Fig. 9).

Obscure Gastrointestinal Bleeding

MDCT is an alternative to more invasive procedures such as conventional angiography when routine workup fails to determine the cause of active intestinal bleeding [44]. According to Hong et al., when combined with advanced 3-D imaging, MDCT (including CT angiography) may have a role in evaluating patients with obscure gastrointestinal bleeding because it can be performed rapidly and noninvasively and can easily identify tumors, inflammatory bowel diseases, and unexpected bleeding foci [44].

Disorders of the Large Bowel

Inflammatory Diseases of Colon

Today, MDCT has a pivotal role in the diagnostic workup of patients suspected of having colitis, as the superb imaging quality of MPRs provides improved visualization of the extent of inflammatory changes in the colon and facilitates surgical planning [19]. This is particularly evident for accurate assessment of the cecum and terminal ileum, where the number of images required for viewing by the clinician can thus be reduced to a minimum [19]. CT allows visualization of the bowel wall as well as adjacent structures and therefore is a very sensitive technique for the detection of intramural disease and its extra-intestinal complications [7].

In ulcerative colitis, the role of MDCT is in defining the extent of the disease. Of particular interest is its ability to depict inflammatory activity (Fig. 5). The changes of chronic ulcerative colitis, particularly the loss of haustrations, giving a lead-pipe colon appearance on barium-enhanced imaging, are well seen on coronal reformations and CT colonographic studies. Wall thickening is also well-demonstrated, with the involvement being diffuse and symmetric in ulcerative colitis, unlike in Crohn's disease where it is eccentric and segmental with skip lesions [7]. The mean wall thickness in Crohn's disease (11–13 mm) is usually greater than

in ulcerative colitis (7.8 mm) [7]. Mural stratification of the thickened bowel wall, as seen in inflammatory bowel disease after contrast administration, is also excellently depicted on MDCT. The fat halo sign of chronic disease and the water halo sign of acute active disease highlight the role of CT in predicting disease activity [7].

In diverticular disease, a common inflammatory condition, CT reveals the colonic wall as well as the surrounding pericolic fat [7]. Diverticulosis appears on CT as small, air-filled outpouchings of the colonic wall, with the wall of the involved segment appearing thickened due to muscular hypertrophy [7]. On CT, diverticulitis appears as enhancing segmental wall thickening with stranding in the surrounding pericolic fat. Conventional CT has a very high detection rate for diverticular disease. The role of MDCT in diverticulitis is in the additional assessment of its complications, such as abscesses and fistulas, and to define the extent of disease, thus assisting in surgical planning. A colovesical fistula is suspected when air is seen in the bladder and there is thickening of the bladder wall adjacent to a diseased segment of bowel (usually the sigmoid) [19]. In diverticulitis, the fistulas tend to occur in the left posterior portion of the urinary bladder due to involvement of sigmoid colon, while in Crohn's disease, because the terminal ileum is diseased, the fistulas are located on the right anterior surface of the urinary bladder [7]. MPRs and 3-D reconstructions have significantly improved the diagnosis of fistulas, which are not clearly visualized on axial slices. It is also useful to keep in mind the superiority of positive contrast agents in the depiction of fistulous communications.

Colorectal Cancer

CT colonography is fast becoming the preferred screening tool for the early detection of polyps. CT colonography will not be dealt in this section as it is beyond the scope of this chapter. MDCT increases the sensitivity of detection of small colon cancers. The MDCT findings of colorectal cancer include a polypoidal mass, irregular mural thickening, irregular stricture, and an exoenteric mass. MDCT evaluates the extent of mural involvement and the pericolic spread of the disease, with accurate evaluation of the lymphnodal spread. Local staging of colon cancer is better with MPRs, which help in accurate evaluation of the extra-enteric component and extension into adjacent organs, thus playing a crucial role in planning treatment and surgery [61]. The advantages over colonoscopy include the ability of CT to visualize the bowel wall beyond the stricture and to identify extramural complications such as fistula formation.

Although it does not have the soft-tissue resolution of magnetic resonance imaging, MDCT can provide accurate staging of rectal carcinoma. The addition of high-resolution MPR images to standard axial images increases the accuracy of T and N staging studies. High-resolution coronal and sagittal MPR images aligned perpendicular to the tumor axis provide greater diagnostic confidence in predicting peri-rectal infiltration and the involvement of adjacent viscera compared with axial images alone, i.e., increased detection of T3 and T4 tumors [62].

Radiation Dose

Despite the fact that MDCT has brought about a radical change in the diagnosis of gastrointestinal lesions, its drawbacks need to be addressed. Surveys have shown that CT examination is the major contributor to medical radiation-dose exposure. Radiation exposure increases by 27–36% with MDCT compared with single-detector CT [63]. Radiation dose is a vital issue that needs serious consideration in applications such as imaging of the abdomen and pelvis of patients with GIT lesions. The major impact of the cumulative radiation dose delivered during the MDCT scans is in pediatric and young patients who must undergo repeated CT scans for chronic conditions such as inflammatory bowel diseases. There are several methods to reduce the radiation dose delivered to a patient, including reducing the tube current milliampere, lowering the tube potential kilovolt peak, using noise filters for processing of images during reconstruction, modifying reconstruction algorithms, and limiting exposure time [64]. These modifications may compromise image quality; however, a fine balance has to be struck between radiation dose and image quality. The issue of radiation dose in MDCT is dealt with in detail elsewhere in this book.

Emerging Trends

Perfusion CT is a functional CT technique that measures perfusion, permeability, and the blood volume of tumors, thereby providing insight into how angiogenesis affects contrast enhancement. This is achieved by measuring the temporal changes in contrast enhancement from a series of CT images acquired over time. This method has been extensively evaluated to study the tumors of the brain and head and neck. The same principles of perfusion CT have been applied to colorectal cancers. Recent studies report promising results regarding the ability of perfusion CT to assess tumor vascularity and changes in perfusion after chemotherapy and radiation therapy [65].

Conclusion

MDCT has opened up innovative opportunities for the radiologist to perform detailed evaluations of the GIT. It not only provides noninvasive assessment of the bowel wall but also yields valuable information on the extra-luminal manifestations of the disease not available with other conventional imaging methods. The increasing use of neutral oral contrast agents due to superior bowel distending capabilities and enhanced wall-to-lumen contrast has ensured more accurate characterization of various GIT pathologies and has thereby facilitated high-quality CT enterography exams. Parallel advances in post-processing techniques have empowered MDCT with the ability to evaluate the GIT in any desired plane using a variety of rendering methods. However, to obtain the maximum benefit from MDCT, it is essential that the radiologist choose the right oral contrast agents and adhere to standard scanning protocols. It is also imperative for him or her to be aware of certain pitfalls, including the radiation dose delivered with MDCT, to ensure optimal utilization of this exciting technology.

References

1. Macari M, Balthazar EJ (2001) CT of bowel wall thickening: significance and pitfalls of interpretation. AJR Am J Roentgenol 176:1105-1116
2. Rydberg J, Buckwalter KA, Caldemeyer KS (2000) Multisection CT. Scanning techniques and clinical applications. Radiographics 20:1787-1806
3. Megibow AJ, Babb JS, Hecht EM et al (2006) Evaluation of bowel distension and bowel wall appearance by using neutral oral contrast agent for multi-detector row CT. Radiology 238:87-95
4. Balfe DM, Koehler RE, Karstaedt M et al (1981) Computed tomography of gastric neoplasm. Radiology 140:431-436
5. Insko EK, Levine MS, Bimbaum BA, Jacobs JE (2003) Benign and malignant lesions of the stomach: evaluation of CT criteria for differentiation. Radiology 228(1):166-171
6. James S, Balfe DM, Lee JKY, Picus D (1987) Small bowel disease: categorization by CT examination. AJR Am J Roentgenol 148:863-868
7. Horton KM, Corl FM, Fishman EK (2000) CT evaluation of the colon: inflammatory disease. Radiographics 20:399-418
8. Fisher JK (1983) Abnormal colonic wall thickening on computed tomography. J Comput Assist Tomogr 7:90-97
9. Macari M, Megibow AJ, Balthazar EJ (2007) A pattern approach to abnormal small bowel: Observations at MDCT and CT enterography. AJR Am J Roentgenol 188:1344-1345
10. Hara AK, Leighton JA, Virender K et al (2005) Imaging of small bowel disease: comparison of capsule endoscopy, barium examination, and CT. Radiographics 25:697-718

11. Thompson SE, Raptopoulos V, Shieman RL et al (1999) Abdominal helical CT: milk as a low-attenuation oral contrast agent. Radiology 211:870-875

12. Paulsen SR, Huprich JE, Fletcher JC et al (2006) CT enterography as a diagnostic tool in evaluating small bowel disorders: review of clinical experience with over 700 cases. Radiographics 26: 641-662

13. Kim JH, Kim AY, Oh ST et al (2005) Gastric cancer staging at multi-detector row CT gastrography: comparison of transverse and volumetric CT scanning. Radiology 236: 879-885

14. Shimizu K, Ito K, Matsunaga N et al (2005) Diagnosis of gastric cancer with MDCT using the water-filling method and multiplanar reconstruction: CT-histologic correlation. AJR Am J Roentgenol 185:1152-1158

15. Chen CY, Wu DC, Kang WY, Hsu JS (2006) Staging of gastric cancer with 16-channel MDCT. Abdominal Imaging 31:514-520

16. Kim HY, Kim HJ, Ha HK (2005) Gastric cancer by multidetector row CT: preoperative staging. Abdom Imaging 30:465-472

17. Raptopoulos V (1989) Technical principles in CT evaluation of the gut. Radiol Clin North Am 27:631-651

18. Jayaraman MV, Mayo-Smith WW, Moyson JS et al (2001) CT of the duodenum: an overlooked segment gets its due. Radiographics 21:147-160

19. Thoeni RF, Cello JP (2006) CT imaging of colitis. Radiology 240(3):623-38

20. Rollandi GA, Curone PF, Biscaldi E et al (1999) Spiral CT of the abdomen after distension of small bowel loops with transparent enema in patients with Crohn's disease. Abdom Imaging 24(6):544-549

21. Grassi R, Di Mizio R, Romano S et al (2000) Multiple jejunal angiodysplasia detected by enema helical CT. Clinical Imag 24(2):61-63

22. Maglinte DDT, Bender GN, Heitcamp DE et al (2003) Multidetector-row helical CT enteroclysis. Radiol Clin N Am 41(2):249-262

23. Romano S, De Lutio E, Rollandi GA et al (2005) Multidetector computed tomography enteroclysis (MDCT-E) with neutral enteral and IV contrast enhancement in tumour detection. Eur Radiol 15:1178-1183

24. Ba-Ssalamah A, Prokop M, Uffmann M et al (2003) Dedicated multidetector CT of the stomach: Spectrum of diseases. Radiographics 23:625-644

25. Lee JH, Jeong YK, Kim DH et al (2000) Two-phase helical CT for detection of early gastric carcinoma: importance of the mucosal phase for analysis of the abnormal mucosal layer. J Comput Assist Tomogr 24:777-782

26. Chen CY, Wu DC, Kang WY, Hsu JS (2006) Staging of gastric cancer with 16-channel MDCT. Abdominal Imaging 31:514-520

27. Takao M, Fukuda T, Iwanaga S et al (1998) Gastric cancer : evaluation of triphasic spiral CT and radiologic-pathologic correlation. J Comput Assist Tomogra 22:288-294

28. Maher MM, Kalra MK, Sahani DV et al (2004) Techniques, clinical applications and limitations of 3D reconstruction in CT of the abdomen. Korean J Radiol 5(1):55-67

29. Horton KM, Fishman EK (2003) Current role of CT in the imaging of stomach. Radiographics 23:75-87

30. Minami M, Kawauchi N, Itai Y et al (1992) Gastric tumors: Radiologic pathologic correlation and accuracy of T staging with dynamic CT. Radiology 185:173-178

31. Hundt W, Braunschweig R, Reiser M (1999) Assessment of gastric cancer: value of breathhold technique and two phase spiral CT. Eur Radiol 9:68-72

32. Takao M, Fukuda T, Iwanaga S et al (1998) Gastric cancer: evaluation of triphasic spiral CT and radiologic-pathologic correlation. J Comput Assist Tomogra 22:288-294

33. Kim AY, Kim HJ, Ha HK (2005) Gastric cancer by multidetector row CT: preoperative staging. Abdom Imaging 30:465-472

34. Chen CY, Wu DC, Kang WY, Hsu JS (2006) Staging of gastric cancer with 16 channel-MDCT. Abomin Imaging 13 (Epub ahead of print)

35. Fishman EK, Wyatt SH, Ney DR et al (1992) Spiral CT of the pancreas with multiplanar display. AJR Am J Roentgenol 159:1209-1215

36. House MG, Yeo CJ, Cameron JL et al (2004) Predicting respectability of periampullary cancer with three dimensional computed tomography. J Gastrointest Surg 8(3):280-288

37. Aufort S, Charra L, Lesnik A (2005) Multidetector CT of bowel obstruction: value of CT processing. Eur Radiol 15:2323-2329

38. Fukuya T, Hawes DR, Lu CC (1992) CT diagnosis of small bowel obstruction: efficacy in 60 patients. AJR Am J Roentgenol 158:765-769

39. Fuchsager MH (2002) The small bowel feces sign. Radiology 225:378-379

40. Jacobs SL, Rozenblit A, Ricci Z (2007) Small bowel feces sign in patients without small bowel obstruction. Clinical Radiology 62:353-357

41. Megibow AJ (1994) Bowel obstruction, Evaluation with CT. Radiol Clin N Am 32: 861-870

42. Balthazar EJ, Bimbaum BA, Megibow AJ (1992) Closed loop and strangulating intestinal obstruction:CT signs. Radiology 185:769-775

43. Zalcman M, Sy M, Donckier V (2000) Helical CT signs in the diagnosis of intestinal ischemia in small bowel obstruction. AJR Am J Roentgenol 175(6):1601-1607

44. Hong SS, Kim AY, Byun JH et al (2006) MDCT of small-bowel disease: value of 3D imaging. AJR Am J Roentgenol 187(5):1212-21

45. Furukawa A, Saotome T, Yamasaki M et al (2004) Cross-sectional imaging in Crohn Disease. Radiographics 24:689-702

46. Nagamata H, Inadama E, Arihiro S et al (2002) The usefulness of MDCT in Crohn's disease. Nippon Shokakibyo Gakkai Zasshi 99:1317-1325

47. Reittner P, Goritschnig T, Petritsch W et al (2002) Multiplanar spiral CT enterography in patients with Crohn's disease using a negative oral contrast material: intial results of a noninvasive imaging approach. Eur Radiol 12:2253-2257

48. Meyers MA, McGuire PV (1995) Spiral CT demonstration of hypervascularity in Crohn disease: "vascular jejunisation of the ileum" or the "comb sign". Abom Imaging 20:327-332

49. Mako EK, Mester AR, Tarjan Z (2000) Enteroclysis and spiral CT examination in the diagnosis and evaluation of small bowel Crohn's disease. Eur J Radiol 35:168-175

50. Gore RM, Marn CS, Kirby DF (1984) CT findings in ulcerative, granulomatous, and indeterminate colitis. AJR Am J Roentgenol 143:279-284

51. Del Campo K, Arribas I, Valbuena M et al (2001) Spiral CT findings in active and remission phases in patients with Crohn disease. J Comput Assist Tomogr 25:792-797

52. Booya F, Fletcher JG, Johnson CD et al (2004) CT enterography: detection of active Crohn's disease during optimal bowel wall enhancement (abstr). In: Radiological Society of North America scientific assembly and annual meeting program. Oak Brook,

III: Radiological Society of North America p. 611
53 Booya F, Fletcher JG, Johnson CD et al (2004) Conspicuity of small bowel inflammation at CT enterography: "enteric" vs "hepatic" phase imaging (abstr). In: Radiological Society of North America scientific assembly and annual meeting program. Oak Brook, III: Radiological Society of North America 611
54. Lee SS, Ha HK, Yang SK et al (2002) CT of prominent pericolic or perienteric vasculature in patients with Crohn's disease: correlation with clinical disease activity and findings on barium studies. AJR Am J Roentgenol 179:1029-1036
55. James S, Balfe DM, Lee JKT et al (1987) Small-bowel disease, categorization by CT examination. AJR Am J Roentgenol 148:863-868
56. Bartnicke BJ, Balfe DM (1994) CT appearance of intestinal ischemia and intramural hemorrhage. Radiol Clin North Am 32:845-860
57. Kim AY, Ha HK (2003) Evaluation of suspected mesenteric ischemia: efficacy of radiologic studies. Radiol Clin North Am 41:327-342
58. Rha SE, Ha HK, Lee SH et al (2000) CT and MRI findings of bowel ischemia from various primary causes. Radiographics 20:29-42
59. Horton KM, Fishman EK (2002) Volume rendered 3D CT of the mesenteric vasculature: normal anatomy, anatomic variants and pathologic conditions. Radiographics 22:161-172
60. Mitsuyoshi A, Obama K, Shinkura N (2007) Survival in nonocclusive mesenteric ischemia: early diagnosis by multidetector row computed tomography and early treatment with continuous intravenous high dose prostaglandin E1. Ann Surg 246:229-235
61. Horton KM, Abrams RA, Fishman EK (2000) Spiral CT of colon cancer: imaging features and role in management. Radiographics 20(2):419-430
62. Sinha R, Verma R, Rajesh A, Richards CJ (2006) Diagnostic value of multidetector row CT in rectal cancer staging: comparison of multiplanar and axial images with histopathology. Clin Radiol 61:924-931
63. Moore HW, Bonvento M (2006) Comparison of MDCT radiation dose: A phantom study. AJR Am J Roentgenol 187:498-502
64. Sahani DV, Kalva SP, Hahn PF, Saini S (2007) 16 MDCT angiography in living kidney donors at various tube potentials: impact on image quality and radiation dose. AJR Am J Roentgenol 188(1):115-20
65. Sahani DV, Kalva SP, Hamberg LM (2005) Assessing tumour perfusion and treatment response in rectal cancer with multisection CT: initial observations. Radiology 234(3):785-792

14

Multi-detector Computed Tomography Urography

Sean E. McSweeney, Owen J. O'Connor, Michael M. Maher

Introduction

The advent of multi-detector computed tomography (MDCT) has enabled evaluation of the entire urinary tract during a single breath-hold, with a concomitant reduction in respiratory misregistration and partial-volume effect. In addition, the acquisition of multiple, thin, overlapping slices of optimally distended and opacified urinary tract potentially provides excellent two-dimensional (2-D) and three-dimensional (3-D) reformations of the urinary tract [1]. The concept of multi-detector CT urography (MDCTU) has emerged from these technical improvements. MDCTU may be defined as MDCT examination of the urinary tract in the excretory phase following intravenous contrast administration [2]. The range of indications for MDCTU has rapidly expanded, and the technique has replaced intravenous urography at many institutions for almost all indications. Refinement of MDCTU protocols remains controversial and is still a work in progress, with a variety of protocols being used at different centres. Protocol design has required input from experts in MDCT technology but also has relied heavily on "old tricks" learned initially by uroradiologists while optimising intravenous urography (IVU) for general usage and for specific indications. Most CT urography protocols resemble those of IVU, providing unenhanced images of the urinary tract for detection of calcifications and subsequent quantification of lesion enhancement following intravenous contrast administration, a nephrographic phase for renal parenchymal evaluation and delayed imaging in the pyelographic phase for evaluation of the urothelium [2].

Indications for MDCTU

Proponents of MDCTU describe it as a comprehensive test that can be performed as a substitute "one-stop" imaging test for a number of imaging studies, thereby saving time, hospital visits and cost and potentially shortening the duration of diagnostic evaluation for urinary-tract pathology [2, 3]. It is widely believed that MDCT is the most sensitive and specific test for the diagnosis of urinary-tract calculi as well as for the detection and characterisation of renal masses [2]. The major controversy surrounding MDCTU is the question of whether this modality is as accurate as IVU for the evaluation of the urothelium in patients presenting with haematuria. In fact, this still represents the final major "hurdle" limiting universal acceptance of MDCTU by radiologists and urologists as a replacement for IVU [2-4]. Unequivocal validation of MDCTU for examining the urothelium in patients with haematuria will promote the use of this technique as a "one-stop" imaging study that simultaneously evaluates the renal parenchyma, ureters and bladder. This, in turn, will eliminate the need for a combination of imaging and other diagnostic tests, as is the case with ultrasound and IVU [4-6]. The second major concern that may limit universal acceptance of MDCTU is the radiation dose associated with the procedure. At the extreme end of the spectrum, radiation dosages between 25 and 35 mSv were reported by Caoili et al. for four-phase MDCTU [7]. This level of radiation dose clearly significantly exceeds that associated with IVU [2, 7]. The radiation dose can be reduced by careful monitoring of the scanning parameters for each phase of MDCTU and by reduction of the number of phases [8, 9].

Imaging Protocol

Non-contrast CT

Non-contrast CT scans are obtained initially to locate the kidneys, visualise anomalies, assess the presence of urinary-tract calcifications including calculi, detect haematoma, and obtain baseline attenuation of renal masses [8]. Unenhanced CT is accepted as the primary imaging investigation to detect urinary-tract calculi [10]. The rationale for the use of unenhanced CT scanning for this indication is its unsurpassed accuracy in detecting urinary-tract calculi [10]. Since Smith's initial report of 97% sensitivity and 96% specificity for the detection of urinary-tract calculi with non-spiral CT, several reports have confirmed these findings, with sensitivities of 98–100% and specificities of 92–100% [5, 11-13]. This compared with much poorer sensitivities of 60% reported for plain radiography and up to 48% of urinary calculi being missed on IVU [8]. Other advantages of MDCT over IVU are the speed at which MDCTU can detect calculi and accurately identify the level of obstruction [10]. With IVU, determining the level of obstruction may involve a delayed in imaging at intervals up to 24 h following contrast injection. MDCT eliminates the need for the administration of iodinated contrast material (required for IVU) in almost all cases and thus eliminates associated risks of nephrotoxicity.

Unenhanced helical CT reliably detects urinary-tract calculi, including those containing uric acid, in the collecting system by direct visualisation, because the calculi are of sufficient density to be visualised by CT [4]. At most institutions, the "stone protocol" component of MDCTU comprises images 3- to 5-mm thick from the upper poles of the kidneys to the symphysis pubis. Oral contrast should be avoided in the evaluation of urolithiasis, as dense oral contrast can make detection of ureteral stones more difficult.

MDCT can detect calculi in unusual positions, such as in caliceal diverticulae, and is more accurate than IVU for detecting the presence, size and location of urinary-tract calculi [4]. The two known exceptions are stones of protease inhibitors, such as indinavir sulphate, or mucoid matrix stones, which are of low attenuation similar to soft tissue and therefore frequently are not visible directly by CT [14, 15].

Following the initial introduction of MDCT to investigate patients with urinary-tract calculi, sceptics argued against the technique because it lacked IVU's advantage of demonstrating physiological information, gained from determination of the degree of delayed excretion, which was considered an index of the severity of obstruction. However, a review of MDCT findings in patients with obstructing urinary-tract calculi showed that it reliably reveals secondary signs of obstructing calculi [4], including hydronephrosis, hydroureter, ipsilateral renal enlargement, perinephric and periureteral fat stranding, perinephric fluid, "ureter rim sign" and ureterovesical oedema [4, 5]. The

combination of hydronephrosis, hydroureter and perinephric stranding has a positive predictive value (PPV) of 90% for obstructing urinary-tract calculi [4]. Recent studies have proposed that the extent of perinephric oedema on unenhanced CT images can be used to accurately predict the degree of acute ureteral obstruction in ureterolithiasis [8, 16]. However, at times, ureteral calculi may be indistinguishable from phleboliths on unenhanced MDCT. The presence of the "soft-tissue rim sign", namely, a circumferential rim of soft-tissue attenuation surrounding an abdominal or pelvic calcification, is a reliable indicator that the calcification in question represents a calculus within the ureter (Fig. 1) [17]. Calculi associated with the soft-tissue rim sign typically have a mean size of 4 mm [18,19]. Conversely, a "comet-tail sign", namely, a linear or curvilinear soft-tissue structure extending from an abdominal or pelvic calcification, has been reported to be an important indicator that a suspicious calcification represents a phlebolith, whereas its absence suggests indeterminate calcification [8, 18-20]. Coll et al. documented the relationship between the spontaneous passage of ureteral calculi and stone size and location, as revealed by unenhanced helical CT. The spontaneous passage rate for ureteric calculi was 76% for 2- to 4-mm calculi, 60% for 5- to 7-mm calculi, 48% for 7- to 9-mm stones and <25% for stones > 9 mm [21].

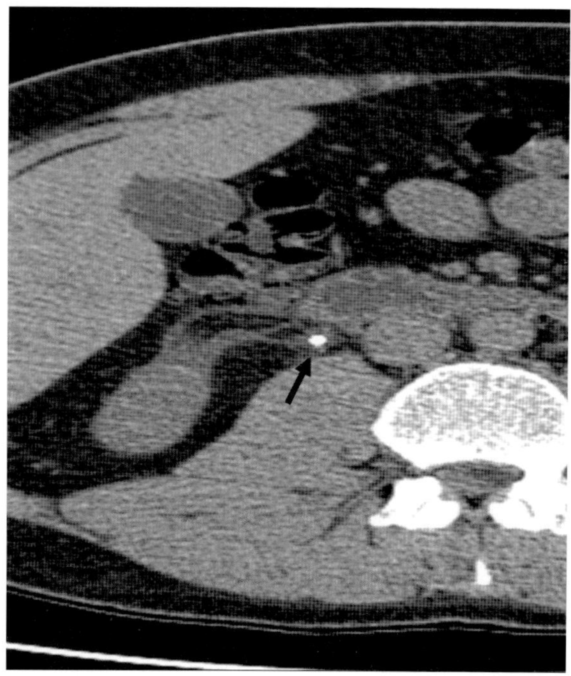

Fig. 1. A 40-year-old man presents with right flank pain. Non-contrast axial image showing calculus within upper third of the right ureter demonstrating the "soft-tissue rim sign" (*arrow*), perinephric fluid and fat stranding

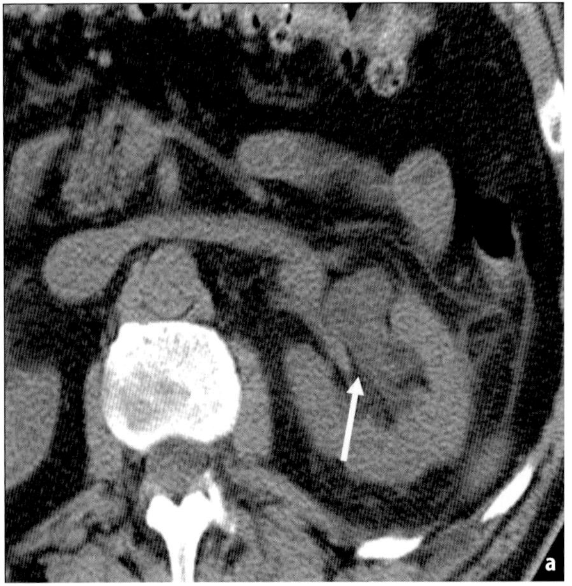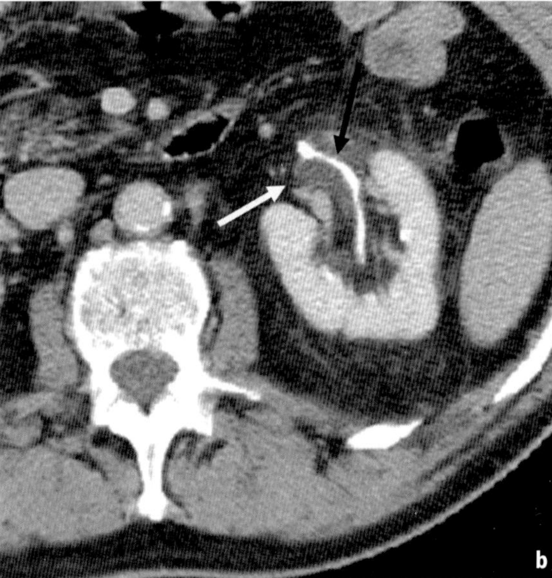

Fig. 2a, b. A 40-year-old man with haematuria. **a** Non-contrast axial computed tomography (CT) image shows a low-attenuation lesion in the left renal pelvis (*arrow*). It was difficult to differentiate hydronephrosis from parapelvic cyst. **b** Multi-detector CT urography (MDCTU) performed in the nephropyelographic phase confirms left parapelvic cyst (*white arrow*) surrounding the proximal left ureter (*black arrow*)

The administration of iodinated contrast is rarely necessary in the investigation of patients with suspected urinary-tract calculi [4]. Rarely, contrast administration followed by imaging in the pyelographic phase may be helpful when uncertainty exits as to whether a calcification is within or external to the urinary tract. Contrast can also be helpful in attempting to distinguish parapelvic cysts from hydronephrosis (Fig. 2), a distinction that may also be difficult on ultrasound examination [4].

Contrast-Enhanced CT

In the 10-year period since the initial description of CT urography, many innovative modifications have been employed to optimise protocols, and currently, there is no consensus as to which of these is the most appropriate [2, 4]. Differences exist at every stage of MDCTU, including:

(a) Techniques of intravenous contrast injection (i.e. a single or "split-bolus" of intravenous contrast)
(b) Number of phases of CT scanning (i.e. single, two-phase, three-phase, or four-phase)
(c) The use of imaging with MDCT alone versus hybrid techniques (i.e. CT combined with conventional intravenous urography or MDCTU supplemented with CT digital radiography images during the excretory phase)
(d) Patient positioning during MDCTU (i.e. prone vs supine vs a combination of both)

(e) The use of compression techniques and the additional administration of saline or low-dose diuretics during the procedure
(f) The timing of CT scanning for pyelographic-phase imaging [2, 4, 22]

Common Protocol Variations

The most commonly used MDCTU protocol comprises three phases that typically consist of an initial unenhanced phase, as described above, a second phase acquired following the administration of non-ionic contrast material (100–150 ml of a 300 mgI/ml solution at a rate of 2–4 ml/s), i.e. the nephrographic phase, which is acquired following a delay of 90–100 s. Typically, during this phase, CT scanning (2.5- to 5-mm slice thickness) is confined to the kidneys and is employed to evaluate the renal parenchyma for masses. The nephrographic phase has been shown to have the highest sensitivity for the detection of renal masses, and unenhanced-phase images must be compared with those from the nephrographic phase in the assessment of unequivocal enhancement within detected renal lesions [4]. In the third phase, the pyelographic phase, the images are typically acquired 5–10 min following contrast administration and serve to evaluate the urothelium from the pelvicaliceal system to the bladder. One of the disadvantages of MDCTU compared with IVU is encountered in patients with asymmetric excretion, most commonly those with unilateral obstruction. In such patients, the lack of sequential imaging with MDCTU can result in suboptimal opacification in the pyelographic phase on the obstructed side [2]. The three-phase protocol is used at most institutions, as it allows thorough evaluation of the urinary tract for the most common causes of haematuria, i.e. urinary-tract calculi, renal neoplasms and urothelial tumours. Caoili et al. described a four-phase protocol (two excretory phases at 5 and 7.5 min) in an effort to optimise ureteric distension and opacification [23]. Subsequently, Caoili's group reverted to the three-phase protocol, with the excretory phase acquired at 12 min [22].

The major disadvantages of three- and four-phase techniques are that they involve a high dose of radiation, are time consuming and yield a larger number of images for review by the radiologist. In an effort to tackle these important issues, which impact patient safety and throughput, Chai et al. proposed a split-bolus technique in place of a single intravenous injection to facilitate a two-phase protocol. This approach results in an unenhanced series of images and a second phase in which nephrographic and pyelographic phases are simultaneously acquired–the "nephropyelographic phase" [24]. After the initial non-contrast examination, 30 ml of non-ionic contrast material (300 mgl/ml) are infused intravenously and the patient is removed from the CT table. If feasible, he or she is encouraged to walk about for 10 min. After 10–15 min, the patient is placed in the prone position on the CT table, and a dynamic contrast-enhanced study is performed following the administration of an additional 100 ml of non-ionic contrast material (300 mgl/ml injected at 2 ml/s) and after a delay of 100 s [4]. Thus, in a single "nephropyelographic- phase" acquisition, the renal parenchyma (nephrographic-phase) and the collecting system, ureters and bladder (pyelographic phase) are assessed (Fig. 3) [4]. A varia-

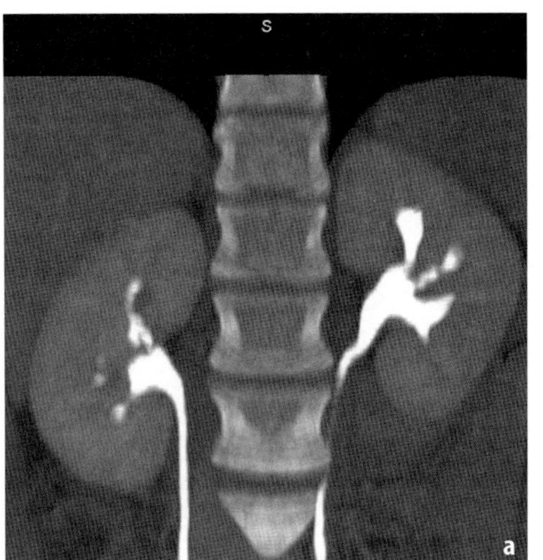
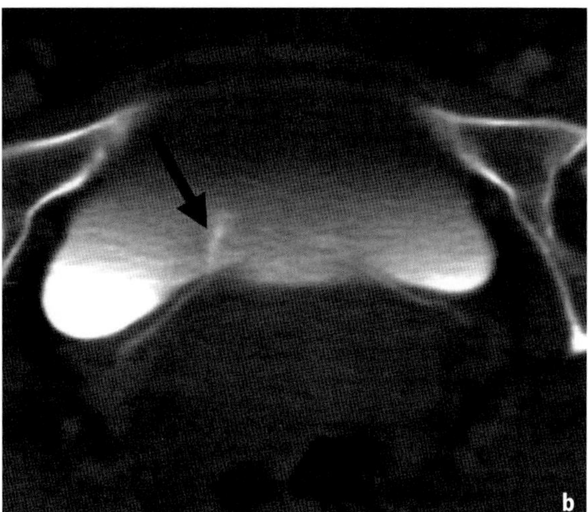
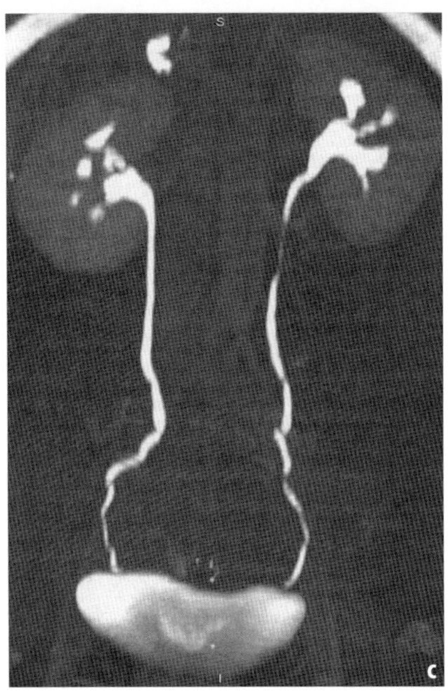

Fig. 3a-c. A 53-year-old patient with microscopic haematuria. Nephropyelographic-phase image showing the normal renal parenchyma, collecting system, ureters, and bladder. **a** Coronal multiplanar reformatted (MPR) image showing normal renal parenchyma, collecting system, and proximal ureters. **b** Axial image during the same acquisition showing opacified distal ureters, ureteric jets (*black arrow*), and bladder. **c** Coronal 3-D maximum intensity projection (MIP) image showing entire urinary tract in a single image

tion of this technique, again using a split bolus to achieve a two-phase technique, was described by Chow et al. [25]. Potential disadvantages of this approach include, (1) the small volume of contrast distending and opacifying the collecting systems and ureters and (2) the potential for streak artefacts from opacified collecting systems during the nephropyelographic phase, which could impact assessment of the renal parenchyma [4, 22, 26]. We have used Chai's technique extensively and have investigated means of optimising opacification and distension of the ureters and collecting system with various manoeuvres, such as supine and prone imaging and additional intravenous administration of saline. Subjective and objective evaluations of the images acquired with these protocols suggested satisfactory technique and the potential disadvantages, noted above, were not encountered [27].

Most experts in the field agree, however, that regardless of the protocol selected, there will always be segments of the ureters that are sub-optimally opacified and distended [4, 8, 22], which may lead to a failure to detect urothelial lesions.

Techniques to Improve Urinary Tract Distension and Opacification

Comprehensive evaluation of the urothelium is widely believed to be dependent on adequate opacification and distension of the pelvicaliceal system and ureters [4]. Consequently, over the past few years, protocol design and modification have focused on these factors [2, 23], with many of the techniques developed for IVU employed as part of these efforts. These are discussed below.

Compression

Lower abdominal compression is a well-established technique in intravenous urography for improving distension of the upper urinary tract [28]. Several authors have shown that compression techniques can be used in CT urography [23, 29, 30] and, again, compression can be incorporated into MDCTU protocols in various ways. One method results in excretory-phase CT scanning being split into two ranges: one from the diaphragm to the iliac crests with compression, and the other (post-release of compression) from the iliac crests to the symphysis [2, 31]. Alternatively, two excretory-phase scans, each including the entire urinary tract, can be acquired: the first with compression, and the second after compression is released [23], but this obviously adds an extra phase and increases the radiation dose, examination time, and number of images for review. External compression is not recommended in patients with abdominal pain or with a history of urinary-tract obstruction, rad-

ical cystectomy, recent surgery, or aortic aneurysm [2]. As to the effectiveness of abdominal compression in improving ureteric distension and opacification, two separate reports by McNicholas et al. and Heneghan et al. suggested a positive impact on the former as a result of abdominal compression [29, 30]. In a subsequent study, Caoili et al. showed that for all segments of the urinary tract, compression resulted in better opacification scores than obtained in controls. However, analysis of the data suggested that the percentage of non-visualised segments reached up to 25% with compression, which was not significantly different from the results achieved by CT urography without compression [23]. We remain unconvinced of the benefits of compression and feel that the benefits are outweighed by the added inconvenience and discomfort for the patient; thus, we have not incorporated compression into our protocol.

Saline Infusion

Another method used to optimise ureteric distension at MDCTU is the addition of intravenous saline infusion to MDCTU protocols. However, theoretically, this can result in reduced opacification of the urinary tract due to saline dilution of the endoluminal iodinated contrast, making this a major disadvantage for IVU [2]. However, with MDCT, because of excellent contrast resolution compared with IVU, over-zealous opacification of the collecting system can result in streak- and beam hardening artefacts; the dilutional effect thus becomes an advantage, since it can counter these effects. Numerous reports have investigated the value of infusing 100–250 ml of saline either before or immediately after the administration of non-ionic contrast [23, 32, 33]. The data from these studies were conflicting, with Caoili et al. and McTavish et al. showing improved opacification following saline infusion; however, the segments in which improved opacification was observed were significantly different in the two studies [23, 32]. Sudakoff et al. found that saline infusion did not significantly improve ureteric distension or opacification [34] and suggested that saline infusion may stimulate ureteric peristalsis in certain cases, thus potentially having the opposite effect. Our group also evaluated the impact of administering 100 ml of intravenous saline on ureteric distension and opacification in the split-bolus two-phase technique described above, and found no significant effect [27]. The ineffectiveness of saline infusion in our study was attributed by some commentators to the fact that 100 ml was an insufficient volume to positively impact ureteric distension and opacification at MDCTU [2].

Diuretic Administration

There are only very few reports describing the effects of intravenously administering a low-dose diuretic to optimise MDCTU. It is currently recommended to administer the diuretic 1 min prior to contrast administration [2]. The addition of an intravenous diuretic has been reported to increase ureteric distension and to dilute contrast. However, as discussed above, because of MDCT's excellent inherent contrast resolution compared with IVU, this may in fact be advantageous.

Patient Positioning

As previously described, distension and opacification of the mid- and especially the distal ureters is frequently suboptimal with MDCTU. McNicholas et al. reported that MDCTU performed with the patient in the prone position achieved higher opacification of the mid- and distal ureters than supine scanning, reaching statistical significance only for the mid-ureters [29]. McTavish et al. found that prone positioning did not significantly impact opacification of the distal ureters [32]. Despite conflicting and equivocal supporting evidence, we routinely employ prone positioning for the nephropyelographic phase of our split-bolus two-phase technique.

Use of High-Concentration Contrast Media

In published studies, MDCTU was carried out with intravenous injections of 100–150 ml of non-ionic contrast material containing approximately 300 mgI/ml, at rates of 2–4 ml/s. As described above, in the majority of protocols, the contrast is administered as a single bolus while two-phase protocols involve split-bolus delivery. In the literature search performed for the purpose of this review, we did not find any reports describing the use of lower volumes of high-concentration contrast medium (HCCM) for MDCTU.

There are theoretical disadvantages to the use of HCCM for MDCTU; most importantly, HCCM requires the delivery of a lower total volume of contrast medium. As described above, the major factors in improving MDCTU for thorough evaluation of the urothelium are distension and opacification. The various manoeuvres to achieve this are the use of saline infusion during MDCTU and the administration of a diuretic. Distension would appear to be the most important factor, as the improved inherent contrast resolution of CT versus conventional intravenous urography means that dense opacification is not as important and dilution can be advantageous by reducing the potential for streak and beam-hardening artefacts. Therefore, with current protocols, it is difficult to see an advantage for HCCM for the pyelographic phase of MDCTU. However, with the split-bolus two-phase technique, a lower volume of HCCM may be useful for the second injection, i.e. the nephrographic component of the nephropyelograhic phase.

Radiation Dose Associated with MDCTU

One of the major concerns that may limit universal acceptance of MDCTU is the radiation dose associated with the procedure. Radiation dosages of between 25 and 35 mSv were reported by Caoili et al. for four-phase MDCTU, which clearly significantly exceeds that of IVU [2, 7]. The radiation dose can be reduced by careful monitoring of the scanning parameters for each phase and by reduction of the number of phases [4, 8, 9]. There is little doubt that the radiation dose can be reduced for the initial non-contrast component, as the inherent image noise associated with the dose reduction is less likely to be problematic with "stone-protocol" MDCT because of the marked difference in density between calculi and the surrounding soft tissue in the kidneys, ureter and bladder. We previously investigated the use of automatic tube-current modulation techniques (z-axis technique) to reduce the radiation dose during stone-protocol MDCT and found that detection of urinary-tract calculi was feasible even with very high noise indices. Significant radiation dose reductions of 43–66% were possible at noise indices of 14 to 20 without compromising stone depiction [35]. Therefore, with consensus emerging regarding protocol design with respect to optimisation of urinary-tract distension and opacification, there is little doubt that future modifications and protocol design will focus on reducing the radiation dose. Based on our previous work, there is cause for optimism that the increased availability of emerging technologies, such as automatic tube-current modulation, will achieve significant dose reductions at least in the initial unenhanced phase. In addition, every effort must be made to reduce the number of imaging phases.

Image Interpretation

As previously discussed, interpretation of MDCTU involves the review of a large number of images, including thorough comparison of unenhanced and enhanced images for the presence of calculi and to assess the degree of contrast enhancement. The latter is particularly important in the characterisation of renal masses. The necessity of state-of-the-art, user-friendly workstations cannot be over-emphasised. When MDCTU was initially introduced, the importance of 3-D reformation was stressed. There is no doubt that 3-D reconstruction was hugely important in convincing urologists of the acceptability of this technique, as 3-D images most closely resembled those produced by conventional IVU. Multi-planar reformatted and maximum-intensity projection images (Fig. 3) are the most commonly used and remain important in evaluations of the ureter and in localising the exact level of the abnormality. These reformats are also useful in the characterisation of urinary-tract anomalies. One other point worth emphasising is that the liberal usage of wide window settings in the evaluation of delayed pyelographic phase images helps to reduce the potential for obscuration of intraluminal filling defects by artefacts from excessively dense endoluminal contrast material within the ureters [4, 8].

Comparison of MDCTU and Magnetic Resonance Urography

One of the main advantages of MDCTU in the evaluation of causes of haematuria is its ability to display the entire urinary tract, including renal parenchyma, pelvicaliceal systems, ureters and the bladder, using a single imaging test [4, 8]. Alternative imaging studies, i.e. ultrasonography, IVU and nuclear medicine alone do not offer equivalent coverage [4]. Magnetic resonance urography (MRU) is the only other option, since with this technique, all the anatomic components of the urinary tract can be thoroughly imaged in a single test [36]. MRU, using either heavily T2-weighted pulse sequences or gadolinium enhanced T1-weighted sequences, has the potential to detect, localise and characterise abnormalities of the collecting system. As neither iodinated intravenous contrast nor ionising radiation is used, the procedure is safe in patients with contraindications to iodinated contrast media as well as in young patients and in the pregnant patient [37]. However, with MRU, contrast is usually required to evaluate the renal parenchyma, especially for renal masses. The main disadvantages of MRU that have hindered its widespread application in the evaluation of the urinary tract is its limited ability to reliably detect urinary-tract calcifications, calculi and air, its limited availability compared with MDCTU and the limited experience in interpretation of the resulting images [36]. With regard to the detection of calcifications and urinary calculi, these appear as filling defects or signal voids on both heavily T2-weighted and gadolinium-enhanced T1-weighted MR urograms. Sensitivities of 94–100% in the diagnosis of ureteral stones in the setting of obstruction were recently reported [37]; however, the visualisation of non-obstructing stones is much more difficult. One of the other disadvantages of MRU is

that the spatial resolution does not approach that of MDCTU or IVU; therefore, subtle ureteric abnormalities could be missed [37]. MRU provides a comprehensive and non-invasive diagnostic tool that can be employed to image all kinds of urinary-tract disorders in adult and paediatric patients. Its use should not be confined to those patients who do not tolerate iodinated contrast agents, as it has become increasingly clear that T1- and T2- weighted MRU techniques are complementary tools that offer several first-choice applications [38].

Current Status of MDCTU in the Evaluation of Patients with Haematuria

There is little doubt that MDCTU is an appropriate imaging test for the detection and characterisation of renal masses [4]. The initial unenhanced CT is obtained to serve as the baseline for measurements of enhancement on nephrographic-phase images [4]. Most renal cell cancers are solid, with attenuation values greater than 20 HU on unenhanced CT [39]. Lesion enhancement greater than 10 HU following intravenous contrast also suggests a solid lesion, while enhancement greater than 20 HU is considered highly suspicious of a malignant lesion [40]. Small lesions (<3 cm) are usually homogeneous in appearance, but large lesions are more likely to be heterogeneous secondary to haemorrhage or necrosis. Confirmation of unequivocal enhancement within a small lesion can be impacted by volume averaging and may be difficult in larger lesions with necrotic components [40].

The location of the tumour may be helpful in the diagnosis and characterisation of solid renal masses. Renal cell carcinoma is frequently located at the periphery or near the corticomedullary junction of the kidney as it originates in the renal cortex, whereas transitional cell carcinoma and other tumours arise from the urothelium. As a consequence, they spread into the kidney from the renal pelvicaliceal system and occur more centrally in the kidney, usually displacing surrounding renal sinus fat [41, 42].

Transitional cell carcinoma is the most common malignant neoplasm of the urothelium [43]. It is 30–50 times more common in the bladder than in the ureters and renal pelvis and is often multifocal [43]. Many urologists believe that intravenous urography is still the gold standard for evaluating the urothelium [37]; however, the detection rate of this technique for urothelial neoplasms is only 43–64% [7]. In the early stages, these neoplasms are seen as subtle filling defects or focal mural thickening (Fig. 4). A filling defect in the renal pelvis or ureter can be due to a neoplasm, cal-

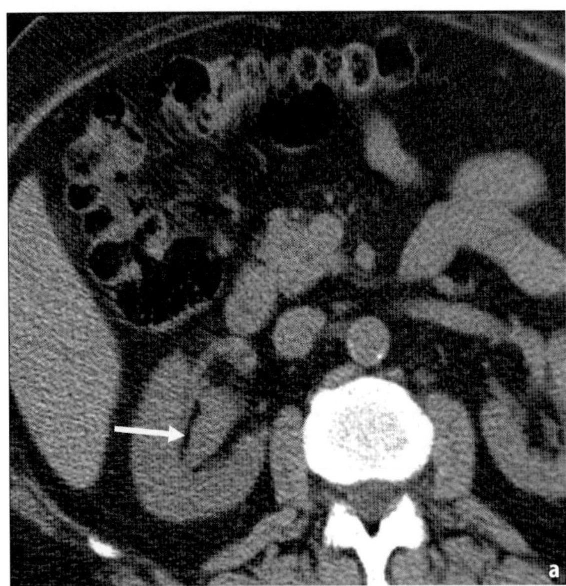

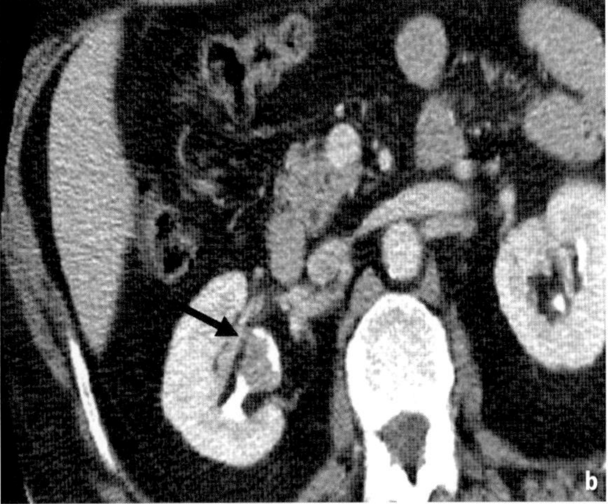

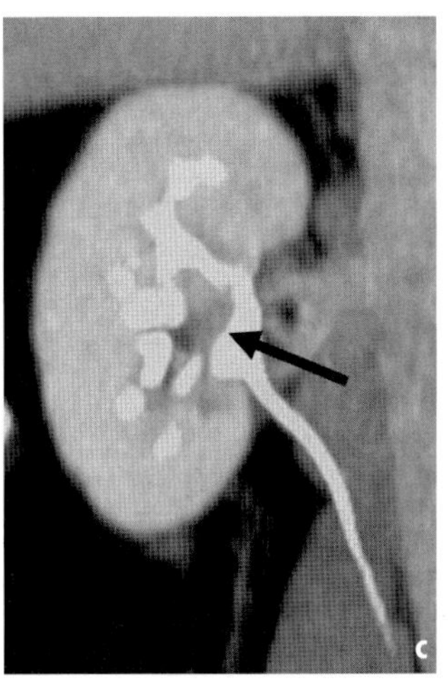

Fig. 4a-c. A 55-year-old man with painless haematuria. **a** Non-contrast axial computed tomography (CT) shows focally dilated right mid-pole calyx (*white arrow*). **b** Multi-detector CT urography (MDCTU) performed in nephropyelographic phase shows filling defect within the right collecting system (*black arrow*). **c** Coronal (poor quality) image during pyelographic phase confirming lesion in collecting system (*black arrow*). This was confirmed at surgery to be transitional cell carcinoma of the collecting system

culus, blood clot, mycetoma or vascular impression. Unfortunately, IVU or retrograde ureterography only demonstrates the lumen of the ureter and does not allow direct visualisation of extrinsic abnormalities that involve the ureter. MDCTU has shown increased sensitivity and specificity for detecting urothelial tumour compared with retrograde ureterography, an imaging test assumed to be superior to IVU in evaluating the collecting system and ureters [44]. One of the main advantages of MDCTU over intravenous urography is the identification and characterisation of intrinsic and extrinsic causes of ureteric obstruction, including mural thickening with short-segment malignant strictures, retroperitoneal masses or lymphadenopathy, retroperitoneal fibrosis, benign ureteric strictures and iatrogenic causes [4, 8].

The ability of MDCTU to detect urothelial tumours in the renal collecting system or in the ureter has not been definitively evaluated or established in the literature [4]. One recent study suggested that MDCTU detects urothelial tumours in up to 89% of cases [45]. Another recent study found MDCT scanning to be an accurate means for the detection and staging of transitional cell carcinoma of the upper urinary tract, with an accuracy for predicting peri-tumoural invasion with PPV and negative predictive values (NPV) of 88.8% and 87.5%, respectively [46]. Cowan et al. validated quantitatively the use of MDCTU for diagnosing upper urinary tract urothelial tumour. They reported a sensitivity of 0.97, a specificity of 0.93, a PPV of 0.79 and a NPV of 0.99 [44]. In the same study, retrograde ureteropyelography (RUP) had a sensitivity of 0.97, a specificity of 0.93, a PPV of 0.79 and a NPV 0.99 [44]. Therefore, MDCTU and RUP share similar diagnostic sensitivities and specificities for the diagnosis of urothelial tumours of the upper urinary tract. Accordingly, it has been recommended that MDCTU replace ul-

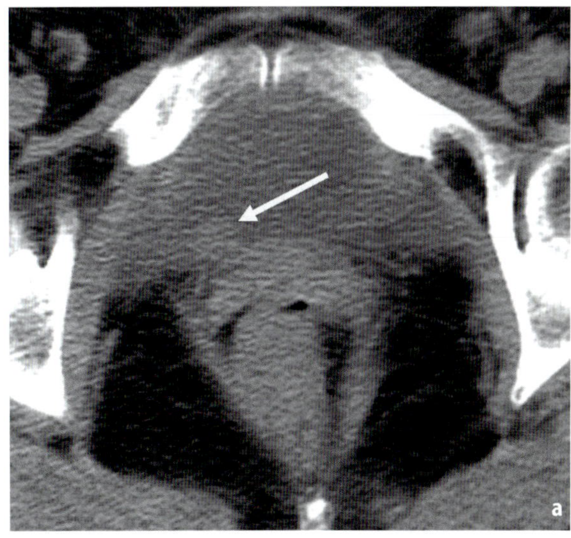
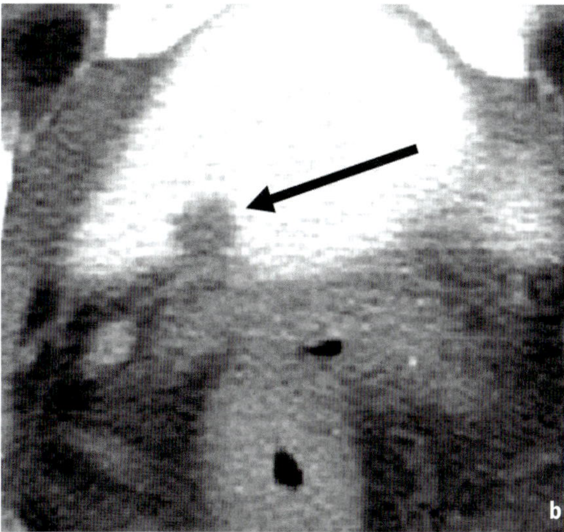

Fig. 5a, b. A 65 year-old woman with haematuria. **a** Non-contrast axial multi-detector computed tomography (MDCT) images through pelvis showing subtle soft tissue attenuation lesion (*white arrow*) in the right side of the bladder. **b** MDCT cystogram confirms lesion in the right side of the bladder (*black arrow*) with subsequent cystoscopy and biopsy confirming transitional cell carcinoma of the bladder

trasound, IVU and RUP for investigating patients with haematuria, and RUP should be reserved for patients in whom MDCTU findings are equivocal and increased radiation is therefore justifiable [44].

Cystoscopy remains the gold standard for evaluation of the urinary bladder, but MDCTU is playing an increasing role in the detection of bladder urothelial neoplasms [47]. As with other urinary-tract tumours, the assessment of bladder tumour requires contrast-enhanced examination with optimum distension and opacification of the urinary bladder for the detection of abnormalities [4]. In patients in whom bladder neoplasm is suspected, the two-phase MDCTU technique can be modified with additional further delayed images (5–10 min post-nephropyelographic phase) to obtain a more densely opacified and more distended bladder [4].

Non-contrast images of the bladder are again important in order to detect focal areas of mural calcification, which can be associated with transitional cell or squamous cell carcinoma of the bladder [4,7]. Other causes of bladder-wall calcification include cyclophosphamide-induced cystitis, prior radiation, schistosomiasis or tuberculosis [8]. Mural filling defects (Fig. 5) or focal bladder-wall thickening, when associated with increased bladder-wall enhancement, also suggests carcinoma, whereas diffuse or uniform bladder-wall thickening is usually secondary to cystitis or changes related to obstructive uropathy [7].

Conclusion

Efforts to optimise contrast opacification and distension have led to refinements of MDCTU protocols in order to allow thorough evaluation of the urothelium in patients with haematuria. Recent studies have shown encouraging data validating MDCTU usage in the evaluation of the urothelium for neoplasms, including transitional cell carcinoma. Future efforts aimed at continued refinement of these protocols must focus on optimisation but also reduction of the radiation dose. The latter will likely be achieved by reducing the number of imaging phases and by using emerging MDCT technologies.

References

1. Chow LC, Sommer FG (2001) Multidetector CT urography with abdominal compression and three-dimensional reconstruction. AJR Am J Roentgenol 177:849-55
2. Nolte-Ernsting C, Cowan N (2006) Understanding multislice CT urography techniques: Many roads lead to Rome. Eur Radiol 16:2670-2686
3. Kawashima A, Vrtiska TJ, LeRoy AJ et al (2004) CT urography. Radiographics 24:S35-54
4. Maher MM, Kalra MK, Rizzo S et al (2004) Multidetector CT urography in imaging of the urinary tract in patients with hematuria. Korean J Radiol 5:1-10
5. Fielding JR, Silverman SG, Rubin GD (1999) Helical CT of the urinary tract. AJR Am J Roentgenol 172:199-206

6. Urban BA (1997) The small renal mass: what is the role of multiphasic helical scanning? Radiology 202:22-23

7. Caoili EM, Cohan RH, Korobkin M et al (2002) Urinary tract abnormalities: initial experience with multi-detector row CT urography. Radiology 222:353-360

8. Kalra MK, Maher MM, Sahani DV et al (2002) Current status of multidetector computed tomography urography in imaging of the urinary tract. Curr Probl Diagn Radiol 31:210-221

9. Nawfel RD, Judy PF, Schleipman AR, Silverman SG (2004) Patient radiation dose at CT urography and conventional urography. Radiology 232:126-132

10. Kenney PJ (2003) CT evaluation of urinary lithiasis. Radiol Clin North Am 41:979-999

11. Smith RC, Verga M, McCarthy S, Rosenfield AT (1996) Diagnosis of acute flank pain: value of unenhanced helical CT. AJR Am J Roentgenol 166:97-101

12. Chen MY, Zagoria RJ (1999) Can noncontrast helical computed tomography replace intravenous urography for evaluation of patients with acute urinary tract colic? J Emerg Med 17:299-303

13. Niall O, Russell J, MacGregor R, Duncan H, Mullins J (1999) A comparison of noncontrast computerized tomography with excretory urography in the assessment of acute flank pain. J Urol 161:534-537

14. Blake SP, McNicholas MM, Raptopoulos V (1998) Nonopaque crystal deposition causing ureteric obstruction in patients with HIV undergoing indinavir therapy. AJR Am J Roentgenol 171:717-720

15. Pfister SA, Deckart A, Laschke S et al (2003) Unenhanced helical computed tomography vs intravenous urography in patients with acute flank pain: accuracy and economic impact in a randomized prospective trial. Eur Radiol 13:2513-2520

16. Boridy IC, Kawashima A, Goldman SM, Sandler CM (1999) Acute ureterolithiasis: nonenhanced helical CT findings of perinephric edema for prediction of degree of ureteral obstruction. Radiology 213:663-667

17. Kawashima A, Sandler CM, Boridy IC et al (1997) Unenhanced helical CT of ureterolithiasis: value of the tissue rim sign. AJR Am J Roentgenol168:997-1000

18. Bell TV, Fenlon HM, Davison BD et al (1998) Unenhanced helical CT criteria to differentiate distal ureteral calculi from pelvic phleboliths. Radiology 207:363-367

19. Guest AR, Cohan RH, Korobkin M et al (2001) Assessment of the clinical utility of the rim and comet-tail signs in differentiating ureteral stones from phleboliths. AJR Am J Roentgenol 177:1285-1291

20. Boridy IC, Nikolaidis P, Kawashima A et al (1999) Ureterolithiasis: value of the tail sign in differentiating phleboliths from ureteral calculi at nonenhanced helical CT. Radiology 211:619-621

21. Coll DM, Varanelli MJ, Smith RC (2002) Relationship of spontaneous passage of ureteral calculi to stone size and location as revealed by unenhanced helical CT. AJR Am J Roentgenol 178:101-103

22. Noroozian M, Cohan RH, Caoili EM et al (2004) Multislice CT urography: state of the art. Br J Radiol 77: S74-86

23 Caoili EM, Inampudi P, Cohan RH, Ellis JH (2005) Optimization of multi-detector row CT urography: effect of compression, saline administration, and prolongation of acquisition delay. Radiology 235:116-123

24. Chai RY, Jhaveri K, Saini S et al (2001) Comprehensive evaluation of patients with haematuria on multi-slice computed tomography scanner: protocol design and preliminary observations. Australas Radiol 45:536-538

25. Chow LC, Kwan SW, Olcott EW, Sommer G (2007) Split-bolus MDCT urography with synchronous nephrographic and excretory phase enhancement. AJR Am J Roentgenol 189:314-322

26. Sussman SK, Illescas FF, Opalacz JP et al (1993) Renal streak artifact during contrast enhanced CT comparison of high versus low osmolality contrast media. Abdom Imaging lS:180-185

27. Maher MM, Jhaveri K, Lucey B et al (2001) Does the Administration of Saline Flush during CT Urography CTU. Improve Ureteric Distension and Opacification? A Prospective Study. RSNA Meeting 2001

28. Hattery RR, Williamson B Jr, Hartman GW et al (1988) Intravenous urographic technique. Radiology 167:593-599

29. McNicholas MMJ, Raptopoulos VD, Schwartz RK et al (1998) Excretory phase CT urography for opacification of the urinary collecting system. AJR Am J Roentgenol 170:1261-1267

30. Heneghan JP, Kim DH, Leder RA et al (2001) Compression CT urography: a comparison with IVU in the opacification of the collecting system and ureters. J Comput Assist Tomogr 25:343-347

31. Chow LC, Sommer FG (2001) Multidetector CT urography with abdominal compression and three-dimensional reconstruction. AJR Am J Roentgenol 177:849-855

32. McTavish JD, Jinaki M, Zou KH, Silverman SG (2000) Multidetector CT urography: analysis of techniques and comparison with IVU. Radiology 27:225

33. Maher MM, Jhaveri K, Lucey BC et al (2000) Does the administration of saline flush during CT urography CTU. improve ureteric distension and opacification? Radiology 221:500

34. Sudakoff GS, Dunn DP, Hellman RS et al (2006) Opacification of the genitourinary collecting system during MDCT urography with enhanced CT digital radiography: nonsaline versus saline bolus. AJR Am J Roentgenol 186:122

35. Kalra MK, Maher MM, D'Souza RV et al (2005) Detection of urinary tract stones at low dose Ct with z-axis automatic tube current modulation: phantom and clinical studies. Radiology 235:523-529

36. Maher MM, Prassad TA, Fitzpatrick JM et al (2000) Spinal dysraphism at MR Urography: Initial experience. Radiology 216:237-241

37. Kawashima A,Glockner JF,King BF Jr (2003) CT urography and MR urography. Radiol Clin North Am 41:945-961

38. Nolte-Ernsting CC, Staatz G, Tacke J, Gunther RW (2003) MR urography today. Abdom Imaging 28:191-209

39. Sheth S, Scatarige JC, Horton KM et al (2001) Current concepts in the diagnosis and management of renal cell carcinoma: role of multidetector CT and three-dimensional CT. Radiographics 21:S237-S254

40. Silverman SG, Lee BY, Seltzer SE et al (1994) Small < or =3 cm. renal masses: correlation of spiral CT features and pathologic findings. AJR Am J Roentgenol 163:597-605

41. Kocakoc E, Bhatt S, Dogra VS (2005) Renal multidector row CT. Radiol Clin North Am 43:1021-1047

42. Zagoria RJ (2000) Imaging of small renal masses: a medical success story. AJR Am J Roentgenol 175:945-955

43. Anderson EM, Murphy R, Rennie AT, Cowan NC (2007) Multidetector computed tomography urog-

raphy MDCTU. for diagnosing urothelial malignancy. Clin Radiol 62:324-332

44. Cowan NC, Turney BW, Taylor NJ et al (2007) Multidetector computed tomography urography for diagnosing upper urinary tract urothelial tumour. BJU Int 99:1363-1370

45. Caoili EM, Cohan RH, Inampudi P et al (2005) MDCT urography of upper tract urothelial neoplasms. AJR Am J Roentgenol 184:1873-1881

46. Fritz GA, Schoellnast H, Deutschmann HA et al (2006) Multiphasic multidetector-row CT MDCT. in detection and staging of transitional cell carcinomas of the upper urinary tract. Eur Radiol 16:1244-1252

47. Dillman JR, Caoili EM, Cohan RH (2007) Multi-detector CT urography: a one-stop renal and urinary tract imaging modality. Abdom Imaging 32:519-529

PET/CT in Abdominal and Pelvic Malignancies: Principles and Practices

Michael Moore, Michael A. Blake

Introduction

Current multi-detector computed tomography (MDCT) allows for rapid acquisition of data sets with accurate anatomic detail and high spatial resolution. This provides valuable multi-planar information regarding the morphologic features and attenuation values of both normal anatomic structures and pathologic lesions. Since its introduction more than 25 years ago, CT has become widely used and can be considered the modality of choice for much cross-sectional imaging, particularly of oncologic entities. A limitation of CT, however, is its reliance on morphologic changes in the size, shape, or attenuation values of a structure to detect pathologic processes. Therefore, CT is less sensitive in the imaging of early disease processes and in the detection of disease recurrence in tissues that are already morphologically abnormal as a result of treatment.

Positron emission tomography (PET) with the fluorine 18 [^{18}F]-labeled glucose analogue [^{18}F]-fluorodeoxyglucose (FDG) allows for the functional imaging of tissues, both normal and diseased. FDG-PET provides both qualitative and quantitative metabolic information that is valuable for diagnosis and management. Furthermore, PET can detect early increases in metabolic activity in otherwise morphologically normal tissue. PET is of value in the differentiation of benign from malignant tumors as well as in follow-up oncologic imaging following surgical, radiation, or chemotherapeutic treatment [1]. However, the sensitivity of PET at detecting hypermetabolic foci with high target-to-background ratios is compromised to a large extent by low-background FDG uptake during attempts at accurate anatomic localization [2]. The lack of readily identifiable and reliable anatomic structures on PET imaging is particularly true for abdominopelvic imaging, which is further complicated by variable physiologic FDG uptake.

One of the most exciting technological imaging advances in recent years is the clinical application of combined PET/CT scanning. Combined imaging with PET/CT scanners enables fusion of the CT-acquired predominantly morphologic information with PET-facilitated functional imaging. Specifically, PET/CT uses the precise morphologic information provided by CT to accurately locate the hypermetabolic foci identified by PET, thereby increasing the diagnostic yield. Furthermore, the information provided by combined PET/CT imaging allows the separation of normal physiologic from pathologic uptake and reduces the incidence of false-negative and false-positive imaging studies. Indeed, it has been shown that PET/CT imaging is more sensitive and more specific for many oncologic entities than either modality alone [3]. In addition, both modalities have individual strengths that are also highly complementary. PET can be used with different radiotracers to provide other useful biologic information, while CT provides valuable multi-planar information regarding the morphologic features and attenuation values of lesions as well as information regarding the behavior of administered contrast material.

Technical Considerations

The earliest attempts at functional and morphologic combination imaging involved software fusion of separately acquired PET and CT data sets. Software manipulation was used to anatomically align results of the two studies. Whereas this was technically easy and successful in the brain, body imaging was more challenging and limited by the temporal separation of the source information. Discrepancies in a number of variables between the two separate scans, including patient position, respiratory motion, bowel peristalsis, and urinary tract distension, frequently resulted in malalignment and subsequent difficulties with interpretation. This stimulated the development of a single machine, a fusion of the PET and CT hardware, able to acquire both data sets as a single study and facilitate subsequent co-registration of the information.

The first PET/CT prototype scanner became functional in 1998 [4]. Following subsequent development, the first commercial scanners appeared in the clinical arena in 2001, and by early 2007, more than 800 combined PET/CT scanners had been installed in clinical institutions worldwide [3]. Although there are technical differences between the different manufacturers, the basic concept is the same: a single unit in which the independent diagnostic PET and CT scanners are physically aligned, usually with a single common patient bed. With this hybrid device, functional and morphologic information can be acquired in a single examination and thereafter be more accurately aligned.

The easier and more accurate co-registration of morphologic and functional data is not the only benefit of hybrid PET/CT machines. Despite the development of new and faster scintillators, such as lutetium oxyorthosilicate and gadolinium oxyorthosilicate, PET-only whole-body scans typically require 45-60 min to complete. One of the biggest contributors to this lengthy scan time is the transmission scan required for attenuation correction, a process that improves the qualitative artifacts and quantitative accuracy of PET [5]. However, CT-based attenuation correction is much faster than traditional transmission methods, provides almost noise-free information, and allows for total PET/CT scanning times of only 20-30 min. This significantly reduces scanning time, enhances patient comfort and convenience, and enables a greater patient throughput. PET scan time may also be reduced by the use of time-of-flight (TOF) technology, which improves scan time and increases signal-to-noise ratio [6]. Recent detector and scintillator developments enable sub-nanosecond coincidence timing resolution, and thus a fast, TOF-based and back-projection-free, 3-D reconstruction algorithm that, coupled with a real-time data acquisition and a fast detector encoding scheme, allows high-precision images to be obtained in real time [7]. FDG-PET also provides quantitative data in the form of the standardized uptake value (SUV) or standardized uptake ratio (SUR). These are uptake measurements that provide a means of comparison of FDG uptake between different lesions. Measurement of SUV requires attenuation correction to avoid the variability in FDG uptake due to differences in tumor depth within the body.

Protocol Considerations

PET/CT is a newly developing and evolving technology, and as such, the optimal protocols are not yet established. There is ongoing debate regarding the most appropriate CT scanning parameters, the use of oral and intravenous contrast material, and the optimal respiratory phase to scan [8-10].

CT-based attenuation correction, as mentioned, provides for faster scan times with significantly less statistical noise than generated with traditional transmission scan attenuation correction. However, with this technique, there is also a potential risk of overestimating the true FDG activity. In normal structures, including bone and soft tissues, this is unlikely to be problematic, although it should be accounted for when comparing results between different PET and PET/CT systems [8]. However, highly attenuating structures on CT, such as metallic prostheses, surgical clips, and intrauterine contraceptive devices, as well as high-attenuation foci of oral and intravenous contrast, can result in overcorrection with subsequent artifact formation. As a consequence, the corresponding photopenic areas on PET may manifest artifactually as hypermetabolic foci. This can usually be recognized by careful review of the non-attenuation-corrected PET images. Furthermore, modifications to the reconstruction algorithms can, to some extent, reduce artifacts related to such high-attenuating substances.

Lesion detection on CT is based on morphologic characteristics, including attenuation differences between the lesion and adjacent structures. Most parenchymal organs and most pathologic conditions have similar attenuation values within a relatively narrow range, typically 30–80 HU. Intravenous CT contrast agents are routinely used to exaggerate the attenuation differences between normal and pathologic tissues and thereby increase the conspicuity of the lesions. However, the higher attenuation values associated with such agents, particularly in vascular structures, are also at risk of artifact production when used to correct attenuation for PET/CT. More recent reports have suggested that such changes in attenuation correction are not statistically or clinically significant [9, 11, 12].

Similarly, oral contrast agents are routinely used to aid in the CT diagnosis of gastrointestinal-tract-related pathologic conditions. Traditionally, these consist of positive, high-attenuating substances including barium and Gastrografin compounds. In practice, the distribution of such agents is variable both in terms of spatial distribution and contrast enhancement and is aggravated by peristalsis-related position changes between the PET and CT components. This again leads to the potential production of erroneous hypermetabolic foci following CT-based attenuation correction. As a result, some authors advocate the use of water-attenuation oral contrast agents [13] or even abstaining from using any oral agent at all. However, oral contrast is clearly desirable for optimal CT evaluation and, as with intravenous contrast agents, there is growing evidence that dilute concentrations of even positive oral contrast agents may not significantly effect attenuation correction [14].

Radiation dose is always an important consideration in CT imaging. A recent, alarming report by Brenner and Hall [15] estimated that 1.5–2% of all cancers in the United States might now be attributable to the radiation from CT studies. Although this estimation is controversial, with many believing the risk to be lower, it nonetheless highlights the potential risk associated with medical ionizing radiation. Modern MDCT scanners allow for the rapid acquisition of high-spatial resolution images, with even isotropic information possible, thus allowing for anatomically perfect multi-planar reconstructions. However, such high-quality imaging has the price of increased patient radiation dose. When integrating a full-dose CT, with a tube current in the order of 100–140 mA, the radiation dose for a scan from the head to the top of the thighs is approximately 15–20 mSv. It has been shown that much lower tube currents, with a range of 10–40 mA, are adequate for CT-based attenuation correction [16]. Such low-dose scans have a significantly lower radiation dose, 3–4 mSv, but it is being currently debated whether such scans are sufficient to allow a CT-based interpretation due to the increased noise level and reduced image quality.

As stated previously, the main advantage of PET/CT over the individual components is the ability to accurately anatomically localize a focus of hypermetabolic activity. The ability to do this is reliant on accurate registration; that is, when the individual PET and CT components are superimposed at the workstation, there is appropriate alignment of the two data sets. The benefit of combined imaging during a single examination minimizes potential misregistration due to patient motion, bowel motility, and urinary tract distention. However, differing respiratory phases are a potential cause of significant misregistration. Standard diagnostic CT studies are performed during a single breath-hold at maximal inspiratory effort, a technique that optimizes pulmonary parenchymal imaging. Although some patients may not be able to breath-hold long enough for a whole-body CT, resulting in motion artifact in the lower parts of the body, modern multi-slice CT scanners, including 64-slice machines, are capable of faster whole-body scan times and enable study completion within a single breath-hold in the majority of patients. Alternatively, PET studies with average acquisition times of 20–30 min, obviously too long for a single breath-hold, are performed during quiet respiration. The two differing techniques might result in widely varying positions of the diaphragm and adjacent organs and thus cause misregistration. The most appropriate CT breathing protocol remains to be determined. During quiet free breathing, the diaphragm spends the majority of time in the position of end-tidal volume, and it has been shown that performing CT during a suspended end-tidal breath hold allows for accurate image registration [17, 18]. This also requires that technologists inform, instruct, and practice the maneuver with the patient so that breathing instructions are understood before the CT component is performed, especially for those patients who might be familiar with the more standard instructions for conventional diagnostic CT. However, other investigators, including those at our institution, have demonstrated that excellent PET and CT alignment is also possible with mid-suspended breath-hold and quiet breathing, as well as end-expiration, without statistical difference [19].

Once the desired PET and CT data sets have been acquired, it is mandatory that the scans are reviewed on a dedicated PET/CT workstation. An accurate interpretation of the study requires the ability to simultaneously review CT data, including multi-planar reconstructions with varied window settings, together with both the non-attenuation-corrected and attenuation-corrected PET scan as well as with the combined co-registered images. All this, along with the ability to compare the results with prior PET or PET/CT studies, is usually beyond the capability of standard photo archiving and communication system (PACS) workstations and requires a dedicated PET/CT workstation.

Protocols in Practice

When one considers the multiple variables involved in the planning of a protocol for an abdominopelvic PET/CT, ranging from low-dose noncontrast CT to a fully diagnostic study employing oral and intravenous contrast, in addition to the limitations and potential artifacts from these various factors, it is readily apparent why a definitive, internationally recognized, and standardized protocol has not yet been agreed upon. In our institution, the practice is to combine the two aforementioned approaches. We first perform a low-dose unenhanced CT, primarily to provide attenuation correction. Thereafter, the PET data are obtained, followed immediately by a fully diagnostic, standard radiation dose, intravenous contrast-agent-enhanced CT with water-attenuation oral contrast. This maximizes the diagnostic information from the study and minimizes the risk of artifacts.

Patients are fasted with no caloric intake for a minimum of 4 h before the test. Water intake is, however, encouraged, together with regular bladder voiding, to aid FDG renal-tract excretion. As FDG is a glucose analogue, its uptake and distribution in tissues are affected by serum glucose and insulin levels, such that low levels of both are desirable. Along with fasting, patients with diabetes should not receive regular insulin within the same 4-h period prior to the study. Serum glucose is measured and should be < 200 mg/dl. If serum glucose is higher, available options include gentle exercise (walking) and then a re-check, administration of subcutaneous insulin and re-checking the serum glucose in approximately 3 h, or re-scheduling the exam.

Once the desired glucose range is confirmed, we administer FDG intravenously at a dose of 140 µCi/kg, and generally within the range of 10-20 mCi. Patients are given 1,350 ml of low-attenuating oral contrast to drink over 45 min. While waiting the 60 min between FDG administration and subsequent imaging, patients are encouraged to rest, and activities including talking, chewing, and walking are restricted. Thereafter, the PET/CT scan is obtained as described above. A sample protocol is shown in Figure 1.

Physiologic and Non-neoplastic Distribution of FDG

Normal physiologic uptake of FDG in the brain, myocardium, brown fat, and skeletal muscle is well understood and relatively predictable. However, FDG uptake in the organs of the abdomen and pelvis is somewhat more variable.

FDG is filtered by the glomerulus but not reabsorbed and consequently is routinely seen in the renal pelvis, ureters, and bladder as a normal excreted product. Hydration and regular bladder voiding are promoted to minimize urinary stasis and the potential for normal physiologic excretion to mask underlying renal-tract malignancy. This is particularly true in the setting of dilated ureters or bladder diverticulae, which may mask retroperitoneal or pelvic FDG uptake by a non-urinary-tract malignancy [20].

The gastrointestinal tract demonstrates more variable FDG uptake [21]. Normal uptake is seen in the stomach wall and can have a variable appearance depending in part on the degree of gastric distension. Physiologic uptake is also seen in the small bowel and colon and is usually identified by its location and linear pattern of uptake. FDG uptake is typically isolated rather than diffuse, but intense uptake can occur, particularly in the right colon. When segmental, small-bowel FDG uptake is usually readily identifiable as representing the

intestine, although very short segments can appear as discrete foci. The precise origin of FDG uptake in the digestive tract is unknown, but theories include active smooth muscle, metabolically active mucosa, lymphocyte concentration, swallowed secretions, or colonic microbial uptake. Increased uptake is also seen in inflammatory bowel disease.

The liver typically demonstrates mild FDG activity, with a uniform mottled appearance. Uptake in the spleen is typically uniform and less active than in the liver. However, intense splenic uptake may be seen in patients undergoing treatment with granulocyte-stimulating factor, a process that may also cause diffuse, intense FDG uptake in the bone marrow [22].

Within the pelvis, FDG uptake in the pre-menopausal endometrium and ovary may be physiologic and varies within the menstrual cycle. Uptake in these organs in the post-menopausal patient is abnormal and suggests malignancy [20].

Non-physiologic, non-neoplastic lesions are a potential source of false-positive hypermetabolic FDG uptake. This can occur in the setting of granulomatous disease, abscess, foreign-body reactions, and acute inflammatory processes, such as diverticulitis, gastritis, and atherosclerosis. Increased FDG uptake is also seen following surgery and radiation therapy, and it is recommended that follow-up imaging to assess for residual tumor or disease recurrence be postponed for at least 6 weeks following such treatment to prevent a false-positive interpretation of persistent post-treatment FDG activity [19].

Gastrointestinal Tract

Esophageal Carcinoma

Although primarily an intrathoracic organ, the incidence of adenocarcinoma of the distal esophagus and gastroesophageal junction has increased dramatically in recent years, currently accounting for the majority of new cases of esophageal cancer [23]. Therefore, imaging of this malignancy will be considered here. In the United States, the guidelines of the Centers for Medicare and Medicaid Services (CMS) approve the use of FDG-PET and thus PET/CT for the diagnosis, staging, and restaging of esophageal cancer, including both squamous cell carcinoma and adenocarcinoma.

Diagnosis of Esophageal Carcinoma

The standard diagnostic tools for esophageal cancer are endoscopic ultrasound (EUS) for local assessment of the T and N statuses and CT for additional staging of distant metastases. Final T stag-

PET/CT for contrast part of PET/CT

64-slice scanner

Neck, chest, ABD/PEL CT for CT part of PET

Patient orientation	Supine – feet first - arms over head
Landmark	OM
IV contrast	Injected at 2.5 ml/s followed by 30 ml saline
Oral contrast	2-3 bottles of low-density contrast (if not possible, H_2O)
Localizer radiograph	Anteroposterior only 120 kVp; 30 mA

Phase	**Non-contrast**	**Post-contrast**	**Additional hi-res chest CT**
Scan parameters			
Breathhold	Quiet breathing/expiration	Quiet breathing/expiration	Inspiration
Range	OM line to upper thigh	OM line to upper thigh	Apex to lung base
Acquisition mode	Helical	Helical	Sequential
kVp	120	140	140
Pitch	1.5	1	Not applicable
Reference mAs	60	200	200
Gantry rotation time	0.5 s	0.5 s	0.5 s
Kernel	B35 medium smooth	B35 medium smooth	B60 (sharp)
Slice thickness/overlap	5 mm/1.5 mm	5 mm/5 mm	1 mm slices at 30-mm interval
		2 mm/2 mm	
DFOV	70 cm	Based on patient's size	Focused to lungs

Non-contrast CT for PET/CT

PET/CT
64-slice scanner

PET Images

Beds need to match topogram

Input how many minutes per bed… up to 200 lbs
2–3 min/bed

200–250 lbs 3–3.5 min/bed

250 lbs over 5 min/bed

Neck, chest, ABD/PEL CT for CT part of PET

Patient orientation	Supine – Feet first - Arms over head
Landmark	OM line
IV contrast	None
Oral contrast	2-3 bottles low-density contrast (450 ml)
Localizer radiograph	AP only (120 kVp, 22 mA)
Kernel	B 35 medium smooth
Breathhold	Quiet breathing/end tidal expiration
Slice thickness	5 mm with 70 cm DFOV
Pitch	1.2
Gantry rotation time	0.5 s
kVp	140 kv
Tube current	4-D automatic tube current modulation
Reconstructed slice thickness (2nd set of images)	2 mm with 50 cm DFOV

Fig. 1. Example of PET/CT protocol

ing is dependent on histopathologic examination of the resected tissue. A review of the published literature has failed to identify any study that evaluates the use of PET or PET/CT for the diagnosis of esophageal cancer, either as a screening modality for undiagnosed tumors or as a diagnostic modality for suspicious esophageal abnormalities found by other means [5]. The reasons PET is not suitable as a screening test for esophageal cancer include radiation dose, cost, and lack of sufficient specificity. However, in studies of patients with known esophageal cancer, PET appears to be accurate for detection of the primary lesion. An early study by Yeung et al. [24] directly compared FDG-PET with CT in the evaluation of patients with esophageal cancer. Of the 67 patients undergoing initial staging, the primary tumor was visible in 66 (99%), with the sole PET-negative lesion measuring 4 mm in size. There was no apparent difference in FDG uptake between squamous cell carcinoma, adenocarcinoma, and carcinomas of other cell types. However, FDG uptake in the esophagus has also been reported in several benign esophageal conditions, which limits the usefulness of PET as a diagnostic modality for esophageal neoplasm. Benign causes leading to FDG uptake include infectious esophagitis, Barrett esophagus without malignancy, inflammatory esophagitis due to reflux disease, and post-procedural changes [3, 5, 25]. No reliable criteria yet exist for the differentiation between benign and malignant esophageal processes on PET images [5].

Initial Staging of Esophageal Carcinoma

Accurate disease staging is vital to appropriate classification of patients as surgical or non-surgical candidates and to determine whether adjuvant therapy is needed. Esophageal carcinoma is most commonly staged according to the American Joint Committee on Cancer (AJCC) staging guidelines, which incorporate the T, N, and M classification. The T descriptor refers to the depth of tumor penetration through the mucosal layers of the esophageal wall, the N descriptor specifies involvement of locoregional lymph nodes, and the M descriptor indicates the presence or absence of distant metastases. The T stage is determined by the extent of invasion by the primary tumor through the mucosal layers of the esophagus and into the adventitia and adjacent organs. A higher T classification is associated with a greater likelihood of nodal metastatic disease and poorer long-term survival [26]. When the primary tumor is confined to the esophageal wall (T1–T2), primary resection is possible. Extension into the periesophageal adventitia signifies a T3 carcinoma, while invasion of tumor into adjacent organs indicates T4 disease. Although most esophageal carcinomas appear FDG avid at PET/CT, the insufficient spatial and contrast resolutions of this technique limit visualization of the anatomic extent of the primary mass and preclude evaluation of the depth of local tumor invasion in most cases. Early stage carcinomas, in particular, may not be detectable at all. A recent study by Little et al. that assessed FDG-PET staging of known superficial esophageal carcinoma reported detection of only 45% of in situ carcinoma (Tis) and 69% of T1 lesions. PET was unable to differentiate between Tis and T1 [27]. Endoscopic ultrasound is the modality of choice for identifying and assessing the depth of penetration of the primary tumor through the esophageal wall at initial staging. One study directly comparing EUS, PET, and

CT in the staging of esophageal carcinoma reported a T-stage accuracy of 42% for CT and for PET with 71% accuracy for EUS [28]. A more recent study by Pfau et al. [29] compared EUS with PET and CT (including PET/CT) in the preoperative staging of esophageal carcinoma. Lesion sensitivity was 80%, 92%, and 100% for CT, PET, and EUS, respectively, and only EUS was able to provide tumor stage. Bar-Shalom et al. [30] assessed the additional benefit of PET/CT over PET alone. They reported PET/CT specificity and accuracy for the detection of esophageal carcinoma of 81% and 90%, respectively, with just 59% and 83% for PET alone.

Staging of nodal metastases in esophageal cancer is either N0 (no malignant lymph nodes) or N1 (lymphatic metastases to locoregional lymph nodes). Locoregional lymph nodes are those that represent the sites of primary lymphatic drainage from the carcinoma and therefore differ depending on tumor location (cervical, intrathoracic, or gastroesophageal). They are normally resected with the primary tumor at the time of surgery. For tumors arising from the gastroesophageal junction, locoregional lymph nodes comprise lower periesophageal and pulmonary-ligament lymph nodes, diaphragmatic lymph nodes (lying on the dome of the diaphragm or in the retrocrural regions), pericardial lymph nodes (located immediately adjacent to the gastroesophageal junction), left gastric lymph nodes, and celiac lymph nodes [26]. Lymphadenopathy just beyond locoregional lymph nodes is regarded as M1a disease, with M1b used to denote distant organ metastases. The nomenclature used for the designation of non-regional lymph nodes depends on the anatomic location of the primary tumor, so that for tumors of the distal esophagus, celiac lymphadenopathy is classified as M1a disease and cervical lymphadenopathy as M1b disease. The designation M1a is used because patients with metastases to non-regional lymph nodes have a much worse outcome than patients with involvement of locoregional lymph nodes only but have a better long-term prognosis than patients with M1b disease. It is important to note that distant lymph node metastases may occur without involvement of intervening locoregional lymph nodes, reportedly in 25% of cases [26].

A meta-analysis of 12 studies reviewing the staging performance of FDG-PET in esophageal carcinoma demonstrated a sensitivity and specificity of 51% and 84%, respectively, for the detection of locoregional lymph node metastases (LNMs) [31]. Lowe et al. [28] compared CT, EUS, and PET; sensitivity and specificity for LNM were 84% and 67% for CT, 86% and 67% for EUS, and 82% and 60% for PET, thus demonstrating similar performance in nodal staging for the three modalities. However, the more recent study by Pfau et al. [29] reported EUS to be more sensitive identifying LNM in a greater number of patients than CT or PET (59%, 27%, and 38%, respectively). This result supports an earlier study by Lerut et al. [32], who reported sensitivity and accuracy for LNM of 22% and 48%, respectively, for PET vs. 83% and 69% for a combination of CT and EUS. However, a more recent study [33] comparing PET with CT for the preoperative staging of esophageal carcinoma found PET to be more sensitive than CT at detection of LNM (71% vs. 29%) and with the same specificity (67%), supporting similar early findings by Flanagan et al. [34]. These mixed results highlight the limited role of PET in detecting LNMs, the cause of which is likely multifactorial. The limited spatial resolution of PET renders FDG uptake within periesophageal lymph nodes that are anatomically close to the primary tumor difficult to differentiate from uptake within the lesion itself. Benign inflammatory processes, including granulomatous infections and sarcoidosis, may on occasion result in false positive results. Furthermore, microscopic metastatic disease within lymph nodes may not demonstrate sufficient FDG uptake for detection with PET [26, 33]. In most studies, the specificity of PET for regional nodal disease is much higher than the sensitivity. PET has been shown to be more specific for disease than CT and EUS, and the presence of discrete focal metabolic activity in periesophageal or regional lymph nodes (RLNs) is highly indicative of nodal metastasis. The usefulness of PET for classification of N stage remains to be defined, but currently the sensitivity does not appear to be sufficient for accurate presurgical staging. Therefore, nodal staging in the patient with esophageal cancer remains a multimodality task, with possible roles for imaging, minimally invasive surgery and intraoperative staging. In clinical practice, nodal status should be determined by a multidisciplinary approach that includes information from EUS, PET, and CT. More recently, a number of studies have demonstrated improved results with combined PET/CT imaging [30]. Yuan et al. [35] directly compared PET/CT with PET in the preoperative detection of LNM in esophageal carcinoma. They reported sensitivity, specificity, and accuracy rates of 82%, 88%, and 86%, respectively, for PET alone and 94%, 91%, and 93% for combined PET/CT imaging (Fig. 2).

The M stage is determined by the presence or absence of metastatic disease and is subdivided into M1a and M1b, as detailed above. Metastatic disease is present in 20–30% of patients with esophageal cancer at initial evaluation [34]. The meta-analysis by van Westreenen et al. reviewing

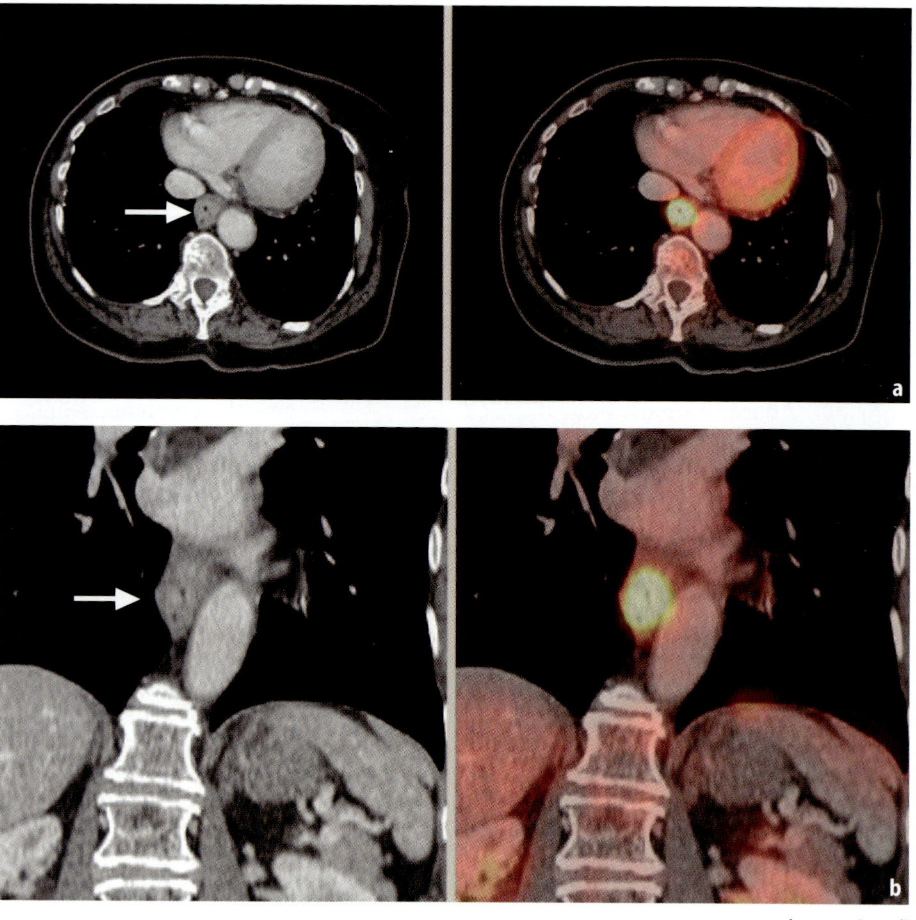

(→ continued)

the staging performance of FDG-PET in esophageal carcinoma demonstrated a sensitivity and specificity of 67% and 97%, respectively, for the detection of distant metastases [31]. PET detects M1a nodal disease significantly better than regional nodal-disease. In a prospective study of 42 patients evaluated with FDG-PET, CT, and EUS, PET was found to be 86% accurate in the evaluation of M1a nodal metas-

tases, with a specificity of 90%. The accuracy and specificity for the combined assessment with CT and EUS were 62% and 69%, respectively [32]. PET has been shown to accurately demonstrate sites of distant metastatic disease, and in most studies, the sensitivity and specificity of PET for M1b disease are higher than those for CT and EUS [28, 29, 32, 34, 36, 37]. This distinction is important because re-

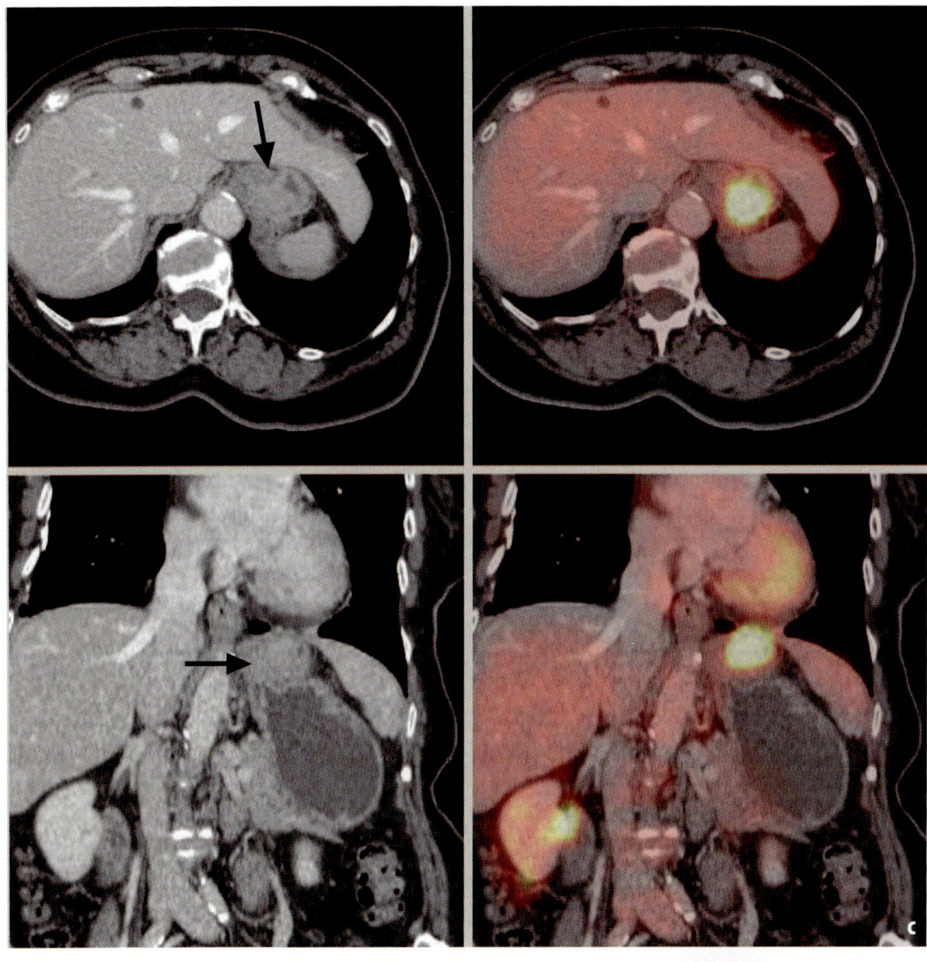

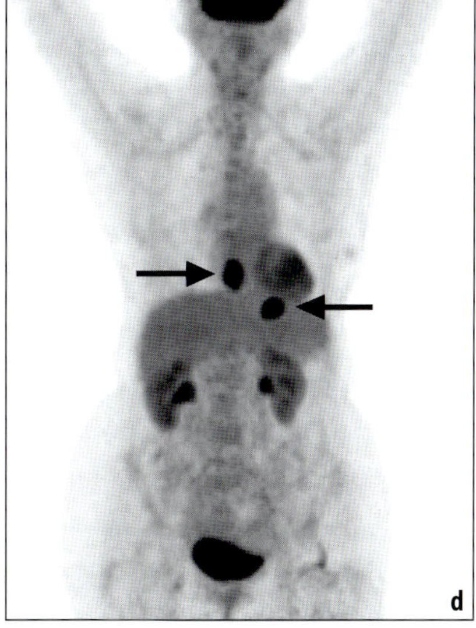

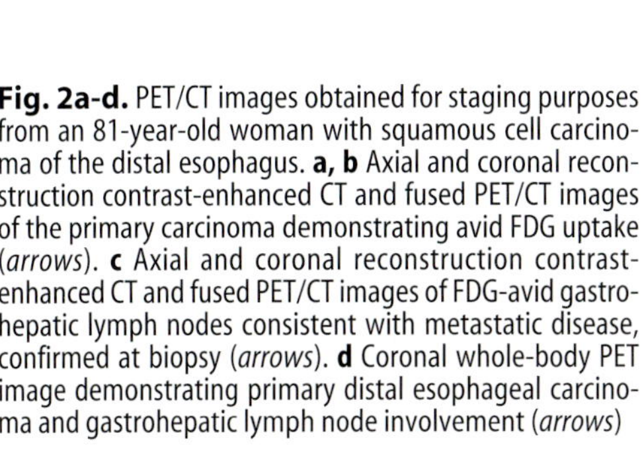

Fig. 2a-d. PET/CT images obtained for staging purposes from an 81-year-old woman with squamous cell carcinoma of the distal esophagus. **a, b** Axial and coronal reconstruction contrast-enhanced CT and fused PET/CT images of the primary carcinoma demonstrating avid FDG uptake (*arrows*). **c** Axial and coronal reconstruction contrast-enhanced CT and fused PET/CT images of FDG-avid gastrohepatic lymph nodes consistent with metastatic disease, confirmed at biopsy (*arrows*). **d** Coronal whole-body PET image demonstrating primary distal esophageal carcinoma and gastrohepatic lymph node involvement (*arrows*)

gional lymphadenopathy adjacent to the esophagus or stomach can be resected and does not preclude curative surgery, whereas distant metastases (liver, lung, bone, supraclavicular lymph nodes, and intraperitoneal spread) are contraindications for radical surgery. In one study, presurgical staging with CT was 65% accurate for the presence of resectable vs. unresectable disease compared with an 88% accuracy of FDG-PET [37]. With combined PET/CT imaging, the functional advantages of PET and the structural advantages of CT combine to improve the detection rate of metastases [30]. If the tumor is anatomically apparent but metabolically inactive, CT will still detect it. If the tumor shows increased metabolic activity but is without CT abnormalities, it will nevertheless be detectable by PET.

The addition of PET to CT and/or EUS in the assessment of patients with esophageal carcinoma frequently results in changes in disease management, usually in the upstaging of patients and the avoidance of unnecessary surgery, and may effect as many as 40% of patients [29, 32, 34, 38]. In addition, the combination of PET/CT changed disease management in 10% of patients compared with PET alone [30]. In patients being evaluated for resection of esophageal carcinoma, a combined approach with the use of both modalities provides the best staging information. Lately, there has been much interest in the role of PET and PET/CT in the planning of radiation treatment. A recent study by Leong et al. [39] comparing PET/CT with CT alone, demonstrated a potential reduction in the undertreatment of tumor when planning was performed with PET/CT.

Restaging of Esophageal Cancer and Evaluation of the Response to Therapy

PET and PET/CT are considered important additions to conventional imaging modalities in follow-up of patients who undergo chemotherapy and radiation therapy, often supplying additional information not otherwise available. Metabolic changes in the tumor usually precede morphologic changes; therefore, FDG-PET of tumor metabolism provides a sensitive means of evaluating response to therapy. A recent study showed that metabolic alterations detected with FDG-PET are sensitive and specific for identifying responders to neoadjuvant therapy [40]. The decrease in FDG uptake after therapy was significantly greater in responders than in non-responders, and the decrease in metabolic activity was closely related to histopathologic outcome. Significant decrease in FDG uptake was also associated with a favorable response to therapy. These findings were echoed by Weber et al. [41] in their study, which also indicated that PET could differentiate responding from non-responding tumors early in the course of therapy and thus may avoid ineffectual and potentially harmful treatment.

In similar fashion to the initial staging of esophageal cancer, a multimodality approach is regularly applied to the detection of recurrent disease in patients after treatment. Endoscopy can be used to assess endoluminal and perianastomotic disease recurrence, and CT is often employed for detection of regional and distant metastatic disease. FDG-PET has been shown to supplement the information provided by those modalities in the evaluation of patients suspected of having disease recurrence.

In a study of 41 patients suspected of having recurrent disease, PET was compared with the conventional diagnostic workup, which included CT, endoscopy, and EUS [42]. Results were compared according to the site of disease recurrence. Of the patients who ultimately proved to have local disease recurrence at the anastomotic site, all were correctly identified at conventional imaging, primarily endoscopy. All local recurrences also showed increased FDG uptake, with 100% sensitivity for local disease recurrence. As discussed previously, however, the specificity of PET for esophageal malignancy is limited because of FDG uptake in benign esophageal conditions, and in this study, the specificity of PET for recurrence was 57%. Specifically, in the post-treatment stage, additional causes of false-positive PET studies include post-balloon dilatation of benign anastomotic strictures and post-radiation therapy. For the diagnosis of regional and distant recurrences, the sensitivity, specificity, and accuracy of PET were 94%, 82%, and 87%, respectively, vs. 81%, 82%, and 81% for conventional diagnostic workup. Sites of distant recurrence included both nodal and extranodal sites of disease. In all, addition of PET to the conventional staging work-up in patients suspected of having disease recurrence provided additional information regarding disease stage in 27% of patients [42].

In a meta-analysis of the published literature addressing the role of CT, EUS, and FDG-PET in the assessment of response to neoadjuvant therapy for esophageal carcinoma, Westerterp et al. [43] reported CT to be significantly inferior to EUS and PET for joint sensitivity and specificity (54%, 86%, and 85%, respectively). A recent study by Guo et al. [44] reported sensitivity, specificity, and accuracy of 93%, 76%, and 87% for the detection of recurrence at all sites by PET/CT in patients with treated esophageal carcinoma. Another prospective trial, with 48 patients, was performed to evaluate CT, EUS, and PET/CT in the assessment of disease response to neoadjuvant chemoradiation. The accuracy for nodal disease was 78% for CT, 78% for EUS, and best at 93% for PET/CT. Complete response was accurately predicted by EUS in 67% and again better by PET/CT in 89% [45].

Colorectal Carcinoma

In the United States, the CMS have approved Medicare coverage for FDG-PET, and thus PET/CT, in the diagnosis, staging, and restaging of colorectal cancer.

Diagnosis of Colorectal Carcinoma

Although FDG-PET is sensitive for detecting primary colorectal carcinoma (95–100%), it has lower specificity than current morphologic imaging modalities at initial staging. Furthermore, PET scanners lack the resolution required to evaluate the depth of tumor penetration through the bowel wall. In clinical practice, FDG-PET is therefore rarely specifically used for the diagnosis of colorectal cancer, although it may make the diagnosis as an incidental finding, particularly as PET, and more specifically PET/CT, become more widely used. At the primary site, however, the negative predictive value (NPV) of PET is greater than the positive predictive value (PPV) due to false-positive FDG-PET findings of inflammatory processes and physiological bowel activity, as previously discussed [46-48].

Staging of Colorectal Carcinoma

The main accepted role of FDG-PET and PET/CT in staging colorectal cancer is the assessment of regional lymph node involvement and distal metastases. In previous studies, FDG-PET was shown to have a low sensitivity of between 22% and 29% for RLN metastases, with CT demonstrating similar low values (29%). However, the specificity of FDG-PET was higher (96% vs. 85%) [47, 48]. False-negative findings in regional metastatic lymph nodes on FDG-PET may be due to microscopic involvement of small lymph nodes or, sometimes, to intense FDG uptake by the primary site, which obscures the immediately adjacent structures.

At the time of initial staging, most patients with colorectal cancer have disease limited to the bowel or to regional pericolic or mesenteric lymph nodes [49]. With early colorectal cancer, surgery is typically performed with the intent to achieve cure, whereas advanced disease often requires the surgical management of complications, including perforation, obstruction, and hemorrhage. Because surgery plays a role in both limited and advanced disease, colorectal cancer staging classifications have been developed on the basis of surgical and pathologic criteria [5].

Currently, the AJCC recommends the standard TNM classification. Due to technical limitations, current imaging modalities are unable to match the diagnostic staging information provided by surgical and pathologic findings. Due to its limited spatial resolution, PET is unable to provide the accurate T-stage determination required for TNM nomenclature, in which precise depth of invasion is the primary determinant. Only in cases of gross serosal penetration and invasion of adjacent structures will PET usually be accurate. CT gives more precise structural information but usually also cannot discriminate the bowel wall layers. Assignment of N stage requires numeric assessment of mesenteric nodes as well as pericolic nodes that are frequently small and lie in close proximity to the primary tumor mass. In addition, pericolic nodes are often involved microscopically by tumor cells, which only become apparent at histopathologic evaluation [5]. Despite the superiority of surgery and histopathology at TNM staging, an attempt to detect nodal or organ metastases is important in directing the general therapeutic approach (i.e., palliation vs. curative tumor resection). PET/CT offers an appealing combination of information that is certainly of use with more advanced local disease.

Metastatic Disease

Disease spread beyond the regional pericolic or mesenteric lymph nodes is considered to represent metastatic disease. Typical lymphatic spread involves internal iliac or retroperitoneal nodes, depending on the location of the primary tumor, whereas hematogenous spread of colorectal cancer usually involves the lung or liver. Metastases to other sites without lung or liver involvement are relatively rare. The main strength of PET and PET/CT imaging is in the detection of these distant metastases [50].

Early identification of liver metastases provides the opportunity for neoadjuvant chemotherapy and resection, which may prolong the survival of patients with colorectal carcinoma [51]. PET and CT accurately identify and delineate metastases to the liver. Contrast-enhanced MDCT is the established primary imaging modality for the detection, localization, and characterization of focal liver lesions [52], with equivocal liver lesions further evaluated with contrast-enhanced magnetic resonance imaging (MRI) in the preoperative setting. In a recent meta-analysis, PET was considered to be superior to older CT technology for the detection of liver metastases [53] but limited in its ability to demonstrate lesions < 1 cm [54]. Kantorová et al. [55] compared PET with CT for the preoperative staging of colorectal cancer. FDG-PET correctly identified 95% of the primary lesions compared with only 49% detected by CT. The sensitivity, specificity, and accuracy of PET for the identification of hepatic metastases were 78%, 96%, and 91%, respectively, compared with 67%, 100%, and 91% for CT. In a recent comparison study at our institution, gadolinium-enhanced MRI outperformed PET in assessing liver metastases from colorectal and pancreatic cancer, again particularly with regard to small lesions [56]. Furthermore, PET as a single modality does not provide sufficient anatomic information for adequate presurgical planning with respect to the precise localization of metastases according to standard hepatic anatomy or to the positioning of lesions in relationship to vessels or gallbladder. Although there are very few studies comparing PET or PET/CT with modern CT or MRI techniques, because PET helps identify metastases and MDCT helps to localize abnormalities, it is possible to foresee an improved effect on patient management with the use of such fusion imaging. In this regard, a recent study by Chua et al. [57] compared PET/CT with standard contrast-enhanced CT for the evaluation of patients with hepatic metastases. In patients with colorectal carcinoma, PET/CT had 94% sensitivity and 75% specificity compared with lower values of 91% and 25%, respectively, for CT. PET/CT imaging may be particularly useful in patients with hypodense or hypoenhancing liver lesions that are not clearly characterized by CT alone, and in patients in whom standard CT fails to detect metastases in the setting of a rising carcinoembryonic antigen (CEA). In these cases, PET/CT has the ability to directly affect patient management by guiding biopsies or directing surgical resections of liver metastases.

The greatest impact of PET imaging in patients with hepatic metastases is in the depiction of extrahepatic sites of disease that would preclude a curative procedure. CT is the standard imaging modality for detection of extrahepatic disease prior to an attempt at cure. However, due to its reliance on morphologic changes to detect disease, CT alone may overestimate the importance of an anatomic abnormality that is unrelated to malignancy or underestimate the significance of a finding because size criteria are not met. Furthermore, the abnormality may indeed be present on CT but overlooked on interpretation, perhaps, on occasion, due to the high volume of CT data to be reviewed. Several investigators have examined the incremental value of PET as a supplement to CT and found that PET offers information beyond that from CT alone and that this information often affects patient care. Investigators have found that when PET is added to CT in preoperative planning for patients with hepatic metastases, additional sites of extrahepatic disease are identified in 11–23% of patients and

can result in improved patient survival following institution of appropriate patient management [58, 59]. This frequently leads to a change in therapeutic management from localized therapy to a more systemic approach with chemotherapy.

FDG-PET can identify previously unrecognized metastases in patients with elevated CEA levels and a negative workup with conventional diagnostic modalities. Indeed, imaging with FDG in patients with colorectal cancer has proven to be a cost-effective technique that often leads to a change in patient management. Valk et al. [60] reported per-patient average savings of $3,003 when PET was added to the diagnostic workup of patients with colorectal cancer before surgery; [^{18}F]-FDG scanning was able to differentiate patients with non-resectable disease from patients with resectable disease, thus avoiding unnecessary surgical procedures. Park et al. [61] reported on the effect of PET/CT imaging preoperatively on patients with primary colorectal carcinoma. PET/CT detected 15 intra-abdominal metastatic lesions, more than abdominopelvic CT scan. PET/CT showed true negative findings in 13 patients. Due to PET/CT results, management plans were altered in 27 patients; nine had inter-modality changes, ten received more extensive surgery, and eight avoided unnecessary procedures. PET/CT correctly altered the management plan in 24% of patients with primary colorectal carcinoma.

Restaging of Colorectal Cancer

Disease recurrence can occur in a variety of sites, most frequently locally or metastatic to the lung or liver. As during the initial staging of colorectal cancer, FDG-PET is sensitive and specific for the presence of metastatic disease and has been reported to be more accurate overall than CT. An early study by Hung et al. [62] compared FDG-PET, CT, and serum CEA in an evaluation of recurrent colorectal disease. The authors reported overall sensitivity and specificity of FDG-PET to be 100% and 83%, respectively, compared with 33% and 86% for CEA. Abdominal CT had a lower sensitivity and specificity of 78% and 61% for detecting local recurrence and detected one lymphatic and one hepatic metastasis. It was concluded that FDG-PET was more accurate than CT and CEA for the detection of recurrent colorectal cancer. Wiering et al. [63] performed a meta-analysis of available studies on the diagnostic accuracy of FDG-PET compared with CT in patients with recurrent colorectal carcinoma. They reported pooled sensitivity and specificity of 88% and 96%, respectively, for FDG-PET in the detection of hepatic metastases compared with lower values of 83% and 84% for CT. With regard to extrahepatic disease, pooled sensitivity and specificity for PET were 92% and 95%, respectively, compared with 61% and 91% for CT. PET findings resulted in the alteration of clinical management in 32% of cases.

The differentiation of the sequelae of prior therapy, including post-operative inflammation and scarring as well as radiation fibrosis, from disease recurrence is a particular challenge in patients with prior colorectal carcinoma. This is most problematic with distal tumors, where presacral scarring and pelvic changes are common. With conventional imaging, serial examinations are frequently required before slowly developing changes can be appreciated. With PET performed 6 months post-surgery–a time frame in which post-surgical change is not hypermetabolic unless there is a leak with persistent inflammation–the presence of metabolic activity in the presacral space is generally indicative of tumor recurrence [5]. PET/CT has been shown to be accurate in the differentiation of benign from malignant presacral changes, with reported sensitivity, specificity, and PPV and NPV of 100%, 96%, 88%, and 100%, respectively [64] (Fig. 3). PET has a further advantage in that only a single study is necessary to make this determination, rather than the usual serial studies required with conventional imaging. The first published study of PET/CT imaging of colorectal cancer reported that the staging and restaging accuracy increased from 78% with PET alone to 89% with PET/CT. The frequency of equivocal and probable lesion characterization was reduced by 50% [65]. Subsequently, the superiority of PET/CT over CT or PET alone has become more established, with a multitude of studies demonstrating improved results [64, 66-68]. In the evaluation of recurrent colorectal carcinoma, Votrubova et al. [67] reported a sensitivity, specificity, and overall accuracy of 82%, 88%, and 86%, respectively, for PET detection of intra-abdominal extrahepatic recurrence compared with higher values of 88%, 94%, and 92% for PET/CT. For extra-abdominal and/or hepatic recurrence, PET/CT had 95% sensitivity, 100% specificity, and 99% accuracy compared with 74%, 88%, and 85%, respectively, for PET. Furthermore, PET/CT imaging as a single study on a hybrid machine is more accurate for recurrent colorectal cancer than subsequent co-registration of separately acquired PET and CT studies [68].

Overall, it is currently believed that PET/CT imaging should be the preferred imaging modality in these patients, because it identifies and localizes the disease in one setting and can appropriately guide diagnostic or therapeutic interventions.

Future Applications for PET/CT in Colorectal Disease

The monitoring of neoadjuvant therapy and the guidance of radiation therapy are other circumstances that may benefit from PET or PET/CT [69]. CT colonography (virtual colonoscopy) is a new approach for the evaluation of patients at risk for colon cancer. It is conceivable that the combination of virtual colonoscopy with [18F]-FDG-PET and combined PET/CT will add specificity to this new method by selectively identifying hypermetabolic polyps, which would be expected to carry a higher risk for malignant degeneration. Recent studies investigating this combined PET/CT colonography approach have reported promising results, showing this modality to be at least equivalent to PET plus CT for the staging of colorectal cancer [70] as well as proving effective at detecting premalignant lesions [71].

Other Gastrointestinal Malignancies

PET and PET/CT have been used in the evaluation of a wide variety of other malignancies associated with the gastrointestinal tract as well as other abdominal organs. Although many of these are not currently covered by the CMS in the United States, the advent of The National Oncologic PET Registry (NOPR) has enabled their use for such diseases and, with time, many of these malignancies may gain full coverage [72]. Several of these will therefore be briefly discussed here.

Gastric Cancer

The majority (> 90%) of gastric cancers are adenocarcinomas, with the remainder comprising uncommon tumors, including leiomyosarcoma and mucosa-associated lymphoid tissue (MALT) lymphoma, as well as carcinoid and squamous cell carcinoma. Microscopically, these cancers are classified according to the Lauren system as being of the intestinal type or diffuse type. Gastric adenocarcinoma most commonly arises from the gastroesophageal junction and is typically staged according to a standard TNM classification. Early stage gastric carcinoma has a relatively good prognosis, but unfortunately, patients usually present late, with advanced disease. As a result, gastric carcinoma is the second leading cause of cancer death worldwide. Where screening for gastric cancer occurs, the prognosis is better, as the disease is detected at an earlier stage [73].

T staging of gastric carcinoma is typically done with EUS, while MDCT has become the standard for N and M staging. The role of FDG-PET and PET/CT remains controversial. An early study by Yeung et al. [74] reported a sensitivity and specificity of 93% and 100%, respectively, for FDG-PET for the detection of primary gastric cancer but on-

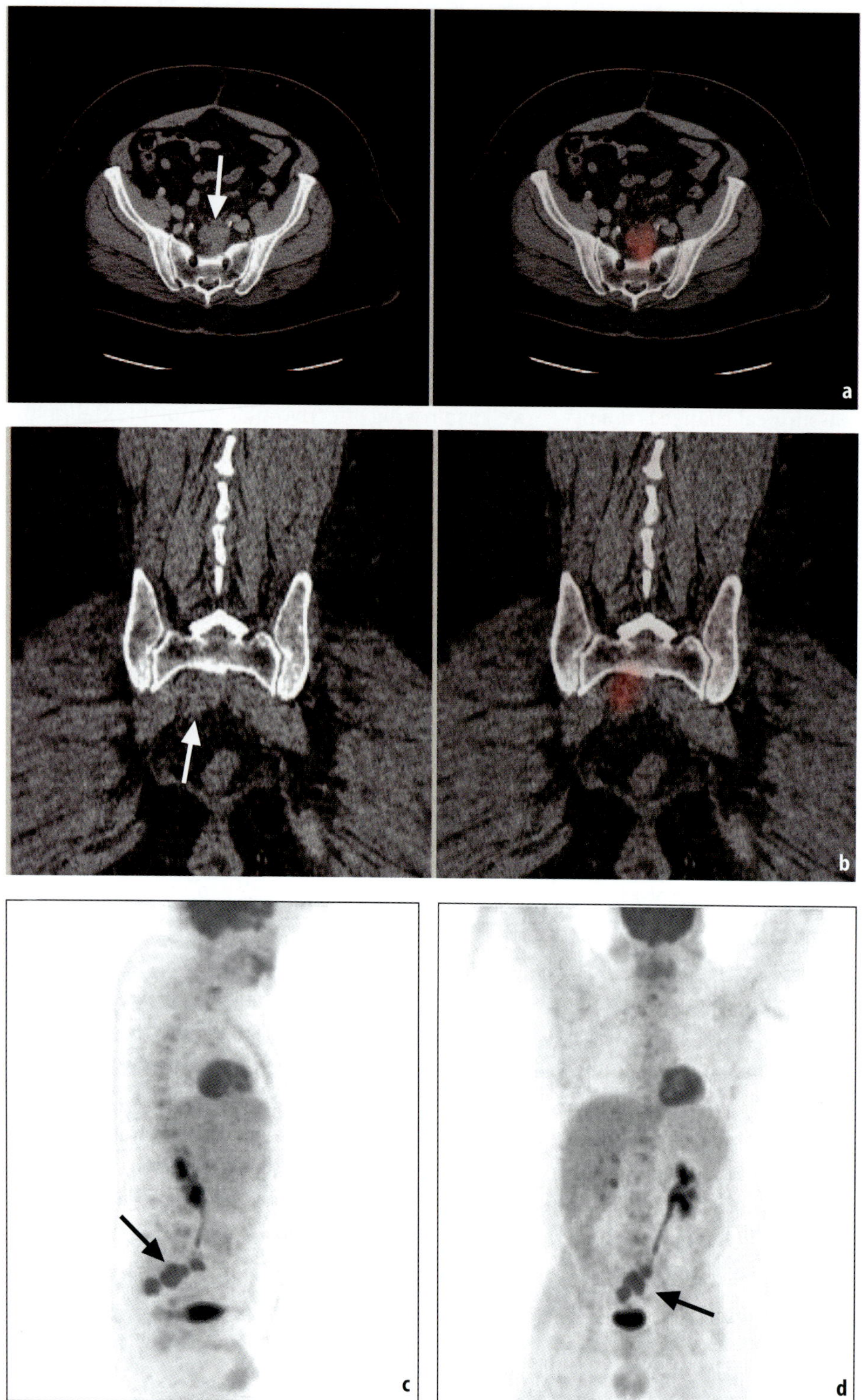

Fig. 3a-d. PET/CT images obtained from a 62-year-old man, 1 year post-treatment for a stage IIIb adenocarcinoma of the sigmoid colon. A non-contrast CT study was performed due to contrast allergy. **a, b** Axial and coronal reconstruction non-contrast CT and fused PET/CT images of new presacral soft-tissue masses demonstrating avid [^{18}F]-fluorodeoxyglucose (FDG) uptake consistent with recurrence (*arrows*). **c, d** Sagittal and coronal whole-body PET images demonstrating the presacral recurrence (*arrows*)

ly 22% and 81% for lymph node metastases. However, other studies have demonstrated inferior rates of primary lesion detection, including a more recent study by Shoda et al. [75] that reported just 10% sensitivity and 99% specificity for early gastric cancer. This has led some authors to conclude that FDG-PET is not an appropriate first-line diagnostic procedure in the detection of gastric cancer and is not helpful in tumor staging [76]. There are a number of reasons for the relatively poor performance of FDG-PET in gastric cancer. Firstly, normal physiologic FDG uptake in the stomach and gastroesophageal junction is variable and can have a focal appearance, especially if the stomach is empty and collapsed, including post-surgical appearances following partial gastrectomy for malignancy. A number of benign inflammatory conditions show increased uptake, which can result in false-positive results. It has been proposed that the sensitivity of PET/CT may be improved upon by having the patient ingest water in order to distend the stomach at the time of scanning [25, 77]. Another explanation for the variable results for FDG-PET in gastric carcinoma is provided by the work of Stahl et al. [78], who reported variable FDG uptake dependent on the histopathologic findings. They reported an overall sensitivity of 60% for the detection of locally advanced gastric cancers. Within this group, the detection rate for intestinal type was 83% vs. just 41% for the diffuse type. The mean SUV was also significantly lower for mucus-containing tumors compared with non-mucus-containing.

Although not proven to be highly accurate in the local staging of disease, it is generally expected that PET/CT can play a valuable role in the detection of distant metastases, such as those of the liver, lungs, adrenal glands, ovaries, and skeleton [79]. FDG-PET may also be helpful in the follow-up of patients undergoing chemotherapy by allowing for the identification of early response to treatment, as reported by Sun et al. [80]. More recently, there has been some interest in PET imaging with different radiotracers. Herrmann et al. [81] reported on a comparison of 3-deoxy-3 [^{18}F]-fluorothymidine (FLT) with FDG for the detection of gastric cancer and reported 100% sensitivity for FLT and 69% for FDG. Further studies are needed to determine the efficacy of FDG and other PET radiotracers in the detection of local nodal metastases and peritoneal dissemination. Nevertheless, the combined use of CT and PET can be helpful in the preoperative staging of stomach cancer and in the therapeutic monitoring of affected patients [76, 79] (Fig. 4).

Small Intestine

Cancer of the small intestine is rare. Adenocarcinoma, although a rare tumor of the small intestine, most commonly occurs in the duodenum. The more typical small intestinal tumors include neuroendocrine tumors and sarcomas, the latter arising most commonly in the jejunum and ileum. Metastatic disease may also occur, e.g., from breast cancer or melanoma, and is frequently detected with PET/CT. PET has been used successfully in the imaging of duodenal tumors, with one study reporting

a 100% sensitivity [82, 83]. PET imaging of neuroendocrine tumors with novel radiotracers yielded positive reports from the use of [^{18}F]-FDG, 6-fluoro-L-dopa (FDOPA), and ^{68}Ga-DOTA-D Phe(1)-Tyr(3)-octreotide (DOTATOC) [84, 85]. FDG-PET has also been useful in the evaluation of sarcomas. One meta-analysis, which included both bone and soft-tissue sarcomas, reported a pooled sensitivity, specificity, and accuracy of 91%, 85%, and 88%, respectively, for the detection of sarcoma [86]. The authors demonstrated the ability of this approach to discriminate between low- and high-grade sarcomas, and it is also expected that combined PET/CT imaging will be of even greater benefit [79].

Gastrointestinal Stromal Tumors

Gastrointestinal stromal tumors (GIST) are rare, accounting for less than 3% of all gastrointestinal neoplasms and less than 6% of all sarcomas. Most (70–80%) GISTs are benign. There is, however, a continuum from benign to malignant that can be predicted, although not absolutely, according to tumor size and mitotic frequency. GISTs can originate anywhere along the gastrointestinal tract but are most commonly located in the stomach and small bowel. They typically arise in the bowel wall, usually from or between the muscularis propria and muscularis mucosa. They may also arise in the mesentery or omentum. Metastatic disease can occur locally by direct invasion of adjacent structures or by the involvement of RLNs. Distant metastatic disease can target the liver, lung, bone, and peritoneum [87].

The role of PET in GIST is not clearly defined, as there appears to be variable FDG uptake by the primary lesion. Hersh et al. [88] performed a retrospective review of the imaging characteristics of GIST in 53 patients. The primary lesion was not identified in four patients due to extensive peritoneal disease. At initial diagnosis before treatment, contrast-enhanced CT identified all of the remaining 49 primary lesions. Eight patients underwent FDG-PET but the primary lesion was identified in just 50% of cases. The false-negative results were in smaller lesions, with a mean diameter of 6 cm, and a homogenous appearance on CT. The PET-positive lesions had an average diameter of 15 cm, were heterogeneous on CT, and all of these patients had metastatic disease. The superior ability of contrast-enhanced CT over FDG-PET in the detection of GIST was confirmed by Goerres et al. [89], who reported variable FDG uptake and a greater sensitivity for contrast-enhanced CT in lesion detection than for PET. Another study assessing FDG-PET and CT in the staging of GIST found little difference between the two modalities [90]. Although the sensitivity and specificity were high-

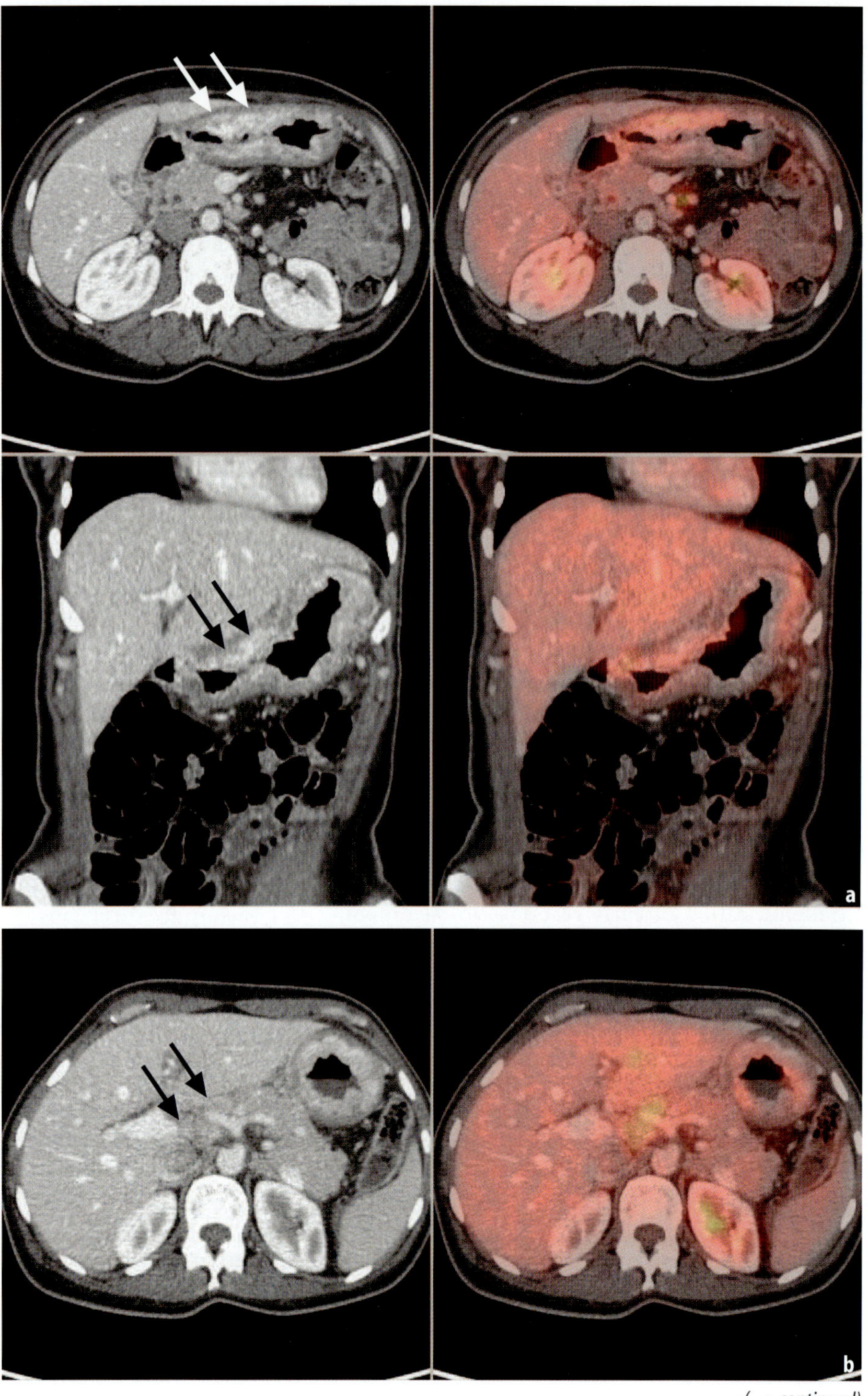

(→ continued)

er with CT than PET (93% and 100%, respectively, for CT vs. 86% and 98% for PET), the difference was not statistically significant. A potential explanation for the varied reported accuracy of PET at GIST staging lies with the varied nature of the neoplasm itself. Although the majority of GISTs are benign, there is a broad histological spectrum between benign and frankly malignant lesions. Previous studies have demonstrated higher FDG uptake in more malignant lesions, and it was proposed that this technique may be used preoperatively to assess malignant potential [91]. Furthermore, lesion size correlates with malignant potential so that benign lesions tend to be smaller in size and therefore demonstrate less FDG uptake. Goerres et al. concluded that single-stage PET/CT imaging was superior to either PET and/or CT [89]. Alberini et al. [92] also reported that PET and CT are

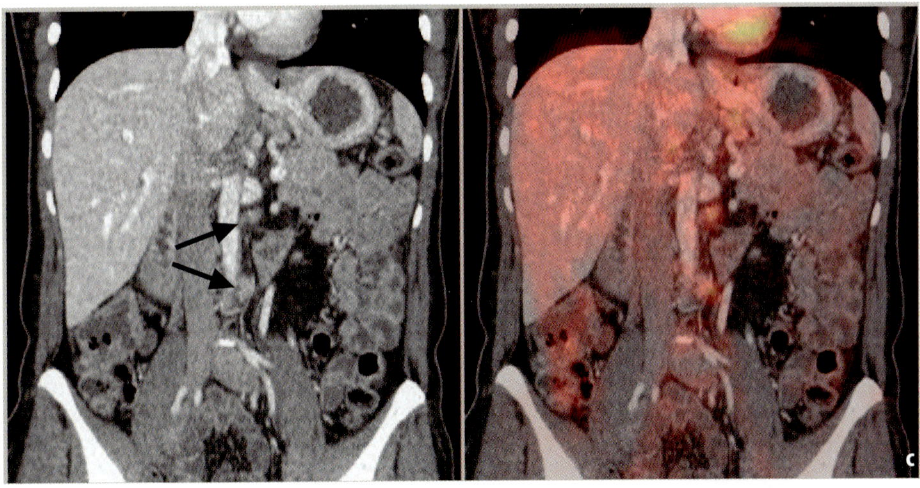

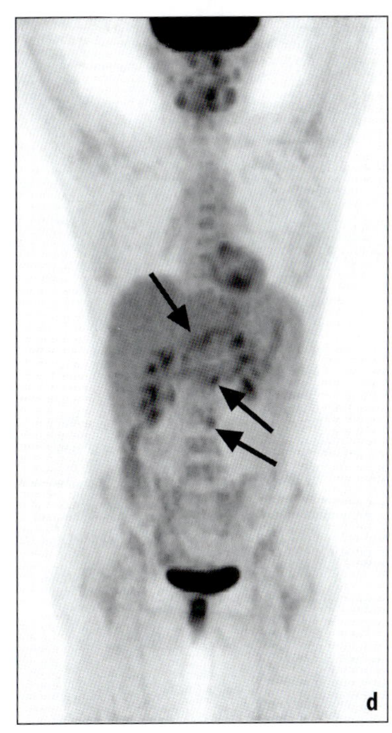

Fig. 4a-d. PET/CT images obtained in a woman with poorly differentiated adenocarcinoma of the stomach. **a** Axial and coronal reconstruction contrast-enhanced CT and fused PET/CT images demonstrating a diffusely thickened gastric wall with markedly increased [¹⁸F]-fluorodeoxyglucose (FDG) uptake, particularly along the lesser curvature (*arrows*). **b** Axial contrast-enhanced CT and fused PET/CT images demonstrating metastatic involvement of periportal lymph nodes, confirmed at biopsy (*arrows*). **c** Coronal-reconstruction contrast-enhanced CT and fused PET/CT images demonstrating metastatic spread to para-aortic lymph nodes (*arrows*). **d** Coronal whole-body PET image demonstrating the primary lesion and metastatic nodal involvement (*arrows*)

complementary and that hybrid PET/CT imaging is useful in GIST.

While complete surgical excision offers the best chance of cure, the high rates of local and distant metastatic disease emphasize the need for effective non-surgical treatment. Despite early disappointing results from chemotherapy, the new tyrosine kinase inhibitor imatinib has yielded good response rates [88]. There has been great interest in the use of FDG-PET as a means to assess the response to imatinib [92]. Heinicke et al. [93] reported that FDG-PET is a valuable method to monitor the response to imatinib as early as 1 week post-therapy. Another study compared separate PET and CT with hybrid PET/CT for the evaluation of disease response to imatinib treatment in patients with GISTs [94]. PET/CT detected 282 lesions compared with 279 with side-by-side PET and CT, 249

with CT, and 135 with PET alone. PET/CT was found to be superior for tumor response characterization, demonstrating 95% accuracy at 1 month and 100% accuracy at 3- and 6-months follow-up. Not only can PET and PET/CT provide information on treatment response rates, it has also been shown that PET results at initial staging and follow-up have important prognostic information [89, 90].

Several characteristics of GIST metastases should be considered in the planning of the CT component of a PET/CT study. Firstly, hepatic metastases from GIST can be isointense to liver on the portal-venous phase of contrast-enhanced CT; therefore, a non-enhanced CT component should be considered for the initial PET/CT staging of GIST. Furthermore, treatment with imatinib may result in liquefaction of hepatic metastases. The appearance of low-attenuation lesions within the liver on subsequent imaging should not be mistaken for new metastatic disease, particularly if the isointense lesions were not appreciated on the initial staging exam. Furthermore, if a pretreatment scan is not available, cystic-appearing metastases on restaging scans should not be misdiagnosed as simple cysts. This internal morphologic change without significant change in lesion size after successful treatment highlights a major limitation of conventional Response Evaluation Criteria in Solid Tumors (RECIST) for assessing such treatment response. Patients who subsequently develop disease recurrence may manifest a new soft-tissue nodule within a liquefied metastasis. This nodule-within-a mass appearance is best appreciated with contrast enhancement, such that intravenous contrast should always be included in the follow-up PET/CT protocol for patients with GIST. Finally, as discussed above, oral contrast for the CT component of a PET/CT study may be either high attenuating (positive) or water attenuating (negative). Peritoneal metastases may also undergo cystic degeneration with imatinib treatment and therefore may be difficult to appreciate and differentiate from bowel loops unless positive contrast is used [95].

Hepatobiliary Tumors

PET and PET/CT use in primary and secondary tumors has produced variable results. The value of PET in metastatic disease is largely dependent on the type of primary tumor. Liver metastases are only likely to be detected if the primary lesion itself is demonstrable with PET. Furthermore, the radiotracer, such as FDG, may itself accumulate in the liver, further reducing the sensitivity of PET. This may be overcome with the use of PET/CT, which can combine morphologic changes with the PET images and therefore increase lesion detection. In addition, the use of PET/CT may more accurately discriminate between superficial but intra-hepatic lesions and true extra-hepatic pathology [79]. The benefit of PET/CT in colorectal hepatic metastases is well established (see Colorectal Carcinoma section). In a study by Böhm et al. [96] comparing FDG-PET, abdominal ultrasound, CT, and MRI for the evaluation of primary and secondary hepatic malignancies, PET was demonstrated to be superior to abdominal ultrasound and CT but not to MRI. The sensitivity, specificity, and PPVs for all hepatic lesions were 82%, 25%, and 96%, respectively, for PET; 63%, 50%, and 96% for ultrasound; 71%, 50%, and 97% for CT; and highest at 83%, 57%, and 97% for MRI. However, PET detected extrahepatic findings in 64% of patients with significantly better sensitivity and specificity than the other modalities. Furthermore, the PET findings had a direct impact on operative management in 18% of patients.

Given the experience with other malignancies, it is reasonable to expect that hybrid imaging of hepatic malignancies with PET/CT will enable more accurate imaging than either modality separately. The recent study by Chua et al. [57] compared PET/CT with contrast-enhanced CT for the detection of hepatic metastases from multiple differing primary malignancies. They reported PET/CT sensitivity and specificity as 96% and 75%, respectively, compared with just 88% and 25% for CT (Fig. 5).

With respect to hepatocellular carcinoma (HCC), the results of studies evaluating FDG-PET have been disappointing. Khan et al. [97] reported sensitivities of 55% and 90% for FDG-PET and CT, respectively. They noted that well-differentiated and low-grade tumors demonstrated lower PET activity than higher-grade tumors, thus concluding that PET helps to assess tumor differentiation. A more recent study reported similar findings and found FDG-PET to have a sensitivity, specificity, and accuracy of just 64%, 33%, and 63%, respectively, in the evaluation of HCC [98]. However, as demonstrated in other areas, PET was better than CT at detecting extra-hepatic disease, and a recent study highlighted the use of PET at detecting extra-hepatic HCC recurrence [99]. Although PET/CT may be expected to perform better than PET alone in the evaluation of HCC, current standard CT imaging of HCC involves triple-phase MDCT. It is therefore important in cases of suspected HCC to tailor the CT component of PET/CT accordingly [79, 95]. In an effort to improve on the performance of PET with respect to HCC, some investigators have looked at other radiotracers. In a small study comparing [^{18}F]-fluorocholine (FCH) with standard FDG, Talbot et al. [100] reported a sensitivity of 100% for the detection of newly diagnosed and recurrent HCC with FCH-PET compared with 56% for FDG-PET. A recent report by Ho et al. [101] evaluated the use of PET/CT employing dual-tracer imaging with standard FDG together with 11-choline-acetate [(11)C-ACT] in the evaluation of metastatic HCC. They reported patient sensitivity and specificity rates of 98% and 86%, respectively, with positive and negative predictive values of 97% and 90%. The overall accuracy was 96%. The authors also demonstrated that dual-tracer imaging was superior to either tracer separately and that combination imaging was complementary.

There has also been great interest in the use of PET and PET/CT in the evaluation of residual or recurrent disease following palliative procedures for the management of inoperable primary and secondary liver tumors, including radiofrequency ablation (RFA) and transcatheter arterial chemo-embolization (TACE). Barker et al. [102] reported that conventional imaging with CT and MRI may result in false-positive results from post-treatment inflammation or hyperemia, resulting in rim en-

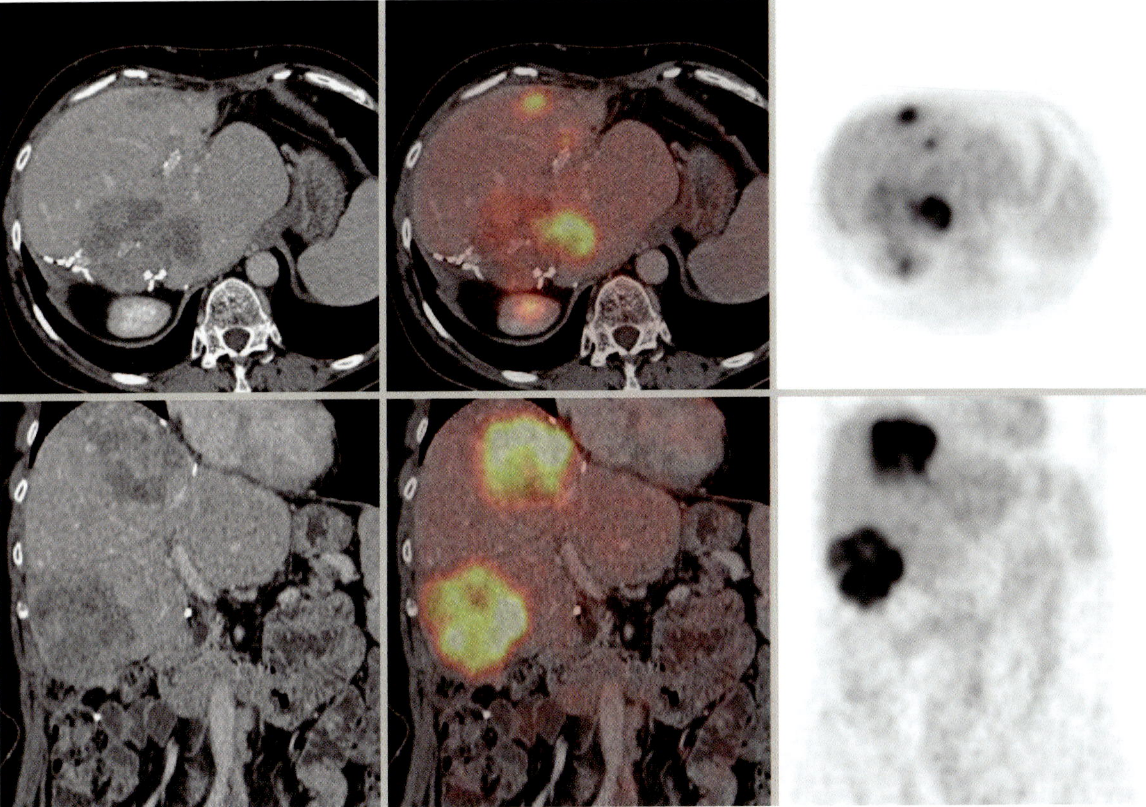

Fig. 5. PET/CT images obtained from a 64-year-old man presenting 5 years following treatment for colorectal carcinoma. Axial and coronal-reconstruction contrast-enhanced CT, PET, and fused PET/CT images demonstrating multiple [^{18}F]-fluorodeoxyglucose (FDG)-avid, hypoenhancing hepatic metastases

hancement of the lesion. Similarly, lesions with no or diffuse enhancement may have focal uptake on FDG-PET, a finding that can be used to direct biopsy. PET and PET/CT with FDG is not affected by scar tissue or the presence of artificial materials [79]. In a study of patients with primary and secondary liver tumors that were treated with RFA, Blokhuis et al. [103] concluded that the use of PET in combination with CT scan at follow-up can lead to earlier detection of tumor recurrence than contrast-enhanced CT alone. A later study comparing PET and PET/CT with CT alone for the detection of residual tumor after RFA demonstrated sensitivity and specificity rates of 65% and 68%, respectively, for PET and PET/CT vs. 44% and 47% for CT [104]. More recently, Prior et al. [105] described a technique of PET/CT-guided RFA of hepatic metastases.

FDG-PET has also been used to evaluate patients with gallbladder carcinoma. Koh et al. [106] reported 75% sensitivity and 88% specificity for FDG-PET in the preoperative detection of gallbladder carcinoma. Similar results were reported by Rodríguez-Fernández et al. [107], who demonstrated 80% sensitivity and 82% specificity as well as PPVs and NPVs of 67% and 90%, respectively. Another study assessed FDG-PET in the post-operative evaluation for residual or recurrent gallbladder carcinoma and demonstrated 78% sensitivity

[108]. The authors reported just 50% sensitivity for extrahepatic metastases; a significant proportion of the false-negative results were in patients with carcinomatosis. In the evaluation of potential gallbladder carcinoma, causes of false-positive results included xanthogranulomatous cholecystitis, tuberculoid granulomatosis, and adenomyomatosis of the gallbladder [107,109]. A false-negative result was reported with mucinous adenocarcinoma [107]. In an effort to improve upon the performance of PET in gallbladder carcinoma, other investigators have assessed the use of delayed or dual-phase PET imaging. Nishiyama et al. [110] performed early and late PET imaging (average 62 and 146 min) after standard FDG administration. They concluded that delayed FDG-PET is more helpful than early FDG-PET for evaluating malignant gallbladder lesions because of increased uptake by the lesion and increased lesion-to-background contrast. A recent study evaluated PET/CT in patients with gallbladder carcinoma and reported 100% sensitivity for primary lesion and the detection of distant metastases [111].

In patients with biliary strictures and suspected cholangiocarcinoma, FDG-PET may have better sensitivity and specificity than CT and is more sensitive than cytological examination of bile. However, false-positive results may occur with primary sclerosing cholangitis and cholecystitis [108, 112, 113]. In the evaluation of cholangiocarcinoma with FDG-PET, Anderson et al. reported 85% sensitivity for the nodular histological subtype and just 18% sensitivity for the infiltrating subtype [108]. Sensitivity for distant metastases was 65% but, similar to patients with gallbladder carcinoma, there was unfortunately a 100% false-negative rate for carcinomatosis. A more recent study by Moon et al. [114] compared PET with CT for the diagnosis and staging of patients with cholangiocarcinoma. They reported the overall accuracy of FDG-PET for discriminating malignant diseases of bile duct from benign conditions to be slightly higher than that of CT scan (89% vs. 82%). The sensitivity of FDG-PET in perihilar cholangiocarcinoma was lower than the value for intrahepatic and common bile duct cancers (83% vs. 91% and 91%). Furthermore, in cases of perihilar cancer, the sensitivity of FDG-PET was lower than that of CT (83% vs. 92%). FDG-PET detected nine distant metastatic lesions not found by other imaging studies and excluded two patients who had potentially resectable conditions, as shown in other imaging studies, from unnecessary laparotomy. In a small study of 22 patients with extra-hepatic bile-duct strictures, PET/CT was used to differentiate benign from malignant causes [115]: 14 patients had histologically

proven cholangiocarcinoma, and the remaining eight had benign disease. Comparison of the SUVs showed a clear cutoff SUV of 3.6 to separate benign and malignant disease. While brush cytology at endoscopic retrograde cholangiography has an average sensitivity of just 50% for the detection of malignant extra-hepatic bile-duct strictures, the authors concluded that PET/CT provides high accuracy for the non-invasive detection of perihilar extra-hepatic cholangiocarcinoma.

Petrowsky et al. [112] compared the use of PET/CT with contrast-enhanced CT in patients with cholangiocarcinoma and reported comparable accuracy for the detection of primary intra- and extra-hepatic lesions. PET/CT had 100% sensitivity for distant metastases with just 25% sensitivity reported for contrast-enhanced CT (Fig. 6). A more recent study by Jadvar et al. [116] assessed the use of PET and PET/CT in the evaluation of recurrent and metastatic cholangiocarcinoma. Overall, the sensitivity and specificity of PET (either alone or combined with CT) was 94% and 100%, respectively, compared with 82% and 43% for CT alone. Finally, the addition of PET and PET/CT to the imaging algorithm for patients with cholangiocarcinoma or gallbladder carcinoma frequently results in alterations in patient management (17–30% of cases), most commonly by the detection of distant

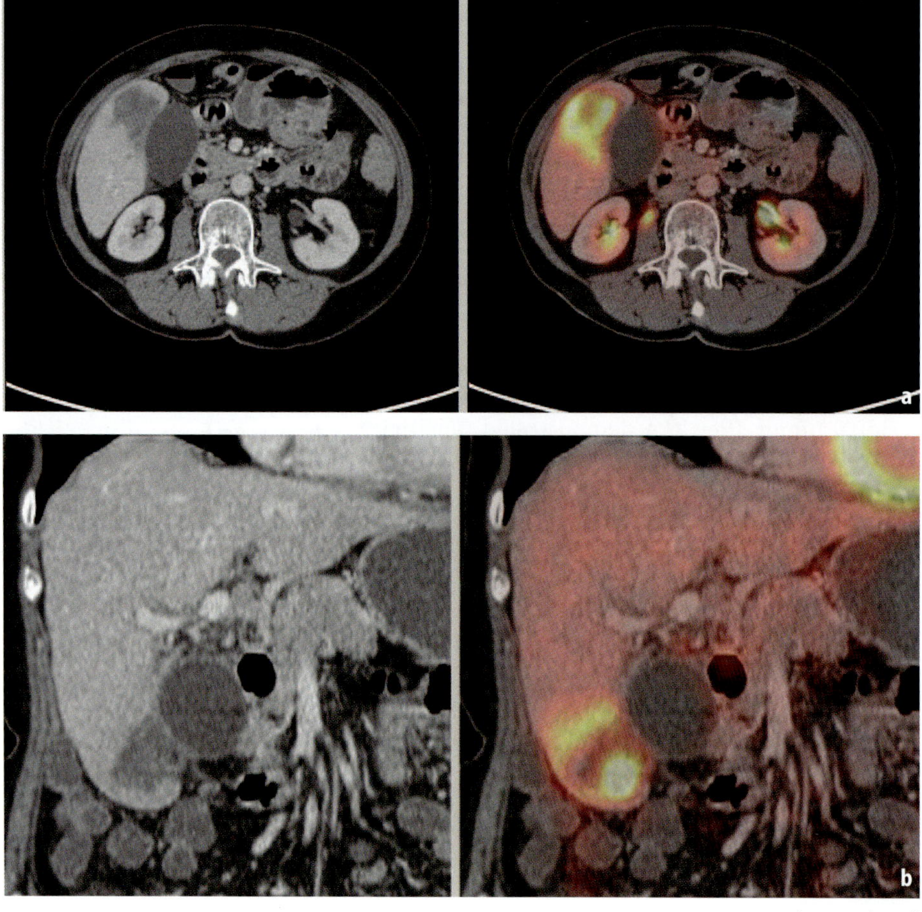

(→ continued)

metastases, and thus changes to the surgical approach [108, 111].

Pancreatic Carcinoma

To date, there have been relatively few studies assessing the role and usefulness of PET, and more specifically of PET/CT, in patients with pancreatic carcinoma. The published reports vary in their conclusions. In the preoperative assessment of pancreatic tumors, Borbath et al. [117] compared MRI, EUS, PET, and staging laparoscopy for the detection and staging of malignant lesions. In the detection of pancreatic adenocarcinoma, EUS was superior to MRI and PET, with respective sensitivities of

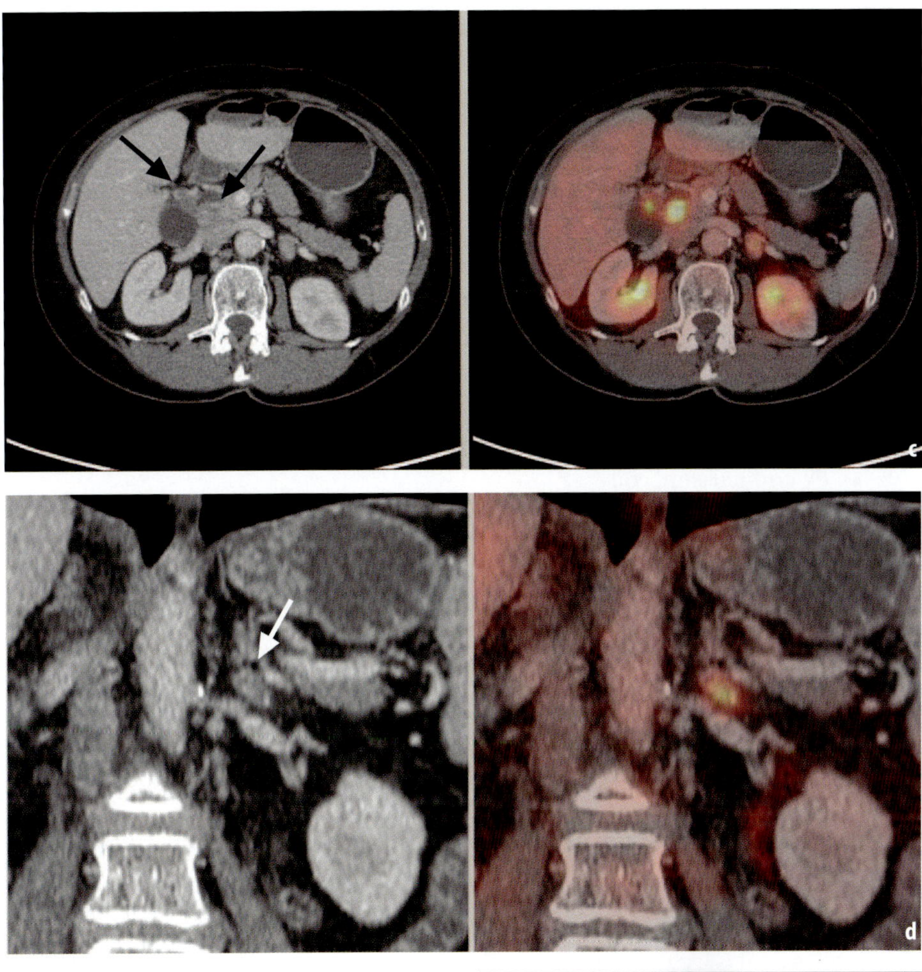

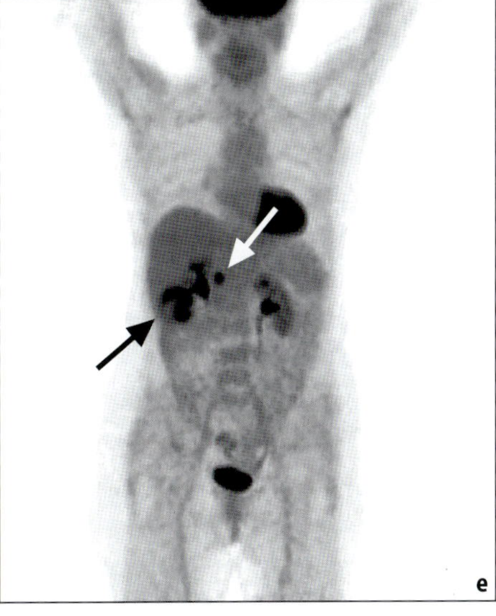

Fig. 6a-e. PET/CT images obtained from a 72-year old woman with poorly differentiated cholangiocarcinoma. **a, b** Axial and coronal-reconstruction contrast-enhanced CT and fused PET/CT images demonstrating the primary lesion as a hypoenhancing [^{18}F]-fluorodeoxyglucose (FDG)-avid mass in segment V. **c** Axial contrast-enhanced CT and fused PET/CT images demonstrating metastatic involvement of periportal lymph nodes (*arrows*). **d** Coronal reconstruction contrast-enhanced CT and fused PET/CT images demonstrating metastatic spread to left para-aortic lymph nodes superior to the left renal artery (*arrow*). **e** Coronal whole-body PET image demonstrating the primary cholangiocarcinoma and metastatic nodal involvement (*arrows*)

98%, 88%, and 88%. MRI was superior at the detection of locoregional staging, i.e., arterial involvement. All modalities had low sensitivities for identifying distant metastases. In a later study by Bang et al. [118], FDG-PET was found to have a diagnostic accuracy of 95% in the diagnosis and staging of patients with suspected pancreatic carcinoma compared with 77% accuracy for CT. PET was also found to be superior to CT in the detection of hepatic metastases. With respect to the evaluation of cystic pancreatic lesions for possible malignancy, one study reported just 57% sensitivity and 85% specificity for FDG-PET [119]. Pancreatic intraductal papillary mucinous neoplasms (IPMNs) are increasingly being recognized, often as incidental findings, especially in people older than 70 and 80 years. Conventional imaging with CT and MRI has proven unreliable in discriminating a benign from a malignant IPMN, prompting Sperti et al. [120] to evaluate the role of FDG-PET in this situation. In a prospective study of 64 patients, increased uptake on $[^{18}F]$-FDG-PET was absent in 13 of 13 adenomas and seven of eight borderline IPMNs, but was present in four of five carcinoma in situ (80%) and in 20 of 21 invasive cancers (95%). By comparison, conventional imaging was only strongly suggestive of malignancy in 40% of cases of carcinoma in situ and 62% of cases of invasive carcinoma. The use of FDG-PET was thus found to influence the surgical decision in patients with malignant IPMN.

As with many other malignancies, it would be expected that combination imaging with CT further improves the accuracy of PET. In an early study by Lemke et al. [121], the retrospective fusion of separately acquired PET and CT studies in patients with suspected pancreatic malignancy led to better results than obtained with either study separately. The sensitivity for malignancy detection was 77% for CT, 84% for PET, and 89% for image fusion. A later study assessed hybrid PET/CT imaging with conventional staging (abdominal CT, chest X-ray and cancer antigen (CA) 19-9 measurement) for the preoperative staging of patients with suspected pancreatic carcinoma [122]. PET/CT had 89% sensitivity and 69% specificity for the detection of malignancy compared with 93% and 21%, respectively, for contrast-enhanced CT. It is worth noting that, in this study, the PET/CT protocol did not include the use of intravenous contrast. PET/CT had a high PPV (91%) but a low NPV (64%) for cancer. False-positive results were caused by an inflammatory pseudotumor, pancreatic tuberculosis, chronic pancreatitis, and focal high-grade dysplasia, which indeed was suspicious for malignancy by brush cytology. RLN metastases were found in 14 of the 25 patients (56%) with histologically proven adenocarcinoma who underwent pancreatic resection. PET/CT detected RLN metastases in only three of these patients, in whom the findings were FDG-positive in two. Sixteen patients had distant metastases, of which standard staging detected nine (56%) and PET/CT detected 13 (81%). In addition, five patients were only diagnosed by PET/CT, resulting in reported sensitivity and specificity of standard staging for distant metastases of 56% and 95%, respectively, compared with 81% and 100% for PET/CT (Fig. 7).

These somewhat varied results were summarized in the review by Pakzad et al. [123], who reported that PET and PET/CT diagnostic sensitivity varied between 90% and 95%, with a specificity ranging between 82% and 100%. For staging, sensitivity varied more widely, between 61% and 100%, with specificity varying between 67% and 100%. The authors concluded that PET and PET/CT are best at diagnosing and staging pancreatic cancer but are relatively inefficient in the detection of nodal disease. Thus, further evidence is required before PET/CT can be considered as a first-line imaging modality.

Adrenal Gland Malignancy

Malignant lesions of the adrenal gland may be primary or secondary, and both PET and PET/CT have been shown to yield excellent results in the evaluation of such lesions. Integrated FDG-PET/CT for adrenal-gland imaging in cancer patients allows early detection and accurate localization of adrenal lesions and differentiation of metastatic nodules from benign lesions. However, a 5% false-positive rate for PET/CT has been reported secondary to a variety of causes, including adrenal adenomas and adrenal endothelial cysts, as well as inflammatory and infectious lesions [124]. Similarly, brown fat with a perinephric distribution represents an important potential pitfall of adrenal PET/CT owing to its increased FDG uptake. Although the characteristic pattern of brown adipose tissue is most commonly recognized in the cervical and supraclavicular regions, it can also be identified in the paraspinal and periadrenal regions, where it can be mistaken for pathologic uptake related to the adrenal gland proper [125]. Moreover, false-negative findings may be seen in adrenal metastatic lesions with hemorrhage or necrosis, small-sized (<10 mm) metastatic nodules, and metastases from pulmonary bronchioloalveolar carcinoma or carcinoid tumors [124].

Metastases to the adrenal glands are common and can have a variety of appearances at CT. The most common primary sites are the lung, breast, skin (melanoma), kidney, thyroid gland, and colon. Most metastases are clinically silent. Up to 50% of adrenal masses in patients with known malignancy may be benign; thus, non-invasive characterization is important in preventing unnecessary biopsy

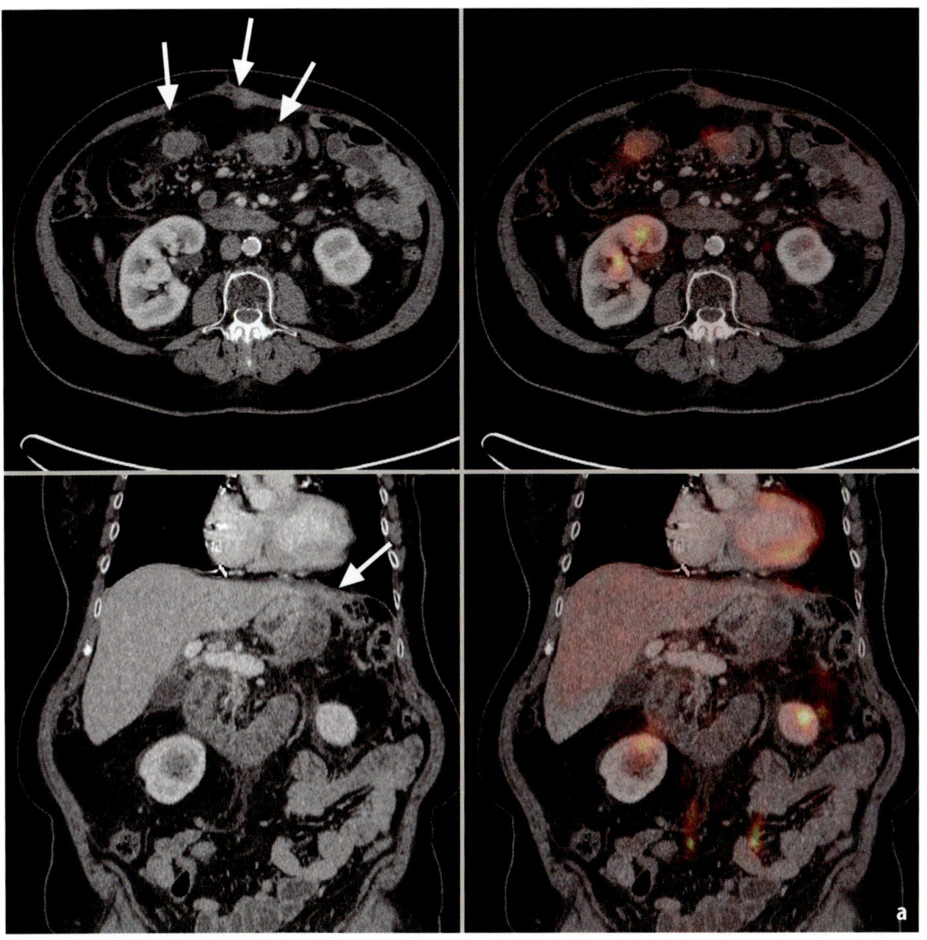

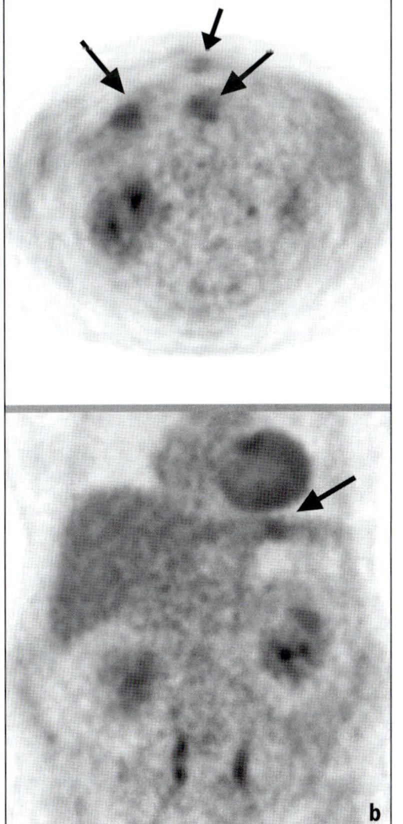

Fig. 7a,b. PET/CT images obtained from a 68-year-old woman 1 year following a distal pancreatectomy for invasive adenocarcinoma. **a**, **b** Axial and coronal reconstruction contrast-enhanced CT, PET, and fused PET/CT images demonstrating multiple enhancing soft-tissue nodules within the mesentery and on peritoneal surfaces, consistent with metastatic disease recurrence (*arrows*)

[125,126]. In one study assessing PET/CT in the characterization of adrenal lesions in patients with suspected or proven malignancy, reported sensitivity, specificity, PPV, and NPV were 100%, 94%, 82%, and 100%, respectively, with an overall accuracy of 95% [127]. In rare instances, the adrenal gland may appear normal or minimally thickened despite the presence of an FDG-avid metastasis, thus making PET/CT useful in detecting otherwise occult disease. Post-treatment PET/CT may be valuable in demonstrating the presence of residual hypermetabolic tumor when anatomic findings alone are equivocal.

Lymphomatous involvement of the adrenal glands in patients with other sites of involvement is rare, reported in only 1–4% of affected patients (Fig. 8). One group took advantage of this low pretest likelihood of adrenal involvement and studied patients with lymphoma to characterize the FDG-PET appearances of normal adrenal glands and demonstrated PET/CT to be superior to PET [128]. PET has been reported as being superior to CT and MRI in the characterization of adrenal lymphoma, including bilateral involvement at presentation [129]. The degree of FDG avidity in adrenal glands involved by lymphoma tends to parallel that in other involved areas, so that the resolution of adrenal gland-uptake often follows that of uptake in other regions. Although rare, one must be cautious in the setting of an adrenal mass in a patient with a history of lymphoma. PET/CT is valuable in distinguishing an incidental nonfunctioning adrenal neoplasm or hyperplasia from lymphomatous involvement [125].

Pheochromocytoma is a rare tumor, uncommonly malignant (10%), and is reported to occur in 0.05–0.2% of hypertensive individuals. Pheochromocytoma may be asymptomatic and may occur in certain familial syndromes, including multiple endocrine neoplasia 2A and 2B, neurofibromatosis, and von Hippel-Lindau disease. CT has an accuracy of 85–95% in detecting adrenal pheochromocytomas ≥1 cm. However, differentiating an adenoma from a pheochromocytoma can be difficult with CT alone, because the two neoplasms may have a similar CT appearance [125]. The procedure of choice in the localization of pheochromocytomas has long been scintigraphy with meta-iodobenzylguanidine (MIBG). Limitations of MIBG include its inconsistent uptake pattern (i.e., not all lesions concentrate the radiotracer) and the fact that MIBG uptake is highly sensitive to the presence of concomitantly administered medications. Shulkin et al. [130] compared FDG-PET with MIBG in the evaluation of patients with pheochromocytoma. They demonstrated 83% sensitivity for MIBG for benign

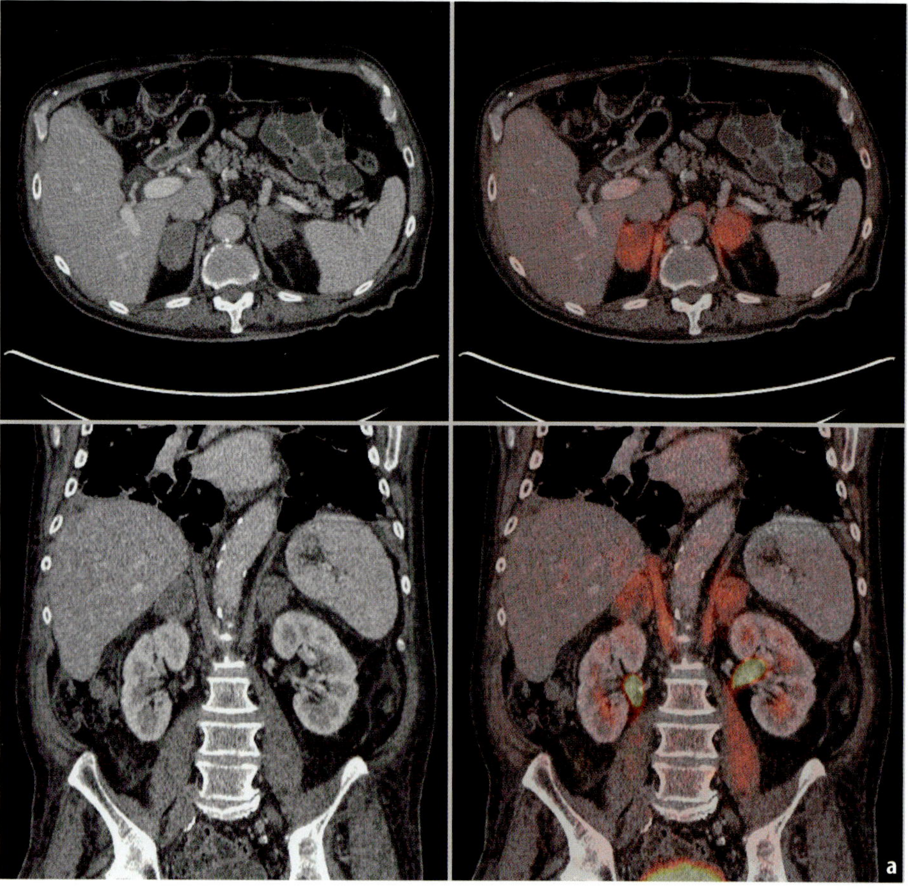

(→ continued)

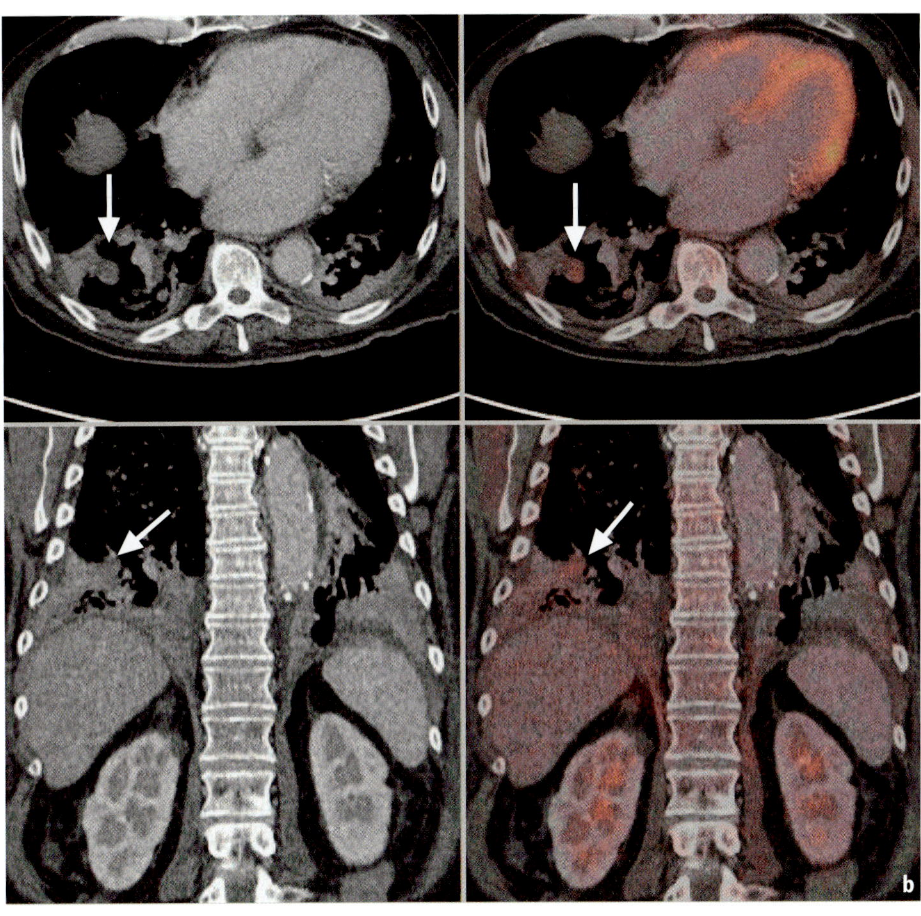

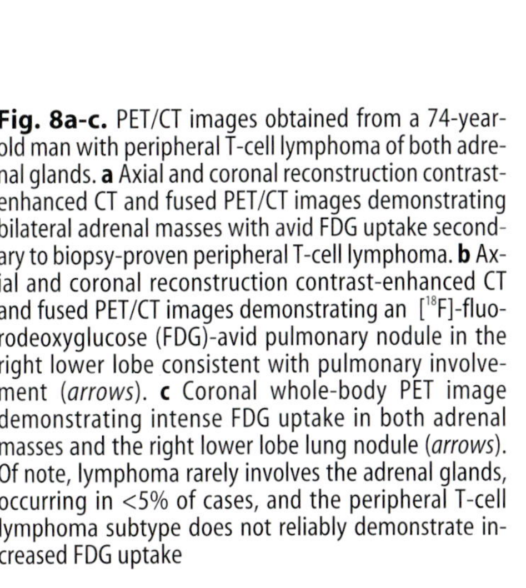

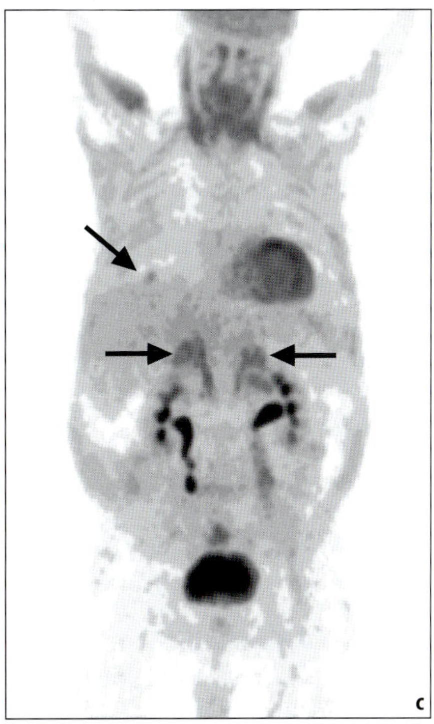

Fig. 8a-c. PET/CT images obtained from a 74-year-old man with peripheral T-cell lymphoma of both adrenal glands. **a** Axial and coronal reconstruction contrast-enhanced CT and fused PET/CT images demonstrating bilateral adrenal masses with avid FDG uptake secondary to biopsy-proven peripheral T-cell lymphoma. **b** Axial and coronal reconstruction contrast-enhanced CT and fused PET/CT images demonstrating an [^{18}F]-fluorodeoxyglucose (FDG)-avid pulmonary nodule in the right lower lobe consistent with pulmonary involvement (*arrows*). **c** Coronal whole-body PET image demonstrating intense FDG uptake in both adrenal masses and the right lower lobe lung nodule (*arrows*). Of note, lymphoma rarely involves the adrenal glands, occurring in <5% of cases, and the peripheral T-cell lymphoma subtype does not reliably demonstrate increased FDG uptake

pheochromocytomas vs. 58% for FDG. For malignant pheochromocytomas, MIBG demonstrated 88% sensitivity vs. 82% for FDG. Although MIBG had better sensitivity, all of the MIBG-negative lesions demonstrated avid FDG uptake. The authors concluded that most pheochromocytomas accumulate FDG, that uptake is found in a greater percentage of malignant than benign pheochromocytomas, and that FDG-PET is especially useful in defining the distribution of those pheochromocytomas that fail to concentrate MIBG.

Adrenocortical carcinoma (ACC) is a rare primary malignant neoplasm of the adrenal gland, accounting for only 0.02–0.2% of all cancer-related deaths. The female:male ratio is approximately 3:1, and two major age peaks are identified: in the first decade of life and again in the fourth to fifth decades. Patients usually present with advanced-stage disease. Radical surgery (when feasible) constitutes the only effective treatment for either local or distant disease. The 5-year survival rate is dismally low, with most patients succumbing within 12 months of diagnosis of advanced-stage disease [125]. Becherer et al. [131] evaluated FDG-PET in patients with known ACC and demonstrated sensitivity and specificity of 100% and 95%, respectively. Additional lesions that went undetected at anatomic imaging alone were identified with the addition of PET in 30% of patients, and the addition of PET modified the management protocol in 20%. A later study evaluating FDG-PET in locally recurrent or metastatic ACC reported 83% sensitivity, with false-negative results occurring in patients with small metastatic lesions (one lung nodule and one hepatic metastasis) [132]. More recently, PET imaging was performed with 11-carbon (^{11}C)-metomidate (MTO), a marker of 11-beta-hydroxylase, for adrenocortical imaging with variable success [133,134]. ^{11}C- and [^{18}F]-fluoro-labeled catecholamines and catecholamine analogs have been used for PET imaging of the adrenal medulla [134].

Renal Tract Malignancies

Multiple studies have assessed the use of PET and PET/CT in the evaluation of renal cell carcinoma (RCC). Although the results have been variable, in general, they have shown RCC to be usually FDG avid [135]. The detection of RCC with FDG-PET is impaired by the normal physiological renal excretion of FDG, although this may partially be overcome by fluid hydration and the administration of diuretics [136]. The variable detection of RCC by FDG-PET is related to the histopathologic characteristics of the tumor, with increased FDG uptake reported in higher-grade than in lower-grade tumors [135,137]. In an early study by Bachor et al.

[138], FDG-PET was used to stage RCC. The reported sensitivity was 77% for RCC detection, with false-positive results occurring with angiomyolipoma, pericytoma, and pheochromocytoma. They also reported higher FDG uptake in dedifferentiated tumors and no false-negative results for the detection of malignant lymph nodes. The sensitivity in this study contrasts with that in the study by Miyakita et al. [137], who reported just 32% sensitivity for RCC detection. A later study by Kang et al. [139] reported on a larger series of patients and compared FDG-PET with conventional CT imaging. For primary RCC, PET had a 60% sensitivity and a 100% specificity compared with 92% and 100%, respectively, for CT. Detection of renal-bed recurrence and/or retroperitoneal lymph node metastases had sensitivity and specificity rates of 75% and 100%, respectively, for PET vs. 93% and 98% for CT. PET was less sensitive than chest CT in the detection of metastatic lung nodules (75% vs. 94%) and less sensitive than isotope bone scan for bone metastases (77 vs. 94%). These results would suggest that hybrid imaging with PET/CT would have better diagnostic performance than PET alone but, to our knowledge, no such study has been conducted (Fig. 9). In another study evaluating the use of PET for distant RCC metastases, sensitivity, specificity, and PPV were 64%, 100%, and 100%, respectively [140]. The mean size of the distant metastases was 2.2 cm for true-positive cases and 1 cm for false-negative cases. This again highlights the limitations of PET at detecting smaller lesions, a problem that would likely be reduced by combination PET/CT imaging.

A more recent study also assessing the use of FDG-PET for metastatic RCC reported 75% sensitivity and 92% PPV. The authors concluded that a positive PET study can be used to modify management decisions but a negative study should not be considered in decision making [141]. Given the limitations incurred by the physiological renal excretion of FDG, there has been some interest in PET imaging with other radiotracers, including [^{11}C]-acetate and [^{18}F]-fluoromisonidazol (FMISO), but without much reported success [135]. However, a more recent study using iodine-124-labeled chimeric antibody G250 (^{124}I-cG250) and PET for imaging clear-cell renal carcinoma produced more promising results. In a phase I trial, the sensitivity of ^{124}I-cG250-PET for clear-cell renal carcinoma was 94%, with a specificity of 100%. NPV and PPV were 90% and 100%, respectively [142].

With respect to bladder cancer, urothelial/transitional cell carcinomas (TCC) account for the majority (90%), while squamous cell carcinoma is the next most common, and adenocarcinoma accounts for just 1%. The issue of physiological renal FDG excretion is even more problematic in the imaging of bladder carcinoma due to the natural ac-

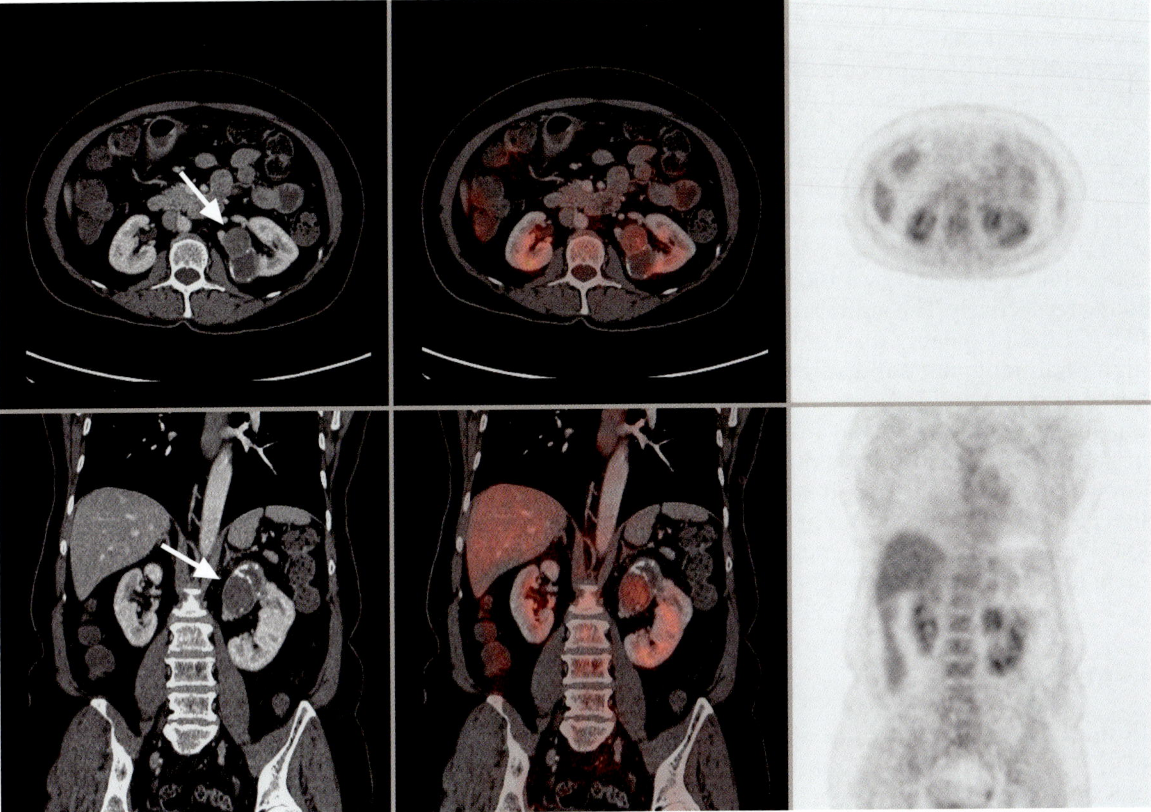

Fig. 9. PET/CT images obtained from a 66-year-old woman with an incidentally-detected left renal mass. Axial and coronal reconstruction contrast-enhanced CT, PET, and fused PET/CT images demonstrating an enhancing, [^{18}F]-fluorodeoxyglucose (FDG)-avid, solid renal mass at the upper pole of the left kidney (*arrows*) anterior to a mildly complex cyst demonstrating rim calcification. Appearances are consistent with a renal cell carcinoma

cumulation of FDG within the bladder. As a result, there have been relatively few studies assessing the use of PET and PET/CT in this area. An early study by Kosuda et al. [143] reported accurate lesion detection in eight of 12 patients but with a 33.3% false-negative rate. FDG-PET detected 100% of distant metastases and two of three RLN metastases. A more recent study by Drieskens et al. [144] used correlated PET and CT images for preoperative staging of invasive bladder carcinoma. They reported 60% sensitivity, 88% specificity, and 78% accuracy for combined metastatic lymph node and distant metastases detection. Median survival time for patients with positive PET/CT studies for metastatic disease was 13.5 months compared with 32.0 months for patients without demonstrable metastases. For lymph node staging with PET, another study reported a sensitivity of 67%, specificity of 86%, and accuracy of 80%, all of which are better than the respective values for CT or MRI [145]. FDG-PET was also used to evaluate metastatic TCC in a comparison before and after chemotherapy. Prior to any treatment, PET had a sensitivity and specificity of 77% and 97%, respectively, for detecting metastatic disease, which fell to just 50% sensitivity for evaluating residual or recurrent disease following systemic chemothera-

py [146]. Other investigators have sought to improve upon the diagnostic accuracy of PET in bladder carcinoma. As with PET imaging in RCC, fluid hydration and diuretics may be used to obtain better image quality. A recent report by Anjos et al. [147] described a technique of delayed pelvic imaging with PET/CT following fluid and furosemide administration, which led to upstaging in 41% of cases. Gofrit et al. [148] reported on the use of PET/CT imaging with [^{11}C]-choline in the preoperative staging of advanced TCC in 18 patients; sensitivity for the primary lesion was 100%. [^{11}C]-choline PET/CT also demonstrated uptake in lymph nodes of six patients, four of whom underwent surgery, with metastatic disease confirmed in three. In the series, there were three patients with carcinoma in situ, all of which were detected. Osseous metastases were detected in four patients who tested normal on CT imaging; the positive results were later confirmed with follow-up imaging.

Spleen

There is very little published data on the use of PET or PET/CT in the evaluation of splenic lesions. FDG uptake is typically increased when there is splenic involvement by lymphoma (see Lymphoma section). Metastatic disease from malignant melanoma has been previously described [149]. Metser et al. [150] reported the largest series; a study of 88 patients, 68 with known malignancies, imaged with PET/CT. The sensitivity, specificity, PPV, and NPV of PET/CT in differentiating benign from malignant solid splenic lesions in patients with and without malignant disease were 100%, 100%, 100%, and 100% vs. 100%, 83%, 80%, and 100%, respectively. The authors demonstrated that PET/CT could reliably discriminate between benign and malignant solid splenic masses in patients with known FDG-avid malignancy. PET/CT was shown to have a high negative predictive value in patients with solid splenic masses and without known malignant disease. It was recommended that FDG-avid splenic masses in patients without a known malignancy be further evaluated, as 80% of them in that study were malignant.

Lymphoma

In the USA, CMS guidelines approve the use of FDG-PET and thus PET/CT for the diagnosis, staging, and restaging of lymphoma. Lymphoma is the fifth most common type of cancer occurring in the USA. It is subdivided into Hodgkin's disease (HD) and non-Hodgkin's lymphoma (NHL). Together, more than 71,000 new cases were expected in the USA in 2007 [151]. The most commonly employed staging system is the Ann Arbor classification, which determines four stages depending on disease location above and/or below the diaphragm as well as nodal vs. extranodal involvement.

Diagnosis of Lymphoma

FDG-PET is rarely employed to make the initial diagnosis of lymphoma, and there are few articles in the published literature directly addressing the diagnosis of unsuspected lymphoma with PET. In our experience, most patients undergo histological diagnosis following percutaneous biopsy or lymph node excision. Furthermore, there are numerous non-lymphomatous causes of increased FDG activity in lymph nodes, leading to difficulty with interpretation and potential false-positive results. The cause of these hypermetabolic lymph nodes includes sarcoidosis, tuberculosis, histoplasmosis and other fungal infections, systemic lupus erythematosus, and Castleman's disease [5,152-155]. In addition, false-negative results may occur in certain low-grade histological subtypes. A recent study comparing FDG-PET with conventional lymphoma imaging found that PET detects 40% more abnormal lymph nodes in follicular lym-

phoma but less than 58% of abnormal lymph node groups in small lymphocytic lymphoma [156]. PET imaging of lymphoma arising in mucosa MALT has produced conflicting results; a recent study showed PET to be unreliable for the detection of the specific subtype of MALT lymphoma without plasmacytic differentiation [157].

Staging of Lymphoma

Until recently, lymphoma staging was predominately performed with CT and 67-gallium-citrate (^{67}Ga) scintigraphy. However, most cell types are FDG avid, and there is now extensive evidence supporting the use of FDG-PET and PET/CT as staging tools in HD and in NHL [158]. Direct comparisons of FDG-PET with ^{67}Ga imaging have shown statistically significantly higher sensitivity, specificity, and accuracy with PET [159-161]. A site sensitivity of 100% vs.71.5% and a patient sensitivity of 100% vs. 80.3% have been reported for PET and ^{67}Ga imaging, respectively [162]. In addition, ^{67}Ga has limited use below the diaphragm due to physiological uptake in the bowel, while PET has been shown to be more sensitive than 67Ga for infradiaphragmatic disease [161].

CT has long been the gold standard for the staging of lymphoma. However, despite the excellent resolution of CT, it remains dependent on morphologic changes in lymph nodes, namely, size > 1 cm or alteration in enhancement pattern, for disease detection. As mentioned previously, PET imaging allows for the detection of increased metabolic activity in otherwise morphologically normal lymph nodes. PET may also reveal enlarged nodes to have low metabolic activity and therefore likely to be reactive rather than malignant. Multiple studies have consistently demonstrated the superiority of PET compared with CT for staging of HD and NHL [163, 164]. Sensitivity rates of 86–100% have been reported for PET compared with 26–100% for CT, together with specificity rates of 92–100% for PET and 50–100% for CT, indicating a wider variability for CT and a more uniform higher performance rate for PET [3].

The accurate detection of extranodal disease is critical for the precise staging of lymphoma, with implications for treatment and prognosis. When imaged with ultrasound and CT, nearly 20% of patients may have undiagnosed infradiaphragmatic disease at staging laparotomy. The sensitivity of CT in these cases was 15–37% for splenic involvement and 19–33% for hepatic involvement [165]. Despite the physiological uptake of FDG by both the liver and spleen, PET is more accurate than CT or ^{67}Ga for the detection of splenic and hepatic lymphoma [161,166] Most patients with lymphoma undergo bone marrow aspiration, typically from the posterior iliac crest. Such random bone marrow biopsies may occasionally miss focal marrow involvement, whereas studies have shown that FDG-PET is accurate in detecting bone marrow involvement. In a study of 78 patients, an 81% sensitivity rate and 100% specificity rate was demonstrated for PET, with only four false negative cases [167]. One important limitation to bone marrow assessment with FDG-PET is in the setting of treatment with granulocyte colony-stimulating factor (G-CSF), the use of which can lead to diffuse increased FDG uptake in the bone marrow and spleen and potentially to a false-positive result [22,168]. It is therefore recommended that PET imaging be postponed for at least 1 month following G-CSF treatment.

In one study directly comparing PET, CT, and ^{67}Ga for the staging of HD and NHL, PET was shown to be at least as good as CT and superior to ^{67}Ga for the detection of nodal and extranodal disease. The study reported PET, CT, and ^{67}Ga sensitivities at nodal detection of 93.3%, 98.9%, and 25.8% with specificities of 100%, 99.1%, and 98.8%. In the same study, extranodal sensitivity was 87.5, 87.5, and 37.5% for PET, CT, and ^{67}Ga, respectively, while specificity for each modality was 100% [169]. The results for CT and PET were comparable and in many respects complementary in the evaluation of lymphoma, highlighting the benefit of combined PET/CT imaging. A number of studies have emphasized the benefits of PET in more accurately staging patients with lymphoma. Compared with conventional imaging, PET findings resulted in changes in clinical stage in 28–44% of patients [170,171]. Staging has been shown to be even more accurate with combined PET/CT imaging, as demonstrated by one group directly comparing PET/CT with PET alone. Accuracy rates for overall staging of 93% for PET/CT and 84% for PET alone were reported [172] (Fig. 10).

Restaging and Treatment Response

Restaging of lymphoma to assess for residual disease is usually undertaken approximately 1 month following completion and cessation of chemotherapy. Patients with intra-abdominal lymphoma frequently present with bulky soft-tissue masses and, following treatment completion, between 40% and 84% have residual masses [173,174]. CT is limited in evaluating these masses for disease activity, as they are already morphologically abnormal, and CT cannot separate post-treatment fibrosis or necrosis from residual disease. Traditional management of such masses includes ^{67}Ga imaging, following these masses with interval CT scans, or biopsy. Between 10% and 18% of such masses are positive for lymphoma at biopsy [175]; however,

biopsy is complicated by residual disease co-existing with fibrotic tissue and necrosis. Moreover, it can be difficult for the treating physician to decide on the most appropriate site for biopsy. A false-negative result may occur as a consequence of a non-representative biopsy. Whereas ^{67}Ga scintigraphy can detect disease activity within these residual masses, it is less sensitive in detecting intra-abdominal and extranodal lymphoma than FDG-PET [160,161,175]. Multiple studies have demonstrated the superiority of FDG-PET over CT in restaging lymphoma [176-178]. One study reported sensitivity, specificity, and accuracy rates of 88%, 83%, and 85%, respectively, for PET and 84%, 31%, and 54% for CT. PET also provides valuable prognostic information in predicting relapse rates. A positive PET scan at treatment completion has a reported 90–100% PPV for disease recurrence. The NPV is not as strong; a relapse rate of 0–18% following a negative PET study was reported [177,178]. To further highlight the complimentary nature of combined PET/CT imaging, one study that directly compared separate PET and CT studies with combination imaging in restaging patients with lymphoma demonstrated patient-based sensitivity rates of 78% for CT alone, 86% for PET alone, and 93% for combined PET/CT imaging. Region-based sensitivities were 61%, 78%, and 96% for CT, PET, and PET/CT, respectively [179].

An alternative to restaging of lymphoma following treatment completion is to assess for treatment response earlier in the treatment regime, after one to three cycles of chemotherapy. Early assessment of therapy is particularly useful in a setting in which there may be a choice of chemotherapeutic regimes. In such cases, early assessment of the treatment response may help to prevent unnecessary side effects of certain chemotherapeutic agents and to avoid excessive expenditures on ineffectual regimes. Several investigators have studied the potential benefit and predictive role of FDG-PET imaging early in chemotherapy regimes for HD and NHL. There is now clear evidence that FDG-PET allows for accurate early assessment of treatment response, enabling ineffective regimes to be adjusted, and also has strong predictive properties for long-term survival [180-183]. One study of 47 patients with classic HD or diffuse large-cell lymphoma used PET imaging after one cycle of therapy. Patients were subsequently followed for a median of 28 months. All 31 PET-negative patients after just one cycle of chemotherapy had sustained complete remission. Of 16 PET-positive patients, 14 had refractory disease or relapsed. The two false-positive results related to one patient with increased uptake at the biopsy site and another patient who had received radiation therapy [182].

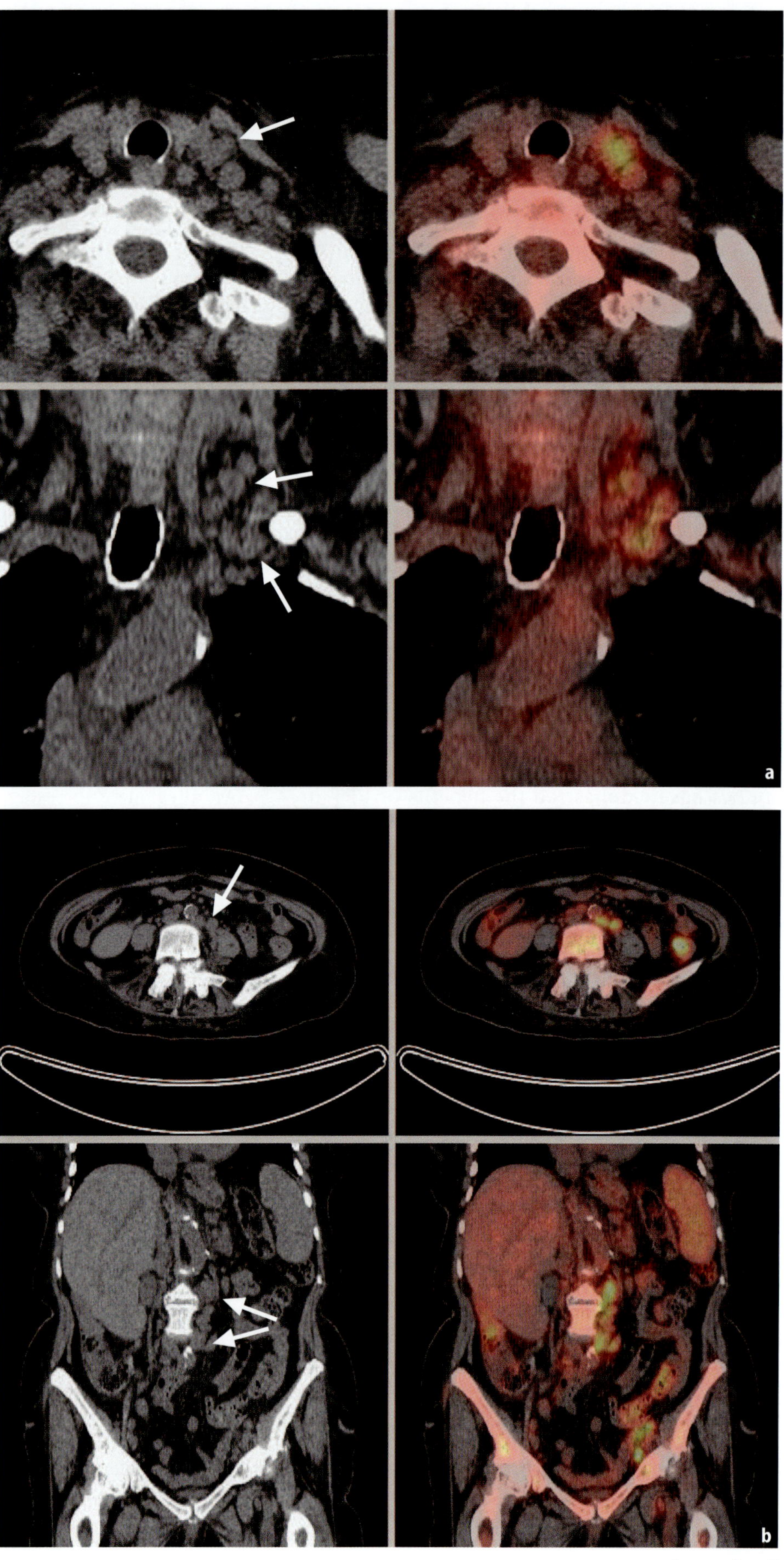

(➝ continued)

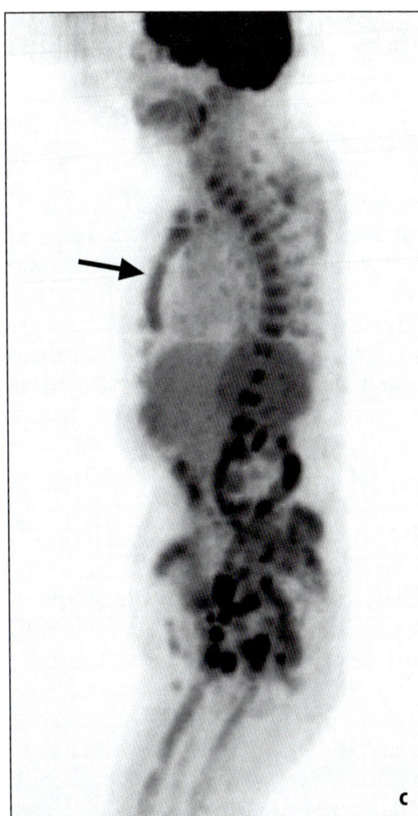

Fig. 10a-c. PET/CT images obtained from an 81-year-old woman for staging of newly diagnosed large B-cell lymphoma. **a** Axial and coronal reconstruction contrast-enhanced CT and fused PET/CT images demonstrating left-sided lower cervical and supraclavicular [^{18}F]-fluorodeoxyglucose (FDG)-avid lymph nodes (*arrows*). **b** Axial and coronal reconstruction contrast-enhanced CT and fused PET/CT images demonstrating multiple FDG-avid left-sided para-aortic lymph nodes (*arrows*). Note also the marked increase in diffuse FDG uptake in the spleen. **c** Sagittal whole-body PET image demonstrating marked increased FDG uptake throughout the bony skeleton, including sternum, multiple vertebrae, and bony pelvis (*arrows*). Although increased splenic and osseous FDG uptake can be seen with granulocyte colony-stimulating factor treatment, in this study performed at initial staging prior to any treatment, the pattern is consistent with diffuse involvement by lymphoma

There is extensive evidence that PET and PET/CT imaging is superior to conventional imaging for the staging and restaging of HD and NHL. Furthermore, PET imaging allows for early assessment of treatment response and has strong predictive qualities for long-term survival when used for both early assessment and at treatment completion.

Malignant Melanoma

In the USA, CMS guidelines approve the use of FDG-PET and thus PET/CT for the diagnosis, staging, and restaging of malignant melanoma. Cuta-

neous malignant melanoma (CMM) accounts for only about 4% of skin-cancer-related cases but is responsible for about 79% of skin-cancer deaths. In the USA, the incidence of CMM is on the rise, and disease-related mortality has dramatically increased by 50% since 1973 [184]. In its early stage, melanoma is curable in up to 85% of patients by means of surgical excision. However, the remaining 15% of patients present with locally advanced or metastatic disease at the time of diagnosis [5]. Apart from certain rare forms, such as choroidal melanoma, the primary lesion is almost always diagnosed clinically at physical exam [3]. Metastatic disease may be local, involving the RLN group, or a variety of distant sites. In addition to the expected sites of hematogenous spread, such as liver, lung, adrenal gland, and bone, melanoma is noted for metastatic disease involving more atypical sites, including gallbladder and spleen [5]. The staging system employed by the AJCC is based upon a standard TNM system that incorporates other factors, i.e., Breslow thickness (tumor depth), Clark level (level of invasion of the skin), ulceration, and involvement of the first node draining the primary tumor, the so-called sentinel lymph node (SLN). In general, malignant melanoma is considered as either early stage (AJCC stages I & II) or advanced stage (AJCC stages III & IV).

Staging

The determination of T stage is based on lesion thickness, with the highest grade, T4, indicating a thickness > 4 mm. Given that the spatial resolution of most PET scanners is, at best, of the order of 5 mm, it is apparent that PET imaging has little to offer in evaluating T stage. The T stage is definitively determined by histopathologic analysis of a punch biopsy or a surgically resected specimen.

The N status is based on the number of involved local RLNs. The most accurate method to determine RLN involvement has proven to be SLN mapping followed by lymphadenectomy. In SLN mapping, a small amount of microfiltered technetium-labeled sulfur colloid is injected intradermally around the primary tumor. The colloid particles are cleared by means of lymphatic drainage, become trapped in the lymph nodes that drain that site, and can then be localized intraoperatively with a gamma probe. Not only has this procedure been shown to be highly accurate for determining the presence of nodal disease, with a sensitivity of 100% and a specificity of 97%, but SLN status has been shown to be the most significant prognostic factor with respect to disease-free survival in patients with stage I or stage II disease [185,186]. Although recurrent metastatic disease may occur without local nodal involvement, it is unusual. In a study of 773 patients with negative SLN biopsy, only 8.9% presented with recurrence within a 3-year period [187]. In a direct comparison of FDG-PET with SLN mapping and biopsy for the detection of local nodal metastases, PET had a16.7% sensitivity and a 50% PPV, albeit with a 95.8% specificity, whereas SLN biopsy had 94.4% sensitivity, 100% PPV, and 100% specificity [188]. Combined imaging with PET/CT has not been shown to be any better at detecting local nodal disease, with a PPV of just 24% in one study [189]. Probably the reason for the poor performance of PET in detecting nodal disease is again related to its spatial resolution. In a study by Wagner et al. [190], 90% sensitivity for RLM detection by FDG-PET required a nodal tumor volume of ≥ 78 mm^3. Median tumor volume in positive SLN basins have been reported as having a volume between 4.3 and 28.3 mm^3 [187,189]. This finding was supported by a later study, which reported sensitivities of 100% for lymph node metastases ≥ 10 mm, 83% for metastases 6–10 mm, and 23% for metastases ≤ 5 mm [191].

Although PET has a limited role in the assessment of T and N status of patients with melanoma, it has been shown to be an important component in the assessment of metastatic disease beyond local RLNs. In on study comparing PET with CT, sensitivity and specificity for PET were 94% and 83%, respectively, as opposed to 55% and 84% for CT [192]. The performance of PET in the detection of distant metastatic disease was reported by Rinne et al. as 100% sensitivity and 94% specificity [193].

The most appropriate imaging protocol for patients with a diagnosis of cutaneous malignant melanoma is a matter of debate. Most authorities would agree that for patients with early disease, as defined as stages I or II, SLN mapping with subsequent lymphadenectomy is sufficient, whereas whole-body FDG-PET is not recommended, as the risk of distant metastatic disease is low [184, 187]. A recent study by Yancovitz et al. [194] assessed the role of imaging studies, including chest X-ray (CXR), CT, and PET, in patients with stage T1b–T3b malignant melanoma. Of the 344 studies performed, only one (0.3%), a PET/CT study, correlated with a confirmed metastatic melanoma. False-positive rates were 71% for CXR, 86% for chest CT, 91% for abdominopelvic CT, 100% for head CT, and 60% for PET/CT. The cost of initial imaging as well as the imaging of abnormal results (mostly false-positives) was estimated as $555,308 for the 158 patients in the study. For patients with higher-risk melanomas, such as primary lesion on the trunk or upper arm, Breslow thickness > 4 mm, or ulceration, imaging with FDG-PET or PET/CT could be reasonably considered [184]. It has been reported that PET/CT should be an integral part in the evaluation of patients with high-risk melanoma prior to selection of the most appropriate therapy [195].

Restaging and Recurrent Disease

The high performance level of FDG-PET in detecting recurrent metastatic malignant melanoma is well established. A meta-analysis of 13 studies by Schwimmer et al. [196] assessing FDG-PET in patients with malignant melanoma revealed an overall sensitivity of 92% and specificity of 90% for recurrent melanoma throughout the body. Furthermore, it was suggested that PET directed a change in management in 22% of patients. As reported with many other malignancies, combined imaging with PET/CT confers advantages over separate PET and CT studies (Fig. 11). Reinhardt et al. [197] compared PET/CT with separate PET and CT studies in 250 patients with malignant melanoma. Imaging was carried out at various time points in the course of the disease. PET/CT detected significantly more visceral and non-visceral metastases than did PET or CT: 99, 89, and 70, respectively. PET/CT accuracy for M staging was 98% compared with 93% for PET and 84% for CT. PET/CT accuracy for N staging was also 98%, with 86% reported for CT. PET/CT resulted in a change in management in 48% of patients. A later study demonstrated combined PET/CT to be superior to side-by-side interpretation of separate PET and CT studies for the evaluation of patients with malignant melanoma [198]. The sensitivity of PET and PET/CT at detecting distant metastatic melanoma includes unexpected and unusual sites, such as gastrointestinal tract, spleen, gallbladder, and testes [149,199-201]. A study by Pfannenberg et al. [202] compared PET/CT with whole-body MRI for the staging of advanced malignant melanoma and found a greater overall accuracy for PET/CT (87 vs. 79%). The greater sensitivity, specificity, and overall accuracy of PET/CT for metastatic melanoma compared with conventional imaging, including PET alone, is such that it frequently results in a change in patient management [197, 202, 203].

Pelvic Malignancy

In the United States, CMS guidelines approve the use of FDG-PET and thus PET/CT for use in staging patients with cervical cancer with CT or MRI findings negative for extra-pelvic metastatic disease. CMS guidelines also approve the use of PET and thus PET/CT for ovarian cancer in limited circumstances. PET and PET/CT has also been used to evaluate patients with endometrial and prostate cancer.

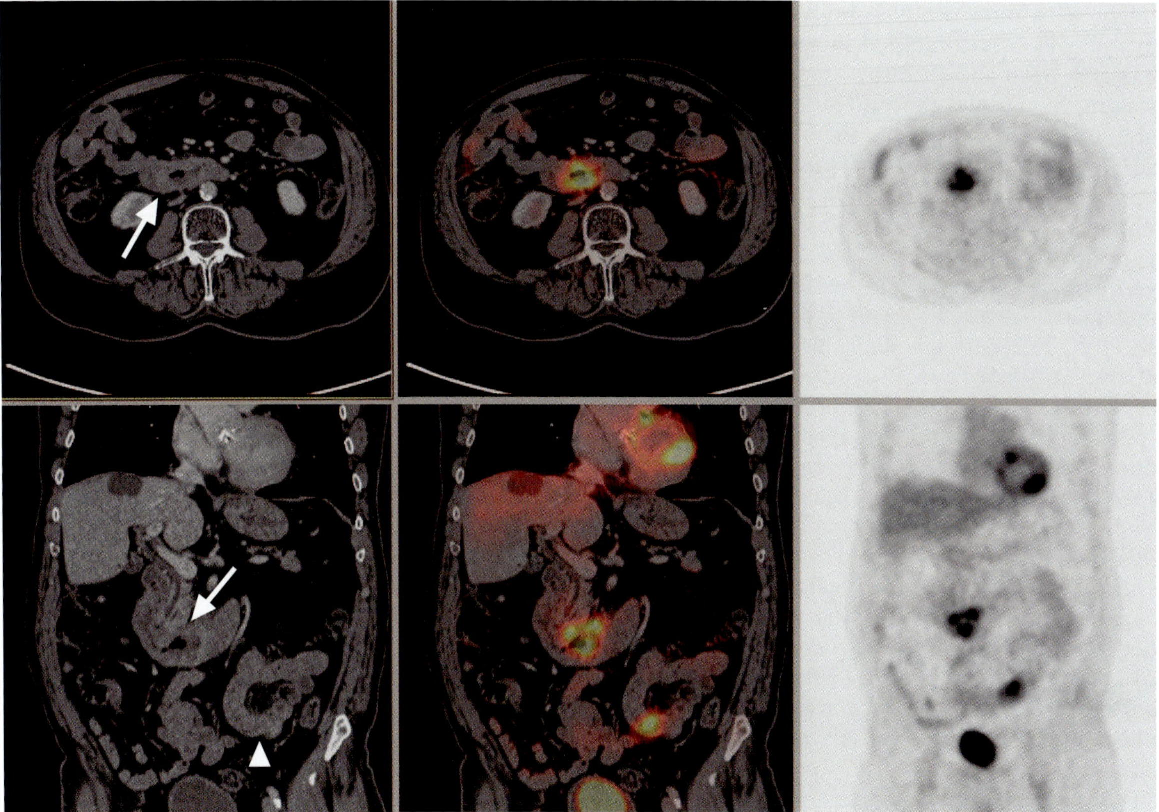

Fig. 11. PET/CT images obtained from a 79-year-old man after primary resection and RLN clearance of malignant melanoma involving the right ear. He later complained of abdominal discomfort. Axial and coronal reconstruction contrast-enhanced CT, PET, and fused PET/CT images demonstrating soft-tissue thickening and increased [^{18}F]-fluorodeoxyglucose (FDG) uptake of the third part of duodenum (*arrow*). There is also a second focus of increased FDG activity in a proximal jejunal loop, without demonstrable abnormality on the CT scan (*arrowhead*). Both lesions were proven at surgery to represent metastatic malignant melanoma

In premenopausal women, the endometrial FDG uptake changes cyclically with menstruation, with increased uptake seen during the ovulatory and menstrual phases. Knowledge of the patient's menstrual history is helpful for informed interpretation, as increased endometrial uptake adjacent to a cervical malignancy does not necessarily reflect tumor invasion. Furthermore, FDG uptake has been demonstrated in uterine fibroids, up to 18% in one series, but only in premenopausal women. Increased ovarian FDG uptake may transiently be seen in premenopausal patients due to uptake in a corpus luteal cyst. Post-menopausal ovarian uptake is not physiological and indicates malignancy [20, 204].

Cervical Cancer

Although the incidence of cervical cancer is decreasing, largely due to efficient screening programs, it is still estimated to be the second most commonly diagnosed malignancy in women worldwide and the third most common gyneco-logic malignancy in the USA [205]. Cervical cancer is staged clinically according to the International Federation of Gynecology and Obstetrics (FIGO) system.

There has been intense interest in the use of PET and PET/CT in cervical malignancy in recent years, and evidence for its beneficial use is emerging with greater frequency, helping to further clarify its role. PET/CT is valuable in the primary staging of untreated advanced cervical cancer, for evaluation of unexplained elevations in tumor markers post-treatment, and for restaging of potentially curable recurrent cervical cancer. However, its value in early stage cervical cancer is limited [206-208]. PET imaging may also prove useful in the evaluation of asymptomatic cervical patients with high levels of tumor markers and negative conventional imaging results [205].

Wong et al. [209] assessed the sensitivity and specificity of PET in the detection of local and distant disease at initial staging and restaging. They reported 100% sensitivity and 100% specificity at initial staging. Restaging sensitivity and specificity rates for local disease were 82% and 97%, respectively, with rates of 100% and 90% reported for distant disease. Combined imaging with PET/CT has also been shown to be accurate in the initial staging of cervical cancer. One prospective study of 120 patients reported a PPV of 75%, a NPV of 96%, sensitivity of 75%, and specificity of 96% for the detection of pelvic lymph node involvement. The PPV, NPV, sensitivity, and specificity rates for para-aortic nodal disease were 94%, 100%, 100%, and 99%, respectively. For the detection of distant metastatic disease, PPV was 63%, NPV 100%, sensitivity 100% and specificity 94% [210]. A meta-analysis of data from 15 studies on FDG-PET in cervical cancer reported a pooled sensitivity and specificity of 84% and 95% respectively for aortic node metastases, and 79% sensitivity and 99% specificity for pelvic node metastases [211].

In the evaluation of cervical cancer recurrence, PET imaging has been shown to be 90.3% sensitive and 76.1% specific for the detection of disease recurrence in patients who otherwise have no evidence of cervical cancer post-treatment [212]. The results for combined PET/CT imaging in the evaluation of disease recurrence are even better, with one study reporting sensitivity, specificity, and accuracy rates of 90.3%, 81.0%, and 86.5%, respectively [213]. The meta-analysis of data from 15 studies on FDG-PET in cervical cancer reported a pooled sensitivity and specificity of 96% and 81%, respectively, for recurrent cervical cancer with clinical suspicion [211].

The use of PET/CT has been shown to alter patient management, by up to 23% of cases in one study [213]. This and other studies have also highlighted the use of PET as a prognostic indicator in cervical cancer. Assessment of para-aortic lymph node metastases is prognostically important and related to progression-free survival in advanced cervical cancer [205]. PET has high sensitivity and specificity and is more sensitive than MRI or CT for the detection of para-aortic lymphadenopathy from advanced cervical cancer [206, 210, 211, 214]. The accuracy of PET in para-aortic lymph node detection has been used for radiation treatment planning. Intensity-modulated radiotherapy (IMRT) helps reduce the radiation dose to adjacent normal structures, and PET/CT has been successfully used to guide IMRT of para-aortic node metastases [215]. Singh et al. reported one study of 47 patients with FIGO stage IIIB cervical cancer. Changes in survival rates with respect to differing nodal disease, as detected with FDG-PET at initial staging before treatment, were assessed. Three-year cause-specific survival was 73% for those with no lymph node metastases, 58% for those with only pelvic nodal disease, 29% for patients with both para-aortic and pelvic nodal involvement, and 0% for those with pelvic, para-aortic, and supraclavicular lymph node metastases [216]. A positive PET study post-treatment was found to be associated with a significantly worse outcome, with subsequent development of metastatic disease and death from cervical cancer [213, 217].

Ovarian Cancer

Ovarian cancer is the second most common gynecologic malignancy. There is no reliable screening tumor marker, and most patients present with advanced disease. With a prevalence of 30–50 per 100,000 women, ovarian cancer is responsible for more than half of the deaths related to gynecologic malignancy. The overall 5-year survival for patients with advanced disease is only 17% [205].

Studies investigating the use of PET and PET/CT in ovarian cancer have produced somewhat mixed results. With respect to initial staging of newly diagnosed ovarian cancer, one study demonstrated CT to have a 53% accuracy rate compared with surgical staging. When the CT studies were evaluated conjointly with FDG-PET, the accuracy rate for combined imaging was 87% [218]. Studies investigating the ability of PET/CT to detect recurrent ovarian cancer have produced variable results, and accuracy rates for the detection of recurrent tumor and nodal recurrence differ. Yen et al. [219] compared FDG-PET with CA-125 levels and conventional imaging with CT or MRI for the evaluation of recurrent ovarian cancer. All three modalities were found to have identical sensitivity rates of 90.9%; however, specificities of 92.3%, 76.9%, and 46.2% were reported for PET, CA-125 levels, and CT/MRI, respectively. The overall accuracy rates were 91.7% for PET, 83.3% for CA-125 level, and 66.7% for CT/MRI. Another study assessed the use of PET/CT in the evaluation of recurrent ovarian tumors with a mass of ≥1 cm. Sensitivity was 83.3%, accuracy 81.8%, and a PPV 93.8% [220]. Pannu et al. [221] also reported on the use of PET/CT for the evaluation of recurrent ovarian cancer. The sensitivity, specificity, and accuracy rates for disease detection on a per-patient basis were 73%, 40%, and 63%, respectively. Although PET/CT detected 100% of nodal recurrence, peritoneal disease was detected in 50% of lesions > 1 cm in size and only 13% of lesions < 1 cm. Despite the 100% nodal detection reported in that study, another study reported just 41% sensitivity rates for retroperitoneal nodal recurrence, with 83% specificity, 69% PPV, and 72% NPV. PET/CT failed to identify microscopic recurrent disease in 59% of pathologically positive nodes [222].

The overall FDG-PET sensitivity in the detection of recurrent ovarian cancer ranges between 45% and 100%, with specificities of 40–99% [205]. Currently, PET imaging is felt to be beneficial for patients with plateaued or increasing abnormal serum CA-125 and for patients with CT- or MRI-defined localized recurrence for whom biopsy is deemed unfeasible [207, 208]. In patients who do not have clinical evidence of disease, second-look laparotomy or laparoscopy is sometimes performed post-treatment to assess disease response, detecting residual disease in 36–73% of such cases [205]. Smith et al. [223] performed a cost analysis comparing FDG-PET with second-look laparotomy. They demonstrated a decrease in unnecessary laparotomies from 70% to 5% with the use of PET and an associated reduction in health care costs. Further studies are required to better clarify the exact role of PET and PET/CT in ovarian cancer.

Endometrial Cancer

Endometrial carcinoma is the most common female pelvic malignancy and fourth most common cancer in women [205]. Surgical staging is definitive, and nodal sampling is performed as part of disease assessment. As adjuvant radiation therapy is given in most cases, with the radiation field including nodal areas, determination of nodal involvement is important. Although not yet approved by the CMS, there is nonetheless some evidence supporting the use of PET and PET/CT in endometrial carcinoma.

One prospective study comparing FDG-PET with CT/MRI for the preoperative evaluation of patients with endometrial carcinoma reported 96.7% sensitivity for PET for the detection of the primary lesion, with just 83.3% sensitivity for CT/MRI. In the evaluation of retroperitoneal lymph nodes, the specificity for PET and CT/MRI was 100% and 85.7%, respectively. However, PET detected none of the five cases of lymph node metastases < 1 cm in diameter. For the detection of extra-uterine lesions, excluding retroperitoneal lymph nodes, PET proved to be 83.3% sensitive as opposed to 66.7% sensitive for CT/MRI. The diagnostic ability of PET was improved when combined with morphologic information from CT/MRI, highlighting the potential benefit of combined PET/CT imaging [224].

Belhocine et al. [225] assessed the usefulness of FDG-PET in the post-therapy surveillance of endometrial cancer and found 96% sensitivity, 78% specificity, and 90% accuracy for the detection of residual or recurrent disease. They reported PPV and NPV of 89% and 91%, respectively. These findings are further supported by another study of post-operative patients with endometrial cancer; PET was found to have 100% sensitivity, 88% specificity, and 93% accuracy for residual or recurrent disease [226]. The same study found PET to be superior to conventional imaging with CT and/or MRI (sensitivity 85%, specificity 86%, and accura-cy 85%) and to tumor marker evaluation (sensitivity 100%, specificity 71%, and accuracy 83%). There were no false negatives with PET. These results have been supported by more recent studies, again highlighting the superior nature of PET over conventional CT imaging or MRI in the detection of recurrent disease [227, 228]. Most of these studies have emphasized that the diagnostic ability of PET is improved upon when combined with a morphologic imaging modality. A recent study of 25 women by Sironi et al. [229] specifically evaluated the role of combined PET/CT imaging in patients with uterine cancer, either cervical or endometrial, for the detection of tumor recurrence. These authors reported patient-based sensitivity, specificity, and accuracy values for the detection of tumor recurrence of 93%, 100%, and 96%, respectively. The PPV and NPV were 100% and 92% (Fig. 12).

These results highlight the potential benefit of PET and PET/CT in endometrial carcinoma, but further trials with larger numbers of patients are required to fully evaluate its role. Early results have shown that the addition of PET to conventional imaging modalities may effect patient management in up to a third of cases and may also have important prognostic capabilities [226].

Prostate Cancer

In the USA, prostate cancer is the most common type of cancer in men and is second only to lung cancer as a cause of cancer-related male deaths [151]. As opposed to many other malignancies, prostate cancer does not display increased glucose metabolism, which reduces the sensitivity of PET imaging with FDG, a glucose analogue [136]. This is further compromised by the normal physiologic renal excretion of FDG that due to its presence in the ureters and accumulation in the bladder, can mask abnormal uptake within the pelvis and retroperitoneum. The limited role of FDG-PET in prostate cancer has been established by numerous studies. A number of them have demonstrated that FDG-PET cannot differentiate between prostate cancer and benign prostatic hyperplasia [230]. Liu et al. [231] assessed FDG-PET in the evaluation of patients with organ-confined prostate cancer and demonstrated just 4% sensitivity. Another group looked at FDG-PET in the setting of metastatic prostatic cancer and found it to be inferior to bone scintigraphy for the detection of osseous metastases, with a sensitivity of 65%. Furthermore, they reported that evaluation of pelvic lymph node metastases was severely limited by FDG accumulation within the bladder [232]. A more recent study evaluating patients with a rise in prostate-specific antigen (PSA) after radical prostatectomy demon-

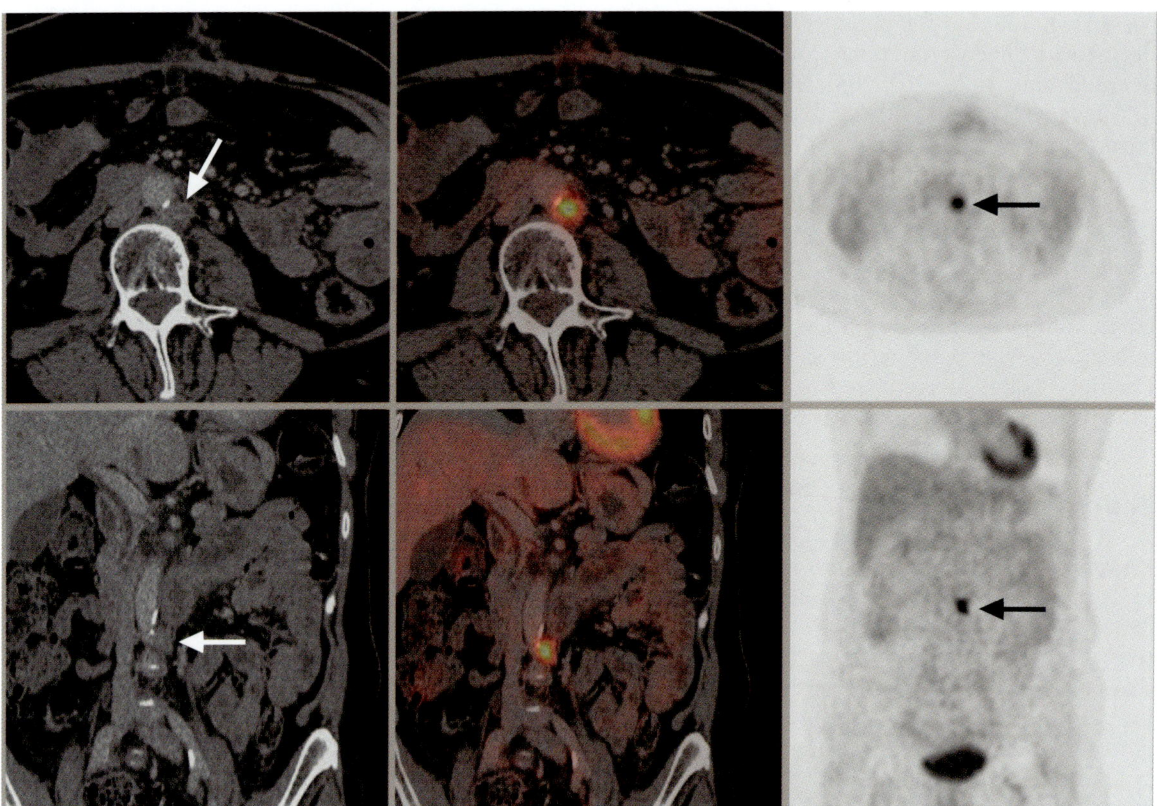

Fig. 12. PET/CT images obtained from a 61-year-old woman 2 years following treatment for a Federation of Gynecology and Obstetrics (FIGO) stage IIIc endometrial carcinoma. Axial and coronal reconstruction contrast-enhanced CT, PET, and fused PET/CT images demonstrating increased FDG activity in a left-sided para-aortic lymph node from biopsy-proven recurrent endometrial adenocarcinoma (*arrows*)

strated FDG-PET to detect only 31% of cases of local or systemic disease [233]. FDG-PET has a proven role in many malignancies in differentiating between residual tumor and post-treatment fibrosis or scar, but it has been shown to be ineffectual in this regard with prostate cancer [230].

Due to the limitations of PET imaging with FDG in prostate cancer, there has been much interest in the development of new PET tracers that are not dependent on glucose metabolism for tracer uptake and do not have renal excretion. Such tracers include [^{11}C]-acetate, [^{11}C]-methionine, [^{18}F]-fluorothymidine, and [^{11}C]- and [^{18}F]-labeled choline [136]. A small study of 22 patients in which [^{11}C]-acetate was compared with FDG-PET imaging demonstrated the former to be more sensitive than FDG for the detection of prostate cancer (100% vs. 79%) as well as at detecting pelvic and osseous metastases [234]. Another study assessing patients with rising PSA levels following treatment found [^{11}C]-acetate to be better at detecting recurrent disease than FDG (30% vs. 9%) [235]. A study of ten patients in which [^{11}C]-choline was compared with FDG in the evaluation of prostate cancer found greater lesion accumulation of radiotracer with [^{11}C]-choline than with FDG; the former was also easier to see, as FDG activity was fre-

quently masked by urinary activity [236]. The combination of the metabolic information provided by PET with the morphologic information provided by CT also enhances the imaging of prostate cancer. Reske et al. [237] reported a study of 26 patients with prostate cancer who were imaged with [^{11}C]-choline PET/CT. This approach was found to be accurate in detecting prostate cancer and differentiating malignant tissue from benign hyperplasia, chronic prostatitis, and normal tissue. PET/CT imaging with [^{18}F]-fluoromethylcholine has also shown promising results. In one study of 100 patients, 54 had positive scans with [^{18}F]-fluoromethylcholine PET/CT, including bone, abdominal lymph node, and pelvic activity, of which all but one were confirmed as malignant disease. Of the 46 patients with negative scans, 89% had serum PSA levels <4 ng/ml and no cases of recurrent disease were proven clinically in a 6-month follow-up period [238]. Overall, it would appear that acetate and choline provide better accuracy than FDG in the detection of local soft-tissue disease, nodal involvement, and distant metastases [239]. However, further studies are required to formally establish the role of PET in the imaging of prostate cancer and to identify the most useful radiotracer(s). A recent study comparing

[^{11}C]-choline PET/CT with MRI and MR spectroscopy in biopsy-proven prostate cancer found PET/CT to have lower sensitivity and accuracy than MR spectroscopy (55% and 67%, respectively, with [^{11}C]-choline PET/CT vs. 81% and 76% with MR spectroscopy) with comparable specificity [240].

Conclusion

PET/CT confers undoubted benefits in the imaging of many abdominopelvic malignancies and has been demonstrated to be the imaging modality of choice for some lesions. Hybrid in-line scanning yields superior diagnostic accuracy compared with separately performed PET and CT tests with subsequent image co-registration. The most appropriate scanning protocols remain to be determined. The development of new radiotracers may help to improve the performance of PET/CT in those tumors that currently are better imaged with more conventional imaging modalities.

References

1. Kapoor V, McCook BM, Torok FS (2005) An introduction to PET-CT imaging. Radiographics 24(2):523-543
2. Wahl RL (2004) Why nearly all PET of abdominal and pelvic cancers will be performed as PET/CT. J Nucl Med 45(Suppl 1):82S-95S
3. Blodgett TM, Meltzer CC, Townsend DW (2007) PET/CT: form and function. Radiology 242(2):360-385. Review
4. Beyer T, Townsend DW, Brun T et al (2000) A combined PET/CT scanner for clinical oncology. J Nucl Med 41(8):1369-1379
5. Rohren EM, Turkington TG, Coleman RE (2004) Clinical applications of PET in oncology. Radiology 231(2):305-332
6. Conti M, Bendriem B, Casey M (2005) First experimental results of time-of-flight reconstruction on an LSO PET scanner. Phys Med Biol 50(19):4507-4026
7. Crespo P, Shakirin G, Fiedler F (2007) Direct time-of-flight for quantitative, real-time in-beam PET: a concept and feasibility study. Phys Med Biol 52(23):6795-67811
8. Nakamoto Y, Osman M, Cohade C et al (2002) PET/CT: comparison of quantitative tracer uptake between germanium and CT transmission attenuation-corrected images. J Nucl Med 43(9):1137-1143
9. Antoch G, Freudenberg LS, Beyer T et al (2004) To enhance or not to enhance? 18F-FDG and CT contrast agents in dual-modality 18F-FDG-PET/CT. J Nucl Med 45(Suppl 1):56S-65S
10. Wong TZ, Paulson EK, Nelson RC et al (2007) Practical approach to diagnostic CT combined with PET. AJR Am J Roentgenol 188(3):622-629
11. Berthelsen AK, Holm S, Loft A et al (2005) PET/CT with intravenous contrast can be used for PET attenuation correction in cancer patients. Eur J Nucl Med Mol Imaging 32(10):1167-1175
12. Yau YY, Chan WS, Tam YM et al (2005) Application of intravenous contrast in PET/CT: does it really introduce significant attenuation correction error? J Nucl Med 46(2):283-291
13. Antoch G, Kuehl H, Kanja J et al (2004) Dual-modality PET/CT scanning with negative oral contrast agent to avoid artifacts: introduction and evaluation. Radiology 230(3):879-885
14. Cohade C, Osman M, Nakamoto Y et al (2003) Initial experience with oral contrast in PET/CT: phantom and clinical studies. J Nucl Med 44(3):412-416
15. Brenner DJ, Hall EJ (2007) Computed tomography—an increasing source of radiation exposure. N Engl J Med 357(22):2277-84
16. Kamel E, Hany TF, Burger C et al (2002) CT vs 68Ge attenuation correction in a combined PET/CT system: evaluation of the effect of lowering the CT tube current. Eur J Nucl Med Mol Imaging 29(3):346-350
17. de Juan R, Seifert B, Berthold T et al (2004) Clinical evaluation of a breathing protocol for PET/CT. Eur Radiol 14(6):1118-23. Epub 2003 Dec 16
18. Goerres GW, Burger C, Kamel E et al (2003) Respiration-induced attenuation artifact at PET/CT: technical considerations. Radiology 226(3):906-910
19. Gilman MD, Fischman AJ, Krishnasetty V et al (2006) Optimal CT breathing protocol for combined thoracic PET/CT. AJR Am J Roentgenol 187(5):1357-1360
20. Blake MA, Singh A, Setty BN et al (2006) Pearls and pitfalls in interpretation of abdominal and pelvic PET-CT. Radiographics 26(5):1335-1353
21. Shreve PD, Anzai Y, Wahl RL (1999) Pitfalls in oncologic diagnosis with FDG-PET imaging: physiologic and benign variants. Radiographics 19(1):61-77
22. Abdel-Dayem HM, Rosen G, El-Zeftawy H et al (1999) Fluorine-18 fluorodeoxyglucose splenic uptake from extramedullary hematopoiesis after granulocyte colony-stimulating factor stimulation. Clin Nucl Med 24(5):319-322
23. Holmes RS, Vaughan TL (2007) Epidemiology and pathogenesis of esophageal cancer. Semin Radiat Oncol 17(1):2-9
24. Yeung HW, Macapinlac HA, Mazumdar M et al (1999) FDG-PET in Esophageal Cancer. Incremental Value over Computed Tomography. Clin Positron Imaging 2(5):255-260
25. Prabhakar HB, Sahani DV, Fischman AJ et al (2007) Bowel hot spots at PET-CT. Radiographics 27(1):145-159
26. Bruzzi JF, Munden RF, Truong MT et al (2007) PET/CT of Esophageal Cancer: Its Role in Clinical Management. Radiographics 27(6):1635-1652
27. Little SG, Rice TW, Bybel B et al (2007) Is FDG-PET indicated for superficial esophageal cancer? Eur J Cardiothorac Surg 31(5):791-796
28. Lowe VJ, Booya F, Fletcher JG et al (2005) Comparison of positron emission tomography, computed tomography, and endoscopic ultrasound in the initial staging of patients with esophageal cancer. Mol Imaging Biol 7(6):422-430
29. Pfau PR, Perlman SB, Stanko P et al (2007) The role and clinical value of EUS in a multimodality esophageal carcinoma staging program with CT and positron emission tomography. Gastrointest Endosc 65(3):377-384
30. Bar-Shalom R, Guralnik L, Tsalic M et al (2005) The additional value of PET/CT over PET in FDG imaging of oesophageal cancer. Eur J Nucl Med Mol Imaging 32(8):918-924
31. van Westreenen HL, Westerterp M, Bossuyt PM et al (2004) Systematic review of the staging performance of 18F-fluorodeoxyglucose positron emission tomography in esophageal cancer. J Clin Oncol 22(18):3805-3812

32. Lerut T, Flamen P, Ectors N, Van Cutsem E, Peeters M, Hiele M, De Wever W, Coosemans W, Decker G, De Leyn P, Deneffe G, Van Raemdonck D, Mortelmans L. et al (2000) Histopathologic validation of lymph node staging with FDG-PET scan in cancer of the esophagus and gastroesophageal junction: A prospective study based on primary surgery with extensive lymphadenectomy. Ann Surg 232(6):743-752

33. Katsoulis IE, Wong WL, Mattheou AK et al (2007) Fluorine-18 fluorodeoxyglucose positron emission tomography in the preoperative staging of thoracic oesophageal and gastro-oesophageal junction cancer. Int J Surg [Epub ahead of print]

34. Flanagan FL, Dehdashti F, Siegel BA et al (1997) Staging of esophageal cancer with 18F-fluorodeoxyglucose positron emission tomography. AJR Am J Roentgenol 168(2):417-424

35. Yuan SH, Yu JM, Yu YH et al (2007) [FDG-PET/CT versus PET alone for pre-surgical detection of lymph node metastasis in esophageal carcinoma] Zhonghua Zhong Liu Za Zhi 29(3):221-224

36. Rice TW (2000) Clinical staging of esophageal carcinoma. CT, EUS, and PET. Chest Surg Clin N Am 10(3):471-485

37. Kole AC, Plukker JT, Nieweg OE, Vaalburg W (1998) Positron emission tomography for staging of oesophageal and gastroesophageal malignancy. Br J Cancer 78(4):521-527

38. Duong CP, Demitriou H, Weih L et al (2006) Significant clinical impact and prognostic stratification provided by FDG-PET in the staging of oesophageal cancer. Eur J Nucl Med Mol Imaging 33(7):759-769

39. Leong T, Everitt C, Yuen K et al (2006) A prospective study to evaluate the impact of FDG-PET on CT-based radiotherapy treatment planning for oesophageal cancer. Radiother Oncol 78(3):254-261

40. Downey RJ, Akhurst T, Ilson D et al (2003) Whole body 18FDG-PET and the response of esophageal cancer to induction therapy: results of a prospective trial. J Clin Oncol 21(3):428-432

41. Weber WA, Ott K, Becker K et al (2001) Prediction of response to preoperative chemotherapy in adenocarcinomas of the esophagogastric junction by metabolic imaging. J Clin Oncol 19(12):3058-3065

42. Flamen P, Lerut A, Van Cutsem E et al (2000) The utility of positron emission tomography for the diagnosis and staging of recurrent esophageal cancer. J Thorac Cardiovasc Surg 120(6):1085-1092

43. Westerterp M, van Westreenen HL, Reitsma JB et al (2005) Esophageal cancer: CT, endoscopic US, and FDG-PET for assessment of response to neoadjuvant therapy-systematic review. Radiology 236(3):841-851

44. Guo H, Zhu H, Xi Y et al (2007) Diagnostic and prognostic value of 18F-FDG-PET/CT for patients with suspected recurrence from squamous cell carcinoma of the esophagus.J Nucl Med 48(8):1251-1258

45. Cerfolio RJ, Bryant AS, Ohja B et al (2005) The accuracy of endoscopic ultrasonography with fine-needle aspiration, integrated positron emission tomography with computed tomography, and computed tomography in restaging patients with esophageal cancer after neoadjuvant chemoradiotherapy. J Thorac Cardiovasc Surg 129(6):1232-1241

46. Gutman F, Alberini JL, Wartski M et al (2005) Incidental Colonic Focal Lesions Detected by FDG-PET/CT. AJR Am J Roentgenol 185(2):495-500

47. Abdel-Nabi H, Doerr RJ, Lamonica DM et al (1998) Staging of primary colorectal carcinomas with fluorine-18 fluorodeoxyglucose whole-body PET: correlation with histopathologic and CT findings. Radiology 206:755-760

48. Mukai M, Sadahiro S, Yasuda S et al (2000) Preoperative evaluation by whole-body 18F-fluorodeoxyglucose positron emission tomography in patients with primary colorectal cancer. Oncol Rep 7:85-87

49. Skibber JM, Minsky BD, Hoff PM (2001) Spread of colorectal cancer. In: DeVita VT, Hellman S, Rosenberg SA, eds. Cancer: principles and practice of oncology. 6th ed. Philadelphia: Lippincott Williams & Wilkins 1229-1230

50. Kamel IR. Cohade C, Neyman E et al (2004) Incremental value of CT in PET/CT of patients with colorectal carcinoma. Abdominal Imaging 29(6):663-668

51. Tanaka K, Adam R, Shimada H et al (2003) Role of neoadjuvant chemotherapy in the treatment of multiple colorectal metastases to the liver. Br J Surg 90:963-969

52. Valls C, Andía E, Sánchez A et al (2001) Hepatic metastases from colorectal cancer: preoperative detection and assessment of resectability with helical CT. Radiology 218(1):55-60

53. Kinkel K, Lu Y, Both M et al (2002) Detection of hepatic metastases from cancers of the gastrointestinal tract by using noninvasive imaging methods (US, CT, MR imaging, PET): A meta-analysis. Radiology 224:748-756

54. Rohren EM, Paulson EK, Hagge R et al (2002) The role of F-18-FDG-PET in preoperative assessment of the liver in patients being considered for curative resection of hepatic metastases from colorectal cancer. Clin Nucl Med 27:550-555

55. Kantorová I, Lipská L, Bělohlávek O et al (2003) Routine (18)F-FDG-PET preoperative staging of colorectal cancer: comparison with conventional staging and its impact on treatment decision making. J Nucl Med 44(11):1784-1788

56. Sahani DV, Kalva SP, Fischman AJ et al (2005) Detection of Liver Metastases from Adenocarcinoma of Colon and Pancreas: Comparison of Mangafodipir Trisodium Enhanced Liver MRI and Whole Body FDG-PET. AJR Am J Roentgenol 185:239-246

57. Chua SC, Groves AM, Kayani I et al (2007) The impact of (18)F-FDG-PET/CT in patients with liver metastases. Eur J Nucl Med Mol Imaging 34(12):1906-1914

58 Huebner RH, Park KC, Shepherd JE, Schwimmer J et al (2000) A meta-analysis of the literature for whole-body FDG-PET detection of recurrent colorectal cancer. J Nucl 41:1177-1189

59. Strasberg SM, Dehdashti F, Siegel BA et al (2001) Survival of patients evaluated by FDG-PET before hepatic resection for metastatic colorectal carcinoma: a prospective database study. Ann Surg 233:293-299

60. Valk PE, Abella-Columna E, Haseman MK et al (1999) Whole-body PET imaging with [18F]fluorodeoxyglucose in management of recurrent colorectal cancer. Arch Surg 134:503-511

61. Park IJ, Kim HC, Yu CS et al (2006) Efficacy of PET/CT in the accurate evaluation of primary colorectal carcinoma. Eur J Surg Oncol 32(9):941-947

62. Hung GU, Shiau YC, Tsai SC et al (2001) Value of 18F-fluoro-2-deoxyglucose positron emission tomography in the evaluation of recurrent colorectal cancer. Anticancer Res 21:1375-1378

63. Wiering B, Krabbe PF, Jager GJ et al (2005) The impact of fluor-18-deoxyglucose-positron emission tomography in the management of colorectal liver metastases. Cancer 104(12):2658-70

64. Even-Sapir E, Parag Y, Lerman H et al (2004) Detection of recurrence in patients with rectal cancer: PET/CT after abdominoperineal or anterior resection. Radiology 232(3):815-822
65. Cohade C, Osman M, Leal J, Wahl RL (2003) Direct comparison of (18)F-FDG-PET and PET/CT in patients with colorectal carcinoma. J Nucl Med 44(11):1797-1803
66. Chen LB, Tong JL, Song HZ (2007) (18)F-DG PET/CT in detection of recurrence and metastasis of colorectal cancer. World J Gastroenterol 13(37):5025-5029
67. Votrubova J, Belohlavek O, Jaruskova M et al (2006) The role of FDG-PET/CT in the detection of recurrent colorectal cancer. Eur J Nucl Med Mol Imaging 33(7):779-784
68. Kim JH, Czernin J, Allen-Auerbach MS et al (2005) Comparison between 18F-FDG-PET, in-line PET/CT, and software fusion for restaging of recurrent colorectal cancer. J Nucl Med 46(4):587-595
69. Ciernik IF, Huser M, Burger C et al (2005) Automated functional image-guided radiation treatment planning for rectal cancer. Int J Radiat Oncol Biol Phys 62(3):893-900
70. Veit-Haibach P, Kuehle CA, Beyer T et al (2006) Diagnostic accuracy of colorectal cancer staging with whole-body PET/CT colonography. JAMA 296(21):2590-2600
71. Gollub MJ, Akhurst T, Markowitz AJ et al (2007) Combined CT colonography and 18F-FDG-PET of colon polyps: potential technique for selective detection of cancer and precancerous lesions. AJR Am J Roentgenol (1):130-138
72. Hillner BE, Liu D, Coleman RE et al (2007) The National Oncologic PET Registry (NOPR): design and analysis plan. J Nucl Med 48(11):1901-1908
73. Yeoh KG (2007) How do we improve outcomes for gastric cancer? J Gastroenterol Hepatol 22(7):970-972
74. Yeung HW, Macapinlac H, Karpeh M et al (1998) Accuracy of FDG-PET in Gastric Cancer. Preliminary Experience. Clin Positron Imaging 1(4):213-221
75. Shoda H, Kakugawa Y, Saito D et al (2007) Evaluation of (18)F-2-deoxy-2-fluoro-glucose positron emission tomography for gastric cancer screening in asymptomatic individuals undergoing endoscopy. Br J Cancer 97(11):1493-1498
76. Lim JS, Yun MJ, Kim MJ et al (2006) CT and PET in stomach cancer: preoperative staging and monitoring of response to therapy. Radiographics 26(1):143-156
77. Imperiale A, Cimarelli S, Sellem DB et al (2006) Focal F-18 FDG uptake mimicking malignant gastric localizations disappearing after water ingestion on PET/CT images. Clin Nucl Med 31(12):835-837
78. Stahl A, Ott K, Weber WA et al (2003) FDG-PET imaging of locally advanced gastric carcinomas: correlation with endoscopic and histopathological findings. Eur J Nucl Med Mol Imaging 30(2):288-295
79. Rosenbaum SJ, Stergar H, Antoch G et al (2006) Staging and follow-up of gastrointestinal tumors with PET/CT. Abdom Imaging 31(1):25-35
80. Sun L, Ye HY, Zhang YH et al (2007) Epidermal growth factor receptor antibody plus recombinant human endostatin in treatment of hepatic metastases after remnant gastric cancer resection. World J Gastroenterol 13(45):6115-6118
81. Herrmann K, Ott K, Buck AK et al (2007) Imaging Gastric Cancer with PET and the Radiotracers 18F-FLT and 18F-FDG: A Comparative Analysis. J Nucl Med [Epub ahead of print]
82. Watanabe N, Hayashi S, Kato H et al (2004) FDG-PET imaging in duodenal cancer. Ann Nucl Med 18(4):351-353
83. Sperti C, Pasquali C, Fiore V et al (2006) Clinical usefulness of 18-fluorodeoxyglucose positron emission tomography in the management of patients with nonpancreatic periampullary neoplasms. Am J Surg 191(6):743-748
84. Plaza P, Montravers F, Aide N et al (2004) [Assessment of a neuroendocrine tumour by 111In-pentetreotid scintigraphy and PET with 18FFDOPA and 18F-FDG]. Rev Esp Med Nucl 23(6):421-424
85. Kowalski J, Henze M, Schuhmacher J et al (2003) Evaluation of positron emission tomography imaging using [68Ga]-DOTA-D Phe(1)-Tyr(3)-Octreotide in comparison to [111In]-DTPAOC SPECT. First results in patients with neuroendocrine tumors. Mol Imaging Biol 5(1):42-48
86. Bastiaannet E, Groen H, Jager PL et al (2004) The value of FDG-PET in the detection, grading and response to therapy of soft tissue and bone sarcomas; a systematic review and meta-analysis. Cancer Treat Rev 30(1):83-101
87. Burkill GJ, Badran M, Al-Muderis O et al (2003) Malignant gastrointestinal stromal tumor: distribution, imaging features, and pattern of metastatic spread. Radiology 226(2):527-532
88. Hersh MR, Choi J, Garrett C, Clark R (2005) Imaging gastrointestinal stromal tumors. Cancer Control 12(2):111-115
89. Goerres GW, Stupp R, Barghouth G et al (2005) The value of PET, CT and in-line PET/CT in patients with gastrointestinal stromal tumours: long-term outcome of treatment with imatinib mesylate. Eur J Nucl Med Mol Imaging 32(2):153-162
90. Gayed I, Vu T, Iyer R, Johnson M et al (2004) The role of 18F-FDG-PET in staging and early prediction of response to therapy of recurrent gastrointestinal stromal tumors. J Nucl Med 45(1):17-21
91. Kamiyama Y, Aihara R, Nakabayashi T et al (2005) 18F-fluorodeoxyglucose positron emission tomography: useful technique for predicting malignant potential of gastrointestinal stromal tumors. World J Surg 29(11):1429-1435
92. Alberini JL, Al Nakib M, Wartski M et al (2007) [The role of PET scan in gastrointestinal stromal tumors] Gastroenterol Clin Biol 31(6-7):585-593
93. Heinicke T, Wardelmann E, Sauerbruch T et al (2005)Very early detection of response to imatinib mesylate therapy of gastrointestinal stromal tumours using 18fluoro-deoxyglucose-positron emission tomography. Anticancer Res 25(6C):4591-4594
94. Antoch G, Kanja J, Bauer S et al (2004) Comparison of PET, CT, and dual-modality PET/CT imaging for monitoring of imatinib (STI571) therapy in patients with gastrointestinal stromal tumors. J Nucl Med 45(3):357-365
95. Kuehl H, Veit P, Rosenbaum SJ et al (2007) Can PET/CT replace separate diagnostic CT for cancer imaging? Optimizing CT protocols for imaging cancers of the chest and abdomen. J Nucl Med 48(Suppl 1):45S-57S
96. Böhm B, Voth M, Geoghegan J et al (2004) Impact of positron emission tomography on strategy in liver resection for primary and secondary liver tumors. J Cancer Res Clin Oncol 130(5):266-272
97. Khan MA, Combs CS, Brunt EM et al (2000) Positron emission tomography scanning in the evaluation of hepatocellular carcinoma. J Hepatol 32(5):792-797
98. Shin JA, Park JW, An M et al (2006) [Diagnostic accuracy of 18F-FDG positron emission tomography

for evaluation of hepatocellular carcinoma] Korean J Hepatol 12(4):546-52

99. Sun L, Guan YS, Pan WM et al (2007) Positron emission tomography/computer tomography in guidance of extrahepatic hepatocellular carcinoma metastasis management. World J Gastroenterol 13(40):5413-5415

100. Talbot JN, Gutman F, Fartoux L et al (2006) PET/CT in patients with hepatocellular carcinoma using [(18)F]fluorocholine: preliminary comparison with [(18)F]FDG-PET/CT. Eur J Nucl Med Mol Imaging 33(11):1285-1289

102. Barker DW, Zagoria RJ, Morton KA et al (2005) Evaluation of liver metastases after radiofrequency ablation: utility of 18F-FDG-PET and PET/CT. AJR Am J Roentgenol 184(4):1096-1102

103. Blokhuis TJ, van der Schaaf MC, van den Tol MP et al (2004) Results of radio frequency ablation of primary and secondary liver tumors: long-term follow-up with computed tomography and positron emission tomography-18F-deoxyfluoroglucose scanning. Scand J Gastroenterol Suppl (241):93-97

104. Veit P, Antoch G, Stergar H et al (2006) Detection of residual tumor after radiofrequency ablation of liver metastasis with dual-modality PET/CT: initial results. Eur Radiol 16(1):80-87

105. Prior JO, Kosinski M, Delaloye AB, Denys A (2007) Initial report of PET/CT-guided radiofrequency ablation of liver metastases. J Vasc Interv Radiol 18(6):801-803

106. Koh T, Taniguchi H, Yamaguchi A et al (2003) Differential diagnosis of gallbladder cancer using positron emission tomography with fluorine-18-labeled fluoro-deoxyglucose (FDG-PET). J Surg Oncol 84(2):74-81

107. Rodríguez-Fernández A, Gómez-Río M, Llamas-Elvira JM et al (2004) Positron-emission tomography with fluorine-18-fluoro-2-deoxy-D-glucose for gallbladder cancer diagnosis. Am J Surg 188(2):171-175

108. Anderson CD, Rice MH, Pinson CW et al (2004) Fluorodeoxyglucose PET imaging in the evaluation of gallbladder carcinoma and cholangiocarcinoma. J Gastrointest Surg 8(1):90-97

109. Maldjian PD, Ghesani N, Ahmed S, Liu Y (2007) Adenomyomatosis of the gallbladder: another cause for a "hot" gallbladder on 18F-FDG-PET. AJR Am J Roentgenol 189(1):W36-38

110. Nishiyama Y, Yamamoto Y, Fukunaga K et al (2006) Dual-time-point 18F-FDG-PET for the evaluation of gallbladder carcinoma. J Nucl Med 47(4):633-638

111. Petrowsky H, Wildbrett P, Husarik DB et al (2006) Impact of integrated positron emission tomography and computed tomography on staging and management of gallbladder cancer and cholangiocarcinoma. J Hepatol 45(1):43-50

112. Sun L, Wu H, Guan YS (2007) Positron emission tomography/computer tomography: challenge to conventional imaging modalities in evaluating primary and metastatic liver malignancies. World J Gastroenterol 13(20):2775-2783

113. Singh P, Patel T (2006) Advances in the diagnosis, evaluation and management of cholangiocarcinoma. Curr Opin Gastroenterol 22(3):294-299

114. Moon CM, Bang S, Chung JB et al (2007) Usefulness of (18)F-fluorodeoxyglucose positron emission tomography in differential diagnosis and staging of cholangiocarcinomas. J Gastroenterol Hepatol 11

115. Reinhardt MJ, Strunk H, Gerhardt T et al (2005) Detection of Klatskin's tumor in extrahepatic bile duct strictures using delayed 18F-FDG-PET/CT: preliminary results for 22 patient studies. J Nucl Med 46(7):1158-1163

116. Jadvar H, Henderson RW, Conti PS (2007) [F-18]fluorodeoxyglucose positron emission tomography and positron emission tomography: computed tomography in recurrent and metastatic cholangiocarcinoma. J Comput Assist Tomogr 31(2):223-228

117. Borbath I, Van Beers BE, Lonneux M et al (2005) Preoperative assessment of pancreatic tumors using magnetic resonance imaging, endoscopic ultrasonography, positron emission tomography and laparoscopy. Pancreatology 5(6):553-561

118. Bang S, Chung HW, Park SW (2006) The clinical usefulness of 18-fluorodeoxyglucose positron emission tomography in the differential diagnosis, staging, and response evaluation after concurrent chemoradiotherapy for pancreatic cancer. J Clin Gastroenterol 40(10):923-929

119. Mansour JC, Schwartz L, Pandit-Taskar N et al (2006) The utility of F-18 fluorodeoxyglucose whole body PET imaging for determining malignancy in cystic lesions of the pancreas. J Gastrointest Surg 10(10):1354-1360

120. Sperti C, Bissoli S, Pasquali C et al (2007) 18-Fluorodeoxyglucose Positron Emission Tomography Enhances Computed Tomography Diagnosis of Malignant Intraductal Papillary Mucinous Neoplasms of the Pancreas. Ann Surg 246(6):932-939

121. Lemke AJ, Niehues SM, Hosten N et al (2004)Retrospective digital image fusion of multidetector CT and 18F-FDG-PET: clinical value in pancreatic lesions-a prospective study with 104 patients. J Nucl Med 45(8):1279-1286

122. Heinrich S, Goerres GW, Schäfer M et al (2005) Positron emission tomography/computed tomography influences on the management of resectable pancreatic cancer and its cost-effectiveness. Ann Surg 242(2):235-243

123. Pakzad F, Groves AM, Ell PJ (2006) The role of positron emission tomography in the management of pancreatic cancer. Semin Nucl Med 36(3):248-256

124. Chong S, Lee KS, Kim HY et al (2006) Integrated PET-CT for the characterization of adrenal gland lesions in cancer patients: diagnostic efficacy and interpretation pitfalls. Radiographics 26(6):1811-1824

125. Elaini AB, Shetty SK, Chapman VM et al (2007) Improved detection and characterization of adrenal disease with PET-CT. Radiographics 27(3):755-767

126. Caoili EM, Korobkin M, Francis IR et al (2002) Adrenal masses: characterization with combined unenhanced and delayed enhanced CT. Radiology 222(3):629-633

127. Blake MA, Slattery JM, Kalra MK et al (2006) Adrenal lesions: characterization with fused PET/CT image in patients with proved or suspected malignancy–initial experience. Radiology 238(3):970-977

128. Bagheri B, Maurer AH, Cone L et al (2004) Characterization of the normal adrenal gland with 18F-FDG-PET/CT. J Nucl Med 45(8):1340-1343

129. Zhang LJ, Yang GF, Shen W, Qi J (2006) Imaging of primary adrenal lymphoma: case report and literature review. Acta Radiol 47(9):993-997

130. Shulkin BL, Thompson NW, Shapiro B et al (1999) Pheochromocytomas: imaging with 2-[fluorine-18]fluoro-2-deoxy-D-glucose PET. Radiology

212(1):35-41

131. Becherer A, Vierhapper H, Pötzi C et al (2001) FDG-PET in adrenocortical carcinoma. Cancer Biother Radiopharm 16(4):289-295

132. Mackie GC, Shulkin BL, Ribeiro RC et al (2006) Use of [18F]fluorodeoxyglucose positron emission tomography in evaluating locally recurrent and metastatic adrenocortical carcinoma. J Clin Endocrinol Metab 91(7):2665-2671

133. Zettinig G, Mitterhauser M, Wadsak W et al (2004) Positron emission tomography imaging of adrenal masses: (18)F-fluorodeoxyglucose and the 11beta-hydroxylase tracer (11)C-metomidate. Eur J Nucl Med Mol Imaging 31(9):1224-1230

134. Gross MD, Avram A, Fig LM, Fanti S et al (2007) PET in the diagnostic evaluation of adrenal tumors. Q J Nucl Med Mol Imaging 51(3):272-283

135. Hain SF, Maisey MN (2003) Positron emission tomography for urological tumours. BJU Int 92(2):159-164

136. Powles T, Murray I, Brock C et al (2007) Molecular positron emission tomography and PET/CT imaging in urological malignancies. Eur Urol 51(6):1511-1520

137. Miyakita H, Tokunaga M, Onda H et al (2002) Significance of 18F-fluorodeoxyglucose positron emission tomography (FDG-PET) for detection of renal cell carcinoma and immunohistochemical glucose transporter 1 (GLUT-1) expression in the cancer. Int J Urol 9(1):15-18

138. Bachor R, Kotzerke J, Gottfried HW et al (1996) [Positron emission tomography in diagnosis of renal cell carcinoma] Urologe A 35(2):146-150

139. Kang DE, White RL Jr, Zuger JH et al (2004) Clinical use of fluorodeoxyglucose F 18 positron emission tomography for detection of renal cell carcinoma. J Urol 171(5):1806-1809

140. Majhail NS, Urbain JL, Albani JM et al (2003) F-18 fluorodeoxyglucose positron emission tomography in the evaluation of distant metastases from renal cell carcinoma. J Clin Oncol 21(21):3995-4000

141. Dilhuydy MS, Durieux A, Pariente A et al (2006) PET scans for decision-making in metastatic renal cell carcinoma: a single-institution evaluation. Oncology 70(5):339-344

142. Divgi CR, Pandit-Taskar N, Jungbluth AA et al (2007) Preoperative characterisation of clear-cell renal carcinoma using iodine-124-labelled antibody chimeric G250 (124I-cG250) and PET in patients with renal masses: a phase I trial. Lancet Onco 8(4):304-310

143. Kosuda S, Kison PV, Greenough R et al (1997) Preliminary assessment of fluorine-18 fluorodeoxyglucose positron emission tomography in patients with bladder cancer. Eur J Nucl Med 24(6):615-620

144. Drieskens O, Oyen R, Van Poppel H et al (2005) FDG-PET for preoperative staging of bladder cancer. Eur J Nucl Med Mol Imaging 32(12):1412-1417

145. Bachor R, Kotzerke J, Reske SN, Hautmann R (1999) [Lymph node staging of bladder neck carcinoma with positron emission tomography] Urologe A 38(1):46-50

146. Liu IJ, Lai YH, Espiritu JI et al (2006) Evaluation of fluorodeoxyglucose positron emission tomography imaging in metastatic transitional cell carcinoma with and without prior chemotherapy. Urol Int 77(1):69-75

147. Anjos DA, Etchebehere EC, Ramos CD et al (2007) 18F-FDG-PET/CT delayed images after diuretic for restaging invasive bladder cancer. J Nucl Med

48(5):764-770

148. Gofrit ON, Mishani E, Orevi M et al (2006) Contribution of 11C-choline positron emission tomography/computerized tomography to preoperative staging of advanced transitional cell carcinoma. J Urol 176(3):940-944

149. van Ufford HM, Zoon PJ, van Waes PF et al (2005) Solitary splenic metastasis in a patient with a malignant melanoma diagnosed with F-18-FDG-PET scanning. Clin Nucl Med 30(8):582-583

150. Metser U, Miller E, Kessler A et al (2005) Solid splenic masses: evaluation with 18F-FDG-PET/CT. J Nucl Med 46(1):52-59

151. Jemal A, Siegel R, Ward E et al (2007) Cancer statistics, 2007 CA Cancer J Clin 57(1):43-66

152. Xiu Y, Yu JQ, Cheng E et al (2005) Sarcoidosis demonstrated by FDG-PET imaging with negative findings on gallium scintigraphy. Clin Nucl Med 30(3):193-195

153. Bakheet SM, Powe J, Ezzat A, Rostom A (1998) F-18-FDG uptake in tuberculosis. Clin Nucl Med 23(11):739-742

154. Fey GL, Jolles PR, Buckley LM, Massey GV (2004) 2-Deoxy-2-[18F]fluoro-D-glucose positron emission tomography uptake in systemic lupus erythematosus-associated adenopathy. Mol Imaging Biol 6(1):7-11

155. Shiozaki A, Otsuji E, Itoi H et al (2005) A case of Castleman's disease arising from the lesser omentum. Hepatogastroenterology 52(62):516-518

156. Jerusalem G, Beguin Y, Najjar F et al (2001) Positron emission tomography (PET) with 18F-fluorodeoxyglucose (18F-FDG) for the staging of low-grade non-Hodgkin's lymphoma (NHL). Ann Oncol 12(6):825-830

157. Hoffmann M, Wöhrer S, Becherer A et al (2006) 18F-Fluoro-deoxy-glucose positron emission tomography in lymphoma of mucosa-associated lymphoid tissue: histology makes the difference. Ann Oncol 17(12):1761-1765

158. Jhanwar YS, Straus DJ (2006) The role of PET in lymphoma. J Nucl Med 47(8):1326-1334

159. Bar-Shalom R, Yefremov N, Haim N et al (2003) Camera-based FDG-PET and 67Ga SPECT in evaluation of lymphoma: comparative study. Radiology 227(2):353-360

160. Yamamoto F, Tsukamoto E, Nakada K, et al (2004) 18F-FDG-PET is superior to 67Ga SPECT in the staging of non-Hodgkin's lymphoma. Ann Nucl Med 18(6):519-526

161. Friedberg JW, Fischman A, Neuberg D et al (2004) FDG-PET is superior to gallium scintigraphy in staging and more sensitive in the follow-up of patients with de novo Hodgkin lymphoma: a blinded comparison. Leuk Lymphoma 45(1):85-92

162. Kostakoglu L, Leonard JP, Kuji I et al (2002) Comparison of fluorine-18 fluorodeoxyglucose positron emission tomography and Ga-67 scintigraphy in evaluation of lymphoma. Cancer 94(4):879-888

163. Stumpe KD, Urbinelli M, Steinert HC et al (1998) Whole-body positron emission tomography using fluorodeoxyglucose for staging of lymphoma: effectiveness and comparison with computed tomography. Eur J Nucl Med 25(7):721-872

164. Jerusalem G, Beguin Y, Fassotte MF et al (2001) Whole-body positron emission tomography using 18F-fluorodeoxyglucose compared to standard procedures for staging patients with Hodgkin's disease. Haematologica 86(3):266-273

165. Munker R, Stengel A, Stäbler A et al (1995) Diagnostic accuracy of ultrasound and computed to-

mography in the staging of Hodgkin's disease. Verification by laparotomy in 100 cases. Cancer 76(8):1460-1466

166. Thill R, Neuerburg J, Fabry U et al (1997) Comparison of findings with 18-FDG-PET and CT in pretherapeutic staging of malignant lymphoma. Nuklearmedizin 36(7):234-239

167. Moog F, Bangerter M, Kotzerke J et al (1998)18-F-fluorodeoxyglucose-positron emission tomography as a new approach to detect lymphomatous bone marrow. J Clin Oncol 16(2):603-609

168. Kazama T, Swanston N, Podoloff DA, Macapinlac HA (2005) Effect of colony-stimulating factor and conventional- or high-dose chemotherapy on FDG uptake in bone marrow. Eur J Nucl Med Mol Imaging 32(12):1406-1411

169. Hong SP, Hahn JS, Lee JD et al (2003) 18F-fluorodeoxyglucose-positron emission tomography in the staging of malignant lymphoma compared with CT and 67Ga scan. Yonsei Med J 44(5):779-786

170. Schöder H, Meta J, Yap C et al (2001) Effect of whole-body (18)F-FDG-PET imaging on clinical staging and management of patients with malignant lymphoma. J Nucl Med 42(8):1139-1143

171. Munker R, Glass J, Griffeth LK et al (2004) Contribution of PET imaging to the initial staging and prognosis of patients with Hodgkin's disease. Ann Oncol 15(11):1699-1704

172. Allen-Auerbach M, Quon A, Weber WA et al (2004) Comparison between 2-deoxy-2-[18F]fluoro-D-glucose positron emission tomography and positron emission tomography/computed tomography hardware fusion for staging of patients with lymphoma. Mol Imaging Biol 6(6):411-416

173. Surbone A, Longo DL, DeVita VT Jr et al (1988) Residual abdominal masses in aggressive non-Hodgkin's lymphoma after combination chemotherapy: significance and management. J Clin Oncol 6(12):1832-1837

174. Zinzani PL, Magagnoli M, Chierichetti F et al (1999) The role of positron emission tomography (PET) in the management of lymphoma patients. Ann Oncol 10(10):1181-1184

175. Kostakoglu L, Agress H Jr, Goldsmith SJ (2003) Clinical role of FDG-PET in evaluation of cancer patients. Radiographics 23(2):315-340

176. Cremerius U, Fabry U, Kröll U et al (1999) [Clinical value of FDG-PET for therapy monitoring of malignant lymphoma-results of a retrospective study in 72 patients] Nuklearmedizin 38(1):24-30

177. Mikhaeel NG, Timothy AR, O'Doherty MJ et al (2000) 18-FDG-PET as a prognostic indicator in the treatment of aggressive Non-Hodgkin's Lymphoma-comparison with CT. Leuk Lymphoma 39(5-6):543-553

178. Zinzani PL, Fanti S, Battista G et al (2004) Predictive role of positron emission tomography (PET) in the outcome of lymphoma patients. Br J Cancer 31;91(5):850-854

179. Freudenberg LS, Antoch G, Schütt P et al (2004) FDG-PET/CT in re-staging of patients with lymphoma. Eur J Nucl Med Mol Imaging 31(3):325-329

180. Mikhaeel NG, Hutchings M, Fields PA et al (2005) FDG-PET after two to three cycles of chemotherapy predicts progression-free and overall survival in high-grade non-Hodgkin lymphoma. Ann Oncol 16(9):1514-1523

181. Hutchings M, Loft A, Hansen M et al (2006) FDG-PET after two cycles of chemotherapy predicts treatment failure and progression-free survival in Hodgkin lymphoma. Blood 107(1):52-59

182. Kostakoglu L, Goldsmith SJ, Leonard JP et al (2006) FDG-PET after 1 cycle of therapy predicts outcome in diffuse large cell lymphoma and classic Hodgkin disease.Cancer 107(11):2678-2687

183. Coleman M, Kostakoglu L (2006) Early 18F-labeled fluoro-2-deoxy-D-glucose positron emission tomography scanning in the lymphomas: changing the paradigms of treatments? Cancer 107(7):1425-1428

184. Belhocine TZ, Scott AM, Even-Sapir E et al (2006) Role of nuclear medicine in the management of cutaneous malignant melanoma. J Nucl Med 47(6):957-967

185. Pu LL, Cruse CW (1999) Lymphatic mapping and sentinel lymph node biopsy for nonmelanoma skin cancers. Surg Oncol Clin N Am 8(3):527-539

186. Gershenwald JE, Thompson W, Mansfield PF et al (1999) Multi-institutional melanoma lymphatic mapping experience: the prognostic value of sentinel lymph node status in 612 stage I or II melanoma patients. J Clin Oncol 17(3):976-983

187. Zogakis TG, Essner R, Wang HJ et al (2005) Melanoma recurrence patterns after negative sentinel lymphadenectomy. Arch Surg 140(9):865-871

188. Wagner JD, Schauwecker D, Davidson D et al (1999) Prospective study of fluorodeoxyglucose-positron emission tomography imaging of lymph node basins in melanoma patients undergoing sentinel node biopsy. J Clin Oncol 17(5):1508-1515

189. Kell MR, Ridge JA, Joseph N, Sigurdson ER (2007) PET CT imaging in patients undergoing sentinel node biopsy for melanoma. Eur J Surg Oncol 33(7):911-913

190. Wagner JD, Schauwecker DS, Davidson D et al (2001) FDG-PET sensitivity for melanoma lymph node metastases is dependent on tumor volume. J Surg Oncol 77(4):237-242

191. Crippa F, Leutner M, Belli et al (2000) Which kinds of lymph node metastases can FDG-PET detect? A clinical study in melanoma. J Nucl Med 41(9):1491-1494

192. Holder WD Jr, White RL Jr, Zuger JH et al (1998) Effectiveness of positron emission tomography for the detection of melanoma metastases. Ann Surg 227(5):764-769; discussion 769-771

193. Rinne D, Baum RP, Hör G, Kaufmann R (1998) Primary staging and follow-up of high risk melanoma patients with whole-body 18F-fluorodeoxyglucose positron emission tomography: results of a prospective study of 100 patients. Cancer 82(9):1664-1671

194. Yancovitz M, Finelt N, Warycha MA et al (2007) Role of radiologic imaging at the time of initial diagnosis of stage T1b-T3b melanoma. Cancer 110(5):1107-1114

195. Iagaru A, Quon A, Johnson D et al (2007) 2-Deoxy-2-[F-18]fluoro-D-glucose positron emission tomography/computed tomography in the management of melanoma. Mol Imaging Biol 9(1):50-57

196. Schwimmer J, Essner R, Patel A et al (2000) A review of the literature for whole-body FDG-PET in the management of patients with melanoma. Q J Nucl Med 44(2):153-167

197. Reinhardt MJ, Joe AY, Jaeger U et al (2006) Diagnostic performance of whole body dual modality 18F-FDG-PET/CT imaging for N- and M-staging of malignant melanoma: experience with 250 consecutive patients. J Clin Oncol 24(7):1178-1187

198. Mottaghy FM, Sunderkötter C, Schubert R et al (2007) Direct comparison of [18F]FDG-PET/CT with PET alone and with side-by-side PET and CT

in patients with malignant melanoma. Eur J Nucl Med Mol Imaging 34(9):1355-1364

199. Kamel EM, Thumshirn M, Truninger K et al (2004) Significance of incidental 18F-FDG accumulations in the gastrointestinal tract in PET/CT: correlation with endoscopic and histopathologic results. J Nucl Med 45(11):1804-1810

200. Rehani B, Strohmeyer P, Jacobs M, Mantil J (2006) Gallbladder metastasis from malignant melanoma: diagnosis with FDG-PET/CT. Clin Nucl Med 31(12):812-813

201. Weng LJ, Schöder H (2004) Melanoma metastasis to the testis demonstrated with FDG-PET/CT. Clin Nucl Med 29(12):811-812

202. Pfannenberg C, Aschoff P, Schanz S et al (2007) Prospective comparison of 18F-fluorodeoxyglucose positron emission tomography/computed tomography and whole-body magnetic resonance imaging in staging of advanced malignant melanoma. Eur J Cancer 43(3):557-564

203. Falk MS, Truitt AK, Coakley FV et al (2007) Interpretation, accuracy and management implications of FDG-PET/CT in cutaneous malignant melanoma. Nucl Med Commun 28(4):273-280

204. Lerman H, Metser U, Grisaru D et al (2004) Normal and abnormal 18F-FDG endometrial and ovarian uptake in pre- and postmenopausal patients: assessment by PET/CT. J Nucl Med 45(2):266-271

205. Pandit-Taskar N (2005) Oncologic imaging in gynecologic malignancies. J Nucl Med 46(11):1842-1850

206. Subhas N, Patel PV, Pannu HK et al (2005) Imaging of pelvic malignancies with in-line FDG-PET-CT: case examples and common pitfalls of FDG-PET. Radiographics 25(4):1031-1043

207. Lai CH, Yen TC, Chang TC (2007) Positron emission tomography imaging for gynecologic malignancy. Curr Opin Obstet Gynecol 19(1):37-41

208. Yen TC, Lai CH (2006) Positron emission tomography in gynecologic cancer. Semin Nucl Med 36(1):93-104

209. Wong TZ, Jones EL, Coleman RE (2004) Positron emission tomography with 2-deoxy-2-[(18)F]fluoro-D-glucose for evaluating local and distant disease in patients with cervical cancer. Mol Imaging Biol 6(1):55-62

210. Loft A, Berthelsen AK, Roed H et al (2007) The diagnostic value of PET/CT scanning in patients with cervical cancer: a prospective study. Gynecol Oncol 106(1):29-34

211. Havrilesky LJ, Kulasingam SL, Matchar DB, Myers ER (2005) FDG-PET for management of cervical and ovarian cancer. Gynecol Oncol 97(1):183-191

212. Ryu SY, Kim MH, Choi SC et al (2003) Detection of early recurrence with 18F-FDG-PET in patients with cervical cancer. J Nucl Med 44(3):347-352

213. Chung HH, Jo H, Kang WJ et al (2007) Clinical impact of integrated PET/CT on the management of suspected cervical cancer recurrence. Gynecol Oncol 104(3):529-534

214. Choi HJ, Roh JW, Seo SS et al (2006) Comparison of the accuracy of magnetic resonance imaging and positron emission tomography/computed tomography in the presurgical detection of lymph node metastases in patients with uterine cervical carcinoma: a prospective study. Cancer 106(4):914-922

215. Esthappan J, Mutic S, Malyapa RS et al (2004) Treatment planning guidelines regarding the use of CT/PET-guided IMRT for cervical carcinoma with positive paraaortic lymph nodes. Int J Radiat Oncol Biol Phys 58(4):1289-1297

216. Singh AK, Grigsby PW, Dehdashti F et al (2003) FDG-PET lymph node staging and survival of patients with FIGO stage IIIb cervical carcinoma. Int J Radiat Oncol Biol Phys 56(2):489-493

217. Grigsby PW, Siegel BA, Dehdashti F et al (2004) Posttherapy [18F] fluorodeoxyglucose positron emission tomography in carcinoma of the cervix: response and outcome. J Clin Oncol 22(11):2167-2171

218. Yoshida Y, Kurokawa T, Kawahara K et al (2004) Incremental benefits of FDG positron emission tomography over CT alone for the preoperative staging of ovarian cancer. AJR Am J Roentgenol 182(1):227-233

219. Yen RF, Sun SS, Shen YY et al (2001) Whole body positron emission tomography with 18F-fluoro-2-deoxyglucose for the detection of recurrent ovarian cancer. Anticancer Res 21(5):3691-3694

220. Bristow RE, del Carmen MG, Pannu HK et al (2003) Clinically occult recurrent ovarian cancer: patient selection for secondary cytoreductive surgery using combined PET/CT. Gynecol Oncol 90(3):519-528

221. Pannu HK, Cohade C, Bristow RE et al (2004) PET-CT detection of abdominal recurrence of ovarian cancer: radiologic-surgical correlation. Abdom Imaging 29(3):398-403

222. Bristow RE, Giuntoli RL 2nd, Pannu HK et al (2005) Combined PET/CT for detecting recurrent ovarian cancer limited to retroperitoneal lymph nodes. Gynecol Oncol 99(2):294-300

223. Smith GT, Hubner KF, McDonald T, Thie JA (1999) Cost Analysis of FDG-PET for Managing Patients with Ovarian Cancer. Clin Positron Imaging 2(2):63-70

224. Suzuki R, Miyagi E, Takahashi N et al (2007) Validity of positron emission tomography using fluoro-2-deoxyglucose for the preoperative evaluation of endometrial cancer. Int J Gynecol Cancer 17(4):890-896

225. Belhocine T, De Barsy C, Hustinx R, Willems-Foidart J (2003) Usefulness of (18)F-FDG-PET in the post-therapy surveillance of endometrial carcinoma. Eur J Nucl Med Mol Imaging. 2002 Sep 29(9):1132-1139

226. Saga T, Higashi T, Ishimori T, Mamede M, Nakamoto Y, Mukai T, Fujita T, Togashi K, Yura S, Higuchi T, Kita M, Fujii S, Konishi J. Clinical value of FDG-PET in the follow up of post-operative patients with endometrial cancer. Ann Nucl Med 17(3):197-203

227. Rebollo-Aguirre AC, Ramos-Font C, Gallego Peinado M et al (2006) [Positron emission tomography with fluordesoxyglucose-F18 in follow-up of endometrial cancer]. Rev Esp Med Nucl 25(6):359-366

228. Chao A, Chang TC, Ng KK et al (2006) 18F-FDG-PET in the management of endometrial cancer. Eur J Nucl Med Mol Imaging 33(1):36-44

229. Sironi S, Picchio M, Landoni C et al (2007) Posttherapy surveillance of patients with uterine cancers: value of integrated FDG-PET/CT in the detection of recurrence. Eur J Nucl Med Mol Imaging 34(4):472-479

230. Hofer C, Laubenbacher C, Block T et al (1999) Fluorine-18-fluorodeoxyglucose positron emission tomography is useless for the detection of local recurrence after radical prostatectomy. Eur Urol 36(1):31-35

231. Liu IJ, Zafar MB, Lai YH et al (2001) Fluorodeoxyglucose positron emission tomography

studies in diagnosis and staging of clinically organ-confined prostate cancer. Urology 57(1):108-111

232. Shreve PD, Grossman HB, Gross MD, Wahl RL (1996) Metastatic prostate cancer: initial findings of PET with 2-deoxy-2-[F-18]fluoro-D-glucose. Radiology 199(3):751-756

233. Schöder H, Herrmann K, Gönen M et al (2005) 2-[18F]fluoro-2-deoxyglucose positron emission tomography for the detection of disease in patients with prostate-specific antigen relapse after radical prostatectomy. Clin Cancer Res 11(13):4761-4769

234. Oyama N, Akino H, Kanamaru H et al (2002) 11C-acetate PET imaging of prostate cancer. J Nucl Med 43(2):181-186

235. Oyama N, Miller TR, Dehdashti F et al (2003) 11C-acetate PET imaging of prostate cancer: detection of recurrent disease at PSA relapse. J Nucl Med 44(4):549-555

236. Hara T, Kosaka N, Kishi H (1998) PET imaging of prostate cancer using carbon-11-choline. J Nucl Med 39(6):990-995

237. Reske SN, Blumstein NM, Neumaier B et al (2006) Imaging prostate cancer with 11C-choline PET/CT. J Nucl Med 47(8):1249-1254

238. Cimitan M, Bortolus R, Morassut S et al (2006)[(18)F]fluorocholine PET/CT imaging for the detection of recurrent prostate cancer at PSA relapse: experience in 100 consecutive patients. Eur J Nucl Med Mol Imaging 33(12):1387-1398

239. Jana S, Blaufox MD (2006) Nuclear medicine studies of the prostate, testes, and bladder. Semin Nucl Med 36(1):51-72

240. Testa C, Schiavina R, Lodi R et al (2007) Prostate cancer: sextant localization with MR imaging, MR spectroscopy, and 11C-choline PET/CT. Radiology 244(3):797-806

MDCT of the Cardiovascular System

16

Imaging Protocols for Cardiac CT

Frank J. Rybicki, Tarang Sheth

The incorporation of multiple detectors into spiral computed tomography (CT) scanners has expanded the clinical role of CT in cardiac imaging, including coronary CT angiography (CTA). Advances in both the speed at which the X-ray source rotates and the number of detectors have improved the ability of CT to resolve smaller anatomic detail and have enabled imaging of the native coronary arterial tree. At present, and for at least the near future, CT is the most robust modality to noninvasively image the coronary arteries. CTA contributes largely to cardiovascular diagnoses, but one of the most important and one of the most promising contributions is its high negative predictive value for coronary artery disease (CAD). That is, using the protocol detailed in this chapter, CAD can be reliably excluded in minutes without arterial catheterization. Moreover, in a single CT acquisition, native coronary imaging can be extended to include the beating myocardium, valve motion, ventricular outflow tracks, and coronary bypass grafts. In this chapter, in addition to detailing a basic cardiac imaging protocol, examples of examinations are illustrated.

Introduction

Protocols for electrocardiogram (ECG)-gated cardiac CT have evolved with rapid improvement in technology. The technique has progressed from early cardiac CT (4-slice multidetector CT [MDCT] with 1-s gantry rotation) to current standards (ECG-gated 64-slice MDCT with gantry rotation times as low as 330 ms). Technology has developed at a rapid rate, fueled primarily by the promise of a robust, noninvasive method of performing diagnostic coronary angiography (Fig. 1). Additional MDCT imaging includes coronary bypass grafts and evaluation of cardiac valves. This chapter fo-

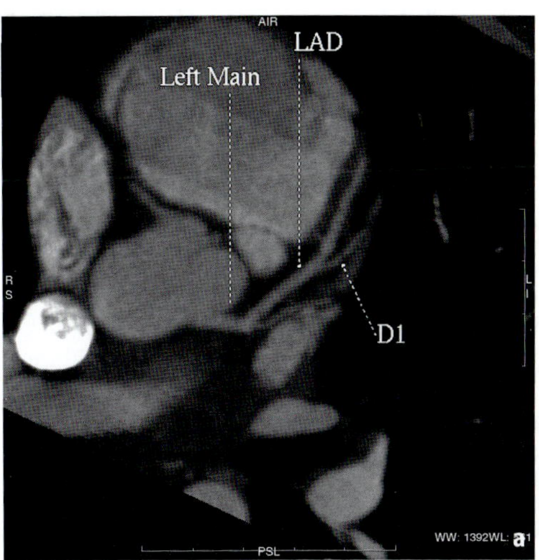

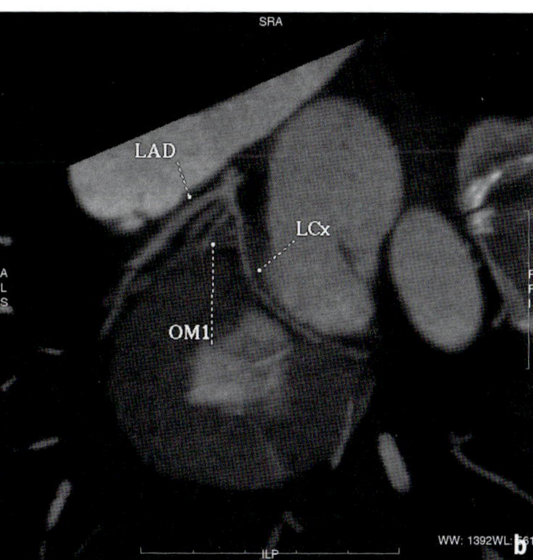

Fig. 1a, b. Multiplanar reformatted CTA images demonstrate the major branches of the left coronary arterial system. This patient presented with atypical chest pain, and coronary artery disease was excluded noninvasively

cuses on the coronary CTA protocol and also describes how the basic protocol can be modified or extended for problem solving.

Temporal Resolution

Successful cardiac imaging by any modality relies on the ability of the technology to produce motion free images or to scan faster than the heart beats. Thus, cardiac CT is founded on (1) imaging faster than the heart beats, or (2) slowing cardiac motion. *Temporal resolution* is the metric that measures imaging speed. For a CT scanner with a single photon source, the temporal resolution is one half of the CT gantry rotation time. This is because image reconstruction requires CT data acquired from one half (180°) of a complete gantry rotation. At the time of publication, all manufacturers have gantry rotation times less than 500 ms, with a minimum of 330 ms. With a 330-ms gantry rotation, an ECG-gated cardiac image can be reconstructed (using single-segment reconstruction described below) with CT data acquired over 165 ms of the cardiac cycle. Thus, the reconstructed images display the average of the cardiac motion over the 165 ms during which the data was acquired. This is how ECG gating enables coronary CTA. Without gating, cardiac images are nondiagnostic because the reconstruction "averages" the motion over the entire RR interval – 1,000 ms for a patient with a heart rate of 60 beats per minute.

Temporal resolution can be improved in single-source scanners by adopting a so-called "multisegment" image reconstruction. The principle underlying multisegment reconstruction is that the acquisition over several heart beats is summed to obtain the one half gantry (i.e., 180°) CT data. For example, in a two-segment reconstruction, two heart beats are used to generate a single axial slice, and thus the temporal resolution is halved. Similarly, if four heat beats are used (four segment reconstruction), only 45° of data are used from each heart beat. This would yield a four-fold reduction in the temporal resolution. Since multiple heart beats are used to fill the 180° of gantry rotation necessary for the reconstruction, stable periodicity of the heart is essential. Moreover, multisegment reconstruction requires a lower CT pitch, resulting in greater data oversampling and a higher radiation dose. Radiation considerations and a simple formula to estimate effective patient dose are given in an upcoming section.

A recent approach to improving temporal resolution involves the use of two independent sources and two independent (64-slice) detector systems (Siemens Definition; Siemens Medical Solutions, Erlangen, Germany). The second X-ray source is positioned 90° from the first X-ray source, and the second detection system is positioned 90° from the first detection system. With respect to temporal resolution, the practical consequence of this CT configuration is that 180° of gantry rotation can be achieved in half the time (e.g., 82.5 ms as opposed to 165 ms). This improvement in the temporal resolution is expected to eliminate the need for multisegment reconstruction. In fact, in patients with a higher heart rate or a heart rate that is difficult to control with beta blockade (described below), the CT pitch can be increased without compromising image quality.

Beta Blockade for Heart-Rate Control

As suggested from the discussion on temporal resolution, beta blockade is an important component of most cardiac CT examinations. A useful rule of thumb for the target heart rate is "the first number is a 5" – i.e., an ideal heart rate between 50 and 59 beats per minute. While this goal is not achieved in every patient, it provides a useful reference frame. IV metoprolol is routinely administered at our institution; with cardiac monitoring, 5-mg increments are given every 5 min up to a total dose of 25 mg. Doses greater than 15 mg are rarely needed. Beta blockade can be safely performed by a radiologist or a cardiologist. An alternative approach involves the use of oral beta blockade. Although this approach has the disadvantage of a longer serum half life, most patients arrive for the study with a heart rate already in the target range. This can simplify patient preparation on site and has the potential to increase patient throughput. The tradeoff is the extra step of premedicating the patient and issues surrounding patient compliance.

In theory, using the multisegment reconstruction approach described above, beta blockade can often be avoided because using multiple heart beats in the reconstruction enables the scanner to have an effective temporal resolution in the range of 40–50 ms. However, when multisegment reconstruction is used, image quality becomes highly dependent on cardiac beat-to-beat variability. In our experience, multisegment reconstruction works well in patients with high heart rates who are being studied for clinical indications where the highest image quality may not be required, for example, coronary bypass graft location and patency. For coronary CT angiography, beta blockade is still recommended.

ECG Gating

ECG gating refers to the simultaneous acquisition of both the patient's ECG tracing and CT data

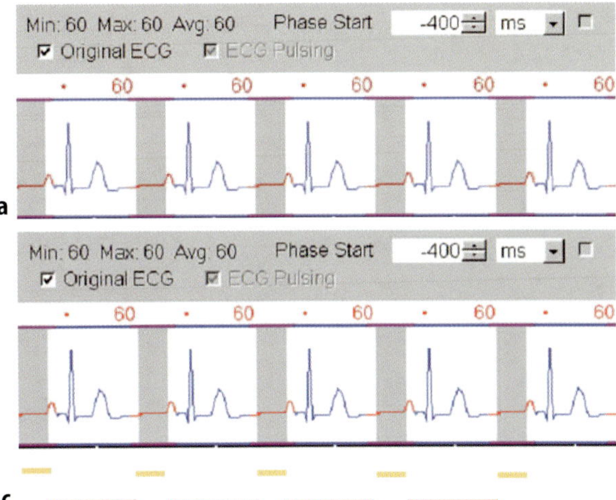

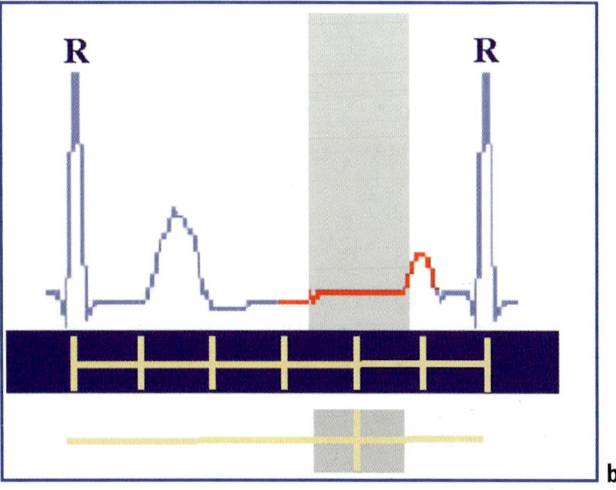

Fig. 2a-c. a Electrocardiogram (ECG) gating as demonstrated on a Somatom Sensation 64 cardiac computed tomography (CT) scanner (Siemens Medical Solutions, Erlangen, Germany). Continuous ECG tracing is displayed on the console. In this case, minimum, maximum, and average heart rate is 60 beats per minute (*top left*). Thus, the width of the RR interval is 1,000 ms. The *gray vertical bars* indicate that portion of the cardiac cycle used in the reconstruction. As discussed in the text, the width of the gray bar is the temporal resolution of the scan. For this single-segment reconstruction, the width is half the gantry rotation time, or 165 ms. The term "–400 ms" refers to the fact that the center of the gray bars is located 400 ms before the second of the two R waves in the RR interval. **b** Enlarged view of a single RR interval. To provide a simple demonstration of how the RR interval is divided, six segments are illustrated. In clinical imaging, CT scanners divide the RR interval into a number of segments between 10 and 20. The gray block at the very bottom emphasizes that each reconstructed image uses only a small portion of the cardiac cycle. The gray block is positioned in diastole; its center is approximately 65% between the R waves, i.e., 650 ms elapse between the first R wave and the center of the block. This reconstruction is the most commonly used to visualize the left coronary arterial system. If this reconstruction does not provide the most optimal images, additional reconstructions, either earlier or later phases, are performed. Since the right and left coronary arterial system are asynchronous, it is sometimes the case that evaluation of the right system is best performed using images closer to systole. **c** ECG-based tube current modulation or ECG pulsing. The ECG tracing is identical to the one illustrated in **a**. *Yellow bars* under the tracing correspond to the gray bars and correlate with where, with current modulation, the optimal tube current (e.g., effective mAs = 650) will be used. *Red lines* show times that correspond to portions of the cardiac cycle where the X-ray CT tube current is minimized. ECG pulsing can reduce patient effective radiation dose by 30–50%

(Fig. 2a, b). By acquiring both pieces of information, CT images can be reconstructed using only a short temporal segment periodically located in the same location of the RR interval over multiple cardiac cycles. The duration of the temporal segment is equal to the temporal resolution of the scanner. Each temporal segment of the RR interval is named by its "phase" in the cardiac cycle; the most commonly used nomenclature is to name the percentage of a specific phase with respect to its position in the RR interval. For example, if a manufacturer enables reconstruction of 20 (equally spaced) phases, they would typically be named 0%, 5%, 10% … 95%, beginning with one R wave and ending with the following R wave. The period in which the heart has the least motion is usually (but not always) in mid diastole, near a phase between 55% and 75%. Thus, under the assumption that the position of the heart remains consistent over the RR intervals during which CT data is acquired, cardiac motion is minimized by producing images from the same phase over multiple cardiac cycles. This explains why ECG gating typically fails to freeze cardiac motion in patients with an irregular rhythm, such as atrial fibrillation. Consequently, atrial fibrillation patients rarely have diagnostic cardiac CT examinations, and it is our policy to not perform coronary CTA in this population.

If only static (as opposed to cine) images are desired, image reconstruction can usually be performed over a small number of phases for which motion is minimized. (This is in contrast to cine imaging where images are reconstructed in all parts of the cardiac cycle and then played, in cine mode, to demonstrate cardiac motion.) The image reconstruction phases used for interpretation must account for differences in movement of the left and right coronary arterial systems. Because coronary arterial motion is not synchronous, the phase of the cardiac cycle that proves best for diagnosis of the left main and left anterior descending artery is often different than the phase that proves most diagnostic for the right coronary artery. Moreover, it is often necessary to view more than one phase to best assess the full extent of an individual artery and its branches (e.g., the left anterior descending and the diagonal branches).

The most complete cardiac CT examinations include cine imaging. In cine cardiac CT, images are reconstructed in periodic phases throughout the cardiac cycle to yield information regarding a

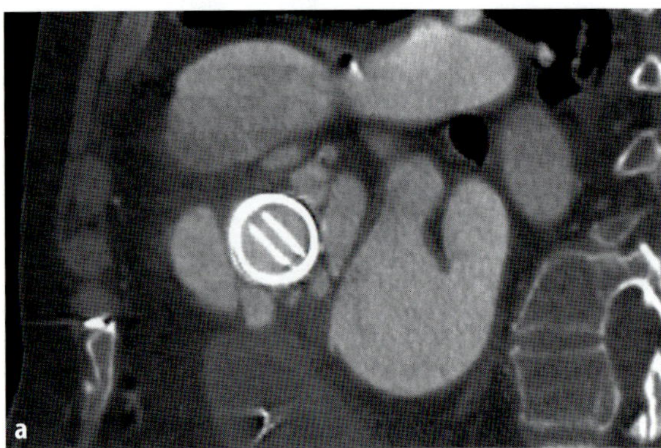
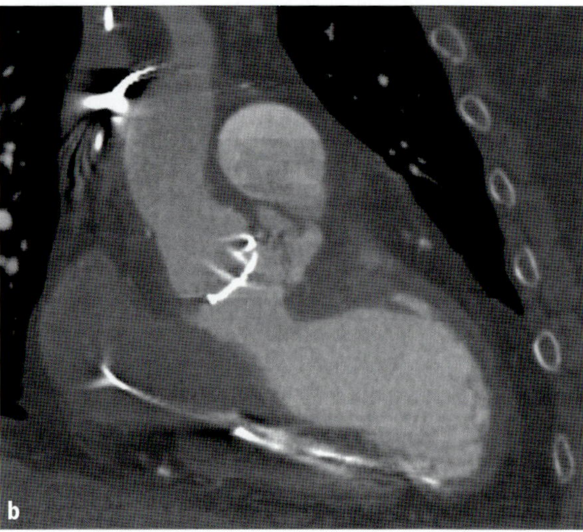

Fig. 3a, b. Reformatted ECG-gated cardiac CT images in a patient status post aortic valve replacement. Note that the patient has a pacemaker (noted by the right heart wires in 3b), and thus magnetic resonance imaging (MRI) was contraindicated. **a** Image through the mechanical valve while it is open demonstrates multiple surrounding collections of contrast, characteristic of pseudoaneurysm. **b** Orthogonal view again demonstrates abnormal contrast to the right of the valve. This patient required emergent surgery with successful placement of a new valve. Images courtesy of Scott Koss, MD

moving structure. For example, cardiac CT offers an outstanding assessment of the aortic valve and aortic root (Fig. 3). In addition to the fact that cine imaging can be used to assess valve motion, CT is by far the best imaging modality to identify and quantify calcification, and thus both structure and function can be well characterized in a single breath-hold CT acquisition. Cine CT can also be used to assess ventricular-wall motion. In comparison with cardiac magnetic resonance (MR), the gold standard for global and regional-wall motion abnormalities, CT has less contrast to noise, and images typically have greater artifact owing to poorer temporal resolution. However, it is important to emphasize that cine CT is not a separate image acquisition. The entire CT data set (coronary, valve, myocardium, pericardium) is acquired in a single breath hold; cine CT is simply part of the image postprocessing. It is also important to note that the most common contraindications for cardiac CT (e.g., impaired renal function as measured by glomerular filtration rate or alternatively by serum creatinine) differ from those for MR (pacemaker), and thus CT can often be used for patients who cannot have MR.

Finally, it is important to note that future CT equipment with up to 256 slices is expected to perform whole-heart coverage with a single half-gantry (180°) rotation. This approach holds the promise of a subsecond cardiac scan. In addition to the fact that patient radiation would be decreased, this would provide the ability to perform multiple scans over the same injection of iodinated contrast material and thus create the opportunity for a host of additional studies (e.g., myocardial perfusion) that are, at present, largely in the domain of cardiac MR and nuclear cardiology.

Patient Irradiation

In some cardiac CT applications, for example, the location and patency of bypass grafts (Figs. 4 and 5), all diagnostic information can typically be obtained from reconstruction of only a single phase of the cardiac cycle in mid diastole. However, as emphasized above, in cardiac CT, image data is acquired throughout the cardiac cycle. Thus, for studies such as bypass graft analyses, the CT data (and the radiation used to acquire that data) in the remaining "unused" phases is wasted.

Because cardiac CT requires ECG gating with a CT pitch less than 1, the patient radiation in cardiac CT is higher than that for CT of any other body part. While dose should be a consideration for all patients undergoing CT, it is essential that discussions regarding CT dose are based on sound principles. The risk most commonly cited as a cause for concern is the development of a fatal radiation-induced neoplasm. While sparse, all human data and anecdotal reports to date support a latency period of no less than 20 years for a radiation-induced neoplasm. For this reason, for the purpose of radiation dose, it is important to sepa-

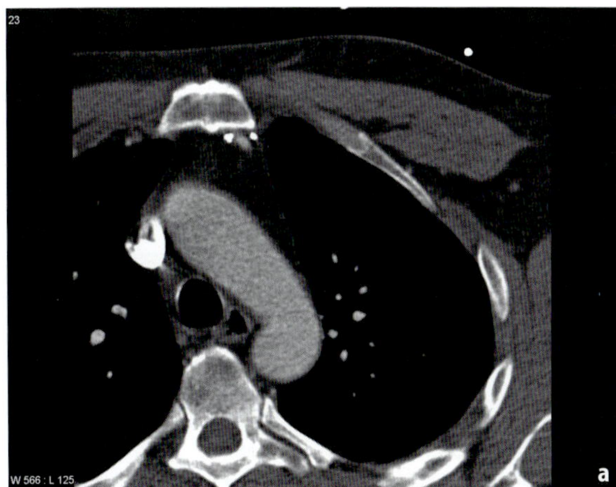

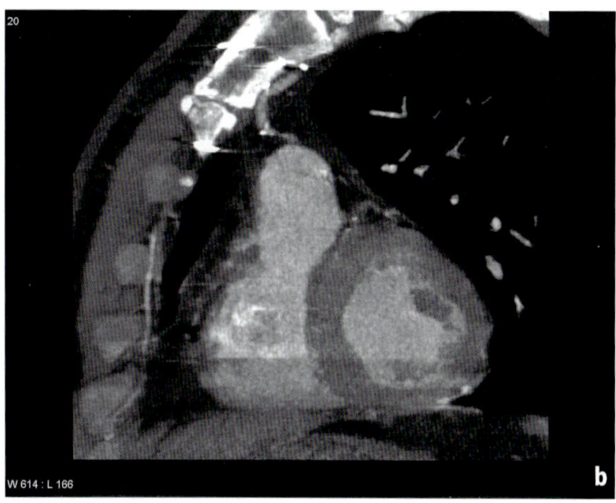

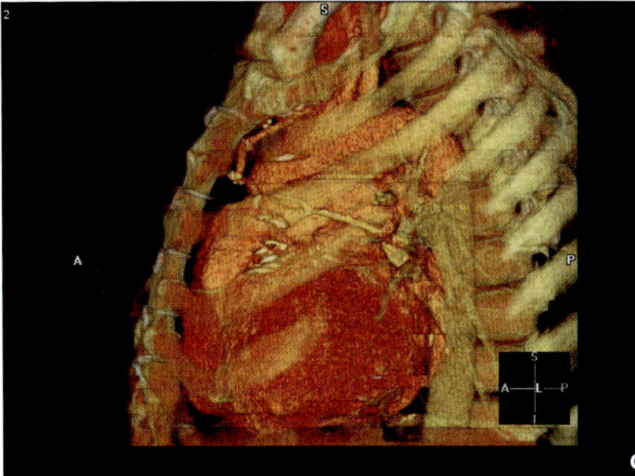

Fig. 4a-c. ECG-gated CT images from a patient status post left internal mammary artery to left anterior descending artery coronary bypass grafting. This patient was scheduled for a repeat bypass graft. CTA with reformatting is now performed routinely to detect cases such as this one where the graft becomes adherent to the posterior table of the sternum. **a** Axial image demonstrates proximity of the internal mammary to the sternum. **b** Sagittal and obliquely reformatted images are essential in the evaluation of these patients. In this case, the graft is demonstrated to be patent and too close to the sternum for a repeat thoracotomy through the sternal incision; an alternate surgical approach was required for this patient. **c** Selected image from a three-dimensional (3-D) volume rendering again demonstrates the course of the graft. Volume rendering is often more appealing to our referring clinicians and can help in the communication of important findings

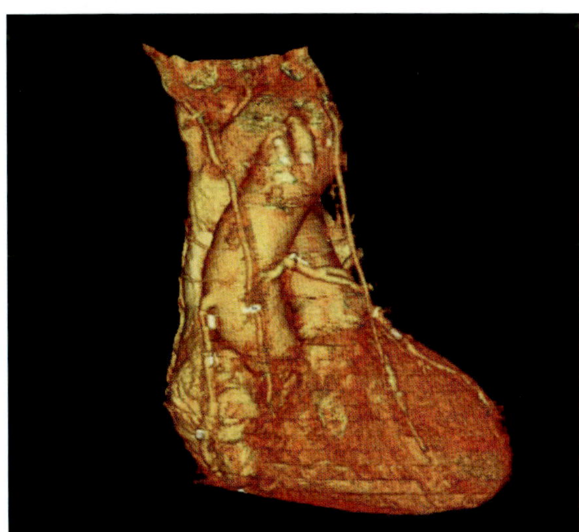

Fig. 5. 3-D volume-rendered image from a patient with normal internal mammary arteries who had undergone saphenous vein coronary bypass grafting. Note that the left-sided vein graft is bifurcated. The vein graft to the right coronary territory is single. In a patient with only saphenous vein grafts, it is essential to image the entire course of the internal mammary arteries since, when normal, they will be used for redo coronary artery bypass

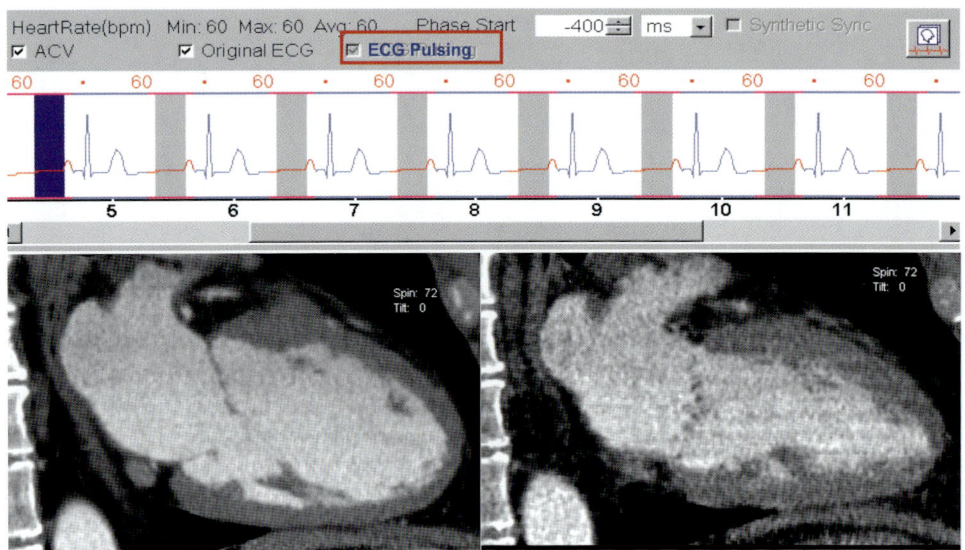

Fig. 6. ECG-based tube current modulation, or ECG pulsing. The *top* demonstrates how the operator selects current modulation from the console of the Somatom Sensation 64 cardiac computed tomography (CT) scanner (Siemens Medical Solutions, Erlangen, Germany). The image on the *left* is a two-chamber view (note the normal mitral valve that is well demonstrated with ECG gating) that is reconstructed at 65% of the RR interval. The *right-hand*, two-chamber view was reconstructed from 10% of the RR interval, where the X-ray CT tube current was dramatically reduced. Subsequently, this image suffers from high noise, the consequence of fewer photons received at the detector

rate patients into two groups: those with a life expectancy of roughly 20 years or less, and those with a longer life expectancy. In the former group, the only dose consideration of any consequence is the radiation that could cause a skin burn (the only short-term complication of any consequence). X-ray skin burns are extremely uncommon, particularly in CT (even for ECG-gated studies), and would be the consequence of multiple exams repeated at short-term intervals. Thus, for this subset of patients, radiation dose should be a lesser consideration in determining a modality for coronary imaging.

For patients with a life expectancy much greater than 20 years, ECG-based tube current modulation (also called ECG pulsing) represents one strategy to lower overall patient radiation by modulating the tube current over the course of the cardiac cycle (Fig. 2c) so that the desired diagnostic tube current is delivered in diastole while the current is reduced for the remainder of the cardiac cycle.

Current modulation is featured on newer CT scanners and is important in many cases (e.g., pediatric patients). However, the decision to incorporate current modulation should be made carefully since the potential drawbacks are significant. First, once current modulation is used, images subsequently reconstructed during phases with low tube current will be noisy (Fig. 6). That is, reducing the tube current results in the production of fewer X-

rays, and subsequently fewer X-rays pass though the patient and reach the detection system. Second, current modulation eliminates the potential to reconstruct high-quality cine imaging since every phase of the cardiac cycle will not have the "full" tube current. Thus, if cine imaging is desired, current modulation cannot be utilized. Another potential drawback concerns the identification of incidental findings (e.g., bicuspid aortic valve) on static imaging acquired with current modulation. In these cases, it is impossible to perform postprocessing of a high-signal cine loop for a more complete evaluation.

While cine cardiac CT can provide a useful adjunct to high spatial resolution anatomic data, CT has poor temporal resolution and ventricular image contrast when compared with steady-state free precession (SSFP) cardiac MR (CMR). For this reason, SSFP cine CMR remains the gold standard to assess cardiac function and to evaluate cardiac masses. However, CT is far more accessible, it is easier to perform, and a cardiac pacemaker is not a contraindication. Moreover, there are many cardiac masses that can be well or better seen on CT (Fig. 7). Hence, CT has become not only an adjunct to cardiac MR but in some cases the diagnostic test of choice (Fig. 8).

Since patient dose in CT is so frequently discussed and has great potential to be misquoted, the fundamentals of CT dose, including the dose from cardiac CT, are described here. There are

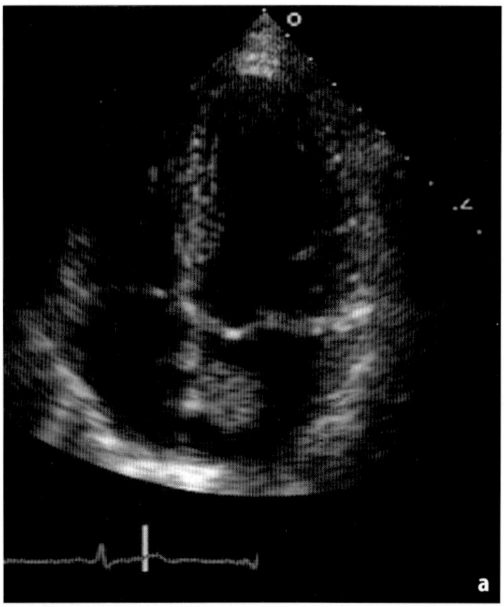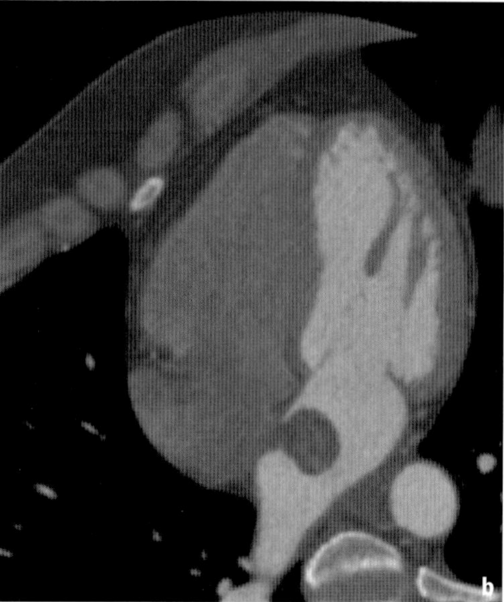

Fig. 7a, b. Left atrial myxoma. **a** Four-chamber echocardiogram demonstrates the round lesion adjacent to the intra-atrial septum. **b** ECG-gated CT shows the mass with higher spatial resolution, well depicting the attachment point of the mass with the intra-atrial septum. Note that the left heart is well opacified with contrast material and the right heart is filled with saline. This is the goal in the timing of the dual injection protocol (contrast followed by saline)

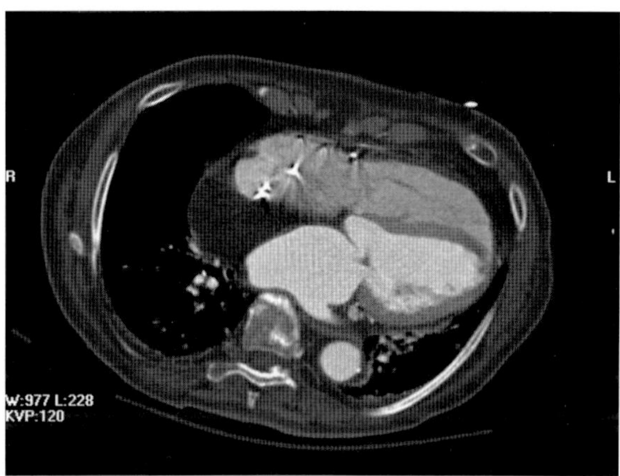

Fig. 8. Axial ECG-gated four-chamber image in a patient with a pacemaker. The patient has a history of renal cell carcinoma, and echocardiography demonstrated an ill-defined echogenic mass. This image from the single 12-s CT acquisition excludes a metastatic deposit as the source of the finding on ultrasound. Fat splays the left and right atria, diagnostic of lipomatous hypertrophy of the intra-atrial septum. CT is the most rapid and accurate imaging modality to demonstrate both fat and calcium

three different parameters used to describe, quantify, and calculate the dose:

1. CT dose index (CTDIvol) [1]. CTDIvol units are milligray (mGy) [3].
2. Dose-length product (DLP) [2]. Units of DLP are mGy × centimeters.
3. Effective dose [3]. Units of effective dose are milliSievert (mSv).

The numerical value for CTDI is determined by measuring dose in a cylindrical phantom. Although the phantom should somehow reflect the attenuation of a human body, the CTDI is not used to make a statement regarding an individual patient's dose. Rather, it is used to compare different scan protocols, optimize scan protocols, and compare protocols used on different CT scanners. In contrast to parameters such as tube current, CTDI values reflect delivered dose since parameters, such as scanner geometry and filtration, are considered.

CTDIvol describes dose for a single rotation. DLP characterizes CT exposure over a complete field of view (FOV); DLP is defined as the product of the CTDIvol and the craniocaudal extent (Z-axis length) of the scan. Even though DLP reflects most closely radiation dose for a specific CT examination, it is important to keep in mind that DLP is a function of patient size (i.e., how much Z-axis coverage is required to complete the CT scan). Therefore, CTDIvol should be used to optimize exam protocols.

While CTDIvol and DLP enable evaluation of

CT scanners and comparison of protocols across manufacturers, these values only characterize the scanner. It is the effective dose, a weighted sum over the organ doses [4], that quantifies patient dose. Since the dose to an individual organ cannot be measured directly, it is difficult to determine the effective dose of a CT scan. However, methods have been described to estimate effective dose from measurable values [5–8]. A simple estimation is that the effective dose is the product of DLP and a conversion factor, E_{DLP} that is specific to a body region. For example, for the chest, the $E_{DLP} = 0.017$ mSv $\times$ mGy$^{-1} \times$ cm^{-1} [2].

As an example of a how this is used in clinical practice, consider the following hypothetical coronary CTA. The user console will give the CTDIvol. A typical value for a high-dose scan without current modulation would be on the order of 60 mGy. Assume that the craniocaudal extent of the scan is 15 cm, a typical value for a normal-sized heart. For this study, the DLP $= 60$ mGy$\times$15 cm $= 900$ mGy$\times$cm. Given that the heart is in the chest, the appropriate conversion factor is $E_{DLP} = 0.017$ mSv$\times$mGy$^{-1}\times$cm^{-1}, and the effective dose for this patient is 60 mGy$\times$15 cm x 0.017 mSv$\times$mGy^{-1} $\times$cm^{-1} ~ 15 mSv. Note that, as discussed above, dose values in gated exams can be reduced with "ECG pulsing". The degree of reduction is a function of the patient's heart rate but is typically 30–50%.

Image Acquisition Time

Improved temporal resolution decreases the time of the CT examination. This is important not only for decreasing the effect of cardiac motion but also for completing the examination in a breath hold. Scan time becomes a factor for cardiac and ascending aorta imaging because of the required ECG gating. The image data must be "oversampled" since, for the reconstruction of each interval, only a small portion of the cardiac cycle is used. Data oversampling for cardiovascular applications differentiates it from all other MDCT scans that can capitalize on undersampling and interpolation in image reconstruction to dramatically decrease scan time.

CT pitch (a unitless parameter) is most accurately characterized as the distance the patient moves through the scanner in a single gantry rotation divided by the width of the X-ray beam used. Because such a small part of the RR interval is used to reconstruct an entire image, significant overlap along the craniocaudal extent of the patient is required, translating into a pitch between 0.2 and 0.35, or an oversampling rate between 5:1 and roughly 3:1. In addition to cardiac imaging, ECG gating is routinely required for CTA of the ascending aorta to eliminate artifacts from aortic motion that can be confused with pathology.

The practical consequence of oversampling is that scan time (craniocaudal imaging over approximately 15 cm) is far greater than nongated scanning of the same Z-axis region of any other body part. This is one great benefit of scanners equipped with a larger number of detectors, which allow coverage of a larger craniocaudal territory per rotation. In the extreme case, craniocaudal coverage can be large enough that the entire heart is covered in a single rotation. The number of detectors and focal spots determines the number of slices obtained per gantry rotation. That is, 64-slice coronary CTA (Figs. 9 and 10) can be achieved with 32 detectors and a dual focal spot or 64 detectors and a single focal spot. The important factors are temporal resolution (determined by gantry rotation time), slice thickness, and quality of the X-ray CT tube.

Increasing either number of slices, thickness of detectors, or both increases "Z-axis coverage" per rotation and thus decreases scan time. For example, for coverage of the heart, a 4-slice scanner may require a 35-s breath hold while a 64-slice acquisition (performed with the same gantry rotation time and detector width) on the same patient may require only 15 s.

While thicker detectors decrease scan time by providing more Z-axis coverage per rotation, increasing detector width for cardiac applications is undesirable since it degrades the *spatial resolution* of the examination. In general, spatial resolution refers to the ability to differentiate two structures. In practical terms, spatial resolution refers to the thinnest axial slices that can be reconstructed from configuration of the detectors. The CT industry, driven by the promise (and the competition) of selling scanners to noninvasively image coronary arteries, has dramatically improved spatial resolution by producing detection systems that can reconstruct submillimeter images. Thinner slices (higher spatial resolution) correspond to longer scan times; however, all imaging applications do not require the highest spatial resolution. For example, myocardial and ascending aortic imaging rarely requires submillimeter slices. In particular, when a patient is expected to have difficulty with breath holding, imaging should be performed with thicker slices to maximize the diagnostic information available.

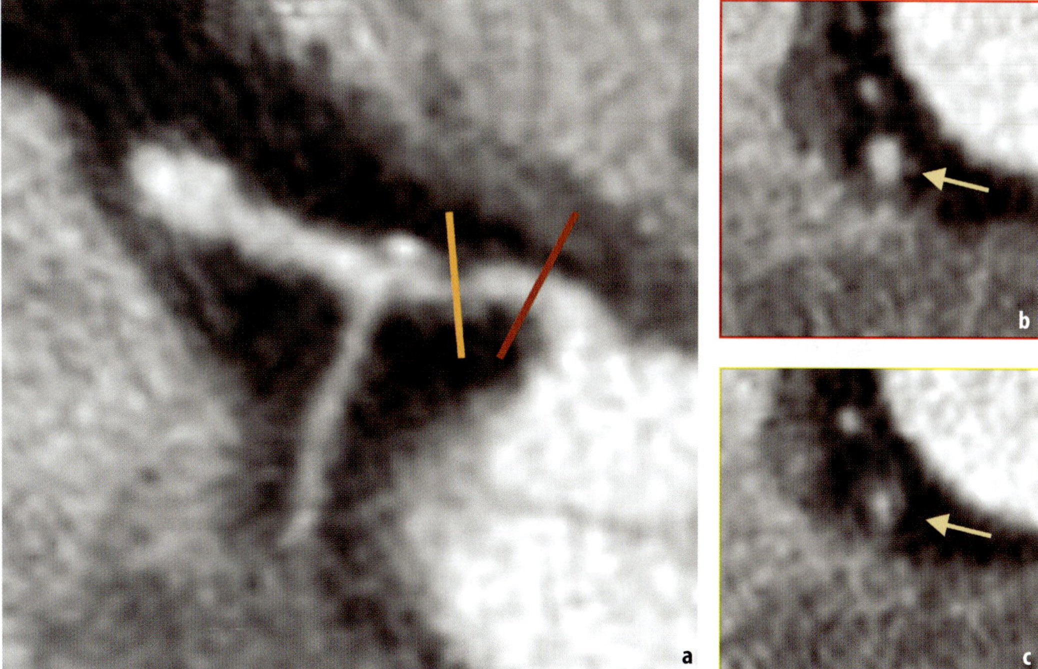

Fig. 9a-c. Diagnostic quality coronary computed tomography angiography (CTA). **a** Oblique multiplanar reformatted image of the proximal right coronary artery. One of the major advantages of coronary CTA in comparison with digital subtraction angiography is the ability to obtain an orthogonal view through any lesion. This is the most important step in image interpretation. **b** The *upper right-hand image* framed in *red* corresponds to the more proximal right coronary artery. There is no coronary artery disease at this level. **c** The *lower right-hand image* framed in *yellow* corresponds to the more distal right coronary artery lesion. This orthogonal view is obtained at the center of the noncalcified (soft) plaque and demonstrates a greater than 70% stenosis

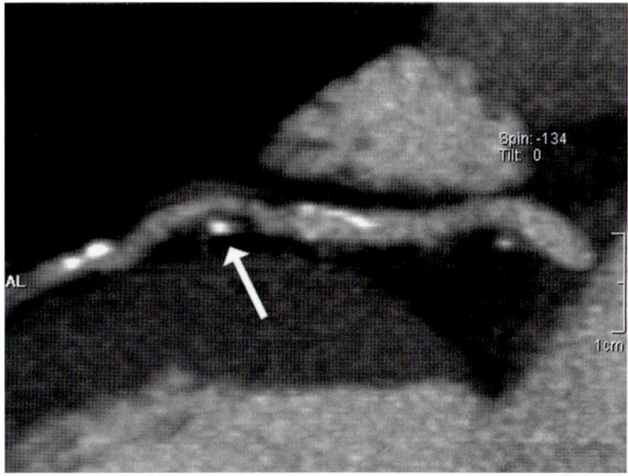

Fig. 10. Curved multiplanar reformatted image of the right coronary artery. Curved multiplanar images track (either automated, semiautomated, or manually) the center of the coronary artery though a long segment of its course and then display this long segment on a single image. While curved multiplanar reformatted images have no added information with respect to multiple short-segment standard reformatted images, they have the advantage that a large amount of data is displayed on a single image. However, it is essential to note that curved multiplanar reformatted images rely heavily on a precise placement of the center line. In our experience, interpretation of curved multiplanar reformatted images created from an imprecise center line is the most common source of error in image interpretation. This image demonstrates a complex (combination of calcified and noncalcified) plaque in the right coronary artery. At the calcified central component (*white arrow*), the stenosis was 50%

Scanning Parameters

As with ECG gating, image data oversampling, and spatial resolution, modern cardiac CT pushes the limits of technology with respect to the X-ray source. The two main scanning parameters that determine the number of photons used are the effective milliampere second (mAs) and kilovolts (kV). Effective mAs is defined as mAs divided by CT pitch and is proportional to X-ray CT tube current and scan time. Effective mAs and kV are set by the operator at the time of image acquisition. Typical values of effective mAs and kV are 550–700

and 120, respectively. However, in order to avoid reconstruction of images with significant noise, larger patients require more photons and thus higher settings. The most common way to maintain diagnostic images is to increase the effective mAs. Cardiac imaging of very obese patients is often limited. All X-ray CT tubes have a "limit" to the number of photons that can be produced, and for a particular application, all methods to decrease image noise (using the tube limit, increasing image thickness, scanning a smaller region) should be considered.

As described above, Z-axis spatial resolution is

determined by image slice thickness. For all modern scanners, the resolution is submillimeter. Although details of image interpretation are beyond the scope of this article, it is important to point out one major advantage of CT in comparison with other imaging modalities, such as catheter angiography, is the ability to perform multiplanar reconstructed images. Quality of reconstructed images is inversely related to image slice thickness, and it is beneficial to reconstruct images on so-called "isotropic data"; that is, CT data sets where spatial resolution is equal in the X, Y, and Z-directions. As an example of the impact of spatial resolution, consider native coronary CTA acquired with perfect ECG gating and no respiratory motion. In this setting, a 3-mm coronary artery reconstructed with 0.4 mm isotropic voxels spans seven or eight high-quality pixels (3 mm/0.4 mm) in any direction. This explains why properly performed CTA can differentiate between <50% and >50% stenosis but cannot grade a stenosis more precisely.

Scan Range and Image Field of View

Scan range in the Z-axis should include the anatomy of interest and allow for variations induced by both breath holding and the possibility that pathology can extend in both the cranial and caudal directions. In coronary imaging, occasionally, the left main and proximal left anterior descending arteries course superiorly over 1–2 cm, after which these vessels follow their usual path. Even in these situations, when imaging the native coronaries, the superior border of the scan should be set at the top of the carina, and the inferior border should scan through the entire inferior wall of the heart. Ideally, the planned field of view (FOV) should include several slices of the liver to account for cardiac displacement during breath holding. Since CT data is acquired in the craniocaudal direction, obtaining a small amount of CT data inferior to the heart does not affect image quality. Extended craniocaudal coverage is required for specific applications (Fig. 11). The most common applications are evaluation of coronary bypass grafts and of chest pain. For bypass grafts, imaging extends cranially to include the origins of the internal mammary arteries from the subclavian arteries. It is important to image the full extent of both sides, as course, caliber, and patency is important in the assessment of patients who have an internal mammary graft as well as those in whom the internal mammary artery is being considered for bypass.

The operator also specifies the FOV in the XY plane for coronary CT reconstruction. Choosing an FOV in the XY plane that is smaller than 24 cm is not recommended, as these images can be noisy. Typical values range between 24 cm and 30 cm, and it is almost always the case that coronary artery reconstruction will include the most important anatomy in the mediastinum.

In every case, complete CT reconstruction with a full FOV should be performed, followed by "skin-to-skin" interpretation in lung, mediastinum, and bone windows. Patients have significant "incidental" findings, including cases of acute pulmonary embolism and lung masses invading the chest wall, that can be the source of chest pain.

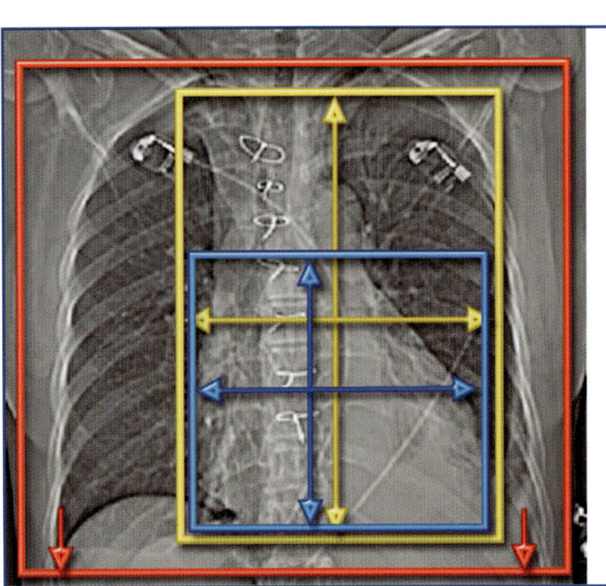

Fig. 11. Topogram of a cardiovascular patient. For imaging of the native coronary arteries (*blue range*), imaging should extend from the top of the carina though the inferior of the heart. Ideally, imaging should include a few slices of the liver to ensure that the inferior of the heart is covered. For bypass graft imaging (*yellow range*), the superior aspect of the range is extended to include both subclavian arteries and the origin of the internal mammary arteries. In chest-pain imaging, the entire chest, as well as the full extent of the aorta, is imaged

Contrast Material

While intravenous contrast can be administered with either a single or a dual injection system, dual injection (iodinated contrast followed by saline) is recommended for coronary CTA. Saline is used to avoid dense opacification of the right heart and potential artifacts that can limit interpretation of the right coronary artery. In addition, the injection of saline after iodinated contrast pushes the iodinated contrast to its anatomic destination and helps to minimize dilution of the contrast as it passes through the central veins.

It is now standard to inject contrast material at rates of at least 5 cc/s, and most centers have an injection rate between 6 cc and 7.5 cc/s. This rate of delivery requires that the IV be placed in the antecubital vein and be at least 20 gauge (usually 18 gauge is required). A right-arm injection is preferred since contrast material injected into the left arm often fills the left brachiocephalic vein at the time of image acquisition, and dense opacification of the brachiocephalic vein can be the source of artifact in the anterior mediastinum. Contrast material volume is determined by contrast injection rate and scan time required to cover the craniocaudal extent of the heart. As an example, consider an 18-s scan of the native coronaries plus bypass grafts. With an injection rate of 5 cc/s, an adequate volume of contrast media would be 90 cc (18 s × 5 cc/s). Since the administration of contrast material after completion of image acquisition is of no benefit, it is important to perform this calculation so that excessive contrast does not fill the right heart and subsequently induce image artifact.

With respect to timing the contrast injection, there are two general methods that can be used: bolus tracking and a test bolus. Both are illustrated in the setting of imaging the native coronary arteries. As previously mentioned, the superior border of the region to be imaged is set at the top of the carina. The axial slice at this position is usually 2–4 cm above the origin of the left main coronary artery. In patients with normal cardiac output, no venous obstruction, and whose arms are positioned over the head and above the right heart, the typical transit time from the right antecubital vein to the ascending aorta at the level of the carina is between 17 s and 23 s. In bolus tracking, the contrast injection begins with the scanner prepared to repetitively image a region of interest (ROI) in the ascending aorta at the axial slice defined by the position of the carina. Roughly 10 s after the contrast injection begins, images of the same slice are acquired while enhancement of the ascending aorta is monitored; that is, the bolus is "tracked" in the ascending aorta just above the coronary ostia. Once enhancement reaches a preset threshold (typically 200 HU above baseline attenuation in the ascending aorta), craniocaudal diagnostic images are acquired, beginning at the axial location where bolus tracking was performed.

A test bolus uses a separate injection to time the diagnostic injection. For an injection rate of 6 cc/s, a typical test bolus would be 12 cc of contrast followed by 30 cc of saline. As with bolus tracking, the ROI is chosen in the ascending aorta at the level of the carina. However, 10 s after the beginning of the test injection, scans separated by 1 s are used to plot enhancement versus time to include the time of peak enhancement (Fig. 12). Once the optimum delay is determined from the plot, the diagnostic images are obtained with a second contrast injection. When using a test bolus, it is important that the test injection mirrors the diagnostic injection. In particular, injection rates should be the same. Also, most centers routinely give nitroglycerin (0.4 mg sublingually) for coro-

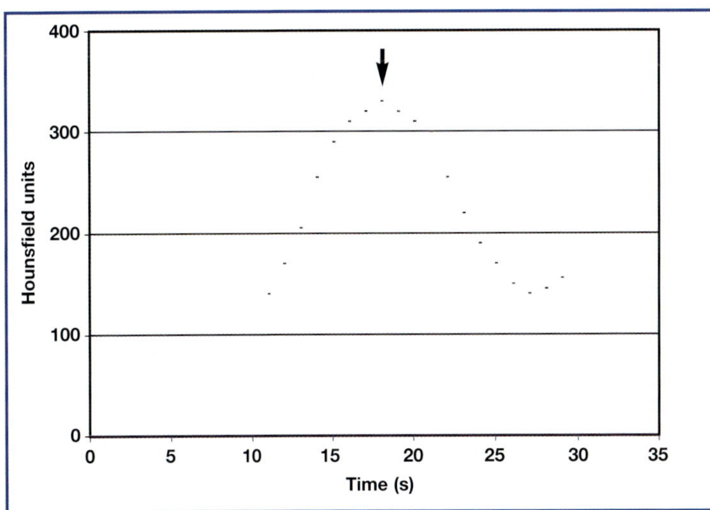

Fig. 12. Typical appearance of timing bolus plot for coronary CTA. The region of interest is approximately 3 cm above the origin of the left main coronary artery. Contrast (12 cc) followed by saline (30 cc) is administered at a rate of 6 cc/s, and images are acquired every second. There are no data points for the first 10 s of the timing bolus since imaging is not performed while the contrast passes from the venous system to the pulmonary arterial system. In this example, the contrast in the ascending aorta peaks at 18 s (*arrow*). The subsequent coronary CTA will use a 21-s delay. The rationale is that the additional 3 s will ensure that the coronary arteries have time to fill with contrast before the CT data are collected

nary vasodilatation to all patients undergoing native coronary CTA. While the effect of nitroglycerin on cardiac output (and thus iodinated contrast transit time) is typically negligible, the nitroglycerin should be administered before the test injection.

While using a test bolus has the disadvantage that a separate injection is required, there are distinct advantages in coronary imaging. First, unlike bolus tracking, when a test bolus is used, actual time to peak enhancement can be obtained. This will better ensure that when the diagnostic contrast injection is performed, peak enhancement will be achieved. Second, the test injection tests the quality of the intravenous access. Finally, since the test bolus can be performed with the breathing instructions that will be used in the diagnostic injection, it allows the patient to "practice" the exam, and it enables the operator to visualize variation in heart rate during a breath-hold IV contrast injection.

Image Reconstruction

Single-segment (one heartbeat) or multisegment (greater than one heartbeat) retrospective image reconstruction can be performed, the later strategy yielding an improvement in temporal resolution at the expense of greater data oversampling and more patient irradiation. In addition to choosing a single- versus multisegment algorithm, the operator can choose a reconstruction kernel for a particular application. Reconstruction with additional kernels is most often done in the evaluation of patients with one or more coronary stents (Fig. 13). At present, stenosis within a stent cannot be quantified reliably. However, sharper imaging kernels (i.e., closer to a bone algorithm than a soft tissue algorithm) can be used to "sharpen" edges and determine that a coronary stent is not occluded. This can provide useful information in patients who present with chest pain post-stent placement.

Another technique that can be used to improve image quality is ECG editing. This refers to the ability to manually modify and/or eliminate a reconstruction phase in one or in a few RR intervals (Fig. 14). ECG editing is most commonly used when a patient has a premature ventricular contraction (PVC) during image acquisition. Since the reconstructed phase of the cardiac cycle is triggered from the high amplitude of the R wave, reconstruction software can mistake a PVC for an R wave. Reconstructed slices that correspond to RR intervals with this error will suffer from severe motion artifact since these slices will be reconstructed over a different part of the cardiac cycle than the remainder of the scan. Since coronary CTA data is oversampled (CT pitch <1), reconstruction can be performed after removal of a PVC, often yielding a dramatic improvement in image quality. This can be a critical step for patients who have a PVC, particularly for those who do not have CAD. Since the high negative predictive value of coronary CTA depends on acquiring diagnostic images through the full extent of the major coronary arteries, elimination of a short segment of severe motion artifact can enable the interpreting physician to determine that a study is normal.

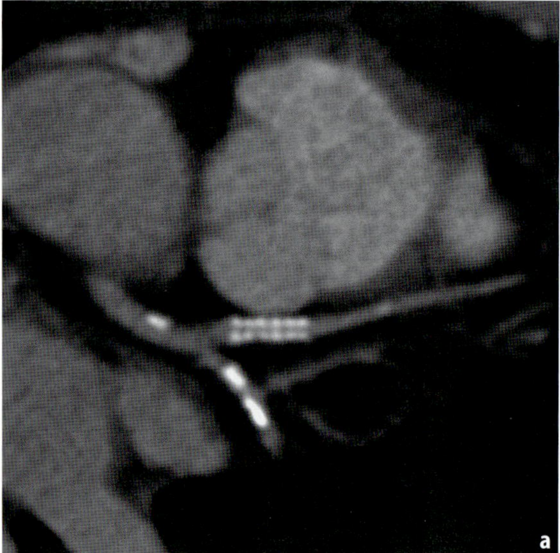

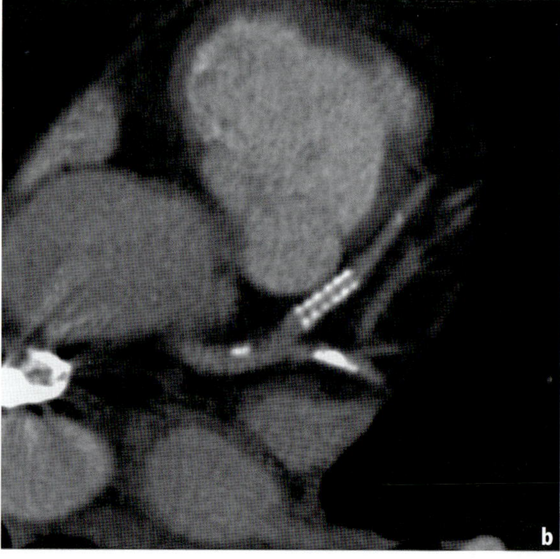

Fig. 13. For patients with coronary artery stents, both image artifacts and the spatial resolution of coronary CTA limit the interpretation. **a** Curved multiplanar reformatted image in a patient with a stent in the proximal left anterior descending artery. This image is reconstructed with a standard coronary imaging kernel. **b** Image reconstructed with a kernel closer to a bone algorithm shows sharper edges and less artifact from the high attenuation stent. The in-stent lumen is better visualized

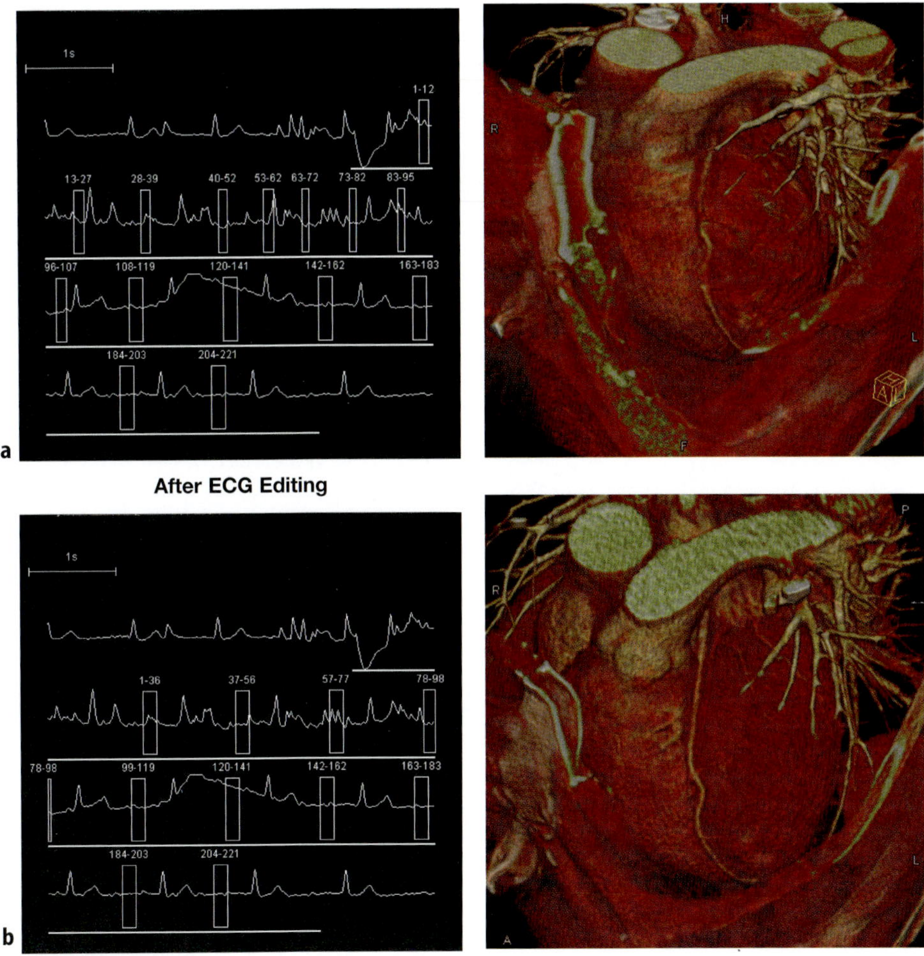

Fig. 14. ECG editing in a patient with suboptimal gating. The *top right* image demonstrates artifact that is explained by the locations (*rectangles* in the *top left image*) in the ECG where reconstruction was performed. Analysis of ECG tracing reveals that for some RR intervals, noise in the ECG is of great enough amplitude that the reconstruction algorithm mistook noise for an R wave. Thus, the different axial levels of the reconstruction reflect different phases of the cardiac cycle, rendering the study nondiagnostic. The *bottom left* image represents the ECG after editing; the location of the reconstruction has been manually placed to correspond with a relatively quiescent period in diastole. The subsequent ECG edited reconstruction (*bottom right image*) showed normal coronary arteries, using the high negative predictive value of coronary CT angiography (CTA) to eliminate coronary artery disease as a source of this patient's chest pain. Image postprocessing courtesy of Melissa Ende, Siemens Medical Solutions

Summary

Imaging protocols for cardiac CT have been revolutionized by recent advances in technology. In addition to the widespread availability of ECG gating, CT equipment with submillimeter resolution, 64 slices per rotation, and gantry rotation times less than one-half second are available from all major vendors. Cardiac imaging protocols are more complicated than CT scanning of other body parts. Strict adherence to the protocol is required to maintain image quality. However, for the clinician familiar with CT, superior diagnostic images can be obtained routinely.

Acknowledgments

The authors gratefully acknowledge useful discussions with Bernhard Schmidt Ph.D., particularly with respect to the section on CT radiation dose.

References

1. International Electrotechnical Commission. Medical electrical equipment. Part 2-44: Particular requirements for the safety of X-ray equipment for computed tomography. IEC publication 60601-2-44 (2002). International Electrotechnical Commission (IEC) Central Office: Geneva. Accessed 17 Jan 2006
2. European Guidelines on Quality Computed Tomography. EUR16262 (2002). http://www.drs.dk/guidelines/CT/quality/index.htm. Accessed 17 Jan 2006
3. Morin R, Gerber T, McCollough C (2003) Radiation dose in computed tomography of the heart. Circulation 107:917–922
4. International Council on Radiation Protection (1991) 1990 recommendations of the International Commission on Radiological Protection. Publication 60. Annals of the ICRP. Pergamon, Oxford
5. Schmidt B, Kalender WA (2002) A fast voxel-based Monte Carlo method for scanner- and patient-specific dose calculations in computed tomography. Physica Medica XVIII(2):43–53
6. Zankl M, Panzer W, Drexler G (1991) The calculation of dose from external photon exposure using reference human phantoms and Monte Carlo methods. Part IV: Organ doses from tomographic examinations. GSF report 30/91. GSF, Neuherberg
7. Kalender WA, Schmidt B, Zankl M, Schmidt M (1999) A PC program for estimating organ dose and effective dose values in computed tomography. Eur Radiol 9:555–562
8. Stamm G, Nagel HD (2002) CT-Expo – ein neuartiges Programm zur Dosisevaluierung in der CT. Fortschr Röntgenstr 174:1570–1576

17

MDCT Angiography of the Thoracic Aorta

Geoffrey D. Rubin, Mannudeep K. Kalra

Introduction

Multidetector computed tomography angiography (MDCTA) is a noninvasive and accurate technique for assessment of many thoracic aortic abnormalities. It offers several advantages over conventional aortography for evaluation of the thoracic aorta. State-of-the-art MDCT scanners, with improved temporal and isotropic resolution, enable volumetric acquisition that provides clear anatomic delineation of thoracic aorta, its tortuous branches, and adjacent aneurysms and pseudo aneurysms. In contrast with the projectional technique of conventional aortography, these frequently overlapping structures can affect visualization and delineation of anatomic relationships. In addition, MDCTA allows simultaneous delineation of true and false luminal flow channels in thoracic aortic dissections, intramural hematomas communicating with the aortic lumen, slow perigraft blood flow around aortic stent grafts, as well as direct visualization of the aortic wall and noncommunicating intramural hematomas. This chapter reviews techniques for acquisition and interpretation of thoracic aortic MDCTA and describes abnormalities in which MDCTA provides valuable information.

Scanning Techniques

Scan Coverage

MDCTA scanning protocol for evaluation of thoracic aorta must extend, at the minimum, from the base of the neck (to assess proximal common carotid and vertebral arteries) to the origin of the celiac axis. Such scan coverage allows evaluation of the supraaortic arterial branches for possible extension of aortic lesions, such as aneurysm and aortic dissection, into these branches. MDCTA of thoracic aorta is often performed to diagnose and lo-

calize aortic disease for planning endovascular and open repair, so inclusion of celiac origin aids in precise localization of lesions affecting distal thoracic aorta. However, in certain abnormalities, such as acute aortic dissection, additional scan coverage may be essential. In dissections, MDCTA is extended to cover the abdomen and pelvis to assess possible diminution of blood flow to the abdominal viscera or lower extremity. In other instances, upper-extremity arterial circulation (to evaluate for sources of embolization to the hands) or entire carotid arterial circulation (for assessing aortic dissection associated with symptoms of cerebral ischemia and large-vessel arteritis) may be included (Fig. 1).

Unenhanced Images

Generally, unenhanced CT images are acquired prior to MDCTA in the setting of suspected bleeding in the chest or aortic wall. These unenhanced images allow visualization of hyperattenuation of the mural crescent corresponding to intramural hematoma in patients with acute chest pain and possible intramural hematoma (Fig. 2). In addition, these images also aid in mapping the location of calcifications around the stent graft, which can simulate an endoleak following contrast administration. We typically use low radiation dose for acquiring these initial images (120 kV, 100 mA, 0.5 s rotation time, 1.3–1.7:1 pitch).

Contrast Media Considerations

For MDCTA of the thoracic aorta, we prefer contrast injection rate of at least 5 mL/s for an injection duration of less than 20 s. Generally, we do not perform MDCTA of thoracic aorta if flow rate is less than 4 mL/s. As a rule, the bolus duration must

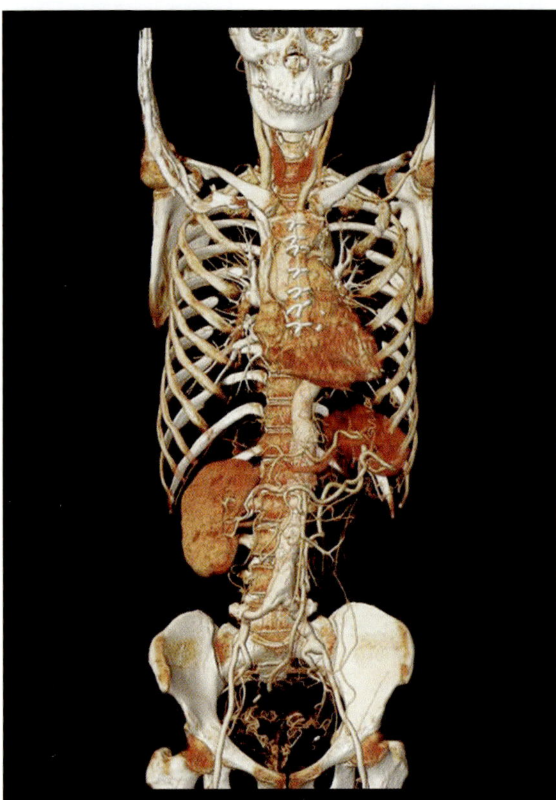

Fig. 1. A 16×1.25-mm multi-detector computed tomography (MDCT) scan acquired in 15 s in a woman with Takayasu arteritis. All arterials beds that might be affected by the disease are imaged from the carotid arteries through the femoral arteries within a single breath hold

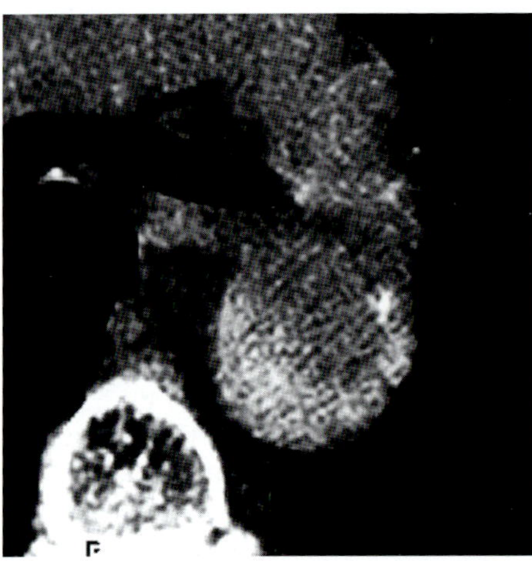

Fig. 2. Unenhanced transverse computed tomography (CT) section demonstrates a hyperattenuated crescent within the aortic wall diagnostic of an intramural hematoma

medium in the veins can affect visualization of adjacent structures, we always administer contrast medium via a right antecubital venous source to avoid opacification of the left brachiocephalic vein which can obscure the origins of the brachiocephalic, left common carotid, and left subclavian arteries.

To obtain optimum enhancement, it is necessary to use appropriate scan delay for contrast administration. We use an automated scan triggering technique for initiating image acquisition of the contrast-enhanced phase of MDCTA. As our MDCT scanners require about 8 s from the time that threshold enhancement is recognized in the descending aorta to the initiation of CTA acquisition, our injection duration is equal to scan duration plus 8 s. We have found that this is the most reliable technique for achieving consistently high-quality MDCTA studies.

Scanning Protocol

MDCTA of the thoracic aorta should be performed with ≤3 mm nominal section thickness and preferably with ≤1.5 mm thickness. The fastest possible gantry rotation time must be used to minimize scan duration and contrast dose. However, a slower gantry rotation time may improve image quality in larger patients by enabling a higher tube current-time product. Alternatively, some MDCT scanners allow use of higher tube current (up to 800 mA). Most MDCTA studies are performed with 120 kVp. We frequently use cardiac gating of MDCTA for evaluation of the ascending aorta and, in particular, coronary arteries [1, 2].

Scanning protocols for MDCTA must allow image acquisition in a single breath hold. If mechanical ventilation or extreme dyspnea does not permit single breath-hold scanning, then one should allow the patient to breathe quietly during image acquisition.

For most MDCTA studies, only arterial phase acquisition is required. However, for evaluation of stent-graft repair of aortic aneurysm, delayed images can be critical for detecting endoleak. These images are acquired about 70 s after initiation of arterial phase acquisition.

Reconstruction Considerations

We generally reconstruct MDCTA images with an interval that is 50% of the effective section thickness. These images are reconstructed with a smaller reconstructed field of view (25–30 cm) to only include the relevant arterial structures. Softer reconstruction algorithms are typically used to minimize noise in thin sections acquired with MDCTA.

be equivalent to image acquisition duration plus any delays by bolus monitoring algorithms. Our experience suggests that an iodinated contrast medium (370 mg of iodine/mL) volume of at least 80 mL is required for reliable opacification. As high CT attenuation values of undiluted contrast

Interpretation Techniques

Image Workstations

Soft copy reading of MDCTA image data sets at a postprocessing or picture archiving and communication system (PACS) workstation is recommended, as it allow scrolling through large number of source images, three-dimensional (3-D) postprocessing, and adjustment of window level and width. Due to variations in aortic enhancement, customization of window width and level settings is important to ensure that discrimination of luminal enhancement from mural calcifications is possible. In addition, very narrow windows are frequently necessary for assessing subtle endoleaks following stent-graft repair on delayed images.

Artifacts in MDCTA

Certain artifacts can affect assessment of patients with suspected aortic dissection. Perivenous streaks and arterial pulsations cause the most interpretative difficulties of MDCTA of thoracic aorta, typically on the visualization of the ascending aorta.

Perivenous streak artifacts result from both beam hardening and motion caused by transmitted pulsation in veins with undiluted contrast medium. Prior studies have recommended modification of scanning techniques to minimize these artifacts. These include the use of dilute contrast medium solutions [3, 4], caudal to cranial scan direction, and femoral venous access [5]. These methods have been abandoned due to the recent availability of dual-chamber contrast medium injectors, enabling the use of a saline chaser bolus to eliminate perivenous shunts (Fig. 3). In most instances, perivenous streaks are seldom misinterpreted as intimal dissection in the ascending aorta due to substantial variation in their orientation from image to image and extension beyond the confines of the aortic wall. However, the difficult area for perivenous streaks is the origin of the supraaortic branches adjacent to a contrast-opacified left brachiocephalic vein, where these artifacts can obscure extension of dissection to these branches as well as occlusive disease caused by atherosclerotic plaque at their origins. The best preventive strategy to avoid this artifact is to ensure peripheral venous access from the right upper extremity.

In addition to perivenous streaks, artifacts from arterial pulsation can also result in a false positive interpretation of aortic dissection. For example, pulsation in the ascending aorta can mimic an intimal flap. With faster acquisition speed and thin overlapping sections provided by MDCT scanners, this artifact may be eliminated. Use of

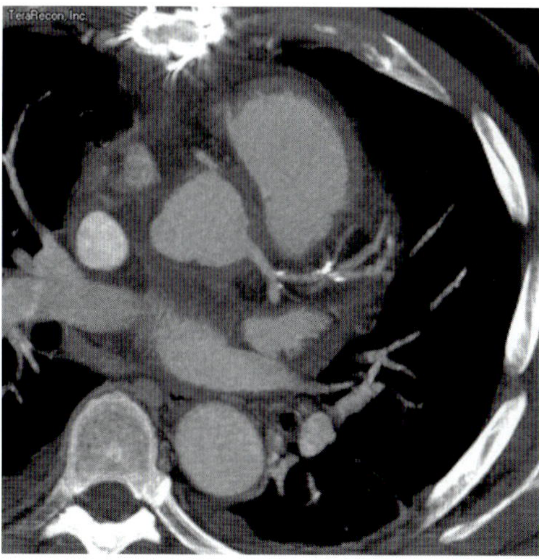

Fig. 3. Transverse multi-detector computed tomography (MDCT) section obtained from a scan acquired with a 50-mL saline chaser bolus demonstrates mild superior vena cava opacification, allowing for artifact-free assessment of the aortic root

wider windows can also help in excluding "artifactual intimal flap" by documenting extension of artifacts beyond aortic walls. Segmented or partial reconstruction of helical scan data can also help in reducing motion artifacts observed on standard reconstructions [6] (Fig. 4). Aortic pulsation, which is particularly more pronounced in thinner patients, results in a serrated appearance to arteries that can simulate fibromuscular dysplasia in blood vessels such as renal arteries, but is rarely a limitation in the chest.

Differential flow of contrast medium in the true and false lumina can simulate appearance of a thrombosed false lumen, particularly when scan delay is triggered on the basis of opacification of the true lumen of the aorta (Fig. 5). Thus, in patients with suspected aortic dissection, bolus tracking must be performed just caudal to the aortic arch, where transverse cross-sections of both the distal ascending as well as proximal descending aorta can be assessed. A region of interest must be placed in both the true and false lumen to obtain two time density curves. Delay time is selected to assure opacification of false lumen. Bolus duration is then increased by the time (seconds) between the true luminal peak and the selected delay time.

Reformation and Rendering

While axial source images remain the mainstay of MDCTA interpretation of the thoracic aorta, multiplanar reformation (MPR) and 3-D rendering techniques can aid in diagnosis. In addition, these techniques can provide an easier and more effec-

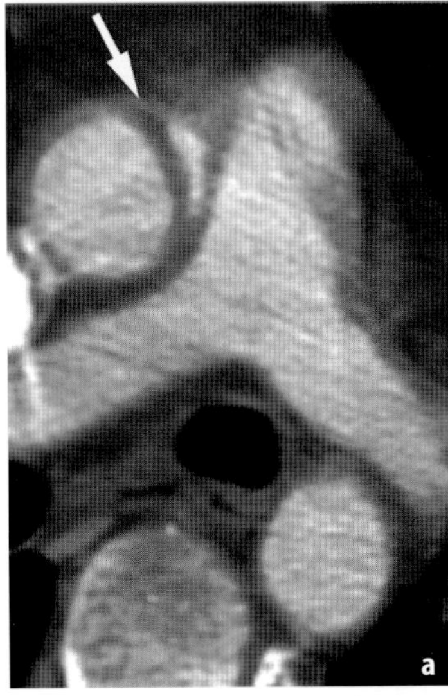
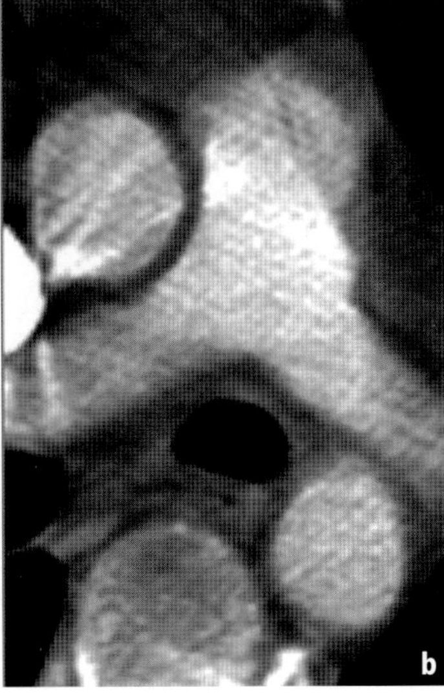

Fig. 4a, b. 3.75-mm transverse-section multidetector computed tomography (MDCT) sections obtained through the ascending aorta in a patient who had been run over by a tractor. Acquisition parameters are 3.75-mm detector width, pitch 1.5, table speed 22.5 mm per rotation, and 0.8 s per rotation. An apparent linear filling defect is present within the ascending aorta (*arrow*). **a** Identical image location from the same CT acquisition reconstructed with a half scan or segmented reconstruction algorithm. The segmented reconstruction requires approximately 220° of data, resulting in an effective temporal resolution of 0.5 s. By reconstructing the section using this algorithm, the apparent linear filling defects are revealed to be motion-related artifacts, and thus there is no suspicion for ascending aortic injury (**b**)

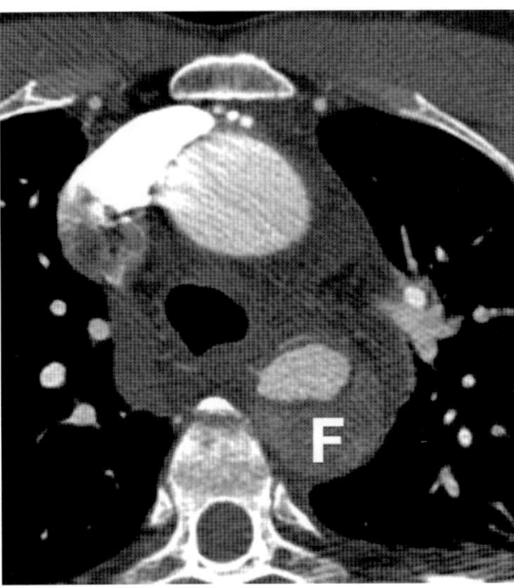

Fig. 5. Transverse section from multi-detector computed tomography angiography (MDCTA) where the scan was triggered using a region of interest placed within the true aortic lumen results in an acquisition that is too early to allow the false lumen to fill, thus leading to the ambiguous appearance of a thrombosed versus a slowly filling false lumen (*F*)

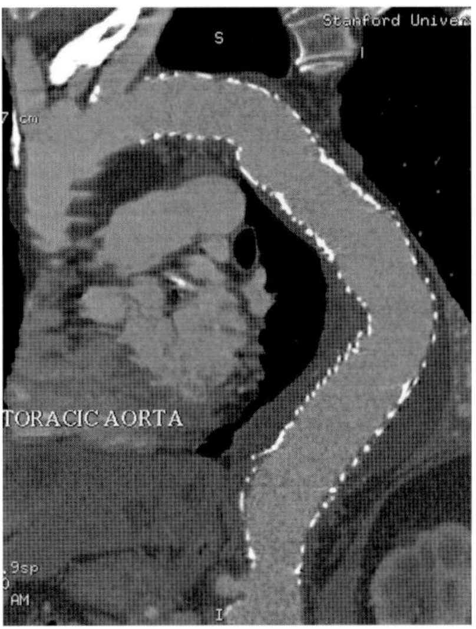

Fig. 6. Curved planar reformation (CPR) through the aortic arch and descending aorta allows clear delineation of the contrast-medium-enhanced aortic lumen, the stent graft, and the thrombosed portions of a descending thoracic aortic aneurysm outside of the stent graft

tive way of explaining critical anatomic relationships to clinicians. The most popular techniques include MPR, maximum-intensity projections (MIP), and volume rendering (VR). In our experience, curved planar reformations (CPR), and VR are the most useful 3-D techniques for assessing the thoracic aorta.

MPR, which also includes CPR and sagittal, coronal, and oblique tomograms, are typically single-voxel-thick tomographic images. The single-voxel-thick MPR, especially the CPR, is the most useful of the MPR techniques [7]. CPR is helpful for visualization of the luminal contents of the aorta or its branches in patients with aortic dissection or aortic stent-graft deployment (Fig. 6). Combining information from adjacent voxels allows thicker MPR images, referred to as a thin-slab, or multiplanar volume rendered (MPVR) images [8]. Thin slabs require no pre-rendering segmentation or editing and help demonstrate vessel origins in different but adjacent planes, such as occurs with branches of the aortic arch.

MIP [9–11] has limited application in evaluation of thoracic aorta. As calcified atheroma is rarely of clinical significance, simultaneous display and distinction of the contrast-enhanced flow lumen and mural calcification with MIP images is not very useful in the thoracic aorta. Besides, in-

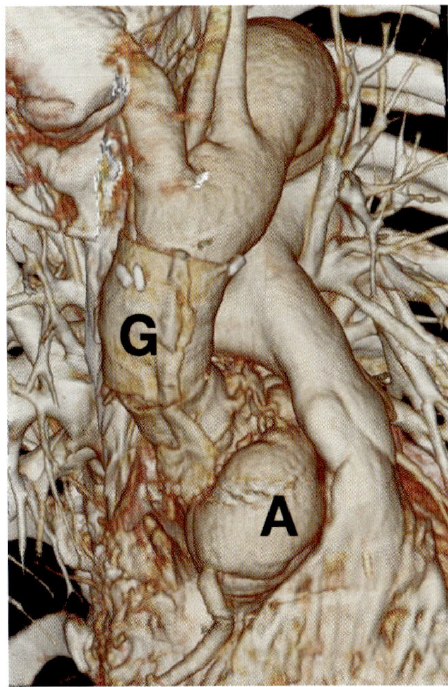

Fig. 7. Volume rendering (VR) allows clear depiction of the ascending aortic interposition graft (*G*) and a root aneurysm (*A*)

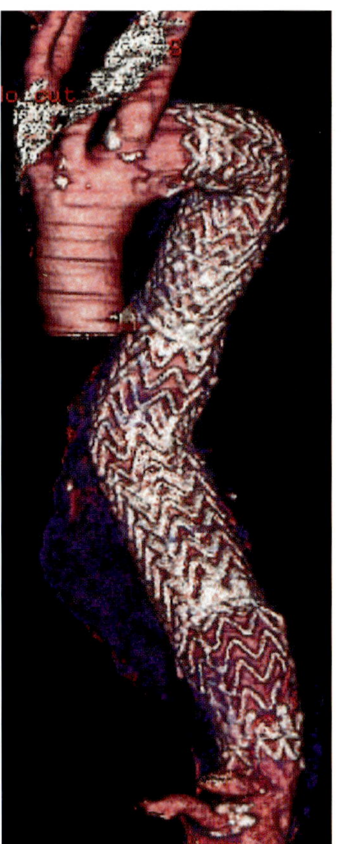

Fig. 8. Volume rendering (VR) demonstrates the metallic stent graft (*white*), the aortic lumen (*pink*), and the thrombosed aneurysm (*blue*) from the same patient as in Figure 6

ability of MIP to discern overlapping vascular anatomy is also a substantial disadvantage.

VR [12–16] is a volumetric 3-D technique that displays complex anatomic relationships, particularly in regions of vessel overlap (Figs. 7–9). With the exception of occlusive diseases, intramural hematomas and some thrombosed false lumina, VR provides the best information about lesion anatomy for surgical planning in most thoracic aortic diseases, such as aneurysms, congenital aberrant branching, and intimal dissection or intramural hematoma.

Clinical Applications of MDCTA of Thoracic Aorta

MDCTA of thoracic aorta provides useful information for congenital anomalies, aneurysms, dissection, aortic trauma, intramural hematoma, and open and endovascular interventions.

Congenital Anomalies

MDCTA of thoracic aorta allows noninvasive diagnosis and characterization of congenital anomalies of the thoracic aorta and aberrant branches of the descending aorta, such as vascular rings, aberrant supraaortic branching, coarctation (Fig. 10), and enlarged bronchial arteries or major arteriopul-

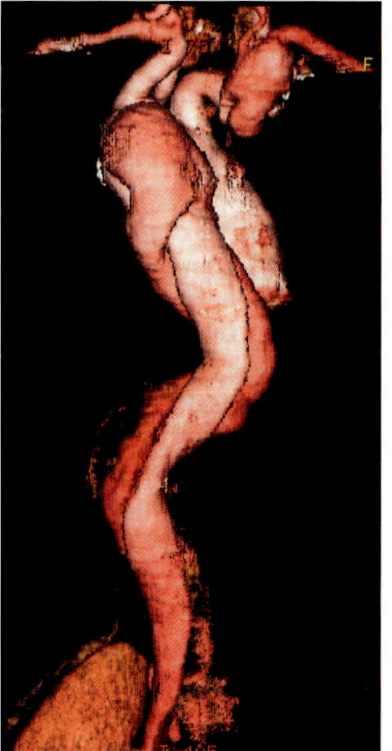

Fig. 9. The complex interrelationship between true and false lumina of the descending aorta are demonstrated with volume rendering (VR)

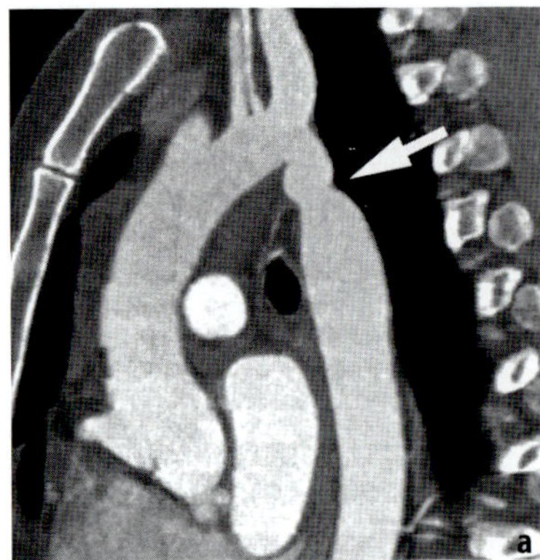
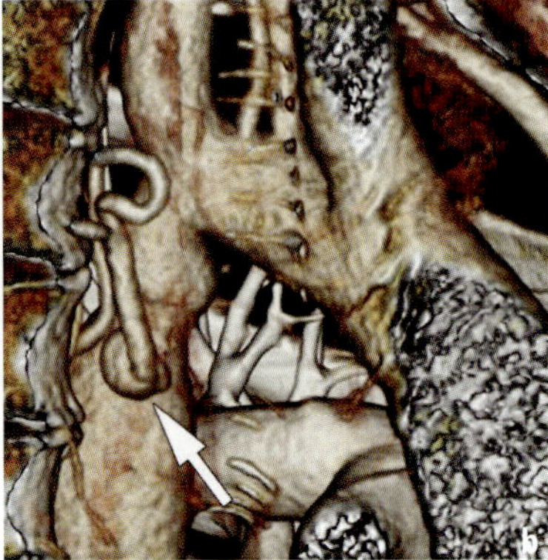
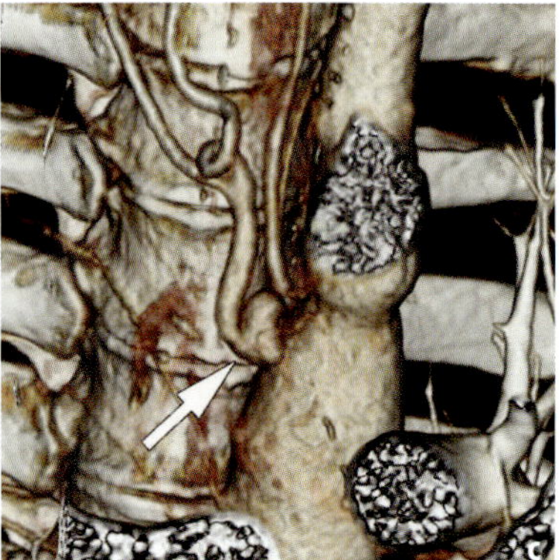

Fig. 10a-c. a Curved planar reformation (CPR) of computed tomography angiography (CTA) in a patient with aortic coarctation (*arrow*). **b** Volume rendering (VR) of the aortic arch and proximal descending aorta viewed from the right demonstrates an aneurysm (*arrow*) at the origin of an enlarged intercostal artery origin, which provides collateral circulation around the coarcted segment. **c** Frontal VR through the descending aorta demonstrates the intercostal artery aneurysm to better advantage (*arrow*)

monary communicating arteries [17, 18] In addition, thin section volumetric MDCTA studies provide information on lesions, such as pulmonary sequestration, as well as depict direct relationship between tracheobronchial narrowing and the presence of aberrant vessels.

Aortic Aneurysm

MDCTA allows accurate evaluation of thoracic aortic aneurysms, including presence of an aneurysm, its extent, size, complications, follow-up evaluation, and prediction of appropriate management [19]. Generally, diagnosis of aortic aneurysms is made from axial-source data, whereas CPR and VR are helpful in determining lesion extent (Figs. 11 and 12). As the thoracic aorta is a tortuous and curved structure, aneurysm size measurement is most accurate when double-oblique MPRs are generated in directions perpendicular to the aortic flow lumen (Fig. 13). This measurement technique for aneurysm sizing is also reproducible for evaluating the rate of aneurysm expansion on follow-up MDCTA studies. It is interesting to note that aneurysm volume allows the most complete measure of aneurysm size. Although volumetric MDCTA data should provide accurate aneurysm volume, the painstaking and time-consuming manual segmentation of patent, thrombosed, and atheromatous elements of the aorta from the adjacent structures is a substantial drawback of aneurysmal volume. To date, there is no data concerning the risk of aneurysm rupture and guidelines for intervention based on aneurysm volume expansion [20, 21].

Generally speaking, thoracic aortic aneurysms >5 cm in cross-sectional dimension have an increased risk for rupture. Surgical repair is often contemplated when thoracic aortic aneurysms

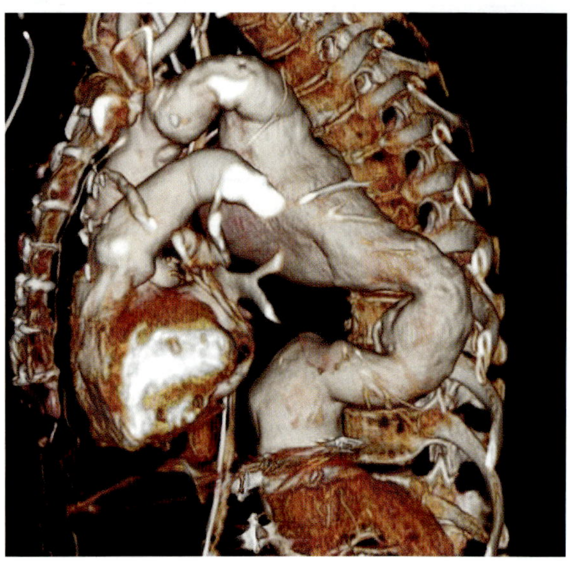

Fig. 11. Volume rendering (VR) of a large descending aortic aneurysm illustrates the tortuous course of the aorta distal the aneurysm

reach a diameter of 5–6 cm [20, 21]. For surgical planning, MDCTA provides a roadmap of aneurysms by depicting the precise anatomic extent of the aneurysm as well as the involvement of aortic branches. A recent study reported 94% accuracy, 95% positive predictive value, and 93% negative predictive value for successful prediction of the need for hypothermic circulatory arrest with transverse and MPR images [19].

Aortic Dissection

Accurate identification and localization (ascending aorta – type A [Fig. 14] or not proximal to the brachiocephalic artery – type B [Fig. 15]) of the in-

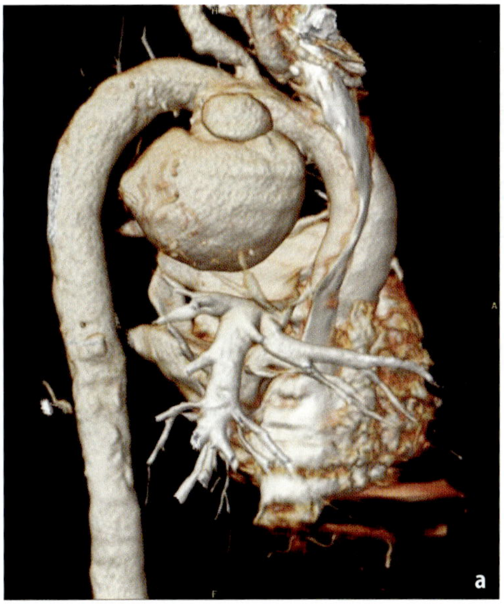
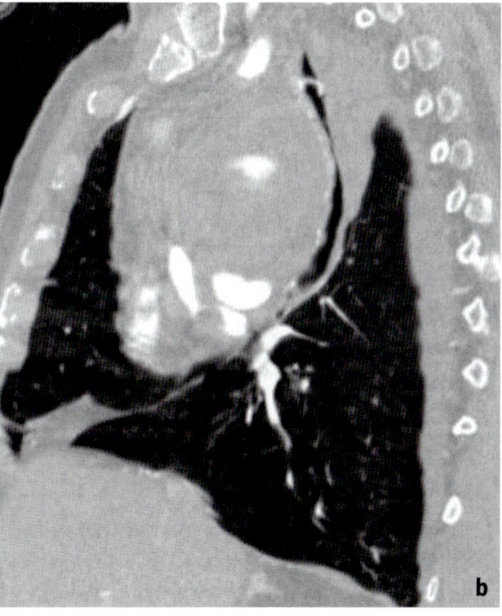

Fig. 12a, b. a The lumen of a large pseudoaneurysm extending from the inferior aspect of the aortic arch is demonstrated with volume rendering (VR). The size of the mural thrombus (not visible) can be inferred from the compression on the superior vena cava. **b** Curved planar reformation (CPR) through the trachea demonstrates the marked compression of the airway by the large aneurysm

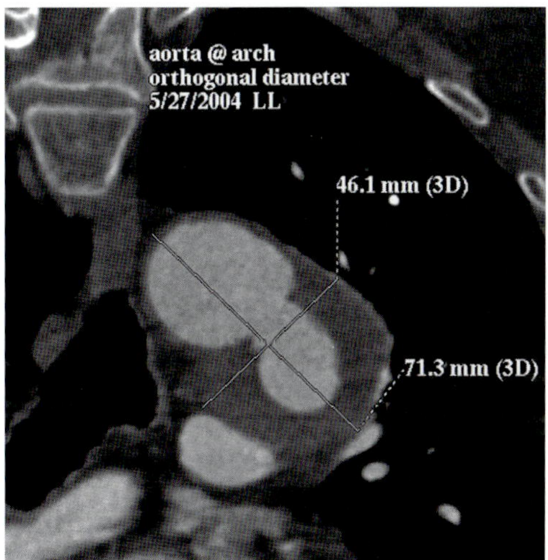

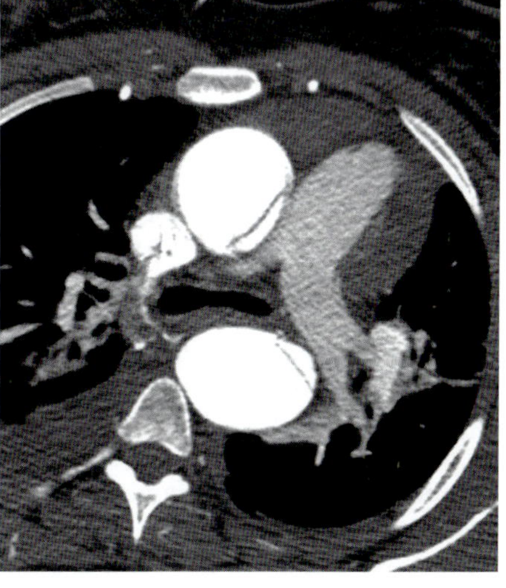

Fig. 13. Measurement of an aortic arch aneurysm using a double oblique view oriented perpendicular to the axis of the aneurysm

Fig. 14. Type A aortic dissection. An intimal flap is observed in both the ascending and descending aorta. Hemopericardium is demonstrated

timal flap is a prerequisite for application of any imaging technique in patients with suspected aortic dissection. Four imaging techniques, conventional angiography, CT scanning, MRI, and transesophageal echocardiography (TEE), can provide this information about aortic dissection and thus aid in decision making for emergent repair.

Although relative accuracy of these imaging modalities is controversial, technologic advances in CT, MRI, and TEE have outpaced the ability of most researchers to compare these techniques in rigorous prospective trials. However, current opinion regards MRI or TEE as the most sensitive tests for aortic dissection [22] although this opinion is based on comparison of state-of-the-art MRI or TEE with relatively primitive conventional CT [23, 24]. Although radiation dose and iodinated contrast medium toxicity are relevant concerns with CT, to the best of our knowledge, no studies have compared state-of-the-art MDCT to either MRI or TEE. Although high-quality TEE offers several advantages over MDCT (on-site performance of TEE in emergency department and identification

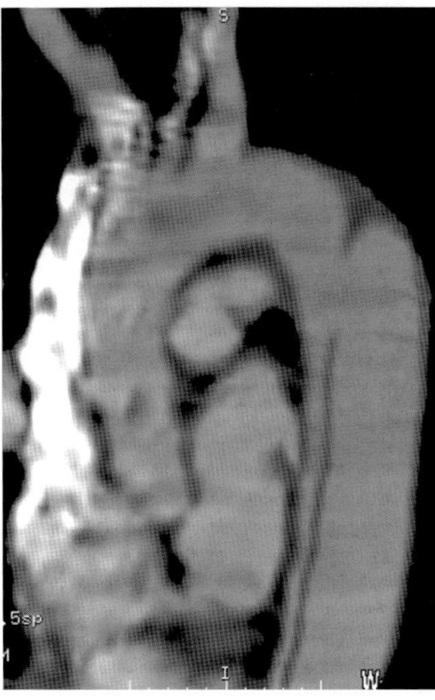

Fig. 15. Type B aortic dissection. The intimal flap originates distal to the brachiocephalic artery

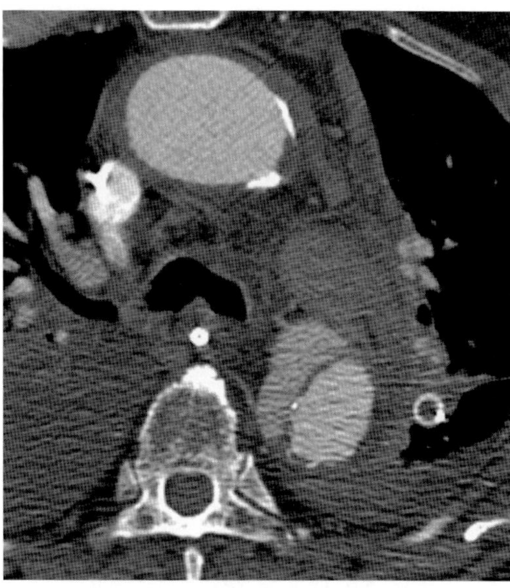

Fig. 16. Rupturing type B aortic dissection. High attenuation blood is present in the mediastinum adjacent to the irregularly enlarged descending aortic false lumen

of aortic valvular insufficiency that requires immediate replacement), when TEE is unavailable, MDCTA will be the most accessible and staffed options to handle potentially hemodynamically unstable patients in most hospitals (Fig. 16).

The primary indication for diagnostic conventional angiography in patients with acute thoracic aortic dissection is in the setting of cardiac arrhythmia or electrocardiographic abnormalities, which suggest possible involvement of coronary artery and myocardial ischemia. However, in expert hands, it is most likely that the accuracy of TEE, MDCTA, and MRI will be nearly identical for diagnosis of aortic dissection.

Certain imaging modalities may be more useful in providing an alternative diagnosis when primary diagnosis is not present. For instance, unlike TEE, MDCTA may provide evidence of other vascular disease (such as coronary artery disease) mimicking aortic dissection. In addition, in patients with chronic or acute aortic dissection that do not require immediate surgical intervention, TEE does not provide sufficient information, such as extension of the intimal flap into aortic branches, true luminal compression by the false lumen that limits blood flow into the abdomen or pelvis, and presence of fenestrations that allow communication between the true and false lumen. However, MDCTA can provide information about extension of intimal flaps into aortic branches. Also, when catheter-based interventions are considered, preinterventional MDCTA can help identification of the best route for achieving access to aortic

branches as well as simultaneous visualization of all aortic lumina to avoid confusion in the angiography suite that results from opacification of only one of three or more lumina in a complex dissection. However, evaluation of thoracic aortic dissection with MDCTA does have pitfalls.

When considering reformation and rendering techniques, CPR is useful for depicting the flap within the center of the vessel (Fig. 17a). VR images demonstrate the interface of the intimal flap with the aortic wall (Fig. 17b). Usefulness of MIP images is limited, as they do not display the intimal flap unless it is oriented perpendicular to the plane of the MIP.

Intramural Hematoma

Several mechanisms have been proposed to explain formation of intramural hematoma, which include spontaneous rupture of the vasa vasorum, intimal fracture at the site of an atherosclerotic plaque, and intramural propagation of hemorrhage adjacent to a penetrating atherosclerotic ulcer. Patients with intramural hematomas exhibit symptoms, physical signs, and risk profiles that are almost identical to typical aortic dissection [25].

Prior studies on CT evaluation of intramural hematomas from penetrating atherosclerotic ulcers have reported that MDCTA aids in visualization of ulcers and intramural hematomas with confirmation of its subintimal location by the observation of displaced intimal calcifications [19, 26, 27] (Fig. 18).

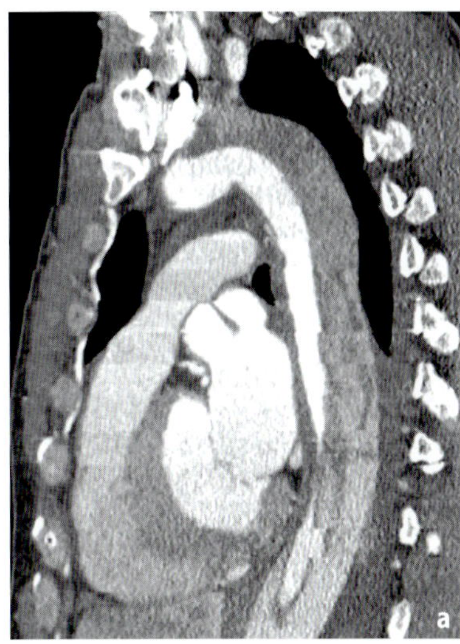

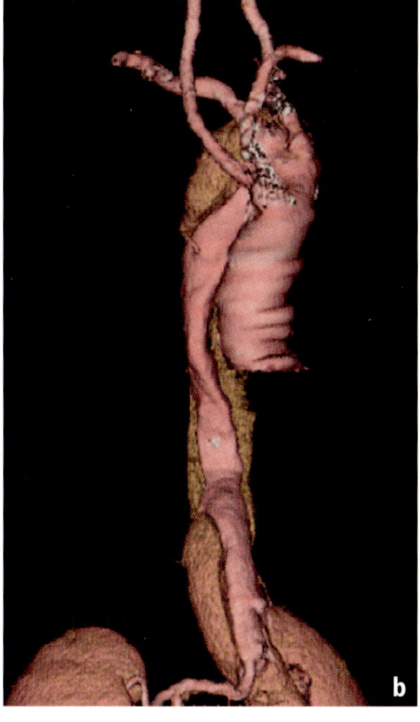

Fig. 17a, b. a Curved planar reformation (CPR) and **b** volume rendering (VR) of a type B aortic dissection. CPR depicts the interior of the lumen while VR demonstrates the interface of the lumen with the aortic wall

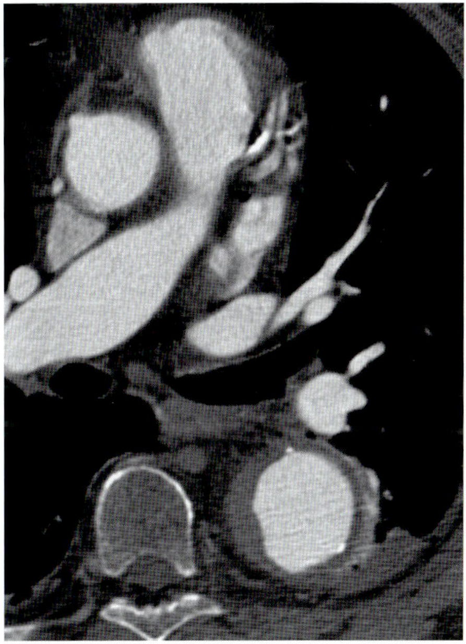

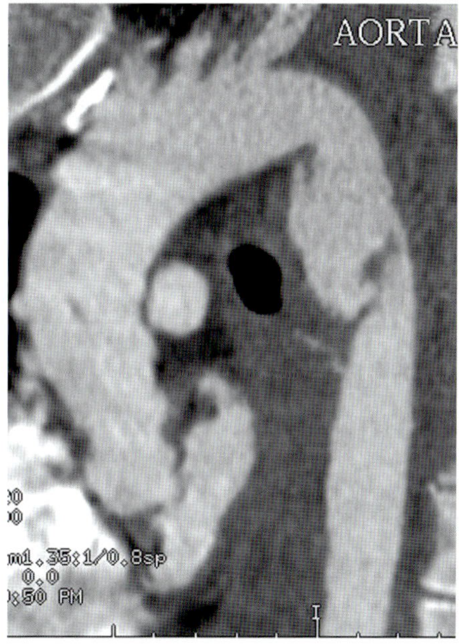

Fig. 18. Transverse section from a multidetector computed tomography angiography (MDCTA) demonstrates an intramural hematoma in the descending aorta. Intimal calcium along the posterior aspect of the aorta is displaced to the luminal surface supporting the conclusion that the mural collection is blood in the wall rather than atheroma within the lumen

Fig. 19. Curved planar reformation (CPR) through the aorta demonstrates a traumatic pseudoaneurysm at the aortic isthmus following high-speed deceleration in a motor vehicle collision

In patients with intramural hematoma, noncontrast images typically reveal a high-attenuation intramural crescent (Fig. 2). In addition, an intense contrast enhancement and thickening of the aortic wall external to the hematoma may be seen on contrast-enhanced images. These findings may represent adventitial inflammatory process.

Aortic Trauma

CT offers an accurate, rapid, and less expensive alternative to conventional aortography for evaluation of patients with suspected thoracic aortic trauma [28]. In such patients, MDCTA allows direct visualization of the aortic tear (Fig. 19). Prior

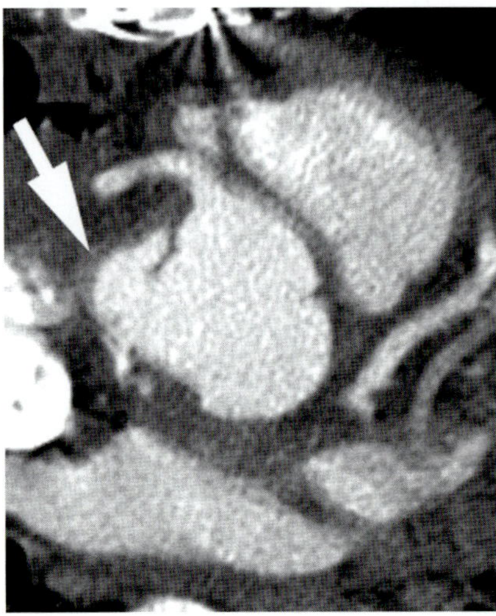

Fig. 20. Anastomotic dehiscence with resulting pseudoaneurysm (*arrow*) at the proximal anastomosis of an ascending aortic interposition graft

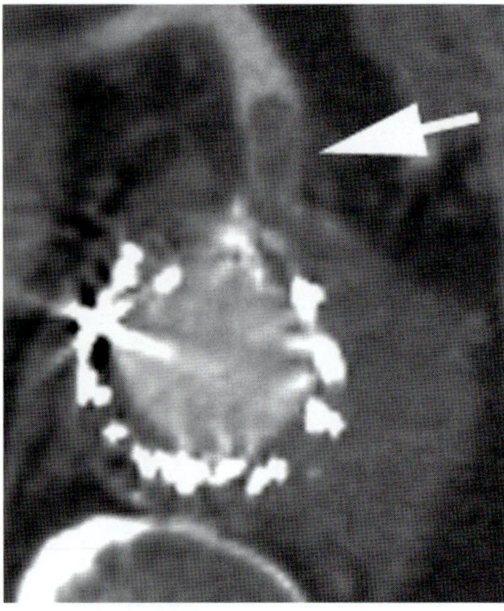

Fig. 21. Thrombotic occlusion of the celiac axis (*arrow*) following inadvertent extension of a thoracic aortic stent graft over the ostium of the celiac axis

studies have shown that helical CTA is a very sensitive technique for detection of aortic injury [29–31]. These studies have also reported that MPR and 3-D reformation do not contribute substantial information to axial source data for identification and characterization of aortic injury [31].

Evaluation of Aortic Interventions

MDCTA can be used for evaluation for assessment of open and endovascular aortic interventions. As vascular clips, sternal wires, and graft materials cause relatively little artifacts on MDCT images, MDCTA allows evaluation of perianastomotic complications following thoracic aortic or coronary artery bypass graft placement (Fig. 20) and complications following placement of access cannulas for cardiopulmonary bypass surgery.

MDCTA has been found useful for the evaluation of endoluminal thoracic aortic stent grafts [32]. It can demonstrate complications of stent grafting such as aortic-branch occlusions (Fig. 21), retroperitoneal hematoma, and iliac artery dissection or occlusion. As regards to imaging evaluation of aortic intervention, it is important to note that complete exclusion of aneurysm following stent-graft deployment determines the success of aneurysm treatment. In absence of complete exclusion of aneurysm, perigraft flow results, which can be very slow and therefore remains undetectable with flush aortography (Fig. 22). As MDCTA depends on intravenous injection of contrast medium for generalized arterial opacification, opacification of perigraft channels are often detected on postdeployment MDCTA, even when conventional aortography suggested complete ex-

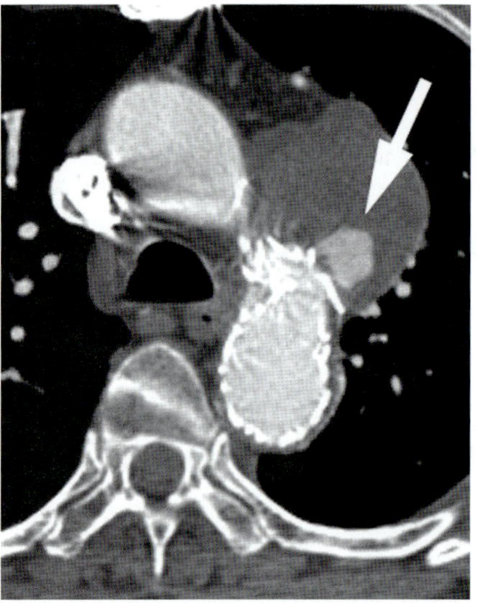

Fig. 22. Small endoleak following stent-graft deployment over an aortic arch aneurysm. The endoleak was not detected with flush aortography

clusion of such flow. MDCTA also helps in depicting the relationship of the aortic stent graft and the brachiocephalic arterial origins.

Conclusion

MDCTA offers a rapid, noninvasive, and accurate "one-stop" technique for evaluation of several thoracic aortic abnormalities [11, 33]. To optimize workflow and interpretation, efficient image postprocessing workstations and software are critical for large MDCTA image datasets [16]. In addition, it is important to update the scanning technique for optimum image acquisition and radiation dose as MDCT scanners evolve from 4-, 16-, 32-, and 40- to 64-slice configurations.

References

1. Lembcke A, Dohmen P, Rodenwaldt J et al (2003) Images in cardiovascular medicine. Recoarctation of the aorta associated with ascending aortic aneurysm demonstrated by ECG-gated multislice CT. Circulation. 107:e80–81
2. Marten K, Funke M, Rummeny EJ, Engelke C (2005) Electrocardiographic assistance in multidetector CT of thoracic disorders. Clin Radiol 60:8–21
3. Remy-Jardin M, Remy J, Wattinne L, Giraud F (1992) Central pulmonary thromboembolism: Diagnosis with spiral volumetric CT with the single-breath-hold technique - Comparison with pulmonary angiography. Radiology 185:381–387
4. Rubin GD, Lane MJ, Bloch DA (1996) Optimization of contrast enhanced thoracic spiral CT. Radiology 201:785–791
5. Prokop M, Schaefer CM, Leppert AGA, Galanski M (1993) Spiral CT Angiography of Thoracic Aorta: Femoral or Antecubital Injection Site for Intravenous Administration of Contrast Material? Radiology 189(P):111
6. Posniak HV, Olson MC, Demos TC (1993) Aortic motion artifact simulating dissection on CT scans: elimination with reconstructive segmented images. AJR Am J Roentgenol 161:557–558
7. Rubin GD, Dake MD, Semba CB (1995) Current status of three-dimensional spiral CT scanning for imaging the vasculature. Radiologic Clinics of North America 33:51–70
8. Napel S, Rubin GD, Jeffrey RB Jr (1993) STS-MIP: A new reconstruction technique for CT of the chest. J Comput Assist Tomogr 17:832–838
9. Rubin GD, Dake MD, Napel S et al (1994) Spiral CT of renal artery stenosis: comparison of three-dimensional rendering techniques. Radiology 190:181–189
10. Keller PJ, Drayer BP, Fram EK et al (1989) MR angiography with two-dimensional acquisition and three-dimensional display. Radiology 173:527–532
11. Napel S, Marks MP, Rubin GD et al (1992) CT angiography with spiral CT and maximum intensity projection. Radiology 185:607–610
12. Drebin RA, Carpenter L, Hanrahan P (1988) Volume rendering. Comput Graphics 22:65–74
13. Levoy M (1991) Methods for improving the efficiency and versatility of volume rendering. Prog Clin Biol Res 363:473–488
14. Rusinek H, Mourino MR, Firooznia H et al (1989) Volumetric rendering of MR images. Radiology 171:269–272
15. Fishman EK, Drebin B, Magid D et al (1987) Volumetric rendering techniques: applications for three-dimensional imaging of the hip. Radiology 163:737–738
16. Rubin GD, Beaulieu CF, Argiro V et al (1996) Perspective volume rendering of CT and MR images: applications for endoscopic imaging. Radiology 199:321–330
17. Katz M, Konen E, Rozsenman J et al (1995) Spiral CT and 3D image reconstruction of vascular ring and associated tracheobronchial anomalies. J Comput Assist Tomogr 19:564–568
18. Hopkins KL, Patrick LE, Simoneaux SF, Bank ER et al (1996) Pediatric great vessel anomalies: initial clinical experience with spiral CT angiography. Radiology 200:811–815
19. Quint LE, Francis IR, Williams DM et al (1996) Evaluation of thoracic aortic disease with the use of helical CT and multiplanar reconstructions: comparison with surgical findings. Radiology 201:37–41
20. Masuda Y, Takanashi K, Takasu J (1992) Expansion rate of thoracic aortic aneurysms and influencing factors. Chest 102:461–466
21. Dapunt L, Galla JD, Sadeghi AM et al (1994) The natural history of thoracic aortic aneurysms. J Thorac Cardiovasc Surg 107:1323–1333
22. Cigarroa JE, Isselbacher EM, DeSanctis RW, Eagle KA (1993) Medical progress. diagnostic imaging in the evaluation of suspected aortic dissection: old standards and new directions. AJR Am J Roentgenol 161:485–493
23. Erbel R, Daniel W, Visser C et al (1989) Echocardiography in diagnosis of aortic dissection. Lancet March 4:457–461
24. Nienaber CA, Kodolitsch Yv, Nicolas V et al (1993) The diagnosis of thoracic aortic dissection by non-invasive imaging procedures. NEJM 328:1–9
25. Nienaber CA, Kodolitsch Yv, Petersen B et al (1995) Intramural hemorrhage of the thoracic aorta: diagnostic and therapeutic implications. Circulation 92:1465–1472
26. Kazerooni EA, Bree RL, Williams DM (1992) Penetrating atherosclerotic ulcers of the descending thoracic aorta: evaluation with CT and distinction from aortic dissection. Radiology 183:759–765
27. Gore I (1952) Pathogenesis of dissecting aneurysm of the aorta. Arch Pathol Lab Med 53:142–153
28. Mirvis SE, Shanmuganathan K, Miller BH et al (1996) Traumatic aortic injury: diagnosis with contrast-enhanced thoracic CT - five year experience at a major trauma center. Radiology 200:413–422
29. Gavant ML, Manke PG, Fabian T et al (1995) Blunt traumatic aortic rupture: detection with helical CT of the chest. Radiology 197:125–133
30. Parker MS, Matheson TL, Rao AV et al (2001) Making the transition: the role of helical CT in the evaluation of potentially acute thoracic aortic injuries. AJR Am J Roentgenol 176:1267–1272
31. Dyer DS, Moore EE, Mestek MF et al (1999) Can chest CT be used to exclude aortic injury? Radiology 213:195–202
32. Armerding MD, Rubin GD, Beaulieu CF et al (2000) Aortic aneurysmal disease: assessment of stent-graft treatment-CT versus conventional angiography. Radiology 215:138–146
33. Rubin GD, Dake MD, Napel SA et al (1993) Abdominal spiral CT angiography: Initial clinical experience. Radiology 186:147–152

18

Pulmonary Embolism Imaging with MDCT

Joseph J. Kavanagh, Douglas R. Lake, Philip Costello

Introduction

The timely and accurate diagnosis of acute pulmonary embolism (PE) is crucial to providing appropriate patient care. Acute PE is a treatable condition with a 3-month mortality rate greater than 15% [1]. Potential complications include cardiogenic shock, hypotension, and myocardial infarction. PE is a relatively common condition, with an estimated overall incidence of about 1 per 1,000 patients within the United States [2]. Of approximately 1,000 computed tomography (CT) studies recently performed to assess for PE at our institution, roughly 10% were found to have PE. Unfortunately, the presenting symptoms of acute PE are relatively nonspecific and may be challenging for the clinician. Symptoms include dyspnea, cough, chest pain, and infrequently, hemoptysis. Chest radiography, electrocardiography (ECG), arterial blood gas measurements, and D-dimer assays all have the potential to suggest PE, but they are nonspecific [3–9]. Radiological imaging plays a crucial role in definitive diagnosis. Many modalities, including pulmonary angiography, ventilation-perfusion scintigraphy (V/Q), compression Doppler sonography, and CT have played important roles in the diagnosis of acute PE.

Over the last 5 years, multidetector CT (MDCT) pulmonary angiography has become the initial diagnostic test of choice in many institutions. Meanwhile, conventional angiography, V/Q scan, and Doppler sonography have been relegated to adjunctive roles [10–12]. Many retrospective and some prospective studies have been completed to prove the accuracy of MDCT for detecting and excluding patients suspected of acute PE. Through this research, there has been a transition from the "gold standard" of pulmonary angiography and V/Q scintigraphy to MDCT as the modality of choice for excluding PE.

Advantages of MDCT

CT has many advantages when compared with other available modalities in the detection of PE. MDCT pulmonary angiography is a rapid test, which can be obtained in a single 10-s breath hold with a 16-slice CT system. CT also has the ability to readily detect other abnormalities that may be contributing to the patient's clinical presentation, including congestive heart failure, pneumonia, interstitial lung disease, aortic dissection, malignancy (Fig. 1), and pleural disease [13, 14].

Due to the relative frequency of PE, its high mortality rate if not treated, and our ability to adequately treat it, the diagnosis of acute PE using CT has been the subject of much research. Multiple studies comparing MDCT with selective pulmonary angiography have shown a negative pre-

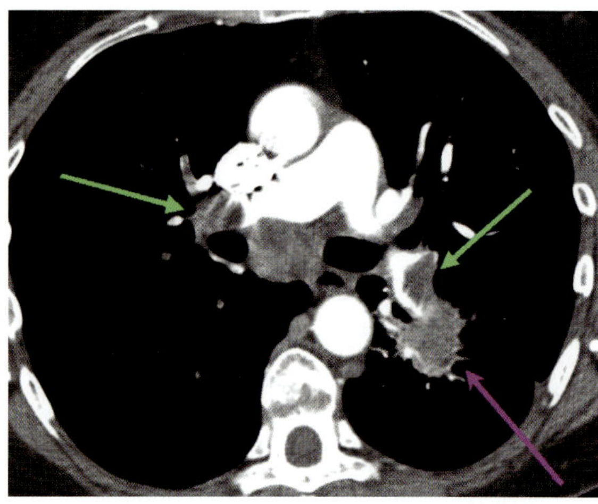

Fig. 1. A 53-year-old woman presented to the emergency department with acute shortness of breath and left-lower-extremity swelling. Multidetector computed tomography (MDCT) pulmonary angiogram axial image demonstrated large pulmonary emboli (*green arrows*) within the left and right main pulmonary arteries as well as an incidentally found left perihilar lung cancer (*purple arrow*)

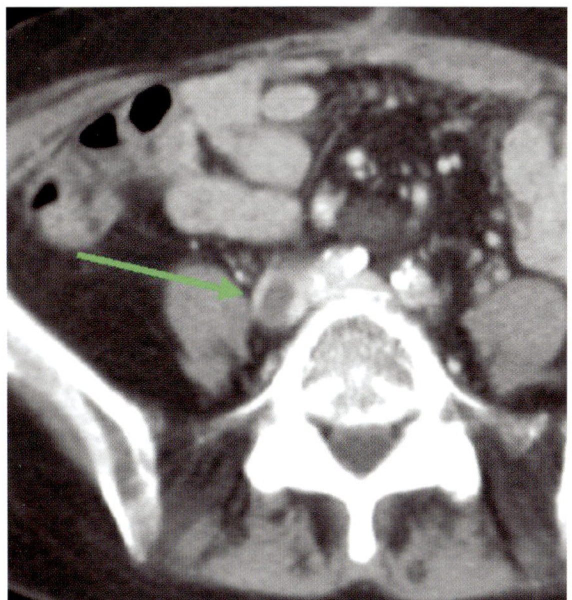

Fig. 2. A computed tomography venography (CTV) exam was performed simultaneously with a CT pulmonary angiogram in a 68-year-old woman with a history of ovarian cancer presenting with dyspnea. Axial CTV image demonstrates a filling defect (*arrow*) within the right common iliac artery consistent with thrombus. Images through the chest failed to demonstrate pulmonary embolism

ative predictive value (NPV) of 99%, which compares favorably with NPVs of conventional pulmonary angiography and greatly exceeds that of V/Q scintigraphy (76–88%) [15, 29–32]. These studies suggest that a negative MDCT pulmonary angiogram does not require any additional radiologic tests to help exclude the presence of acute PE. Because of its high sensitivity and specificity, MDCT can be both a screening and confirmatory study. Use of CT would help decrease additional and unnecessary imaging tests and limit the time between clinical presentation and effective treatment. More recently, the greater spatial resolution of MDCT has permitted the detection of small subsegmental emboli in sixth- and seventh-order arterial branches with a high degree of interobserver agreement [33–35]. Selective pulmonary angiography has low interobserver agreement rates, ranging from 45–66% [36, 37]. Similarly, V/Q scintigraphy has not only poor interobserver agreement rates but also poor specificity of low probability studies (10%). Additionally, up to 73% of V/Q scans are reported as intermediate probability [15, 30].

dictive value greater than 96% for both single-slice [15–21] and MDCT [22, 14, 23–27] in PE detection. A large prospective study by Perrier et al. [28] showed that patients with a negative D-dimer and a negative MDCT pulmonary angiogram had less than a 1% chance of having a lower-extremity deep venous thrombosis and a 3-month follow-up thromboembolic risk of only about 1.5%. A meta-analysis of 3,500 patients with a negative CT study who did not receive anticoagulation showed a neg-

In addition to imaging the pulmonary arterial system, CT venography (CTV) may be performed to assess for venous thrombosis within the pelvis and lower extremities. Delayed venous-phase images from the pelvis through the knees are obtained 180 s following intravenous contrast injection. CTV is able to detect venous thrombosis in the pelvis veins, which is typically not possible during Doppler sonography due to overlying bowel gas (Fig. 2). Acute deep venous thrombosis (DVT) on CTV is detected as a filling defect within the vein (Fig. 3). Other signs include perivenous stranding, mural enhancement, and vein enlargement [38]. A study by Cosmic et al. [39] showed that up to 11% of patients with a negative chest CT

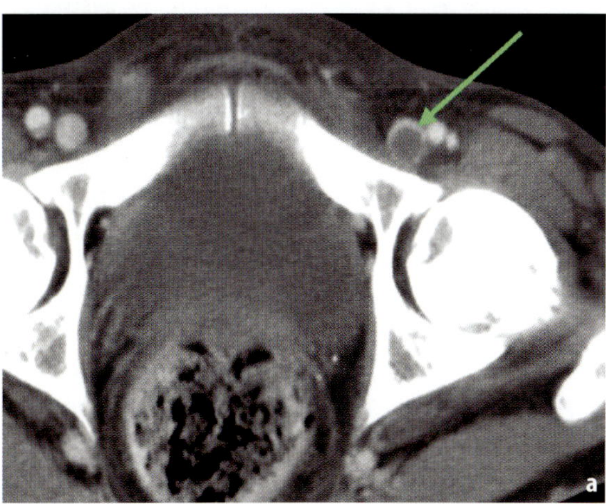

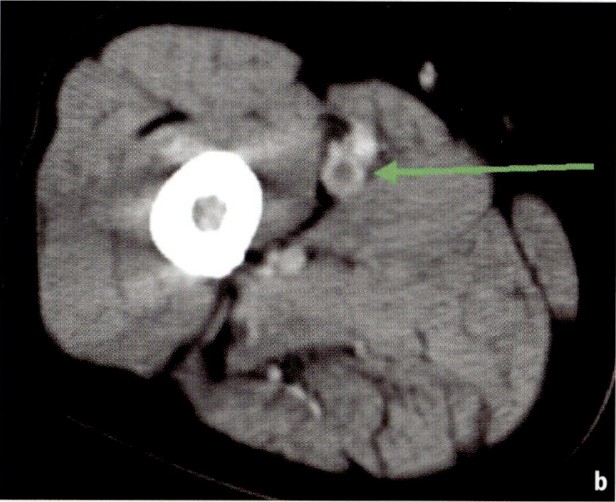

Fig. 3a, b. Axial computed tomography venography (CTV) images in two different patients presenting for CT pulmonary angiography demonstrate filling defects surrounded by intravenous contrast consistent with deep venous thrombosis (DVT) (*arrows*) in both the left common femoral vein (**a**) and right superficial femoral vein (**b**)

demonstrated venous thrombosis on CTV. Although this study did not take into account D-dimer levels, it proved the efficacy of imaging both the pelvis and lower-extremity venous structures following CT of the pulmonary arteries.

PE Findings Using MDCT

Most commonly, PE presents on CT as a filling defect within a pulmonary artery surrounded by a thin rim of contrast. These emboli often lodge at bifurcation points, extending into peripheral arteries (Fig. 4). When viewed in the transverse plane, the emboli may be described as having a "polomint" or "lifesaver" appearance (Fig. 5). When seen longitudinally, these filling defects may present as a "railway-track" sign, with the clot surrounded by contrast material within the vessel lumen (Fig. 6).

Occasionally, an abrupt arterial cutoff may be encountered, with complete obstruction of the pulmonary artery [40–43].

Secondary signs of acute PE are often present and may clue the radiologist to the presence of an embolus. On lung windows, small, wedge-shaped and peripheral areas of consolidation or ground glass opacity are seen in approximately 25% of patients [44]. These opacities mostly represent areas of pulmonary hemorrhage that clear within 4–7 days, but some represent pulmonary infarcts (Fig. 7). Pulmonary infarcts on CT appear as wedge-shaped peripheral opacities often characterized as a "Hampton hump" (Fig. 8). With larger emboli, there may be regions of localized oligemia and redistribution of blood flow (mosaic perfusion) in the involved portions of lung (Fig. 9). Frequent but nonspecific signs of PE include subsegmental atelectasis and small pleural effusions.

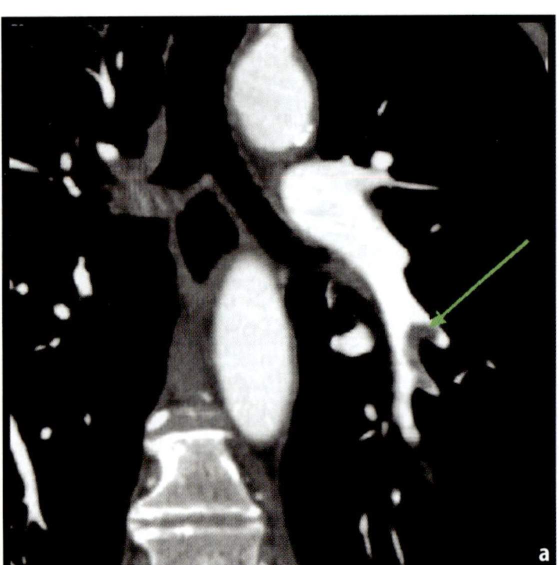

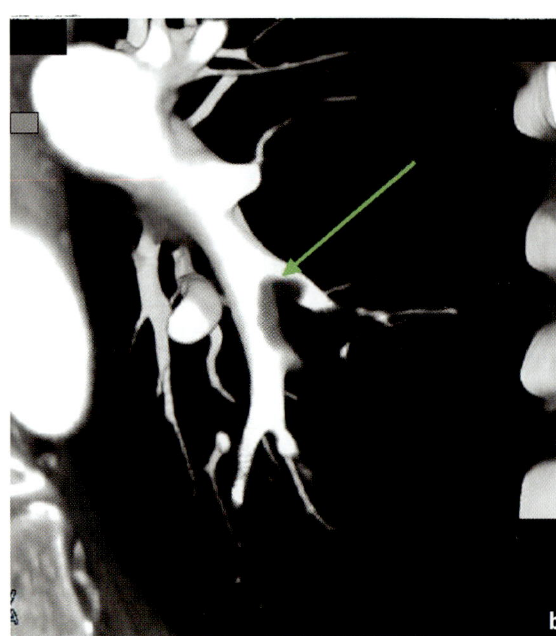

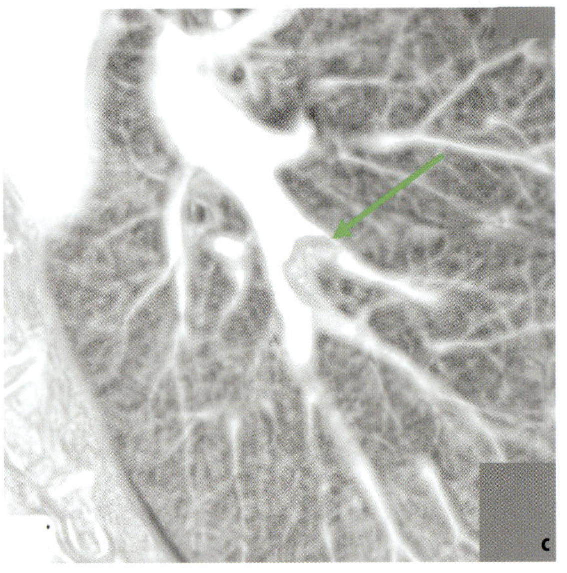

Fig. 4a-c. Sagittal multiplanar reformation (MPR) images (**a**) from a multidetector computed tomography (MDCT) pulmonary angiogram obtained in a patient with metastatic pancreatic cancer and shortness of breath demonstrate a filling defect at a branching point within the left lower lobe pulmonary artery, with extension into the segmental arterial branches (*arrow*). Three-dimensional (3-D) volume-rendered displays (**b, c**) help demonstrate the full extent of this embolus (*arrows*)

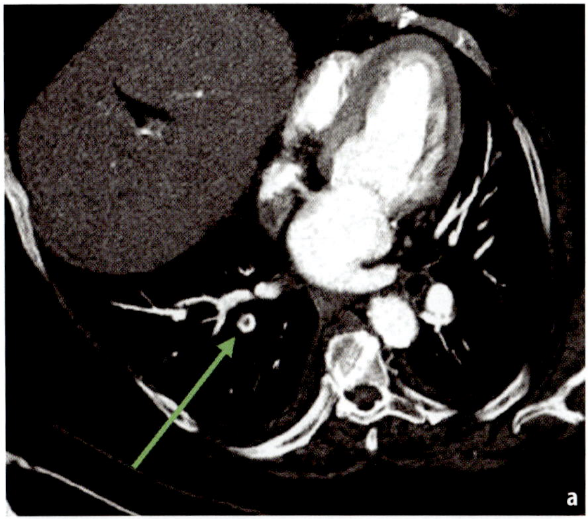

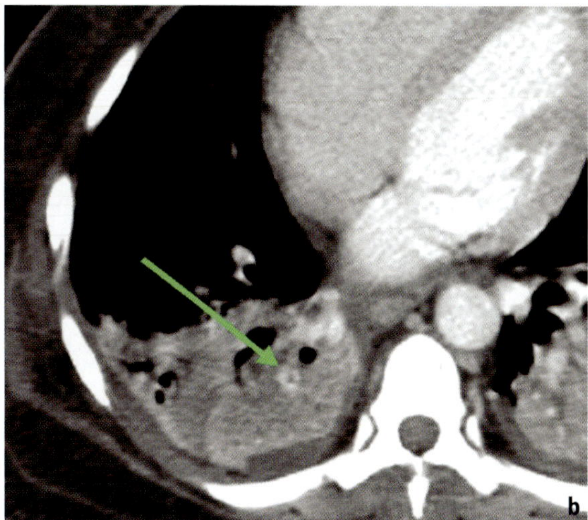

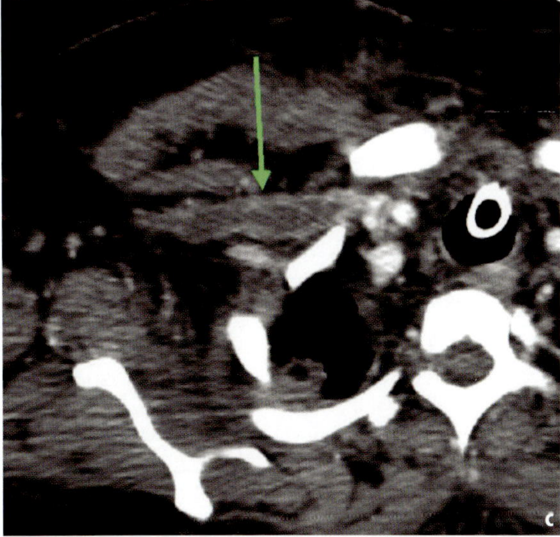

Fig. 5a-c. Multidetector computed tomography (MDCT) images of the "lifesaver" or "polo-mint" sign indicating pulmonary emboli visualized in the transverse plane. Oblique multiplanar reformation (MPR) images from an MDCT data set (**a**) demonstrate a filling defect within a right lower lobe segmental pulmonary artery (*arrow*). Axial MDCT images from a different patient, a 44-year-old woman with tachypnea and tachycardia following a motor vehicle collision (**b**), demonstrate a small subsegmental right lower lobe pulmonary artery filling defect surrounded by atelectatic lung (*arrow*). Axial images from higher in her chest (**c**) incidentally discovered thrombus in the right subclavian vein (*arrow*)

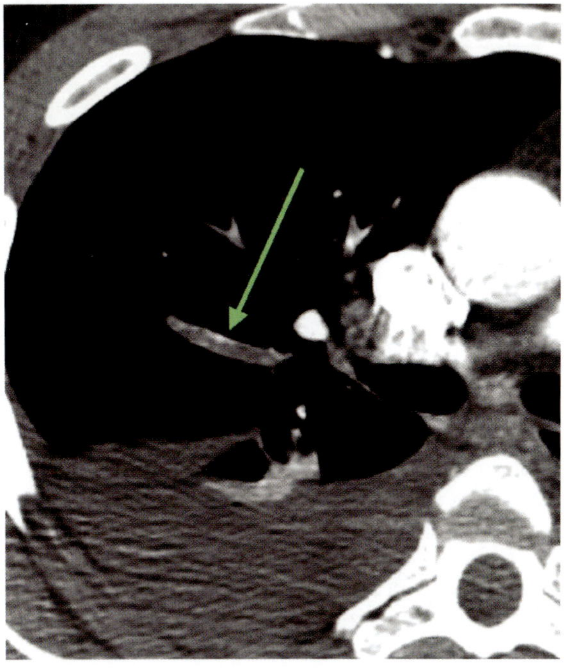

Fig. 6. Multidetector computed tomography (MDCT) images from CT pulmonary angiography in the axial plane demonstrate thrombus tracking longitudinally through a right middle lobe pulmonary artery feeding the lateral segment (*arrow*) with a characteristic "railway-track" appearance

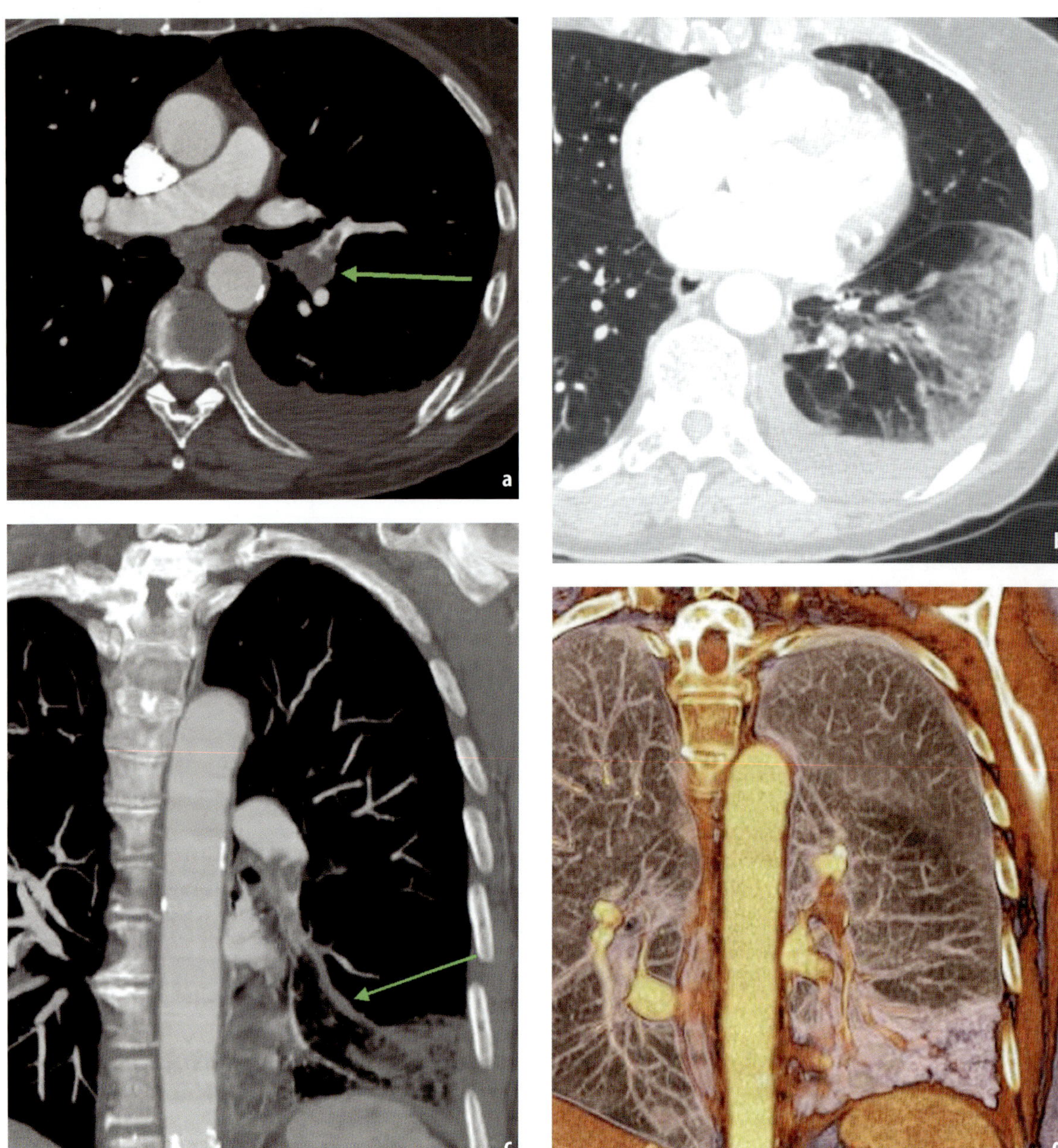

Fig. 7a-d. An 80-year-old woman presented with chest pain on the left with deep inspiration. Single-axial contrast-enhanced image (**a**) demonstrates a large embolus within the left main pulmonary artery extending into the left lower lobe pulmonary artery (*arrow*). Axial slice examined using lung windows (**b**) demonstrates a wedge-shaped region of ground-glass opacity in the periphery of the left lower lobe consistent with hemorrhage. Coronal multiplanar reconstruction (MPR) image (**c**) shows thrombus extending into the area of hemorrhage (*arrow*). Coronal three-dimensional (3-D) volume rendering (**d**) again demonstrates the large embolus and area of hemorrhage

Prognostic Value of CT in PE Patients

In addition to diagnosing emboli and other potential etiologies of dyspnea and chest pain, CT may provide some insight into the prognosis of patients with PE. There are cardiac findings on CT that may portend a worse clinical prognosis or warrant more emergent care in an intensive care unit and possible catheter intervention, thrombolysis, or surgical embolectomy, in addition to anticoagulation. Poor prognostic factors relate to the degree of right ventricular dysfunction and include the degree of right ventricular enlargement (Fig. 10), pulmonary artery thrombus load, enlargement of the main pulmonary artery, reflux of contrast into the hepatic veins (Fig. 11), and bowing of the ventricular septum toward the left ventricle.

Patients with a right ventricular diameter to left ventricular diameter (RVD/LVD) ratio of

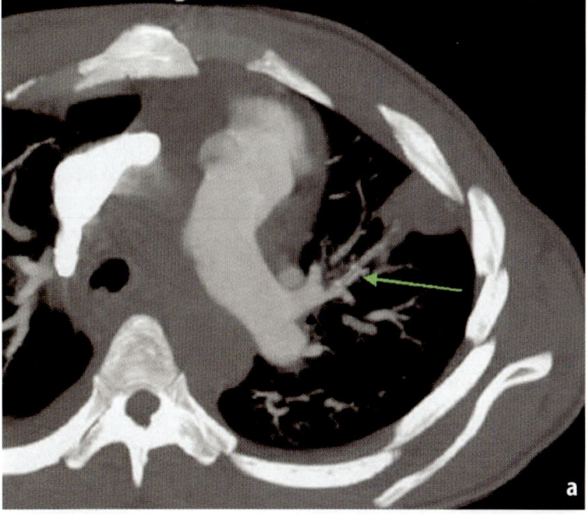

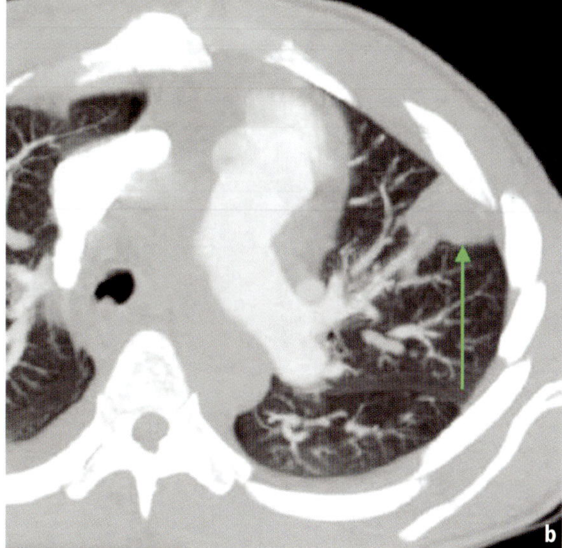

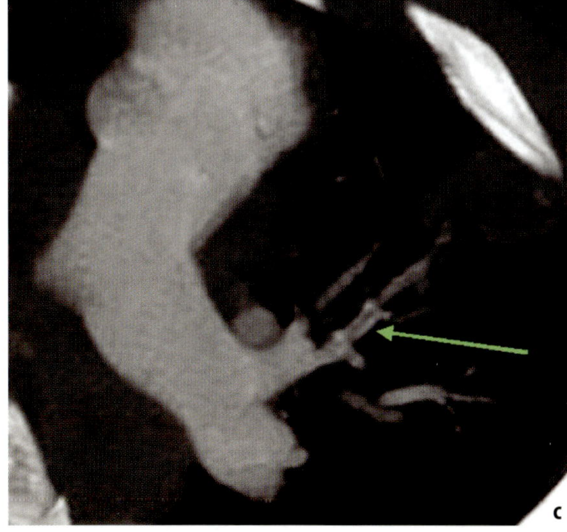

Fig. 8a-c. Axial image (**a**) from a computed tomographic (CT) pulmonary angiogram demonstrates a segmental embolus within the left upper lobe extending to a peripheral area of dense consolidation (CT Hampton hump) (*arrow*). Axial image obtained using lung windows (**b**) clearly defines the wedge-shaped region of infarcted lung (*arrow*). Magnified axial view of the embolus (**c**) demonstrates the "railway-track" appearance of the thrombus in the longitudinal plane (*arrow*)

greater than 0.9 have a significant increase in mortality and a much greater likelihood of major complications [45–47]. One study showed a positive predictive value for PE-related mortality of 10.1% within the first 3 months after the diagnosis of PE with right ventricular enlargement (RVD/LVD ratio greater than 1.0). Perhaps more significantly, in those patients with a RVD/LVD ratio less than 1.0, there was a negative predictive value of 100% for an uneventful course [48]. Therefore, those patients without right ventricular enlargement are less unlikely to have an adverse outcome and are more likely to survive. Therefore, signs of right heart strain should be mentioned in the report and discussed with the referring physician, as they represent important prognostic factors that could assist in treatment planning and patient placement.

Studies have also shown a relationship between the percentage of pulmonary vascular bed obstruction and 3-month mortality. A scoring system based upon the number and degree of vascular obstructions was utilized. The highest possible score of 40 indicates complete obstruction of the pulmonary trunk [49]. Patients with a degree of vascular obstruction of greater than 40% have an 11% increased risk of dying from PE within the first 3 months. The negative predictive value in patients with a less than 40% degree of obstruction was 99%; indicating a very low rate of PE-related mortality [48, 50].

PE Protocol Using MDCT

Protocols employed for the detection of PE have evolved with rapid advances in CT technology.

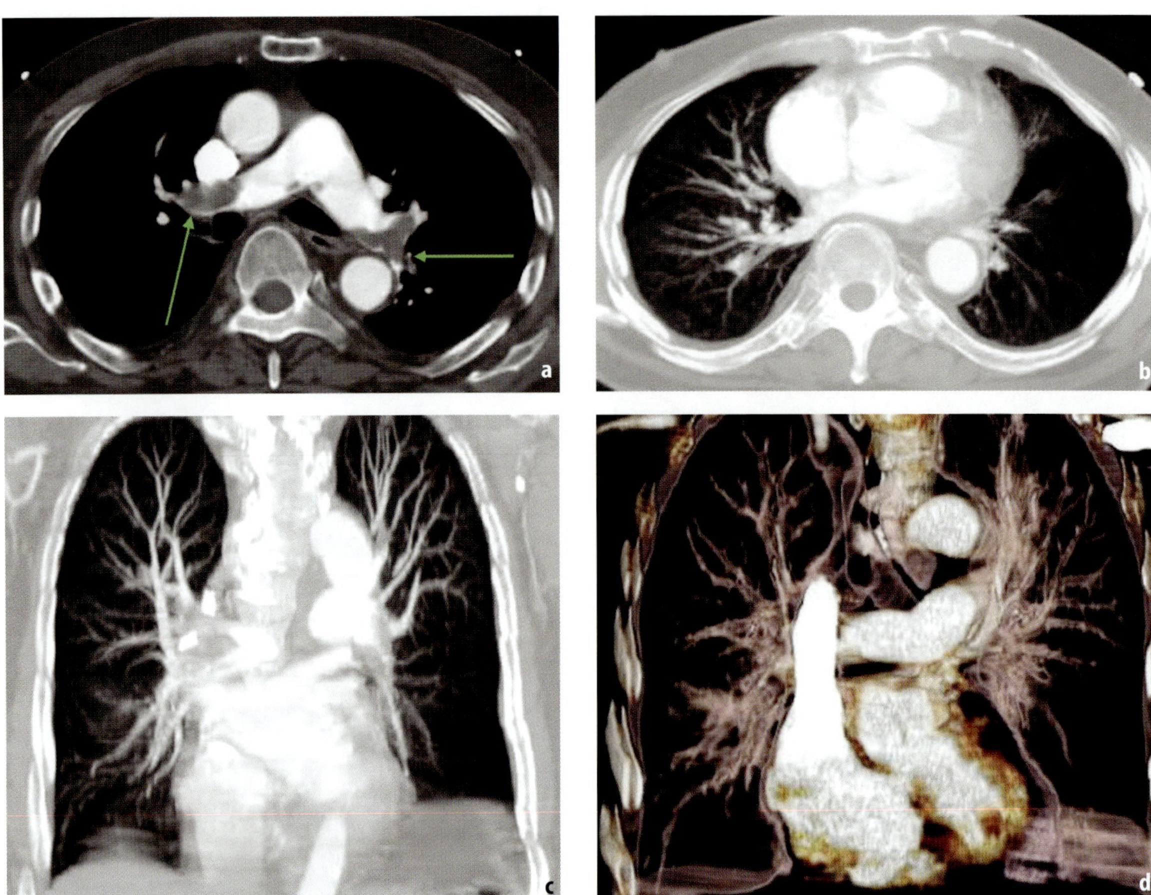

Fig. 9a-d. Axial image from a multidetector computed tomography (MDCT) pulmonary angiogram (**a**) demonstrates bilateral pulmonary emboli in a patient with acute shortness of breath and right lower extremity swelling (*arrows*). Axial image through the lower lobes using lung windows (**b**) demonstrates oligemia in the left lower lobe (CT Westermark sign). Coronal multiplanar reconstruction (MPR) image (**c**) again demonstrates the asymmetric hypovascularity in the left lower lobe. Three-dimensional (3-D) volume rendering in the coronal plane (**d**) more clearly defines the region of oligemia

Current MDCT scanners are capable of providing image resolution of less than 1 mm. Patient respiratory motion artifacts have decreased dramatically over the last few years as acquisition of the entire thorax can be obtained in under 10 s using a 16-slice scanner and in less than 5 s with 64-slice units.

The quality of enhancement of the pulmonary arteries relies on several parameters: the amount and concentration of contrast agent used, the injection rate, and the delay between injection and scanning. To ensure adequate opacification of the pulmonary arteries, images are obtained 20 s following intravenous administration or, preferably, by using bolus tracking software to determine peak contrast delivery to the pulmonary arteries (Table 1).

Scan delay is obtained by injecting 15 ml of contrast material and placing a region of interest over the main pulmonary artery. Using a high concentration contrast agent, such as Isovue-370, and a rapid flow rate of up to 4 ml/s ensures ideal vascular opacification. Injection of contrast media is typically via an 18- or 20-gauge peripheral intravenous line, preferably through the antecubital vein. A saline chaser may be used to decrease the amount of beam-hardening artifact caused by dense opacification of the superior vena cava and to decrease the amount of iodinated contrast needed to adequately opacify the pulmonary arteries [51–53]. While shorter scan times decrease respiratory motion and associated artifacts, timing the delivery of contrast becomes very critical with 16- and 64-slice protocols (Table 1).

In patients who are physically larger than average, 2.0–2.5 mm acquisitions can be used to decrease quantum mottle [43]. ECG gating has been recently implemented in some institutions to elim-

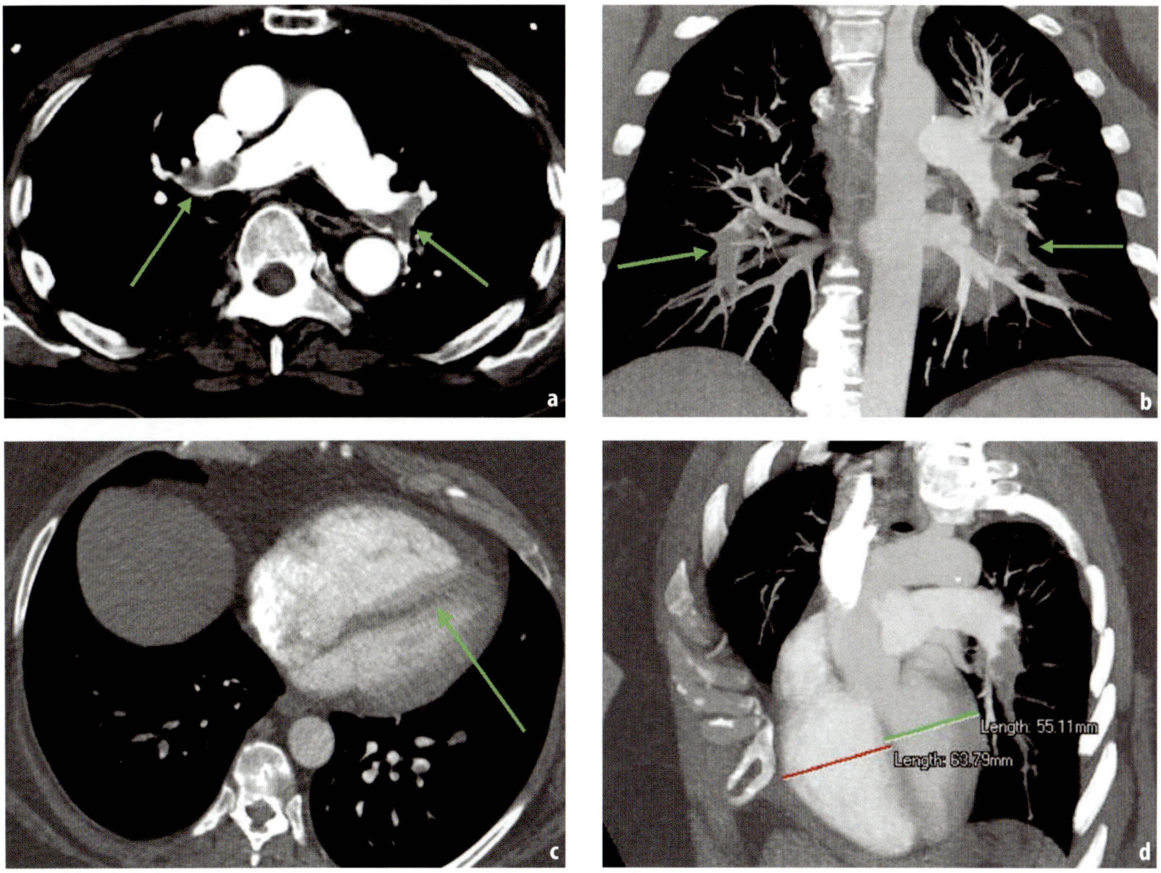

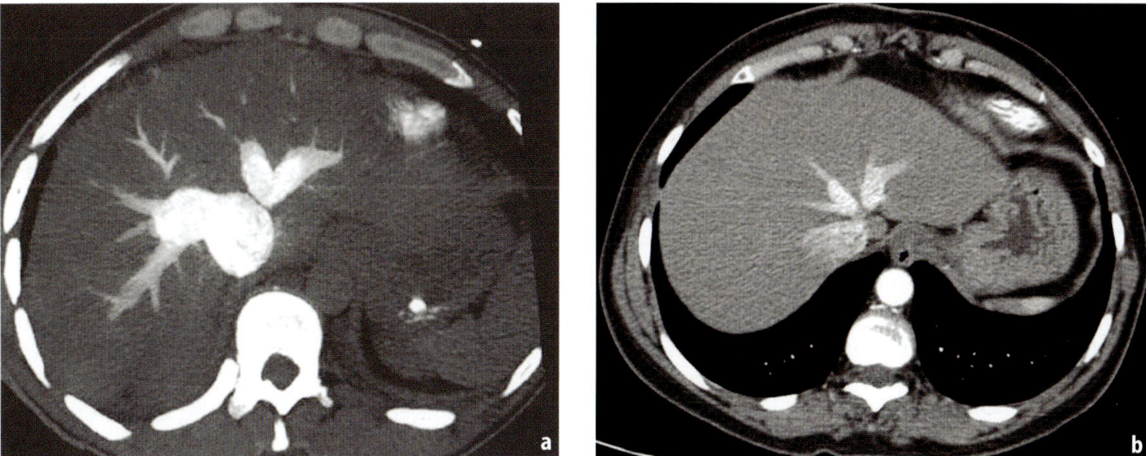

Fig. 10a-d. Computed tomographic (CT) pulmonary angiogram performed in a 49-year-old woman with chest pain and shortness of breath. Axial image through the pulmonary arteries (**a**) demonstrates large emboli within the left and right pulmonary arteries (*arrows*). Coronal multiplanar reconstruction (MPR) image (**b**) more clearly demonstrates the extent of the emboli (*arrows*). Axial image through the ventricular septum (**c**) reveals straightening of the septum and dilation of the right ventricle (*arrow*). Further evaluation with oblique MPR (**d**) clearly shows a right ventricular diameter (*red line*) that is larger than the left ventricular (*green line*) diameter (RVD/LVD ratio >1) consistent with right ventricular dysfunction

Fig. 11a, b. Axial images (**a, b**) obtained during multidetector computed tomography (MDCT) pulmonary angiography in two different patients show reflux of intravenous contrast into the hepatic veins, which is a sign of right ventricular dysfunction. The first image (**a**) also demonstrates distention of the hepatic veins. Both patients had large pulmonary emboli

Table 1. Computed tomography (CT) protocols: CT pulmonary angiography

Scanner type	4-slice	16-slice	64-slice
Collimation		16 × 0.75	64 × 0.6
Reconstruction (mm)	1.25	1.00	0.75
Rotation time (s)	0.8	0.5	0.33
Contrast volume (370 mgI/ml)	100 ml	100 ml	75–100 ml
Saline flush		50 ml	50 ml

inate cardiac pulsation artifacts seen in small vessels adjacent to the heart; however, this technique requires a longer breath hold and increased radiation exposure. When viewing the pulmonary arterial system, window and level settings should be placed around 700 and 1,000 Hounsfield units (HU), respectively [43, 54].

Currently employed MDCT yields very large numbers of axial images – up to 1,000 with some newer systems. This can result in difficulties for the interpreting radiologist due to the sheer number of images to review. Two potential solutions include display tools and computer-aided diagnosis (CAD), which allow for rapid production of maximum intensity projection (MIP) images, multiplanar reconstructions (MPR), and three-dimensional (3-D) reformations. These reformations and reconstructions of the source images allow improved visualization of distal subsegmental pulmonary arterial branches with reconstruction of fewer overall images, without sacrificing PE detection sensitivity. CAD tools are under development and may be used as a second reader, potentially reducing study reading times. Preliminary experience in a small study population showed CAD tools can detect segmental emboli but are currently inaccurate for subsegmental emboli [55].

Disadvantages to MDCT

Approximately 3% of the CT scans completed for PE at our institution are inadequate for accurate interpretation [56]. Most problems relate to technical factors, including poor bolus timing and poor venous access. Correctly applied bolus tracking with density measurements over the pulmonary artery provides scan-precise delay times and optimal enhancement of the pulmonary arteries. Beam-hardening artifacts from dense contrast bolus within the superior vena cava may obscure small emboli in adjacent vessels (Fig. 12), particularly in the right main and right upper lobe pulmonary arteries [43]. Saline bolus chasing follow-

ing initial contrast injection with a dual-head injector can eliminate these artifacts completely. Abrupt loss of pulmonary artery opacification caused by the mixing of unopacified blood from the inferior vena cava may occur. This pulmonary artery flow artifact, also known as a "stripe sign," occurs during inspiration and results in loss of the contrast column in the pulmonary arteries; thus mimicking emboli [57, 58].

Patient factors that may hinder PE interpretation most often involve a large patient body habitus, leading to increased quantum mottle or an inability to breath hold for the desired length of time, resulting in motion artifact. Additional diagnostic pitfalls include partial volume averaging from hilar lymph nodes and mucous-filled bronchi. By utilizing a combination of workstation analysis, MIP, and MPR, both lymph nodes and mucous-filled bronchi can be distinguished from adjacent pulmonary arteries [59].

Radiation dose considerations with CT require careful evaluation when developing protocols. During a typical CT pulmonary angiogram, the effective patient dose ranges from 4-8 mSv, with an absorbed breast dose of 21 mGy [60]. As a comparison, the absorbed breast dose during a screening mammogram is only 2.5 mGy [60]. However, the risk-to-benefit ratio of using CT for diagnosing PE typically weighs heavily in favor of performing the study. CT pulmonary angiography using a single-slice scanner utilizes a radiation dose five times less than that of conventional angiography [61]. Performing CT examinations in young or pregnant women requires special considerations. In a young woman with a negative chest radiograph and low-to-moderate clinical suspicion, a V/Q scan might be considered as a more appropriate option. However, many patients undergo a subsequent CT study, so additional radiation burden to the female breast should be carefully evaluated. In pregnant patients with suspected PE, CT is recommended over V/Q scintigraphy, as the absorbed radiation dose to the fetus is 1–2 mGy for V/Q scans versus 0.1-0.2 mGy for CT [62, 63].

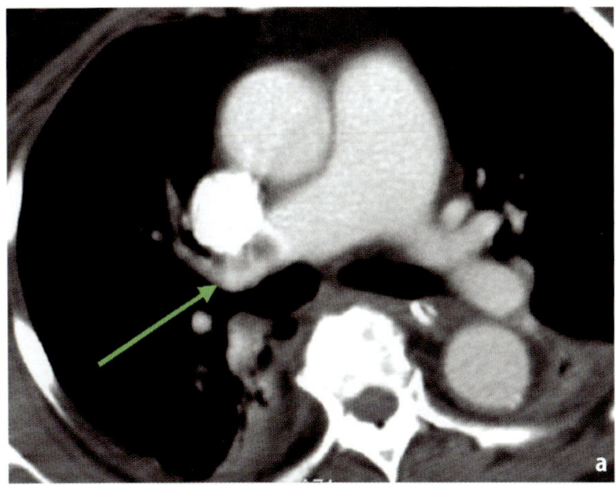
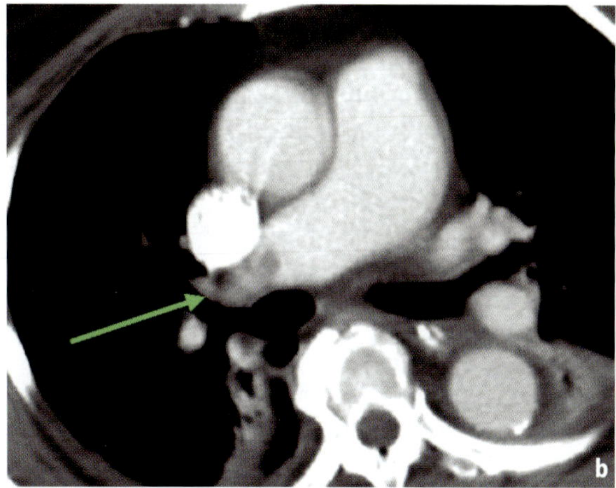

Fig. 12a, b. A 76-year-old woman who was postoperatively day 1 from a bilateral salpingooophorectomy presented with decreased breath sounds in the right lung base, decreased oxygen saturation, and increased A-a gradient. Subsequent axial images from a contrast-enhanced multidetector computed tomography (MDCT) study (**a, b**) demonstrate beam-hardening artifact almost completely obscuring a large thrombus within the right main pulmonary artery (*arrows*). A saline chaser following injection of the iodinated contrast would have eliminated this artifact

Role of D-Dimer

D-dimer enzyme-linked immunosorbent assays (ELISA) play an important role in the workup for possible PE. D-dimer is a highly sensitive test (97%) with a negative predictive value of 99.6% [4]. This inexpensive measurement is an effective screening test in the outpatient setting for suspected PE. As a result, further diagnostic tests would be unnecessary in patients with a negative D-dimer assay, as there would be a very low likelihood of PE [64, 65]. Taking this one step further, Perrier et al. [28] showed that patients have a very low likelihood of having any adverse affects related to PE when there is a negative CT angiogram and a negative D-dimer assay. Therefore, these patients are not only unlikely to have a PE, but they are also unlikely to suffer any adverse events secondary to venous thromboembolism within 3 months of the negative diagnostic tests. Unfortunately, the D-dimer assay is highly nonspecific and is of limited value within the inpatient setting. Other etiologies resulting in elevated D-dimer assays include cancer, myocardial infarction, pneumonia, sepsis, and pregnancy.

Future of MDCT

With continued technological improvements, MDCT pulmonary angiography will continue to be the test of choice for the diagnosis of PE. It is likely that these advances will center not only on hardware but also on the software used to reformat the large amount of acquired data during the CT examination. With slice thickness under 1.00 mm, there may be up to 1,000 axial images for the radiologist to evaluate. Unfortunately, small pulmonary emboli may be "overlooked" by having to individually examine each acquired image. In retrospect, these "perceptual errors" may be readily detectable: 60% of missed diagnoses occur because the embolus was simply not seen on first examination [66, 67]. CAD for PE has shown potential for limiting these perceptual errors [68, 69].

Advancements in the software used to create 2-D and 3-D reformations of the axial CT data will continue to improve our ability to detect emboli in obliquely oriented pulmonary arteries (Fig. 13) [70]. One promising technique involves performing "paddle wheel" reformations of the pulmonary arteries. A horizontal axis centered at the lung hila is used as a pivot point to image the pulmonary arteries. This type of multiplanar volume reformation helps prevent the "slicing" of pulmonary arteries into small fragments that are seen on coronal and sagittal reformations. Presumably, this will not only improve visualization of the pulmonary arterial tree but also decrease the overall number of images for the radiologist to review to accurately diagnose PE [71, 72].

Studies are also underway to assess the possibility of using a single, contrast-enhanced, ECG-gated CT scan to assess patients with chest pain for coronary artery disease, pulmonary disease, and aortic disease [73]. Results of PIOPED II, which prospectively compared V/Q scanning, Doppler sonography for DVT, digital subtraction pulmonary angiography, and contrast venography with MDCT for the detection of venous thromboembolism [41], may provide practice guidelines.

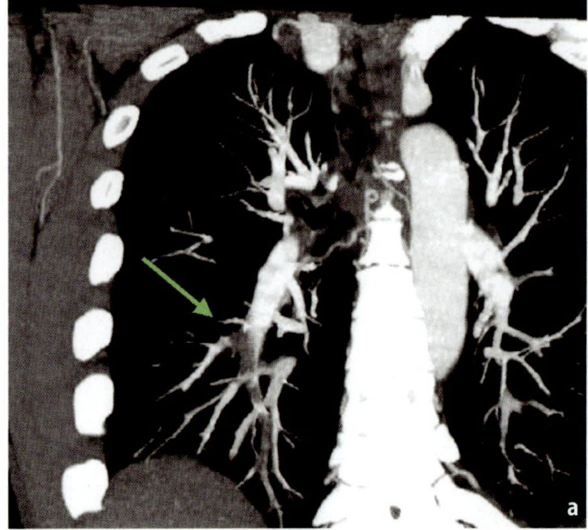
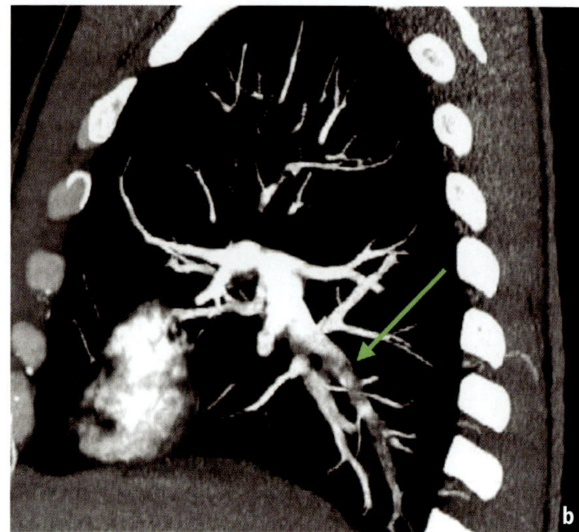
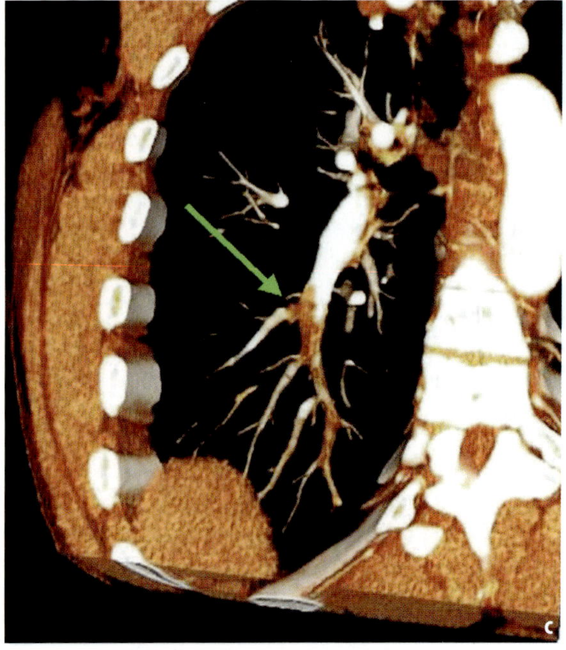

Fig. 13a-c. Computed tomographic (CT) pulmonary angiogram was obtained in a 42-year-old man presenting with chest pain and shortness of breath. Coronal (**a**) and sagittal (**b**) oblique multiplanar reproduction (MPR) images through the right lower lobe pulmonary artery demonstrate extensive thrombus extending almost the entire length of the artery (*arrows*). A three-dimensional (3-D) volume rendering of the multidetector computed tomography (MDCT) data set (**c**) more clearly demonstrates the mass-like nature and extent of the embolus (*arrow*)

Conclusion

CT pulmonary angiography has become the imaging modality of choice for the detection of acute PE. MDCT has proven sensitivity and specificity for detecting small pulmonary emboli in distal subsegmental pulmonary arteries with high interobserver agreement and cost effectiveness. Additionally, CT allows for the detection of other etiologies that may or may not be contributing to the patient's clinical presentation. When combined with CT venography, MDCT now provides a standalone test for excluding venous thromboembolism. High-risk patients with right ventricular dysfunction are also readily identifiable with CT pulmonary angiography, allowing for more appropriate management. Furthermore, continued improvements in postacquisition reformations and CAD will continue to enhance the ability to detect pulmonary emboli with an accuracy far exceeding that of other modalities.

References

1. Carson JL, Kelley MA, Duff A et al (1992) The clinical course of pulmonary embolism. N Engl J Med 326(19):1240–1245
2. Goldhaber SZ, Elliott CG (2003) Acute pulmonary embolism: part I: epidemiology, pathophysiology, and diagnosis. Circulation 108(22):2726–2729
3. Daniel KR, Courtney DM, Kline JA (2001) Assessment of cardiac stress from massive pulmonary embolism with 12-lead ECG. Chest 120:474–481
4. Dunn KL, Wolf JP, Dorfman DM et al (2002) Normal D-dimer levels in emergency department pa-

tients suspected of acute pulmonary embolism. J Am Coll Cardiol 40:1475–1478

5. Elliott CG, Goldhaber SZ, Visani L et al (2000) Chest radiographs in acute pulmonary embolism. Results from the international cooperative pulmonary embolism registry. Chest 118:33–38

6. Ferrari E, Imbert A, Chevalier T et al (1997) The ECG in pulmonary embolism: predictive value of negative T waves in precordial leads: 80 case reports. Chest 111:537–543

7. Kucher N, Walpoth N, Wustmann K et al (2003) QR in V1: an ECG sign associated with right ventricular strain and adverse clinical outcome in pulmonary embolism. Eur Heart J 24:1113–1119

8. Stein PD, Goldhaber SZ, Henry JW (1995) Alveolar-arterial oxygen gradient in the assessment of acute pulmonary embolism. Chest 107:139–143

9. Stein PD, Goldhaber SZ, Henry JW et al (1996) Arterial blood gas analysis in the assessment of suspected acute pulmonary embolism. Chest 109:78–81

10. Prologo JD, Glauser J (2002) Variable diagnostic approach to suspected pulmonary embolism in the ED of a major academic tertiary care center. Am J Emerg Med 20:5–9

11. Prologo JD, Gilkeson RC, Diaz M et al (2004) CT Pulmonary angiography: A comparative analysis of the utilization patterns in emergency department and hospitalized patients between 1998 and 2003. AJR Am J Roentgenol 183:1093–1096

12. Stein PD, Kayali F, Olson RE (2004) Trends in the use of diagnostic imaging in patients hospitalized with acute pulmonary embolism. Am J Cardiol 93:1316–1317

13. Kim KI, Muller NL, Mayo JR (1999) Clinically suspected pulmonary embolism: utility of spiral CT. Radiology 210:693–697

14. Kavanagh EC, O'Hare A, Hargaden G (2004) Risk of pulmonary embolism after negative MDCT pulmonary angiography findings. AJR Am J Roentgenol 182:499–504

15. Blachere H, Latrabe V, Montaudon M et al (2000) Pulmonary embolism revealed on helical CT angiography: comparison with ventilation-perfusion radionuclide lung scanning. AJR Am J Roentgenol 174:1041–1047

16. Bourriot K, Couffinhal T, Bernard V et al (2003) Clinical outcome after a negative spiral CT pulmonary angiographic finding in an inpatient setting from cardiology and pneumology wards. Chest 123:359–365

17. Garg K, Sieler H, Welsh CH et al (1999) Clinical validity of helical CT being interpreted as negative for pulmonary embolism: implications for patient treatment. AJR Am J Roentgenol 172:1627–1631

18. Goodman LR, Lipchik RJ, Kuzo RS et al (2000) Subsequent pulmonary embolism: risk after a negative helical CT pulmonary angiogram – prospective comparison with scintigraphy. Radiology 215: 535–542

19. Lomis NN, Yoon HC, Moran AG et al (1999) Clinical outcomes of patients after a negative spiral CT pulmonary arteriogram in the evaluation of acute pulmonary embolism. J Vasc Interv Radiol 10:707–712

20. Ost D, Rozenshtein A, Saffran L et al (2001) The negative predictive value of spiral computed tomography for the diagnosis of pulmonary embolism in patients with nondiagnostic ventilation-perfusion scans. Am J Med 110:16–21

21. Tillie-Leblond I, Mastora I, Radenne F et al (2002) Risk of pulmonary embolism after a negative spiral CT angiogram in patients with pulmonary disease: 1-year clinical follow-up study. Radiology 223: 461–467

22. Gottsater A, Berg A, Certergard J et al (2001) Clinically suspected pulmonary embolism: is it safe to withhold anticoagulation after a negative spiral CT? Eur Radiol 11:65–72

23. Krestan CR, Klein N, Fleischmann et al (2004) Value of negative spiral CT angiography in patients with suspected acute PE: analysis of PE occurrence and outcome. Eur Radiol 14:93–98

24. Musset D, Parent F, Meyer G et al (2002) Diagnostic strategy for patients with suspected pulmonary embolism: a prospective multicentre outcome study. Lancet 360:1914–1920

25. Nilsson T, Olausson A, Johnsson H et al (2002) Negative spiral CT in acute pulmonary embolism. Acta Radiol 43:486–491

26. Qanadli SC, Hajjam ME, Mesurolle B et al (2000) Pulmonary embolism detection: prospective evaluation of dual-section helical CT versus selective pulmonary arteriography in 157 patients. Radiology 217:447–455

27. Swensen SJ, Sheedy PF II, Ryu JH et al (2002) Outcomes after withholding anticoagulation from patients with suspected acute pulmonary embolism and negative computed tomographic findings: a cohort study. Mayo Clin Proc 77:130–138

28. Perrier A, Pierre-Marie R, Sanchez O et al (2005) Multidetector-row computed tomography in suspected pulmonary embolism. N Engl J Med 352:1760–1768

29. Henry JW, Stein PD, Gottschalk A et al (1996) Scintigraphic lung scans and clinical assessment in critically ill patients with suspected acute pulmonary embolism. Chest 109:462–466

30. PIOPED Investigators (1990) Value of the ventilation/perfusion scan in acute pulmonary embolism JAMA 95:498–502

31. Quiroz R, Kucher N, Zou KH et al (2005) Clinical validity of a negative computed tomography scan in patients with suspected pulmonary embolism – a systematic review. JAMA 293:2012–2017

32. van Beek EJ, Reekers JA, Batcherlor DA et al (1995) Feasibility, safety and clinical utility of angiography in patients with normal pulmonary angiograms. Chest 107:1375–1378

33. Ghaye B, Szapiro D, Mastora I et al (2001) Peripheral pulmonary arteries: how far in the lung does multi-detector row spiral CT allow analysis? Radiology 219:629–636

34. Patel S, Kazerooni EA, Cascade PN (2003) Pulmonary embolism: optimization of small pulmonary artery visualization at multi-detector row CT. Radiology 227:455–460

35. Schoepf UJ, Holzknecht N, Helmberger TK et al (2002) Subsegmental pulmonary emboli: improved detection with thin-collimation multi-detector row spiral CT. Radiology 222:483–490

36. Diffin DC, Leyendecker JR, Johnson SP et al (1998) Effect of anatomic distribution of pulmonary emboli on interobserver agreement in the interpreta-

tion of pulmonary angiography. AJR Am J Roentgenol 171:1085–1089

37. Stein PD, Henry JW, Gottschalk A (1999) Reassessment of pulmonary angiography for the diagnosis of pulmonary embolism: relation of interpreter agreement to the order of the involved pulmonary arterial branch. Radiology 210:689–691

38. Washington L (2005) Venous thromboembolism: epidemiologic, clinical, and imaging perspectives. Cardiopulmonary imaging, categorical course syllabus. American Roentgen Ray Society 41–51

39. Cosmic MS, Goodman LR, Lipchik RJ et al (2002) Detection of deep venous thrombosis with combined helical CT scan of the chest and CT venography in unselected cases of suspected pulmonary embolism. Am J Respir Crit Care Med 165:A329

40. Ghaye B, Remy J, Remy-Jardin M et al (2002) Non-traumatic thoracic emergencies: CT diagnosis of acute pulmonary embolism-the first 10 years. Eur Radiol 12:1886–1905

41. Gottschalk A, Stein PD, Goodman LR et al (2002) Overview of prospective investigation of pulmonary embolism diagnosis II. Semin Nucl Med 32:173–182

42. Washington L, Goodman LR, Gonyo MB (2002) CT for thromboembolic disease. Radiol Clin North Am 40:751–771

43. Wittram C, Maher MM, Yoo AJ et al (2004) CT angiography of pulmonary embolism: diagnostic criteria and causes of misdiagnosis. Radiographics 24:1219–1238

44. Shah AA, Davis SD, Gamsu G et al (1999) Parenchymal and pleural findings in patients with and patients without acute pulmonary embolism detected at spiral CT. Radiology 211:147–153

45. Quiroz R, Kucher N, Schoepf UJ et al (2004) Right ventricular enlargement on chest computed tomography: prognostic role in acute pulmonary embolism, Circulation 109:2401–2404

46. Reid JH, Murchison JT (1998) Acute right ventricular dilation: a new helical CT sign of massive pulmonary embolism. Clin Radiol 53:694–698

47. Schoepf UJ, Kucher N, Kipfmueller F et al (2004) Right ventricular enlargement on chest computed tomography: a predictor of early death in acute pulmonary embolism. Circulation 110:3276–3280

48. Van der Meer RW, Pattynama PM, van Strijen MJ et al (2005) Right ventricular dysfunction and pulmonary obstruction index at helical CT: prediction of clinical outcome during 3-month follow-up in patients with acute pulmonary embolism. Radiology 235:798–803

49. Qanadli SD, El Hajjam M, Vieillard-Baron A et al (2001) New CT index to quantify arterial obstruction in pulmonary embolism: comparison with angiographic index and echocardiography. AJR Am J Roentenol 176(6):1415–1420

50. Wu AS, Pezzullo JA, Cronan JJ et al (2004) CT pulmonary angiography: quantification of pulmonary embolus as a predictor of patient outcome – initial experience. Radiology 230:831–835

51. Cademartiri F, Mollet N, van der Lugt A et al (2004) Non-invasive 16–row multislice CT coronary angiography: usefulness of saline chaser. Eur Radiol 14:178–183

52. Dorio PJ, Lee FT, Henseler KP et al (2003) Using a saline chaser to decrease contrast media in abdominal CT. AJR Am J Roentgenol 180:929–934

53. Haage P, Schmitz-Rode T, Hubner D et al (2000) Reduction of contrast material dose and artifacts by a saline flush using a double power injector in helical CT of the thorax. AJR Am J Roentgenol 174: 1049–1053

54. Storto ML, Di Credico A, Guido F et al (2005) Incidental detection of pulmonary emboli on routine MDCT of the chest AJR Am J Roentgenol 184: 264–267

55. Schoepf UJ, Schneider AC, Das M et al (2005) Pulmonary embolism: computer aided detection at multi-detector row spiral CT. Radiology (*in press*)

56. Schoepf UJ, Savino G, Lake DR et al (2005) The age of CT pulmonary angiography. J Thorac Imaging 20(4):273–279

57. Gosselin MV, Rassner UA, Thieszen SL et al (2004) Contrast dynamics during CT pulmonary angiogram: analysis of an inspiration associated artifact. J Thorac Imaging 19:1–7

58. Yoo AJ, Wittram C (2003) CTPA pulmonary artery flow artifact: pitfall in the diagnosis of pulmonary embolism Radiology 352(P):233

59. Gruden JF (2005) Pulmonary embolism: MDCT technique and interpretative pitfalls. Cardiopulmonary imaging, categorical course syllabus. American Roentgen Ray Society 53–60

60. Wiest PW, Locken JA, Heintz PH et al (2002) CT scanning: a major source of radiation exposure. Semin Ultrasound CT MR 23(5):402–410

61. Resten A, Mausoleo F, Valero M, Musset D (2003) Comparison of doses for pulmonary embolism detection with helical CT and pulmonary angiography. Eur Radiol 13:1515–1521

62. Huda W (2005) When a pregnant patient has a suspected pulmonary embolism, what are the typical embryo doses from a chest CT and a ventilation/perfusion study? Pediatr Radiol 25:25

63. Winer-Muram HT, Boone JM, Brown HL et al (2002) Pulmonary embolism in pregnant patients: fetal radiation dose with helical CT. Radiology 224(2):487–492

64. Abcarian PW, Sweet JD, Watabe JT et al (2004) Role of a quantitative D-dimer assay in determining the need for CT angiography of acute pulmonary embolism. AJR Am J Roentgenol 182:1377–1381

65. Kline JA, Wells PS (2003) Methodology for a rapid protocol to rule out pulmonary embolism in the emergency department. Ann Emerg Med 42: 266–275

66. Berlin L (1996) Malpractice issues in radiology. Perceptual errors. AJR Am J Roentgenol 167:587–590

67. Renfrew DL, Franken EA Jr, Berbaum KS et al (1992) Error in radiology: classification and lessons in 182 cases presented at a problem case conference. Radiology 183:145–150

68. Peldschus K, Herzog P, Wood SA et al (2005) Computer-aided diagnosis as a second reader: Spectrum of findings in computed tomography studies of the chest interpreted as normal. Chest 128:1517–1523

69. Wittram C, Meehan MJ, Halpern EF et al (2004) Trends in thoracic radiology over a decade at a large academic medical center. J Thorac Imaging 19: 164–170

70. Remy-Jardin M, Remy J, Cauvain O et al (1995): Diagnosis of central pulmonary embolism with helical

CT: role of two-dimensional multiplanar reformations. AJR Am J Roentgenol 165:1131–1138

71. Chiang EE, Boiselle PM, Raptopoulos V et al (2003) Detection of pulmonary embolism: comparison of paddlewheel and coronal CT reformations – initial experience. Radiology 228:577–582

72. Simon M, Chiang EE, Boiselle PM (2001) Paddle-wheel multislice helical CT display of pulmonary vessels and other lung structures. Radiol Clin North Am 41:617–626

73. Schoepf UJ, Becker CR, Ohnesorge BM et al (2004) CT of coronary artery disease. Radiology 232:18–37

19

MDCT Angiography of Peripheral Arterial Disease

Geoffrey D. Rubin, Mannudeep K. Kalra

Introduction

Greater scan coverage and faster scanning with multi-detector row computed tomography (MDCT) has provided a unique opportunity for noninvasive and accurate imaging of vascular diseases of lower extremities [1]. This chapter describes scanning parameters, contrast medium administration features, image postprocessing techniques, and clinical applications of MDCT angiography (MDCTA).

Scanning Parameters

For an average-size patient, we use 120 kV and 300 mA for peripheral MDCTA. A lower tube current and/or tube potential can be used for smaller patients, greater current and potential can be used for obese patients. Alternatively, automatic exposure control techniques can also be used to adapt tube current to patient size. Using the greater trochanter as a bony landmark, a small to medium imaging field of view is used for section reconstruction. For reconstruction of CT angiography (CTA) images, we use a soft or medium reconstruction kernel.

For peripheral CTA, the patient is placed supine and feet first on the CT table, with careful alignment of the patient's knees and feet positioned close to the gantry isocenter [2, 3]. The anatomic scan length for a typical lower-extremity CTA study is 110–130 cm and extends from the renal artery origins at T12 vertebra to the patient's feet. Compared with the 4- and 8-row MDCT scanners, 16- and 64-row MDCT scanners allow acquisition of thinner sections at faster speed. With these latter scanners, it is also possible to acquire submillimeter, isotropic images of the entire peripheral arterial tree. These "thinner" image data sets can improve visualization of small vessels (Fig. 1). This maximum spatial reso-

lution may translate into improved visualization and treatment planning of patients with advanced peripheral arterial occlusive disease. For most routine CTA of the entire peripheral arterial tree, we reconstruct images at 1.25- to 1.5-mm section thickness for 8- and 16-row scanners, and 1-mm section thickness with 64-row MDCT scanners while maintaining constant image quality with use of automatic exposure control techniques.

Contrast Medium

Oral contrast is not administered to patients undergoing peripheral CTA. Although the same principles for contrast medium injection for CTA (relationship of injection flow rate and injection duration with arterial enhancement) apply to peripheral CTA, the latter is more complex due to the need for acquiring optimum enhancement of the entire lower extremity arterial tree in a single CT acquisition.

For peripheral CTA studies, we inject 1–1.5 g of iodine per second for an average person (75 kg) and make patient-weight-based adjustment to the contrast volume and injection flow rate for heavier (>90 kg) or smaller (<60 kg) subjects. In peripheral CTA studies, attenuation values are usually lowest in the abdominal aorta and peak at the level of the infrageniculate popliteal artery [4]. This can be explained on the basis of continuous arterial enhancement with a continuous and prolonged intravenous injection of contrast media (e.g., 35 s) [5]. Thus, biphasic injections may result in more uniform enhancement over time, particularly for longer scan and injection times (>25–30 s) [6].

In addition to volume and injection for contrast media, an optimum scan delay for peripheral CTA is also critical. Contrast medium transit time ($tCMT$), the time interval between the beginning of an intravenous contrast medium injection and arrival of the bolus in the aorta, varies considerably between

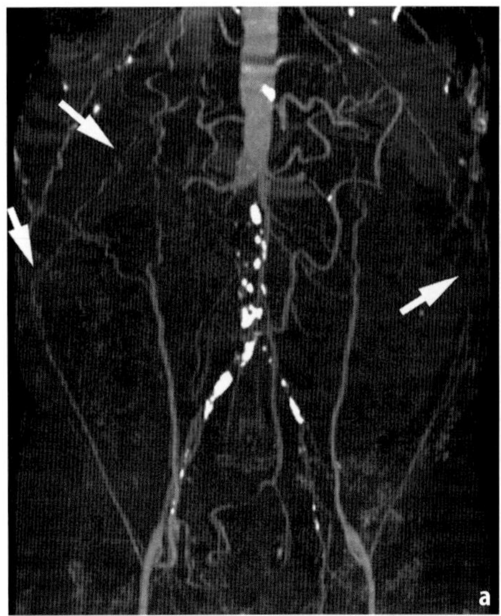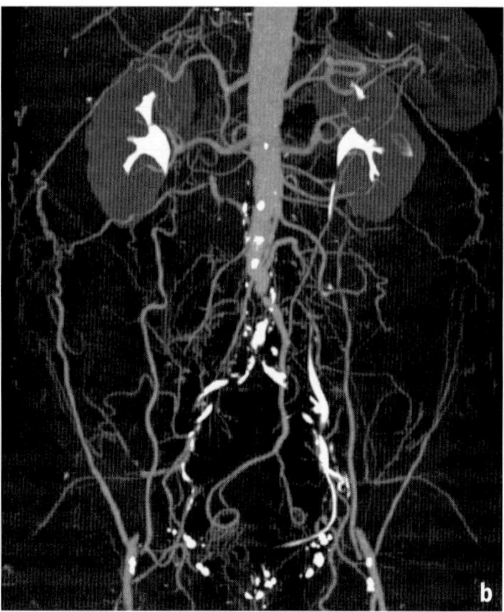

Fig. 1a, b. a Maximum intensity projection (MIP) from a multidetector computed tomography (MDCT) angiogram acquired with 4×2.5-mm-thick sections demonstrates an occlusion of the aorta and common iliac arteries. Collateral arteries connecting intercostal and lumbar arteries with deep lateral circumflex iliac arteries are not seen throughout their entire course and appear blurred (*arrows*). **b** MIP from an MDCT angiogram acquired in a different patient with 8×1.25-mm-thick sections demonstrates distal abdominal aortic and bilateral common and external iliac arterial occlusions. Similar collateral arteries are present, as in (**a**), but the thinner sections allow them to be visualized with less blurring

patients with coexisting cardiovascular diseases and may range from 12–40 s. Therefore, individualization of scanning delay (or determination of the individual's *t*CMT) is recommended in peripheral CTA with the help of either a small test-bolus injection or automated bolus triggering techniques. These techniques help the choice of scanning delays that may equal to the *t*CMT or exceed *t*CMT by being chosen at a predefined interval (e.g., "*t*CMT+5 s" implies that the scan starts 5 s after contrast medium has arrived in the aorta).

Contrast medium injection protocols in peripheral CTA are also complicated since arterial stenosis, occlusions, or aneurysms anywhere between the infrarenal abdominal aorta and the pedal arteries can substantially delay downstream arterial enhancement [7, 8] (Fig. 2). In fact, patients with peripheral arterial occlusive disease, transit times of intravenous (IV) contrast medium from the aorta to the popliteal arteries can range from 4 s (at transit speed of 177 mm/s) to 24 s (at a transit speed of 29 mm/s) [9]. This is particularly important with the use of faster acquisition speeds, as the scanner table may move faster than the intravascular contrast medium, and the scanner may thus outrun the bolus. It is important to note that this phenomenon of "outrunning" has only been reported at a table speed of 37 mm/s in one study on peripheral CTA [10], but it has not been reported at table speeds of 19-30 mm/s in other studies [10-14]. Thus, we categorize injection strategies for peripheral CTA into those for "slow" acquisitions (at a table speed of ≤ 30 mm/s) and those for "fast" ac-

quisitions (at a table speed of > 30 mm/s).

For slow acquisitions, table speed usually translates into a scan time of approximately 40 s for the entire peripheral arterial tree. As data acquisition follows the bolus from the aorta to the feet, injection duration can be about 5 s shorter than the scan time (e.g., 40-s acquisition = 35-s injection duration). At a constant injection rate of 4 ml/s, this translates to 140 ml of contrast medium. If the beginning of data acquisition is timed closely to contrast arrival time in the aorta (using a test bolus or bolus triggering), biphasic injections achieve more favorable enhancement profiles with improved aortic enhancement.

In patients with peripheral arterial occlusive disease, fast acquisition protocols (>30 mm/s table speed) may be faster than contrast medium transit times through the peripheral arterial tree. In order to prevent CT acquisition from outrunning the bolus, the bolus should be given a "head start" by combining fixed injection duration of 35 s to fill the arterial tree and a delay of the start of CT acquisition relative to *t*CMT. The faster the acquisition, the longer "diagnostic delay" should be. We employ such a strategy with both a 16-row scanner with a 16×1.25-mm protocol, beam pitch 1.375:1, and 0.6-s gantry rotation period (table speed 45 mm/s) and a 64-row scanner with a 64×0.6-mm, beam pitch 1.0:1, and 0.5-s gantry rotation period, and table speed 45 mm/s. Our diagnostic delay is typically 15–20 s in these cases.

As there is a possibility of even more delayed arterial opacification than accounted for with the

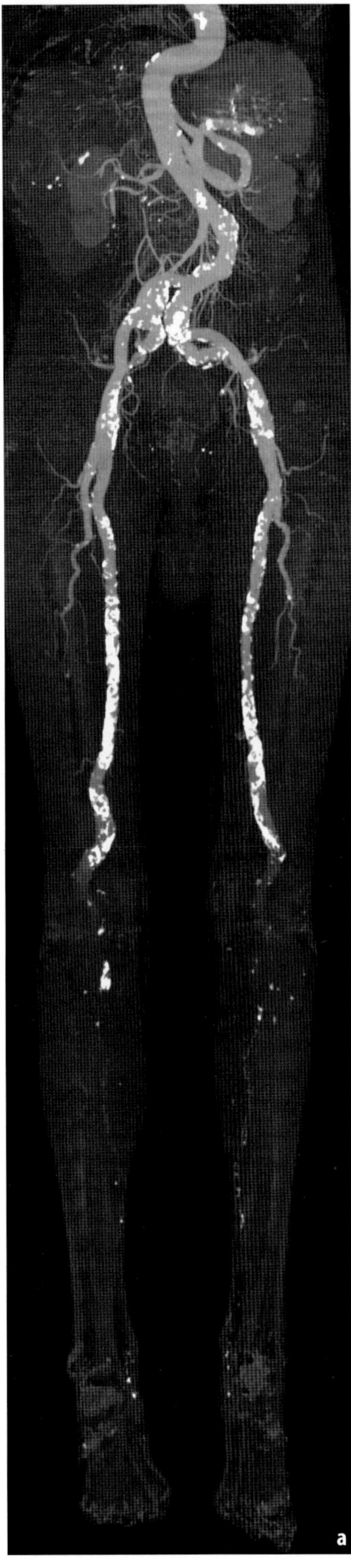

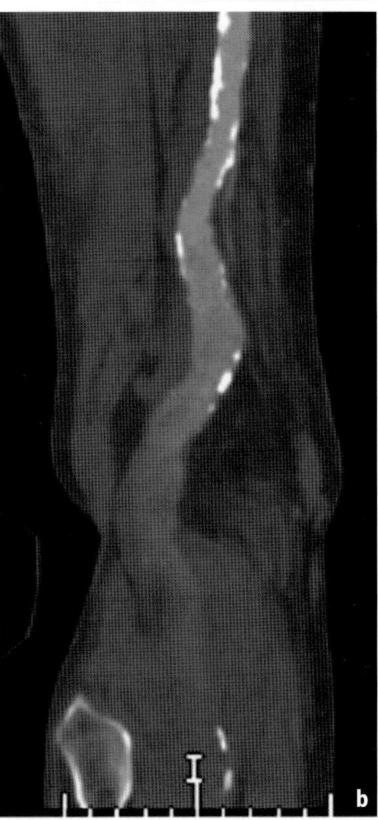

Fig. 2a, b. a Multidetector-row computed tomography angiogram (MDCTA) obtained with 32×1.0-mm-thick sections and a table speed of 80 mm/s immediately after arrival of contrast medium into the abdominal aorta. Arteriomegaly is present throughout but most notably in the iliofemoral arteries. Arterial opacification ceases in the popliteal artery, resulting in a nondiagnostic examination of the popliteal, crural, and pedal arteries. **b** A curved planar reformation through the proximal right popliteal artery demonstrates the presence of a popliteal artery aneurysm. The slow-flow characteristic of patients with large arteries results in a CT angiogram where the CT table is moving faster than the blood flow and the scanner thus overruns contrast medium bolus

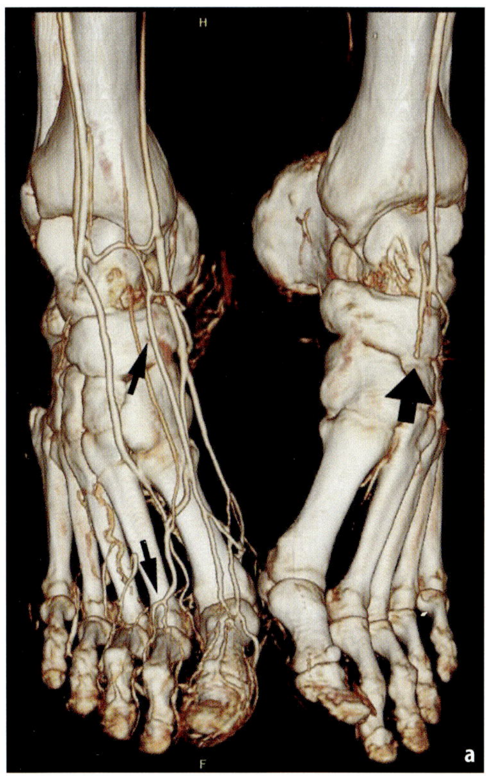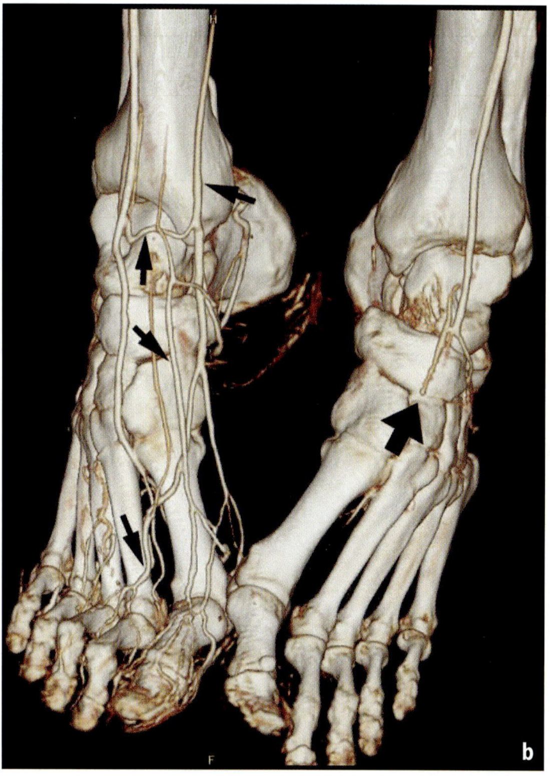

Fig. 3a,b. Two volume-rendered (VR) views of the feet in a patient with right-foot cellulitis. Extensive venous opacification (*narrow arrows*) complicates analysis of the right foot while arteries only are opacified in the left foot, allowing clear visualization of a dorsalis pedis arterial occlusion (*wide arrow*)

slow acquisition protocol [9], a second CTA acquisition (covering the popliteal and infrapopliteal vasculature) must be preprogrammed into the scanning protocol and can be initiated by CT technologists if they do not see any contrast medium opacification in the distal vessels. Opacification of deep and superficial veins cannot be completely avoided in some patients with rapid arteriovenous transit times [4, 15] and is more likely to occur with longer scan times and in patients with active inflammation, e.g., from infected or nonhealing ulcers (Fig. 3). However, stronger arterial enhancement with correct injection timing [4], along with adequate anatomic knowledge and postprocessing tools, can help to avoid diagnostic problems from venous enhancement.

Visualization Techniques

Despite the availability of state-of-the-art two- (2-D) and three- (3-D) dimensional image postprocessing techniques, transverse CT images are indispensable for assessment of nonvascular abdominal and/or pelvic abnormalities. These source images can also be used to analyze findings on 2-D or 3-D images that suggest artifactual lesions. For some vascular lesions, transverse images may provide an initial impression or may provide all the required information, for example, in patients with or without only minimal disease, trauma, or suspected acute occlusions. However, for most patients with peripheral vascular disease, review of large number of transverse images is time consuming and less accurate [11] than alternative 2-D and 3-D visualizations.

Three dimensional overview techniques with at least one 2-D technique are generally used for atherosclerotic peripheral vascular diseases. Our protocol for peripheral MDCTA comprises curved planar reformations (CPRs), thin-slab maximum intensity projections (MIPs) through the renal and visceral arteries, and interactive exploration of volume renderings (VRs) of the abdomen, pelvis, and each leg. These 2-D and 3-D techniques enable faster and easier interpretation of huge data sets of axial images. MIP and VR techniques facilitate assessment of vascular structures by providing "angiographic maps" of the arterial tree. Being closest to the angiographic map, MIP images are suitable for illustrating abnormalities to the requesting physicians and can serve as a vascular map for patient management in the catheter angiography suite or operating rooms (Fig. 4). However, the need for time-consuming bone removal from image data, inadvertent removal of vascular structures adjacent to

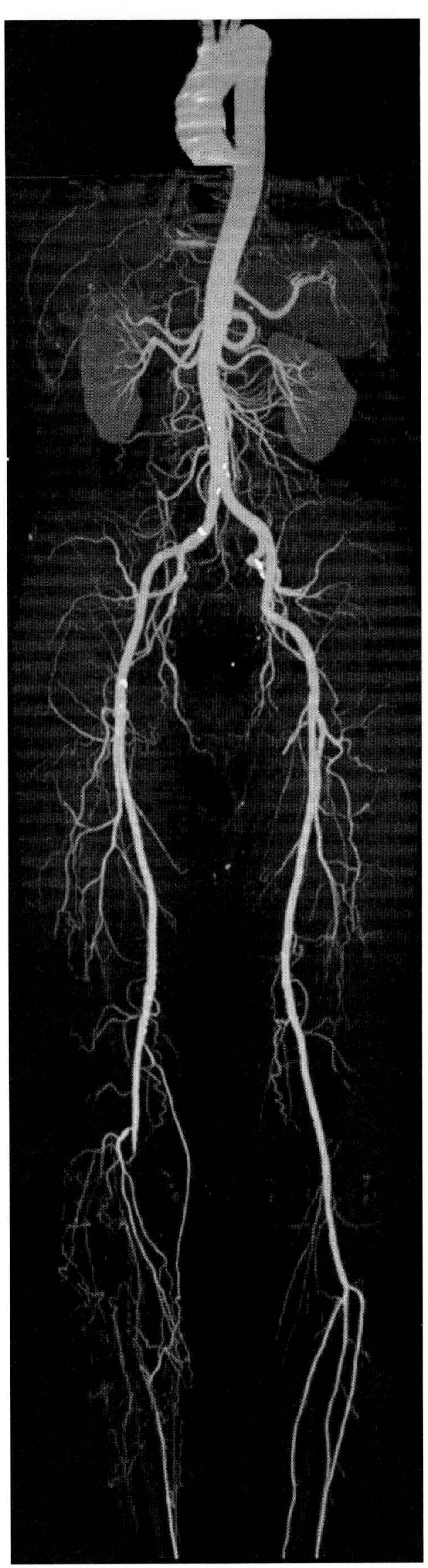

Fig. 4. Frontal maximum projection intensity (MIP) of computed tomography angiography (CTA) comprising the entirety of the aorta, iliac arteries, and runoff performed to assess for a source of distal embolization. This full-volume MIP requires preliminary removal of the bones to allow visualization of the arterial anatomy. There is an occlusion of the proximal right popliteal artery with robust collateralization reconstituting the posterior tibial artery

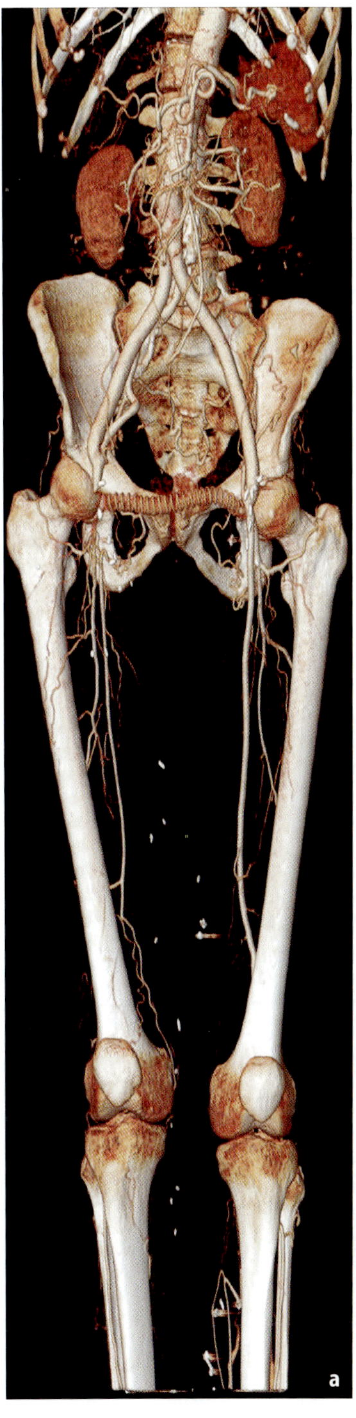
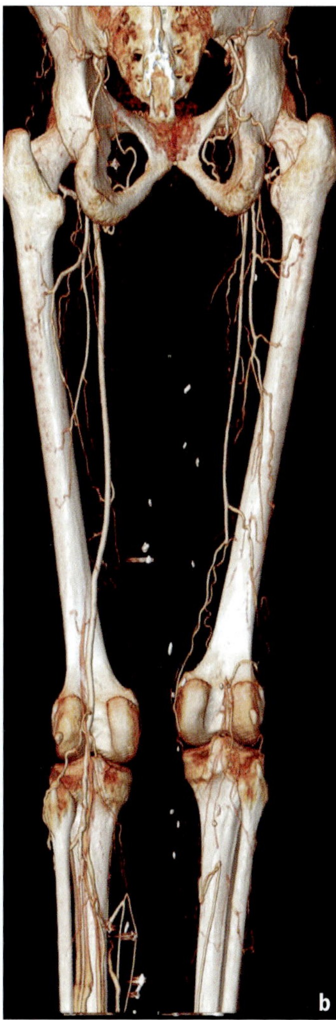

Fig. 5a, b. Anteroposterior **a** and posteroanterior volume renderings (VRs) **b** in a patient with an aortobifemoral bypass graft and an occluded femorofemoral bypass graft. The right femoral artery and distal right superficial femoral arteries are occluded. VRs allow visualization of complex, overlapping arterial channels without the need for preliminary bone removal, providing an excellent overview of the complex anatomy

bony structures, and lack of depth information are some of the limitations of the MIP technique. On the other hand, VR techniques maintain 3-D depth information, and bone removal is not essential (Fig. 5). VR is an ideal technique for rapid and interactive viewing and exploration of peripheral CTA data sets. The main limitation of both MIP and VR is that vessel calcifications and stents may completely obscure the vascular flow channel. This precludes its exclusive use in up to 60% of patients with peripheral arterial occlusive disease [16].

In the presence of calcified plaque, diffuse vessel-wall calcification, or endoluminal stents, cross-sectional views such as transverse source images, sagittal, coronal, or oblique multiplanar reformations in conjunction with VR are important for assessing luminal contrast flow. Alternatively, longitudinal cross-sections along a predefined vascular centerline (CPR) can be created with either manual or (semi) automated tracing of the vessel centerlines for the most comprehensive cross-sectional display of luminal pathology [17, 18] (Figs. 6 and 7).

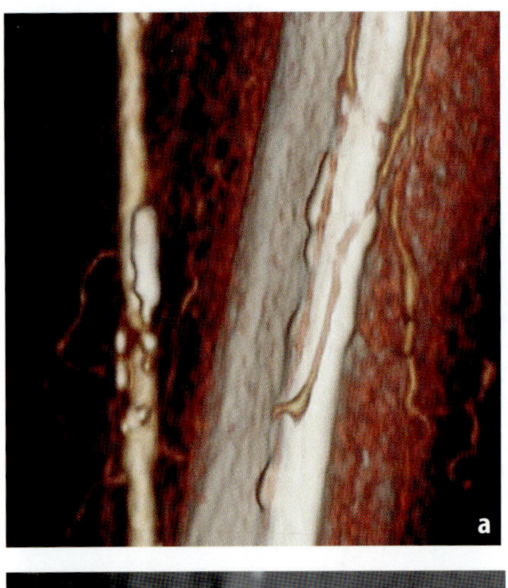
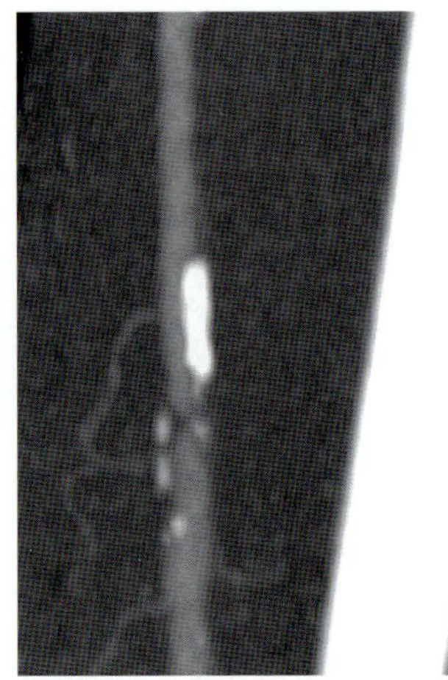
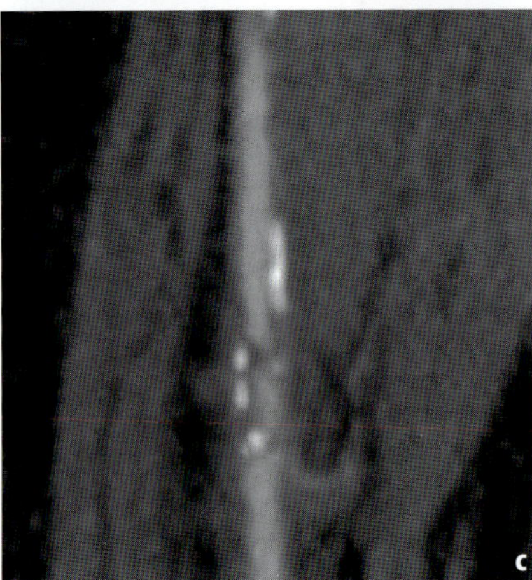

Fig. 6a-c. a Volume rendering (VR), **b** maximum intensity projection (MIP), and **c** curved planar reformation (CPR) through a mid superficial femoral artery lesion. All images demonstrate a >75% stenosis distal to a large calcified plaque. The lumen adjacent to the calcification is partially obscured on VR and MIP. The CPR (**c**) establishes that there is only minimal luminal narrowing as a result of this calcified plaque

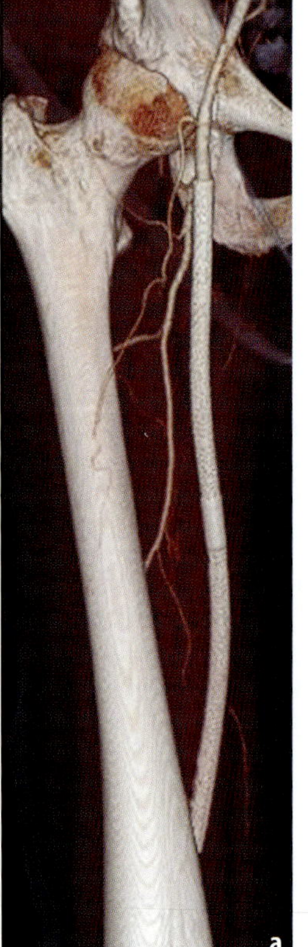
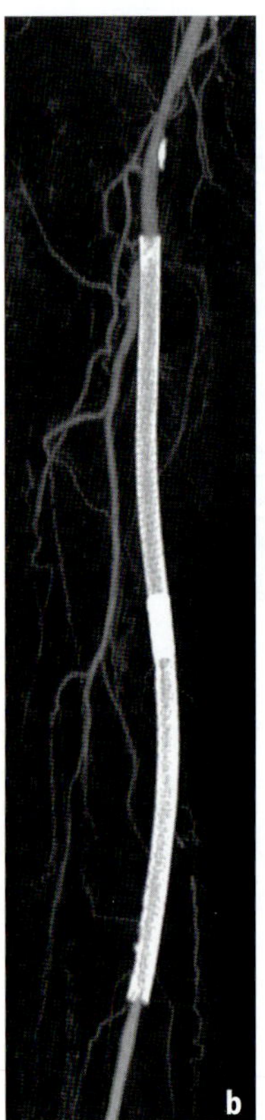
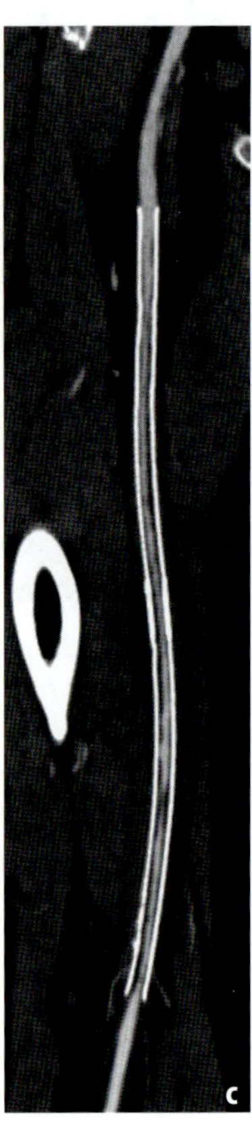

Fig. 7a-c. a Volume rendering (VR), **b** maximum intensity projection (MIP), and **c** curved planar reformation (CPR) through a stented segment of the superficial femoral artery. The lumen of the stent is obscured on both VR and the MIP. The CPR (**c**) demonstrates the lumen of the stent with irregular neointimal hyperplasia. (Images courtesy of Justus Roos, MD and Dominik Fleishmann MD, Department of Radiology, Stanford University School of Medicine, Stanford, CA, USA)

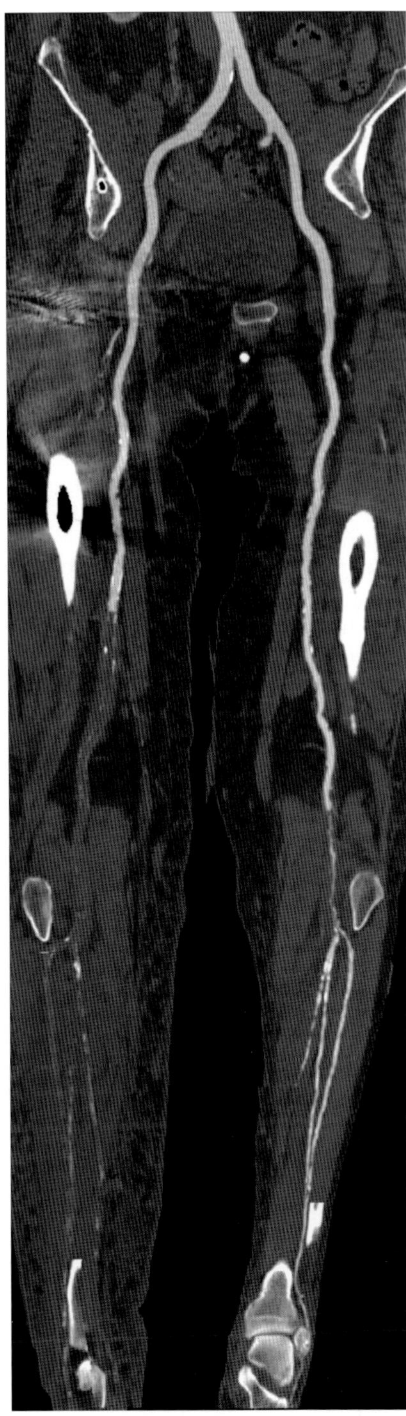

Fig. 8. Multipath curved planar reformation (CPR) demonstrates all iliac, femoral, and crural arteries bilaterally in a single image. Six traditional CPRs would be required to demonstrate all of the arterial lumina shown on this single view. There is extensive thrombus in the mid right superficial femoral artery (SFA) extending inferiorly to involve all three crural arteries. There is a high-grade stenosis of the left popliteal artery and occlusion of the mid left anterior tibial artery. Reprinted from [2], with permission from Lippincott Williams & Wilkins

At least two orthogonal CPRs per vessel segment (e.g., sagittal and coronal views) are required for complete evaluation of eccentric disease. One problem of (single) CPRs in the context of visualizing the peripheral arterial tree is their limited spatial perception. Unless clear annotations are present, the anatomic context of a vascular lesion may be ambiguous. In this context, multipath CPRs provide simultaneous longitudinal cross-sectional views through the major blood vessels without obscuring vascular calcifications and stents while maintaining spatial perception [18] (Fig. 8).

Despite remarkable improvements in 3-D image postprocessing, no algorithms allow fully automated detection of vessel centerlines, automated segmentation of bony structures, and detection (and subtraction) of vessel-wall calcification for peripheral CTA studies. Although it is reasonable to expect further improvements in computer-assisted segmentation and visualization in the not too distant future, it appears unlikely that expert user interaction (radiologist or 3-D technologist) can be completely avoided for creating clinically relevant and representative peripheral CTA images.

Clinical Applications

Several noninvasive imaging techniques, such as ultrasound, CTA, and magnetic resonance angiography (MRA) are available for evaluating clinical conditions involving the lower-extremity vascular structures. Peripheral CTA with state-of-the-art MDCT scanners has the advantages of high spatial resolution, relative freedom from operator dependence, and widespread (and increasing) availability. As a result, peripheral CTA is increasingly used in many imaging centers for a wide range of clinical indications. However, only sparse original data on its accuracy in patients with peripheral arterial occlusive disease, particularly for 16- or 64-row MDCTA, are available when compared with conventional angiography [4, 10–13]. Published studies suggest that peripheral CTA has a high diagnostic accuracy relative to conventional angiography [10–13]. Reported sensitivities and specificities range from 88% to 100%. In general, sensitivity and specificity are greater for arterial occlusions than for detection of stenoses. Accuracies and interobserver agreement are also higher for femoropopliteal and iliac vessels when compared with infrapopliteal arteries. Pedal arteries have not been specifically analyzed in the literature. At least in patients with intermittent claudication, peripheral CTA has the potential to be cost effective [19].

Intermittent Claudication

Surgical or endovascular revascularization is performed when medical management of patients with claudication fails to improve the symptoms. Factors that influence choice of treatment include lesion morphology (degree of stenosis/occlusion and lesion length) [20], location, and, most importantly, status of runoff vessels, specifically the calf arteries, which can predict long-term patency rates after intervention [21]. Peripheral CTA provides complete delineation of both the femoropopliteal segment and inflow and outflow arteries, including lesion number, length, stenosis diameter and morphology, adjacent normal arterial caliber, degree of calcification, and status of distal runoff vessels. These findings help in planning the procedure with respect to route of access, balloon selection, and expected long-term patency after femoropopliteal intervention. Compared with catheter angiography, peripheral CTA provides better estimates of the effects of eccentric stenoses on luminal diameter reduction [22]. In addition, collateral vessels can be evaluated with MIP and VR images, and arterial segments distal to long-segment occlusions are well visualized (Fig. 9). It is also expected that peripheral CTA is more cost effective than digital subtraction angiog-

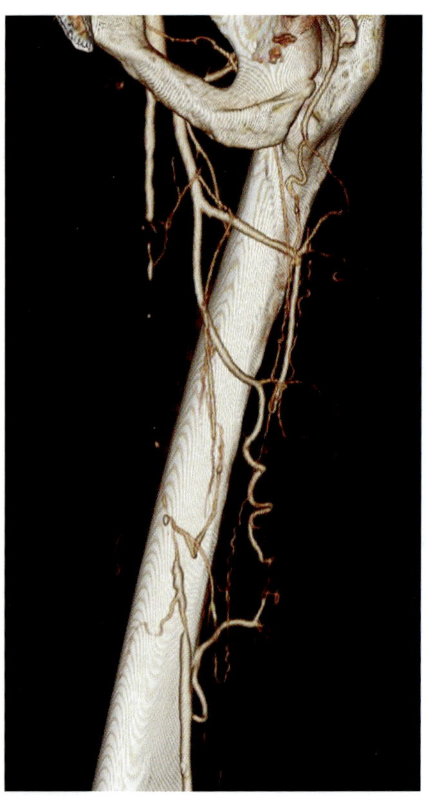

Fig. 9. Volume rendering (VR) of an occluded superficial femoral artery (SFA) in a patient with calf claudication. Computed tomography angiography (CTA) demonstrates the site of occlusion and associated collateral arteries that reconstitute the SFA via the profunda femoris

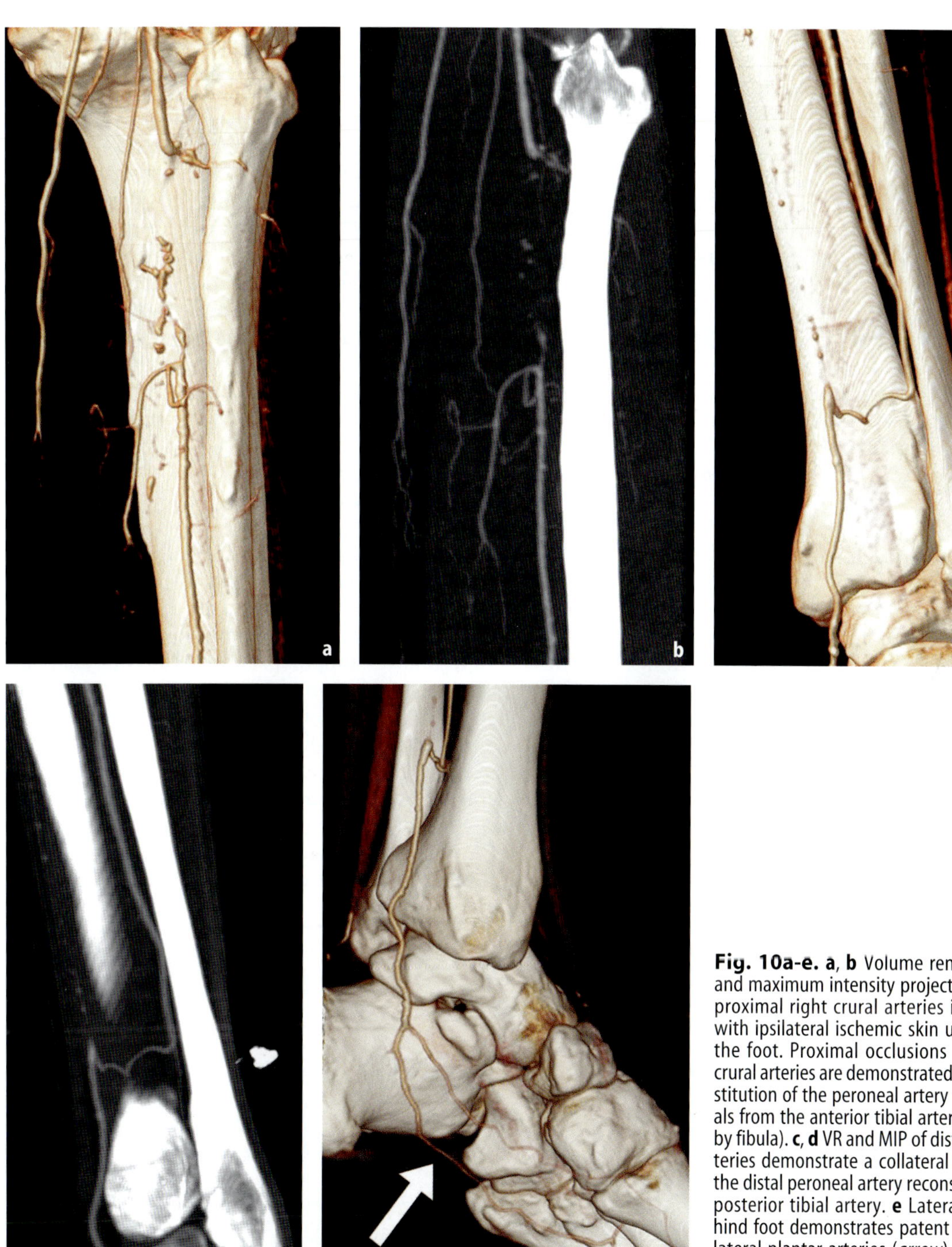

Fig. 10a-e. a, b Volume rendering (VR) and maximum intensity projection (MIP) of proximal right crural arteries in a patient with ipsilateral ischemic skin ulceration in the foot. Proximal occlusions of all three crural arteries are demonstrated with reconstitution of the peroneal artery via collaterals from the anterior tibial artery (obscured by fibula). **c, d** VR and MIP of distal crural arteries demonstrate a collateral artery from the distal peroneal artery reconstituting the posterior tibial artery. **e** Lateral VR of the hind foot demonstrates patent medial and lateral plantar arteries (*arrow*). These normal distal arteries represent excellent bypass graft candidates for pedal revascularization

raphy (DSA) for preprocedure evaluation of patients with claudication [23, 24].

Chronic Limb-Threatening Ischemia

In patients with chronic limb-threatening ischemia, the principal goal of treatment is prevention of tissue loss and need for amputation, assessment, and promotion of blood flow through the calf arteries. An accurate roadmap to lesions amenable to percutaneous transluminal angioplasty or other endovascular techniques and delineation of patent, acceptable target vessels for distal bypass are the challenges of vessel analysis in this advanced disease group (Fig. 10). In this respect, "isotropic" image data sets (<1 mm) and optimum contrast-medium delivery, especially with the state-of-the-art 64-row MDCT scanners, may provide improved visualization of small crural and pedal vessels in patients with chronic limb-threatening ischemia.

Acute Ischemia

For evaluation of acute lower-extremity ischemia, catheter angiography appears to be the most appropriate evaluation technique if urgent percutaneous (thrombolysis, etc.) or surgical intervention is planned [25]. However, in some situations, peripheral CTA may guide the choice of percutaneous or surgical intervention and help in preprocedural planning. For example, CTA can determine the extent and location of thrombosis and whether thrombus or emboli involves all trifurcation vessels, a previously patent bypass graft, or resides within a popliteal aneurysm, and whether thrombolytic therapy may be most efficacious [26] (Fig. 8). In addition, demonstration of thrombus in locations not accessible to embolectomy may direct treatment to catheter-based techniques. In the subacute ischemic population for whom surgical intervention may be best, peripheral CTA can provide a comprehensive map of the affected vascular territories for surgery planning. CTA may provide rapid and adequate evaluation for patients who refuse catheter angiography and/or thrombolysis. It is important to remember that in these settings, an additional CTA acquisition in a delayed phase immediately after the initial arterial phase is often helpful to differentiate patent but slowly flowing vessels from thrombus.

Aneurysms

Peripheral CTA is a noninvasive and cost-effective alternative to DSA for detection and characterization of lower-extremity aneurysms. It provides detailed information about aneurysm size, presence, and amount of thrombus, presence of distal embolic disease, associated significant proximal and distal steno-occlusive disease, and coexistent abdominal or iliac aneurysms. Three-dimensional volumetric analysis provides accurate measurement of aneurysm volume as well as luminal dimension.

Follow-Up and Surveillance After Percutaneous or Surgical Revascularization

Ultrasound is the first choice for routine bypass graft surveillance or serial follow-up evaluation after intervention (e.g., in research protocols)

[27, 28]. However, peripheral CTA is an important problem-solving tool for the workup of patients with nondiagnostic (limited access due to skin lesions, wounds, draping, or obesity) or equivocal ultrasound studies. In these settings, CTA provides rapid, noninvasive, and accurate evaluation of peripheral arterial bypass grafts and stents and detects related complications, including stenosis, aneurysmal changes, and arteriovenous fistulae [29] (Fig. 7). CTA can also demonstrate the results of percutaneous interventions and reveal residual disease and both vascular and extravascular complications. Peripheral CTA has replaced catheter DSA completely at our institution in these settings and is used to decide upon further management.

Vascular Trauma

CTA provides rapid and accurate demonstration of traumatic arterial injuries, relationship of arterial segments to adjacent fractures, bone fragments, and soft tissue injuries, hematoma, associated vascular compression, or pseudoaneurysm. CTA can be performed in combination with CT of other organ systems (abdomen, chest, etc.) for complete delineation of the distribution and severity of injuries in each individual organ system [30]. Transverse source images are usually sufficient for interpretation, although MPRs may improve rapidity of analysis. VR images can improve depiction of the anatomic relationship between arteries and adjacent bony/soft tissue injuries and foreign bodies (Fig. 11).

Vascular Mapping

Peripheral CTA data sets can be used to generate vascular maps for subsequent surgical intervention. Prior to MDCTA, catheter angiography was used to generate these vascular maps. Peripheral CTA in the trauma setting is useful if subsequent surgical reconstruction is planned. Likewise, preoperative knowledge of vascular anatomy is also important for plastic surgery reconstruction for various diseases. Fibular free-flap procurement requires preoperative assessment of the limb to prevent ischemic complications and flap failure and to exclude variant peroneal artery anatomy and occlusive disease, which could alter the surgical procedure [31]. CTA allows high-resolution 3-D evaluation of arteries, veins, and soft tissues [32–34] with less risk and at lower cost than catheter angiography [34]. Vascular mapping with CTA is also useful for character evaluation and vascular supply of musculoskeletal tumors [30] and evaluation of suitability of the thoracodorsal and internal mammary arteries prior to trans-

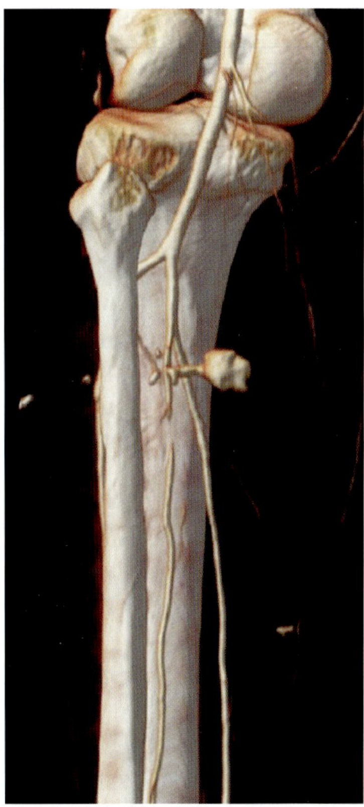

Fig. 11. Volume rendering (VR) of a 16-year-old male following a gunshot wound to the left calf demonstrates a pseudoaneurysm of the peroneal artery with distal occlusion due to peroneal arterial spasm

overcome the learning curve and avoiding interpretation pitfalls associated with visual perception and interpretation of vascular abnormalities in a new and different format (such as VR or CPR images).

Commonly, pitfalls related to interpretation of peripheral CTA studies can occur with use of narrow viewing-window settings in the presence of arterial wall calcifications or stents. Blooming artifacts related to these high-attenuation structures leads to overestimation of a vascular stenosis or suggest spurious total occlusion, even at relatively wide window settings. Thus, we use a much higher window width of at least 1,500 HU for evaluating luminal patency at the site of a calcified lesion or a stent. Some vendors (Siemens Medical Solutions) recommend use of special higher spatial resolution reconstruction kernels in the presence of stents. Despite these measures, peripheral CTA studies may not resolve luminal diameter in the presence of extensive atherosclerotic or media calcification within small crural or pedal arteries, such as those found in diabetic patients and in patients with end-stage renal disease.

Pitfalls related to image interpretation can also result from misinterpretation of editing artifacts (inadvertent removal of vascular structures in MIP images) and pseudostenosis and/or occlusions due to inaccurate centerline definition (in CPR images). These pitfalls underscore the importance of reviewing source images, additional views, or complimentary imaging modalities.

verse rectus abdominis muscle flap reconstruction.

Miscellaneous Applications

Peripheral CTA can provide important information about many other vascular conditions affecting the lower extremity, such as vascular malformations, arterial compression by adjacent masses, vasculitides, inflammatory/infective processes of soft tissue and bone affecting adjacent vessels, adventitial cystic disease, and popliteal entrapment syndrome [30, 35]. Image acquisition at rest and with provocative maneuvers (e.g., active plantarflexion against resistance) in patients with popliteal entrapment syndrome allows anatomic delineation of the medial head of the gastrocnemius as well as the dynamic degree of arterial obstruction.

Pitfalls

It is important to review peripheral CTA studies in the context of a patient's symptoms, disease stage, and available therapeutic options. This can help

Conclusion

In conclusion, state-of-the-art MDCT scanners with 16 and 64 detector rows enable acquisition of high spatial resolution peripheral CTA, which helps in noninvasive imaging and treatment planning of peripheral arterial disease.

References

1. Rubin GD, Schmidt AJ, Logan LJ et al (1999) Multi-detector row CT angiography of lower extremity occlusive disease: a new application for CT scanning. Radiology 210(2):588
2. Fleischmann D, Hallett RL, Rubin GD (2006) CT angiography of peripheral arterial disease. J Vasc Interv Radiol 17(1):3–26
3. Fleischmann D, Rubin GD, Paik DS et al (2000) Stair-step artifacts with single versus multiple detector-row helical CT. Radiology 216(1):185–196
4. Rubin GD, Schmidt AJ, Logan LJ, Sofilos MC (2001) Multi-detector row CT angiography of lower extremity arterial inflow and runoff: initial experience. Radiology 221(1):146–158
5. Fleischmann D, Hittmair K (1999) Mathematical analysis of arterial enhancement and optimization

of bolus geometry for CT angiography using the discrete fourier transform. J Comput Assist Tomogr 23(3):474–784

6. Fleischmann D, Rubin GD, Bankier AA, Hittmair K (2000). Improved uniformity of aortic enhancement with customized contrast medium injection protocols at CT angiography. Radiology 214(2):363–371

7. Bron KM (1983) Femoral arteriography. In: Abrams HL (ed) Abrams angiography: vascular and interventional radiology, 3d edn. Little, Brown, Boston. pp 1835–1875

8. Versteylen RJ, Lampmann LE (1989) Knee time in femoral arteriography. AJR Am J Roentgenol 152(1):203

9. Fleischmann D, Rubin GD (2005) Quantification of intravenously administered contrast medium transit through the peripheral arteries: implications for CT angiography. Radiology 236(3):1076–1082

10. Martin ML, Tay KH, Flak B et al (2003) Multidetector CT angiography of the aortoiliac system and lower extremities: a prospective comparison with digital subtraction angiography. AJR Am J Roentgenol 180(4):1085–1091

11. Ofer A, Nitecki SS, Linn S et al (2003) Multidetector CT angiography of peripheral vascular disease: a prospective comparison with intraarterial digital subtraction angiography. AJR Am J Roentgenol 180(3):719–724

12. Ota H, Takase K, Igarashi K et al (2004) MSCT compared with digital subtraction angiography for assessment of lower extremity arterial occlusive disease: importance of reviewing cross-sectional images. AJR Am J Roentgenol 182(1):201–209

13. Catalano C, Fraioli F, Laghi A et al (2004) Infrarenal aortic and lower-extremity arterial disease: diagnostic performance of multi-detector row CT angiography. Radiology 231(2):555–563

14. Portugaller HR, Schoellnast H, Hausegger KA et al (2004) Multislice spiral CT angiography in peripheral arterial occlusive disease: a valuable tool in detecting significant arterial lumen narrowing? Eur Radiol 14(9):1681–1687

15. Milne EN (1967) The significance of early venous filling during femoral arteriography. Radiology 88(3):513–518

16. Koechl A, Kanitsar A, Lomoschitz E et al (2003) Comprehensive assessment of peripheral arteries using multi-path curved planar reformation of CTA datasets. In: European Congress of Radiology, p 268

17. Kanitsar A, Fleischmann D, Wegenkittl R et al (2002) Curved planar reformation. In: Moorehead R, Gross M, Joy KI (eds) Proceedings of the 13th IEEE Visualization 2002 Conference, Boston, 27 October–11 November 2002. IEEE Computer Society, Piscataway, pp 37–44

18. Raman R, Napel S, Beaulieu CF et al (2002) Automated generation of curved planar reformations from volume data: method and evaluation. Radiology 223(1):275–280

19. Visser K, Kock MCJM, Kuntz KM et al (2003) Cost-effectiveness targets for multi-detector row CT angiography in the work-up of patients with intermittent claudication. Radiology 227:647–656

20. Surowiec SM, Davies MG, Eberly SW et al (2005)

21. Clark TW, Groffsky JL, Soulen MC (2001) Predictors of long-term patency after femoropopliteal angioplasty: results from the STAR registry. J Vasc Interv Radiol 12(8):923–933

22. Hirai T, Korogi Y, Ono K et al (2001) Maximum stenosis of extracranial internal carotid artery: effect of luminal morphology on stenosis measurement by using CT angiography and conventional DSA. Radiology 221(3):802–809

23. Visser K, de Vries SO, Kitslaar PJ et al (2003) Cost-effectiveness of diagnostic imaging work-up and treatment for patients with intermittent claudication in The Netherlands. Eur J Vasc Endovasc Surg 25(3):213–223

24. Rubin GD, Armerding MD, Dake MD, Napel S (2000) Cost identification of abdominal aortic aneurysm imaging by using time and motion analyses. Radiology 215(1):63–70

25. Rutherford RB, Baker JD, Ernst C et al (1997) Recommended standards for reports dealing with lower extremity ischemia: revised version. J Vasc Surg 26(3):517–538

26. Costantini V, Lenti M (2002) Treatment of acute occlusion of peripheral arteries. Thromb Res 106(6):V285–V294

27. Mills JL, Harris EJ, Taylor LM Jr et al (1990) The importance of routine surveillance of distal bypass grafts with duplex scanning: a study of 379 reversed vein grafts. J Vasc Surg 12(4):379–386; discussion 387–389

28. Moody P, Gould DA, Harris PL (1990) Vein graft surveillance improves patency in femoropopliteal bypass. Eur J Vasc Surg 4(2):117–121

29. Willmann JK, Mayer D, Banyai M et al (2003) Evaluation of peripheral arterial bypass grafts with multidetector row CT angiography: comparison with duplex US and digital subtraction angiography. Radiology 229(2):465–474

30. Karcaaltincaba M, Akata D, Aydingoz U et al (2004) Three-dimensional MSCT angiography of the extremities: clinical applications with emphasis on musculoskeletal uses. AJR Am J Roentgenol 183(1):113–117

31. Whitley SP, Sandhu S, Cardozo A (2004) Preoperative vascular assessment of the lower limb for harvest of a fibular flap: the views of vascular surgeons in the United Kingdom. Br J Oral Maxillofac Surg 42(4):307–310

32. Karanas YL, Antony A, Rubin G, Chang J (2004) Preoperative CT angiography for free fibula transfer. Microsurgery 24(2):125–127

33. Chow L, Napoli A, Klein MB et al (2005) Vascular mapping with multidetector CT angiography prior to free-flap reconstruction. Radiology 237(1):353–360

34. Klein MB, Karanas YL, Chow LC et al (2003) Early experience with computed tomographic angiography in microsurgical reconstruction. Plast Reconstr Surg 112(2):498–503

35. Takase K, Imakita S, Kuribayashi S et al (1997) Popliteal artery entrapment syndrome: aberrant origin of gastrocnemius muscle shown by 3D CT. J Comput Assist Tomogr 21(4):523–528

20

Coronary CTA in Acute Chest Pain

Ian S. Rogers, Udo Hoffmann

Introduction

It has been estimated that over 5 million patients present to emergency departments (EDs) in the United States with acute chest pain each year [1], Although rapid triage of these patients is crucial for optimizing treatment and improving prognosis, an effective strategy for diagnosis remains elusive in a majority of these patients. The current strategies for triage of the large subset of patients who present with acute chest pain but have normal or unchanged electrocardiograms (ECG) and negative initial cardiac enzymes provide inadequate risk stratification. This stems from the fact that the predictive value of symptom history [2] as well single variables such as patient age, sex, cardiac risk factors, and biochemical markers for adverse outcomes is limited [3, 4]. Moreover, symptoms of chest pain from cardiac etiologies are often similar to those from non-cardiac etiologies, further complicating accurate diagnosis [5].

As a result of the inadequate risk stratification, it has been estimated that 2–4% of acute coronary syndromes (ACS) are missed in the ED, leading to a twofold increase in mortality [6, 7]. Missed ACS also accounts for 20% or more of the losses in ED malpractice dollars [4]. ED physicians have responded to the potentially fatal consequences and high malpractice costs of missed ACS by practicing with a very low threshold for hospital admission for patients presenting with chest pain or atypical cardiac symptoms.

Approximately 60% of patients who are eligible for early discharge are instead admitted to the hospital [8]. Consequently, almost 3 million Americans are admitted to the hospital each year with chest pain, resulting in an estimated, US $8 billion dollars in health care costs [9], although most of these patients are at very low risk for ACS [10, 11]. The numbers of potentially avoidable hospital days per 1,000 patients range from 65 in New Zealand to 839 in Germany [12].

The sensitivities and specificities of 64-slice cardiac multi-detector computed tomography (MDCT) are between 91 and 100% for the detection of significant coronary artery stenosis, compared to invasive angiography [13, 14]. MDCT is also highly sensitive (84–92%) for detecting coronary atherosclerotic plaque compared with intracoronary ultrasound [15]. Given that the majority of ACS events are caused by underlying coronary artery disease (CAD) [16] and that MDCT has shown to be safe in patients with acute chest pain [17], MDCT scanned with high-concentration contrast media represents a noninvasive method that quickly and accurately excludes the presence of CAD, thus providing incremental value to standard cardiovascular risk factors and standard clinical risk assessment.

Patient Selection

As a result of the high sensitivity and negative predictive value (NPV) of MDCT, it is helpful to assess a patient's pretest likelihood of angiographically significant CAD when considering the use of this modality in a patient with acute chest pain. This is distinct from the above-mentioned risk assessment for ACS. Just as a patient with a lower pretest likelihood of CAD might present with a high-risk constellation of symptoms, a patient with known CAD might present with a low-risk constellation of symptoms. While MDCT may be very useful in demonstrating the absence of plaque or stenosis in the patient with a lower pretest likelihood of CAD, it will likely be of limited value in patients with established disease.

Patients with known CAD also introduce the element of evaluation of coronary stents and coronary artery bypass grafts. Even studies conducted by very experienced researchers indicate that the evaluability of stents for restenosis can be limited, and that limitation is usually correlated with stent diameter. Rixe et al. reported an evaluability rate of 8% for stents < 3.0 mm, 58% for stents = 3.0 mm, and 78% for stents ≥3.5 mm with 64-slice MDCT [18]. Cademartiri et al. presented evaluability rates between 90% and 94.3% and a NPV of 98.7% in their study with 64-slice MDCT and stents ≥2.75 mm. The overall positive predictive value (PPV) to detect in-stent restenosis ≥50% was just 44.2% [19].

The diagnostic accuracy of 64-slice MDCT for the detection of graft stenosis has been evaluated in a number of relatively small, single-center feasibility studies. In general, these studies indicated that most grafts are evaluable, even in unselected patients. Excellent accuracy data exist for the evaluation of venous grafts, with a slightly lower sensitivity and specificity for arterial grafts. In one trial, assessment of 57 arterial grafts yielded a sensitivity, specificity, PPV, and NPV of 100% and assessment of 64 venous grafts yielded a sensitivity of 100%, specificity of 96%, PPV of 97.5%, and NPV of 100% [20]. Unfortunately, MDCT often has a limited ability to assess the native coronary arteries in patients with bypass grafts due to the heavily diseased state of these vessels. As a result, it is not possible to exclude CAD as the etiology of chest pain in these patients.

Thus, the ability of MDCT to exclude CAD as the etiology of a patient's acute chest pain is greatest in patients with a low to intermediate pretest likelihood of CAD, following a negative or non-diagnostic EKG and initial cardiac enzymes. MDCT can potentially reduce unnecessary hospital admissions in these patients through enhanced triage and cost-effectiveness. Most investigators agree that patients with a high pretest likelihood of CAD or with known CAD are best evaluated with myocardial perfusion imaging or with invasive angiography [21, 22]. Similarly, the costs and risks associated with MDCT almost always outweigh the benefits in patients with a very low likelihood of CAD, who would already be safely discharged directly from the ED.

The Correlation Between CAD and ACS

Information regarding the presence and extent of CAD, which is easily obtainable with MDCT, can substantially improve the clinical care and management of patients with acute chest pain. These findings significantly expand upon the standard clinical evaluation and are obtained in a rapid and non-invasive manner. Trials have shown that risk stratification can be improved in patients with acute chest pain through the detection of a significant stenosis [23].

While the discovery of a coronary stenosis has been shown to correlate with the incidence of ACS, a causal relationship cannot necessarily be established. Previous trials with invasive coronary angiography have identified a significant coronary stenosis in 80–94% of patients presenting with an unstable angina syndrome or non–ST-segment-elevation myocardial infarction [24-26]. However, observational trials also found that a myocardial infarction also may occur in patients with < 50% stenosis [27, 28].

Several studies conducted with intravascular ultrasonography found a distinct morphology to many coronary atherosclerotic lesions that led to acute events, including a thrombus, small residual vessel lumen, greater plaque burden, and more pronounced positive remodeling [29-31]. Initial studies found similar characteristics of plaques in patients with ACS [32]. As such, patients at risk for ACS can be identified by the detection and characterization of in situ coronary atherosclerotic plaque.

Clinical Trials

Observational Double-Blinded Trial

The Rule Out Myocardial Infarction using Computer Assisted Tomography (ROMICAT) trial was conducted as a prospective double-blinded observational cohort study of consecutive adult patients presenting to the ED with acute chest pain. The results of the first 103 patients in this trial were published in 2006 [22]. All patients had a low to intermediate risk of ACS and had an inconclusive initial ED evaluation, including a negative EKG and a normal initial set of cardiac biomarkers; based on the overall clinical presentation, these patients were awaiting admission to the hospital for further evaluation. Patients underwent 64-slice MDCT while in the ED and then received standard clinical care to rule out ACS during their index hospitalization. All physicians, including those in the ED, that were involved in the clinical care of the subjects were blinded to the result of the MDCT. The design enabled the assessment of the prevalence of CT angiographic patterns of CAD and, more importantly, an unbiased assessment of the safety of several diagnostic thresholds for immediate discharge of patients.

The presence of any coronary atherosclerotic plaque was excluded in 41 patients (40%), none of whom was determined to have ACS (NPV, 100%). In 62 patients, plaque was detected, including all 14 patients with ACS (PPV, 23%). The presence of a significant coronary artery stenosis (> 50% luminal narrowing) was excluded in 73 patients (71%), none of whom had ACS (NPV, 100%). In 13 patients, a significant stenosis was detected; eight of these patients had ACS. In 17 patients, the presence of a significant stenosis could not be excluded because of factors such as heavy calcification or previously placed stents. Six of these patients had ACS. Thus, a significant stenosis either was detected or could not be excluded in 30 patients (29%), corresponding to a specificity of 82% and a PPV of 47%. These initial data therefore suggested that the absence of any CAD is a safe triage criterion and such patients may be discharged directly from the ED. These findings provide the basis for the development of a decision-making tool for ED physicians.

Diagnostic Trials

Goldstein et al. [33] conducted a single-center randomized trial to compare the efficiency of MDCT with rest-stress myocardial perfusion single-photon-emission computed tomography (SPECT) imaging for assessment of very-low-risk acute chest pain patients. In that study, 197 ED patients with completely normal initial ECG and normal serial cardiac biomarkers were enrolled and randomized to MDCT vs. SPECT. Patients in the MDCT group were classified as "normal" if no plaques were found that caused > 25% stenosis ($n = 72$), as "intermediate" if plaques were found that caused 26–70% stenosis or if the MDCT was non-diagnostic ($n = 24$), or as "severe" if plaques were found that caused > 70% stenosis ($n = 0$).

There were no events (myocardial infarction, unstable angina pectoris) in the entire study population during the index hospitalization or after 6-month follow-up. However, the study found that the rate of invasive angiographies tripled in the MDCT group compared with those receiving standard care ($n = 11$ vs. $n = 3$, respectively). Moreover, 24 patients (24.2%) were scored as "intermediate" or "non-diagnostic" and were nonetheless referred for SPECT. The investigators were courageous to perform this study despite the lack of preliminary data. Remarkably, discharge rates were higher in the standard-care group, although time to diagnosis and length of hospital stay were significantly reduced in the MDCT arm. Most likely, this can be attributed to the access to the tests rather than the diagnostic value of MDCT or SPECT.

Rubinshtein and colleagues used a registry-like approach in which two study cardiologists in consensus provided a presumptive diagnosis or exclusion of ACS for each subject, as well as suggested a plan of care, which was either discharge, admit for further evaluation, or admit for an early invasive angiography. All patients then underwent 64-slice MDCT, and the cardiologists were asked to reassess and revise, if necessary, their diagnosis or

exclusion of ACS for each subject as well as their suggested plan of care [34].

Using this theoretical approach, based upon MDCT findings, the diagnosis of ACS was "revised" in 18 of 41 patients (44%; 16 normal MDCT/widely patent stents, 2 alternative diagnoses), planned hospitalization was canceled in 21 of 47 patients (45%; 13 normal MDCT/patent stent, 8 minor branch vessel disease), and planned early invasive strategy was altered in 25 of 58 patients (43%; unnecessary in 20 of 32, advisable in 5 of 26 others). One discharged patient had an event during a 15-month follow-up period. Although MDCT was thought to have reduced the diagnosis of ACS and need for admission with statistical significance, MDCT did not decrease the number of angiograms performed.

Beyond the Angiogram

Although the power of MDCT to non-invasively detect coronary plaque and stenosis is the driving force behind the technology, research is emerging to validate the use of functional and perfusion data as incremental information to the angiogram. In retrospectively gated studies, the improved temporal resolution of 64-slice and dual-source 64-slice scanners provides for the acquisition of an accurate multiphasic data set throughout the cardiac cycle, which can be reconstructed and viewed in cine to evaluate for global and regional left ventricular (LV) function. In the acute chest pain scenario, this capability is useful given previous research conducted with echocardiography, SPECT, and cardiac magnetic resonance imaging (MRI) to detect ACS in ED patients [35-37].

In the study by Kwong et al., 161 patients who presented to the ED with chest pain within the prior 12 h underwent cardiac MRI as soon as feasible in their evaluation [37]. Only patients with ST-segment elevation myocardial infarctions (STEMI) were excluded; patients with a known history of CAD were not. Both a quantitative (e.g., absolute wall thickening) and qualitative (e.g., visually detectable regional wall motion abnormalities) analysis of LV function was conducted. Absolute wall thickening provided the best overall accuracy in detecting ACS (82%), STEMI (89%), and ischemic heart disease (98%). In fact, wall motion was the single most powerful element of the study for detecting ACS.

A number of studies have shown the very good to excellent correlation between LV function assessment with cardiac MRI and cardiac MDCT, such as the study conducted by Fischbach et al. In that trial comparing LV function between the modalities, 95% of normal segments and 88% of segments with decreased wall motion were correctly identified by MDCT, yielding a sensitivity of 88% and specificity of 95% for identification of wall motion abnormalities [38]. Given this agreement, an initial subanalysis from the ROMI-CAT trial was performed to evaluate the ability of resting regional LV function to predict ACS on MDCT [39]. The specificity (96%) and NPV (96.6–100%) for the detection of ACS was excellent. Further analysis on the incremental value of LV functional analysis to angiographic findings is forthcoming.

In addition to LV functional analysis, there is preclinical and preliminary clinical evidence that MDCT can provide assessment of myocardial perfusion. Myocardial perfusion defects from acute and chronic infarcts can be detected on MDCT reconstructions. Acute infarcts appear as areas of relative hypoenhancement on early reconstructions, measured in one study as an average of 53.7 ± 33.5 Hounsfield units (HU) compared with 122.3 ± 25.5 HU in remote myocardium [40]. Initial evidence suggests that 5-mm, thick multi-planar reconstruction (MPR) and 5-mm minimal intensity projection (MinIP) images allow for the best visualization of the infarcts [41]. In preclinical animal models of infarction compared with gross pathology, Lardo et al. demonstrated excellent agreement of infarct size in the setting of acute infarction and chronic myocardial scar [42]. Gerber et al. found similar results in 16 and 21 patients with acute and chronic infarction, respectively [43].

In summary, MDCT data already acquired for reconstruction of an angiogram can also provide useful information on global and regional LV function as well as demonstrate perfusion defects and other changes consistent with acute and chronic infarcts, without the need for any additional contrast or radiation exposure. However, further research regarding the incremental value of this information in the evaluation of patients with acute chest pain is still necessary.

The Comprehensive Thoracic CT Evaluation of Chest Pain

Despite the many potential etiologies that may cause a patient to present to the ED with chest pain, thorough history and physical examination are able to focus the differential diagnosis in the majority of patients. However, a small subset of patients present with an undifferentiated chest pain or chest pain with a component of dyspnea such that these patients are often evaluated with multiple examinations to exclude the presence of the three most feared etiologies of chest pain: CAD, pulmonary embolus (PE), and aortic dissection (AD).While contrast-enhanced spiral CT angiography has become a standard procedure in the

evaluation of the presence of PE [44] and AD [45], it was only recently that non-invasive detection of coronary artery stenosis with MDCT became feasible. As the technology continues to advance, the logical progression in some minds is a study protocol that excludes all three of these potential killers.

Several observational case series have suggested the feasibility of such a comprehensive thoracic MDCT (CT-MDCT) protocol to simultaneously evaluate the coronary arteries, thoracic aorta, and pulmonary arteries [46, 47]. In addition, a recently presented study demonstrated that an individually tailored ECG-gated 64-slice MDCT protocol with a single contrast injection can indeed permit simultaneous visualization of the coronary arteries, thoracic aorta, and pulmonary arteries with excellent image quality using 130 ml of contrast and 17 mSv radiation exposure [48]. However, the principal limitation to a 64-slice protocol is that patients in whom all three conditions comprise the differential diagnosis rarely have low heart rates, and beta-blockade is relatively contraindicated in patients in whom PE is suspected. As such, the temporal resolution (165 ms) of standard 64-slice MDCT would not be expected to be sufficient.

With the advent of dual-source 64-slice CT (DSCT) and the accompanying improvement in temporal resolution to 83 ms, it has been hypothesized that a comprehensive protocol can be achieved without beta-blockade and without a reduction in image quality. In one trial by Johnson et al. [49], 109 patients who presented with acute chest pain underwent comprehensive DSCT without prior administration of a beta-blocker. Adequate contrast enhancement was achieved in the pulmonary arteries, the coronary arteries and the aorta in 94.5% (103/109) of scans. Sensitivity for identification of the etiology of the chest pain was 98% and the sensitivity and NPV for coronary stenosis was 100% compared with invasive angiography. The median radiation exposure was 15.1 mSv.

In another trial, by Schertler et al. [50], 60 consecutive patients with acute chest pain underwent comprehensive DSCT in the ED, also without beta-blocker administration. The image quality of the thoracic aorta was diagnostic in all 60 patients, that of the pulmonary arteries was diagnostic in 59, and for the coronary arteries image quality was diagnostic in 58 patients. The coronary arteries were scored as non-diagnostic in one patient due to ECG-gating-related artifacts and in another patient due to obesity. Mean scan time was 12 s.

As such, comprehensive thoracic DSCT offers significant promise for the simultaneous exclusion of CAD, PE, and AD in the small subset of patients in whom a thorough history and physical examination is unable to focus the differential diagnosis.

The impact of such a comprehensive protocol will require further evaluation.

Conclusion

Overall, cardiac MDCT may improve early ED triage of patients with acute chest pain. After the safety of CT findings on plaque and stenosis for immediate patient discharge has been confirmed in larger observational blinded studies, randomized trials may clarify whether this information will be used by ED physicians in a way that decreases hospital admissions. Furthermore, these trials need to answer questions related to the possible adverse effects of cardiac CT, such as a potential increase in the use of additional diagnostic tests during index hospitalization (e.g., number of invasive angiograms), the effect of the detection of incidental findings, and the cumulative radiation exposure. Nonetheless, the long-term benefits stemming from the new information on the presence of CAD also need to be explored.

References

1. McCaig LF, Burt CW (2004) National Hospital Ambulatory Medical Care Survey: (2002 emergency department summary. Adv Data 340:1–34
2. Swap CJ, Nagurney JT (2005) Value and limitations of chest pain history in the evaluation of patients with suspected acute coronary syndromes. JAMA 294:2623–2629
3. Ornato JP (2003) Management of patients with unstable angina and non-ST-segment elevation myocardial infarction: update ACC/AHA guidelines. Am J Emerg Med 21:346–351
4. Limkakeng A Jr, Gibler WB, Pollack C et al (2001) Combination of Goldman risk and initial cardiac troponin I for emergency department chest pain patient risk stratification. Acad Emerg Med 8:696–702
5. McCarthy BD, Beshansky JR, D'Agostino RB (1993) Missed diagnoses of acute myocardial infarction in the emergency department: results from a multicenter study. Ann Emerg Med 22:579–582
6. Pope JH, Aufderheide TP, Ruthazer R et al (2000) Missed diagnoses of acute cardiac ischemia in the emergency department. N Engl J Med 342: 1163–1170
7. Lee TH, Rouan GW, Weisberg MC et al (1987) Clinical characteristics and natural history of patients with acute myocardial infarction sent home from the emergency room. Am J Cardiol 60:219–224
8. Gibbons RJ, Chatterjee K, Daley J et al (1999) ACC/AHA/ACP-ASIM guidelines for the management of patients with chronic stable angina: executive summary and recommendations. A Report of the American College of Cardiology/American Heart Association Task Force on Practice Guidelines (Committee on Management of Patients with Chronic Stable Angina). Circulation 99:2829–2848
9. Tosteson AN, Goldman L, Udvarhelyi IS, Lee TH (1996) Cost-effectiveness of a coronary care unit versus an intermediate care unit for emergency department patients with chest pain. Circulation 94:143–150
10. Lee TH, Goldman L (2000) Evaluation of the patient with acute chest pain. N Engl J Med 342: 1187–1195
11. Goldman L, Cook EF, Johnson PA et al (1996) Prediction of the need for intensive care in patients who come to emergency departments with acute chest pain. N Engl J Med 334:1498–1504
12. Kaul P, Newby LK, Fu Y et al (2004) International differences in evolution of early discharge after acute myocardial infarction. Lancet 363:511–517
13. Leschka S, Alkadhi H, Plass A et al (2005) Accuracy of MSCT coronary angiography with 64-slice technology: first experience. Eur Heart J 26:1482–1487
14. Mollet NR, Cademartiri F, van Mieghem CA et al (2005) High-resolution spiral computed tomography coronary angiography in patients referred for diagnostic conventional coronary angiography. Circulation 112:2318–2323
15. Leber AW, Knez A, von Ziegler F et al (2005) Quantification of obstructive and nonobstructive coronary lesions by 64-slice computed tomography: a comparative study with quantitative coronary angiography and intravascular ultrasound. J Am Coll Cardiol 46:147–154
16. Roe MT, Harrington RA, Prosper DM et al (2000) Clinical and therapeutic profile of patients presenting with acute coronary syndromes who do not have significant coronary artery disease: the Platelet Glycoprotein IIb/IIIa in Unstable Angina: Receptor Suppression Using Integrilin Therapy (PURSUIT) Trial Investigators. Circulation 102:1101–1106
17. Hoffmann U, Nagurney JT, Moselewski F et al (2006) Coronary multidetector computed tomography in the assessment of patients with acute chest pain. Circulation 114(21):2251-2260
18. Rixe J, Achenbach S, Ropers D et al (2006) Assessment of coronary artery stent restenosis by 64-slice multi-detector computed tomography. Eur Heart J 27(21):2567-2572
19. Cademartiri F, Schuijf JD, Pugliese F et al (2007) Usefulness of 64-slice multislice computed tomography coronary angiography to assess in-stent restenosis. J Am Coll Cardiol 49(22):2204-2210
20. Malagutti P, Nieman K, Meijboom W et al (2007) Use of 64-slice CT in symptomatic patients after coronary bypass surgery: evaluation of grafts and coronary arteries. Eur Heart J 28(15):1879-1885
21. Berman DS, Hachamovitch R, Shaw LJ et al (2006) Roles of nuclear cardiology, cardiac computed tomography, and cardiac magnetic resonance: Noninvasive risk stratification and a conceptual framework for the selection of noninvasive imaging tests in patients with known or suspected coronary artery disease. J Nucl Med 47(7):1107-1118
22. Hendel RC, Patel MR, Kramer CM et al (2006) ACCF/ACR/SCCT/SCMR/ASNC/NASCI/SCAI/SIR (2006 appropriateness criteria for cardiac computed tomography and cardiac magnetic resonance imaging: a report of the American College of Cardiology Foundation Quality Strategic Directions Committee Appropriateness Criteria Working Group, American College of Radiology, Society of Cardiovascular Computed Tomography, Society for Cardiovascular Magnetic Resonance, American Society of Nuclear Cardiology, North American Society for Cardiac Imaging, Society for Cardiovascular Angiography and Interventions, and Society of Interventional Radiology. J Am Coll Cardiol 48(7):1475-1497
23. Hoffmann U, Nagurney JT, Moselewski F et al (2006) Coronary multidetector computed tomography in the assessment of patients with acute chest pain. Circulation 114:2251-2260

24. Wallentin L, Lagerqvist B, Husted S et al (2000) Outcome at 1 year after an invasive compared with a non-invasive strategy in unstable coronary-artery disease: the FRISC II invasive randomised trial. FRISC II Investigators. Fast revascularisation during instability in coronary artery disease. Lancet 356:9–16

25. Wallentin L (2002) Non-ST-elevation acute coronary syndrome: fuel for the invasive strategy. Lancet 360:738–739

26. Roe MT, Harrington RA, Prosper DM et al (2000)Clinical and therapeutic profile of patients presenting with acute coronary syndromes who do not have significant coronary artery disease. The Platelet Glycoprotein IIb/IIIa in Unstable Angina: Receptor Suppression Using Integrilin Therapy (PURSUIT) Trial Investigators. Circulation 102:1101–1106

27. Ambrose JA, Tannenbaum MA, Alexopoulos D et al (1988) Angiographic progression of coronary artery disease and the development of myocardial infarction. J Am Coll Cardiol 12:56–62

28. Falk E, Shah PK, Fuster V (1995) Coronary plaque disruption. Circulation 92:657–671

29. Nakamura M, Nishikawa H, Mukai S et al (2001) Impact of coronary artery remodeling on clinical presentation of coronary artery disease: an intravascular ultrasound study. J Am Coll Cardiol 37:63–69

30. Ehara S, Kobayashi Y, Yoshiyama M et al (2004) Spotty calcification typifies the culprit plaque in patients with acute myocardial inarction: an intravascular ultrasound study. Circulation 110:3424–3429

31. Maehara A, Mintz GS, Bui AB et al (2002) Morphologic and angiographic features of coronary plaque rupture detected by intravascular ultrasound. J Am Coll Cardiol 40:904–910

32. Hoffmann U, Moselewski F, Nieman K et al (2006) Noninvasive assessment of plaque morphology and composition in culprit and stable lesions in acute coronary syndrome and stable lesions in stable angina by multidetector computed tomography. J Am Coll Cardiol 47(8):1655-1662

33. Goldstein JA, Gallagher MJ, O'Neill WW et al (2007) A randomized controlled trial of multi-slice coronary computed tomography for evaluation of acute chest pain. J Am Coll Cardiol 49(8):863-871

34. Rubinshtein R, Halon DA, Gaspar T et al (2007) Impact of 64-slice cardiac computed tomographic angiography on clinical decision-making in emergency department patients with chest pain of possible myocardial ischemic origin. Am J Cardiol 100:1522–1526

35. Kontos MC, Arrowood JA, Jesse RL et al (1998) Comparison between 2-dimensional echocardiography and myocardial perfusion imaging in the emergency department in patients with possible myocardial ischemia. Am Heart J 136(4 Pt 1):724-733

36. Sabia PJ, Powers ER, Jayaweera AR et al (1992) Functional significance of collateral blood flow in patients with recent acute myocardial infarction. A study using myocardial contrast echocardiography.Circulation. 85(6):2080-2089

37. Kwong RY, Schussheim AE, Rekhraj S et al (2003) Detecting acute coronary syndrome in the emergency department with cardiac magnetic resonance imaging. Circulation 107:531-537

38. Fischbach R, Juergens KU, Ozgun M et al (2007) Assessment of regional left ventricular function with multidetector-row computed tomography versus magnetic resonance imaging. Eur Radiol 17:1009–1017

39. Rogers IS, Seneviratne SK, Bamberg F et al (2007) Resting regional left ventricular function as assessed using cardiac 64-slice computed tomography to predict acute coronary syndrome in patients with acute chest pain. Circulation 116(Suppl II):II-562

40. Nikolaou K, Sanz J, Poon M et al (2005) Assessment of myocardial perfusion and viability from routine contrast-enhanced 16-detector-row computed tomography of the heart: preliminary results. Eur Radiol 15:864-871

41. Rogers IS, Cury RC, Shapiro MD et al (2007) Evaluation of cardiac multidetector computed tomography reconstruction modalities for the detection of perfusion defects in patients presenting with acute ST Segment elevation myocardial infarction. J Cardiovasc Comput Tomogr 1(1 Supp):S31

42. Lardo AC, Cordeiro MA, Silva C et al (2006) Contrast-enhanced multidetector computed tomography viability imaging after myocardial infarction: characterization of myocyte death, microvascular obstruction, and chronic scar. Circulation 113:394–404

43. Gerber BL, Belge B, Legros GJ et al (2006) Characterization of acute and chronic myocardial infarcts by multidetector computed tomography: comparison with contrast-enhanced magnetic resonance. Circulation 113:823–833

44. Kruip MJ et al (2006) A simple diagnostic strategy in hospitalized patients with clinically suspected pulmonary embolism. J Intern Med 260(5):459-466

45. Yoshida S, Akiba H, Tamakawa M et al (2003) Thoracic involvement of type A aortic dissection and intramural hematoma: diagnostic accuracy—comparison of emergency helical CT and surgical findings. Radiology 228(2):430-435

46. White CS, Kuo D, Kelemen M et al (2005) Chest pain evaluation in the emergency department: can MDCT provide a comprehensive evaluation? AJR Am J Roentgenol 185(2):533-540

47. Raptopoulos VD, Boiselle PB, Michailidis N et al (2006) MDCT angiography of acute chest pain: evaluation of ECG-gated and nongated techniques. AJR Am J Roentgenol 186(6 Suppl 2):S346-356

48. Shapiro MD, Dodd J, Wittram C et al (2007) A novel imaging protocol to visualize the coronary artery tree, thoracic aorta, and pulmonary artery vasculature with a single contrast bolus and twenty second scan duration using ECG-gated 64-slice MDCT. Meeting: RSNA 2007, November 27, 2007, Chicago, Abstract SS G19-03

49. Johnson TR, Nikolaou K, Becker A et al (2007) Dual-source CT for chest pain assessment. Eur Radiol [Epub ahead of print]

50. Schertler T, Scheffel H, Frauenfelder T et al (2007) Dual-source computed tomography in patients with acute chest pain: feasibility and image quality. Eur Radiol 17(12):3179-3188

21

Coronary CTA for Stent Evaluation

Gopi Kiran Reddy Sirineni, Stefan Tigges, Arthur E. Stillman

Introduction

Stent placement is commonly used for the treatment of obstructive coronary artery disease. Initially, bare-metal stents were deployed to maintain vessel patency, but 21–36% of these stents developed in-stent re-stenosis (ISR) due to neointimal hyperplasia [1, 2]. Neointimal hyperplasia is a normal reparative process that occurs after stent deployment and is usually not extensive enough to cause hemodynamic significant narrowing [3]. However, if there is sufficient cellular proliferation, hemodynamic stenosis may be significant enough to bring about recurrent ischemia [3].

The newer drug-eluting stents have made ISR a much less common problem. These stents are coated with agents that prevent cellular proliferation such that re-stenosis rates are as low as 7–8%–a marked improvement compared with the rates with bare-metal stents [1, 2]. However, long-term follow up of patients with these newer stents, especially Paclitaxel stents, suggests a higher incidence of stent thrombosis than occurs with bare-metal stents [4]. Thus, patients with either stent type may require imaging to determine stent patency.

At present, catheter angiography is the procedure of choice for the evaluation and follow-up of stent patency. However, this procedure is invasive, with a low but important rate of intra- and post-procedural complications and a fairly long recovery period [5, 6]. Noninvasive imaging options such as magnetic resonance imaging (MRI) [7–9], and electron-beam computed tomography (EBCT) [10, 11] have had poor success in evaluating ISR. Susceptibility artifacts from the metallic stents degrade MRI quality, precluding a reliable MRI study. The low spatial resolution of EBCT makes visualization of the stent lumen difficult. Nuclear imaging studies, such as single photon emission computed tomography (SPECT) and positron emission tomography (PET), provide very little anatomical information about the location of the culprit stenosis. Before the advent of multi-detector-row computed tomography (MDCT) technology, CT imaging of the heart was considered impractical (with the exception of EBCT) due to low temporal resolution. Attempts at evaluating stent stenosis with earlier generations of 4-slice MDCT scanners were disappointing [12]. Studies on stent patency involving new-generation 16-slice [13] and 64-slice [14–16] MDCT scanners showed improving results, but stent evaluation is limited by the blooming and beam-hardening artifacts [17] resulting from the high X-ray attenuation of the stent struts. MDCT imaging of stents is also susceptible to motion artifacts and is dependent on the temporal resolution of the scanner. The latest MDCT technologies, such as dual-source MDCT, are expected to further improve accuracy-as they have a higher temporal resolution [18].

Stent-Related Artifacts

Blooming, beam hardening, and motion all produce artifacts that degrade the evaluation of coronary stents.

Blooming

Blooming occurs because of partial volume averaging. This, in turn, is due to the high attenuation of strut metal along the inner diameter of the stent, which results in a spuriously increased density of the adjacent stent lumen [19]. Artifactual luminal stenosis of the stent arises from the effect of blooming on the stent interior (Fig. 1). The effect on the stent's external diameter is similar: partial volume averaging of the outer diameter metal with the adjacent vessel wall causes the stented vessel to appear larger than the adjacent native

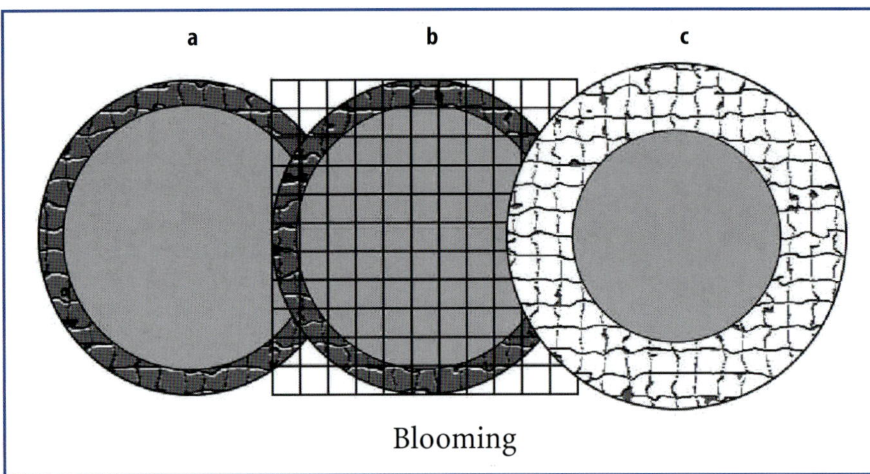

Fig. 1. Blooming. The true stent dimensions are represented in (**a**). When a computed tomography (CT) scan of this stent is performed; the resultant image is constructed based on attenuation values in voxel grid (**b**). The high attenuation of the metallic stent causes an increase in the attenuation of adjacent voxels due to partial voluming, such that the stent appears spuriously larger, and the stent lumen spuriously narrower (**c**)

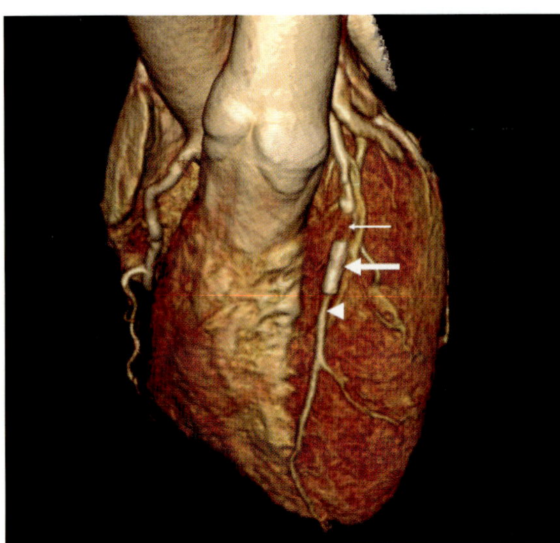

Fig. 2. Blooming. A volume-rendered image of the heart and coronary arteries showing a stent (*thick arrow*) in the left anterior descending artery (LAD). This stent appears artifactually larger than the native vessel lumen (*arrowhead*), although in reality it is within the vessel lumen. This is due to the effect of blooming, caused by the high density of the stent strut material. Note that the portion of the LAD just proximal to the stent shows an occlusive plaque (*thin arrow*), depicted here in a color different from that of the contrast-filled lumen

vessel (Fig. 2). Blooming artifacts increase with strut thickness and the density of the strut material and decreases with improving spatial resolution of the scanner. The tube potential (kVp) inversely affects the amount of blooming artifact, although to a lesser extent in the medical range of exposures [20, 21]. With current MDCT technology, visualization of the luminal diameter of the stent at best represents 50–70% of the true value [20, 22].

Beam Hardening

The X-rays produced by MDCT scanners are poly-chromatic. When polychromatic X-rays pass through high-density structures, such as a metallic stent, calcium, and bone, lower-energy photons are more likely to be deflected than photons of higher energy, resulting in an increase in the mean energy of the X-ray beam [19, 23]. This higher-energy beam can more easily penetrate adjacent structures, resulting in an artifactual decrease in the attenuation of tissues next to high-density material (Fig. 3). In the case of a stent, the lumen that is immediately adjacent to the metal strut appears artifactually darker (hypodense), making it difficult to differentiate true neointimal hyperplasia from artifact. Use of higher kVp as well as filters to maintain beam uniformity may reduce these artifacts. Newer methods for differential energy weighting and iterative reconstruction algorithms may be helpful in reducing the effects of these artifacts [24–26].

Motion Artifacts

Coronary and respiratory motions degrade the image quality of CT coronary angiography. The patient's heart rate is usually lowered by the administration of beta-blockers [27]. For single-source 64-slice MDCT scanners, a regular heart rhythm with a heart rate of 60–65 beats per minute (bpm) is preferred for optimum image quality [28]. Such stringent control of heart rate is not required for the newer dual-source MDCT scanners [29, 30].

Imaging Parameters

The acquisition phase for MDCT imaging in stent evaluation is the same as for routine coronary CT angiography. For image reconstruction, a sharper kernel with high spatial frequency is used. The standard imaging protocol employed at our institution is shown in Table 1. Certain protocol varia-

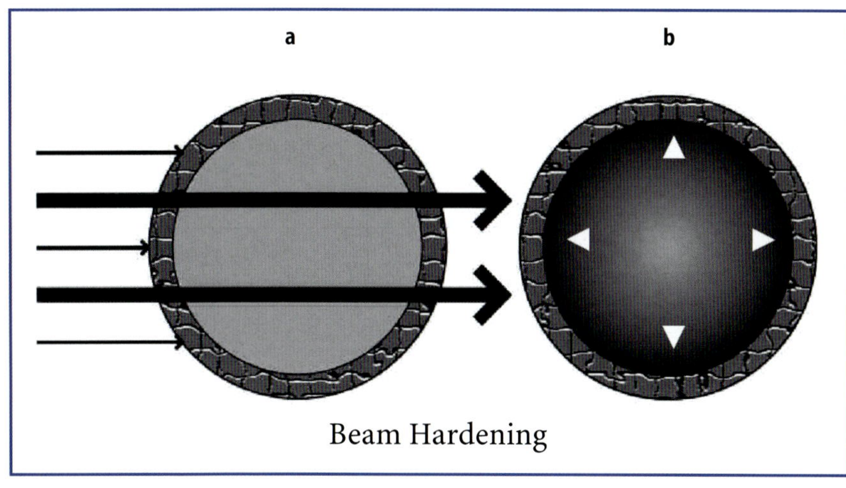

Fig. 3. Beam hardening. The X-ray beam from the computed tomography (CT) scanner source is polychromatic in nature, consisting of photons of higher (*thick arrows*) and lower (*thin arrows*) energies. The metallic stent strut absorbs the lower-energy photons, causing the beam to consist predominantly of higher-energy photons that pass through the stent, a process known as beam hardening. This causes relative darkening (*arrowheads*) of the stent lumen adjacent to the stent strut. This artifact mimics a plaque, making it difficult to differentiate true vs. artifactual plaque

Table 1. Protocol for 64 slice single and dual-source MDCT: The typical protocol used in our institution for single-source and dual-source scanners in the evaluation of stents

Detector collimation	64×0.6
Slice thickness	0.75 mm
Reconstruction interval	0.5 mm
Pitch	0.2:1 For single-source automatic adjustment by scanner, for a dual source based on heart rate
Reconstruction kernel	B46 or sharp or bone kernel in addition to the standard or medium smooth reconstructions
kVp	120
Rotation time	0.33 s
Effective mAs	850–900
ECG gating	Retrospective
ECG pulsing	50–80% R-R for single source
	30–70% R-R for dual source; usually this is automatically adjusted by the scanner based on the patient's heart rate
FOV	~200 mm
Contrast injection	Test bolus: 20 ml of nonionic iodinated contrast 350% at 5 ml/s followed with saline chase of 20 ml at 5 ml/s. ROI in the ascending aorta. Peak enhancement calculated. 80 ml of nonionic iodinated contrast 350 mgI/mL or higher at 5 ml/s followed with 40 ml of saline at 5 ml/s. Scan delay is calculated as peak enhancement time +4 s
Phase reconstructions	65% and 75% when heart rate is < 65 bpm; 45% and 55% at higher heart rates

tions may be useful on a case-by-case basis, and it is essential to know the effects of the various imaging parameters on stent visualization.

Effects of Imaging Parameters on Stent Visualization

Tube Potential (kVp)

An increase in kVp theoretically causes less blooming and beam-hardening effects and should thus improve stent visualization [21]. However, kVp cannot be increased beyond 140 kV on medical scanners since higher levels increase the patient radiation dose. An in vitro coronary stent CT study confirmed that there is improved visualization of stent luminal diameter when kVp is increased from 120 to 140 kV, but the difference was not enough to warrant the routine use of this technique [20]. An increase in kVp may be useful when stents with thicker struts and smaller luminal diameters are imaged. A tradeoff is the reduced attenuation of contrast material with higher kVp.

Contrast Concentration

The concentration of iodinated contrast agent in the stent lumen influences estimations of stent diameter. Lower concentrations of contrast agent result in more accurate diameter measurements; likewise, a non-contrast study provides the best estimate of stent luminal diameter [20, 31]. However, a drastic reduction in the concentration of contrast agent is not advisable because very dilute concentrations limit the evaluation of plaque within the stent and elsewhere in the coronary arterial tree. Estimation of the true luminal diameter of the stent is not critical for assessing stent patency.

Reconstruction Kernel

The reconstruction kernel has the greatest impact on visualization of the stent lumen and the evaluation of stent patency. Use of a high spatial frequency reconstruction algorithm optimizes stent evaluation by improving stent diameter measurement and providing a more reliable contrast density within the stent lumen [32, 33] (Figs. 4, 5). Many CT vendors have included dedicated stent reconstruction kernels in their cardiac software [32, 33]; however, these kernels are usually available on all scanners in some form or another. If these kernels are not available, other high-spatial-reconstruction algorithms, such as a bone reconstruction algorithm or a high-resolution CT (HRCT) reconstruction algorithm, can be used.

Spatial Resolution

Acquisition of images at the highest possible spatial resolution improves visualization of the stent lumen by decreasing partial volume effects. Early studies performed on the 4-slice MDCT scanners demonstrated poor visualization because the spatial resolution of these scanners was low [12]. The spatial resolution of scanners has progressively increased from 4 slices to 16 and 64 slices. With the new 64-slice scanners, a spatial resolution of 0.4–0.625 mm can be achieved. The spatial resolution is dependent on detector thickness and collimation; hence, the thinnest possible detector collimation and thickness should be selected to get good results in stent evaluation. The near isotropic nature of MDCT data sets makes multiplanar reconstructions more reliable for measuring the stent lumen.

Effects of Stent Type

Stent type and diameter are probably the most important factors affecting lumen visualization. Stents made of high-density material such as tantalum and gold have such severe blooming artifacts that lumen visualization is almost impossible. In an in vitro study performed on 68 different stents, only 3.3% of the actual stent luminal diameter of a tantalum stent was visible [22]. Similarly, stents with thicker struts cause greater artifactual luminal narrowing than stents with thinner struts [34]. For patients with these types of stents, evalu-

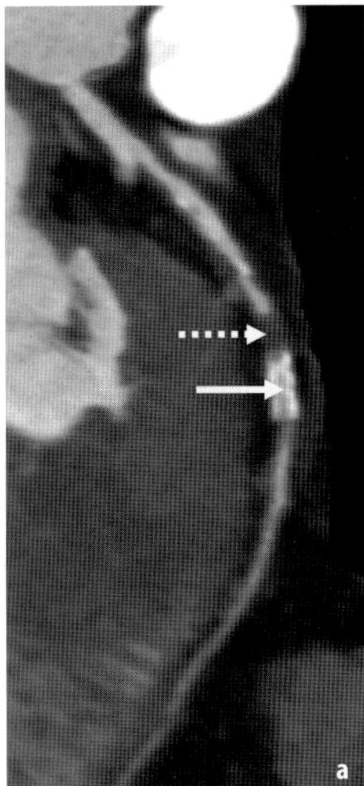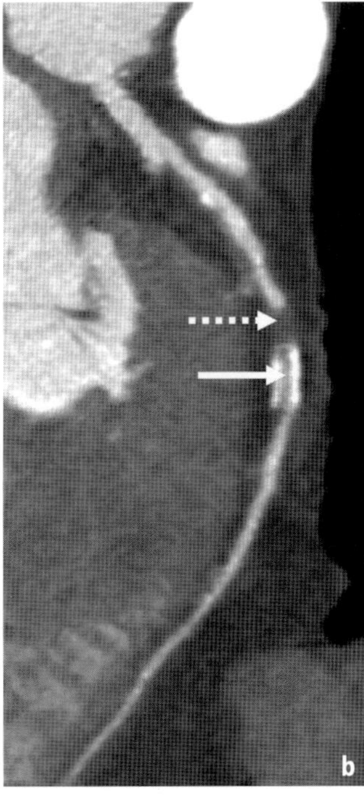

Fig. 4a, b. Reconstruction kernel. Curved reformats showing a stent in the mid-LAD. Standard medium smooth reconstruction is shown in (**a**). The stent lumen is not clearly visualized with this reconstruction (*solid arrow*). Note that the occlusive plaque just proximal to the stent is clearly visualized (*dotted arrow*). Reconstruction of the same acquisition using a sharp kernel (**b**) results in good visualization of the stent lumen (*solid arrow*) without adversely affecting visualization of the proximal plaque (*dotted arrow*)

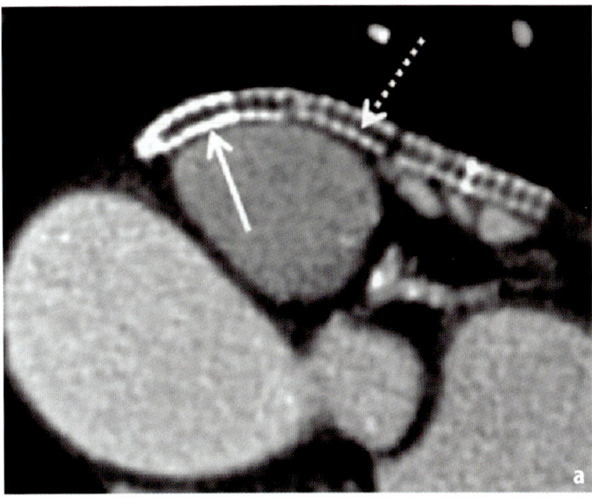
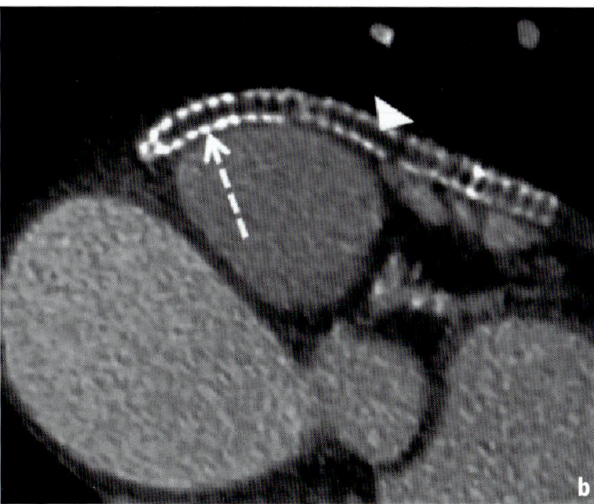

Fig. 5a, b. Reconstruction kernel. Multi-planar images of three stents in an occluded saphenous vein graft (SVG) reconstructed with a standard smooth kernel (**a**) and a sharper kernel (**b**). Visualization of the stent struts (*solid arrow*) and the stent lumen (*dotted arrow*) is limited when a standard smooth reconstruction kernel is used. The individual stent struts (*dashed arrow*) can be clearly identified using a sharper reconstruction kernel, with improvement in stent luminal (*arrowhead*) visualization. All the stents are totally occluded, with no intraluminal contrast

ation of stent patency with MDCT is a wasteful exercise. However, in most of the stents evaluated in the study by Maintz et al. [22] lumen visibility was > 50% of the actual diameter. The likelihood of encountering such favorable stents for MDCT imaging is high. The same study reported that lumen visualization in stents made with Nitinol was as high as 73% of the stents' actual diameters [22]. Finally, high-density stents have artifactually increased and non-uniform stent luminal attenuation.

Coronary Stent Imaging

Like all coronary CT imaging, multi-planar reformatted images are the workhorse of coronary stent evaluation. Curved reformats and transverse images are particularly useful in the visualization of the stent lumen. Since 64-slice MDCT data sets are near isotropic, measurements on any type of reformats are expected to produce consistent and reliable results. However, as discussed above, artifacts from stent struts make estimation of in-stent stenosis difficult.

It seems intuitive that larger stents with diameters > 3–4 mm are better evaluated by MDCT [35] than smaller stents, but a recent study found no such difference in the evaluability of stent patency based on stent diameter [36]. Although debatable, it is reasonable to assume that stent material composition and thickness have a greater effect on stent evaluation than stent luminal dimensions.

On average, 7–12% of stents may be non-evalu-

able because of stent-related artifacts or cardiac and respiratory motion[16, 37]. Current literature reports for 64-slice MDCT evaluation of in-stent stenosis indicate a sensitivity of 92–95%, a specificity of 81–93%, a positive predictive value of 63–77%, and a negative predictive value of 98–99% compared with invasive coronary angiography [37, 38]. These results indicate that MDCT is best used to exclude stenosis, rather than as a tool for detecting and grading stenosis, because of the substantial false-positive rate [37, 38].

The contrast enhancement pattern in the vessel lumen proximal to a stent, within a stent lumen, and distal to the stent are important considerations in patency evaluation. A stent can be considered occluded when the stent lumen is darker than the contrast-enhanced vessel proximal to the stent or when no contrast is present at the distal end of the stent. Such totally occluded stents can be identified readily. Reduced or absent distal runoff usually indicates a significantly occluded stent. Nonetheless, the converse is not true. Normal distal runoff does not necessarily indicate a significantly occluded stent because of potential collateral filling of the distal vessel.

Cross-sectional or end-on views are important in the evaluation of partial stenoses. A significant stent stenosis is present if ≤ 50% of the cross section is enhanced with contrast. Any stent luminal obstruction ≥ 50% is considered significant and may warrant further study. As noted above, beam-hardening artifacts cause darkening of the stent lumen and simulate neointimal hyperplasia. These artifacts are usually close to the stent strut and fade toward the center of the lumen. Beam-hardening artifacts are also darker and regular, with highly negative attenuation values. However, it may not be possible to differentiate these artifacts from true plaque. This translates into a high number of false-positive results, decreasing the specificity of MDCT as a test for evaluation of in-stent stenosis. The presence of calcium may also complicate stent evaluations.

MDCT does not yet rival invasive catheter angiography in the detection and grading of in-stent stenosis, but no other imaging modalities currently challenge MDCT in accurate anatomical localization of the stent. This is particularly useful in immediate post-percutaneous coronary intervention (PCI) localization of stent deployment and assessment of the anatomical relationship of the stent to the coronary ostia. Such accurate localization may be especially useful in interventions involving coronary bypass graft stents. Volume-rendered images are most helpful in depicting the global anatomy of the coronary arteries and the stents. On these images, stents appear as thickened structures over the coronary vessel due to the blooming effect of the struts.

It is likely that combining perfusion imaging under hyperemic conditions (e.g., adenosine) with CT angiography will improve the diagnostic accuracy of in-stent stenosis evaluation by CT.

Summary

Coronary stent evaluation by MDCT is limited by many artifacts inherent to CT technology. Despite these limitations, reasonable accuracy in detecting in-stent stenosis can be achieved with 64-slice MDCT. A high negative predictive value for MDCT means that significant stent stenosis can be reliably excluded, thus making CT a suitable alternative to invasive coronary angiography in excluding significant ISR. Although the data are limited, the newer dual-source scanners may further reduce artifacts, especially those related to coronary motion.

References

1. Moses JW, Leon MB, Popma JJ et al (2003) Sirolimus-eluting stents versus standard stents in patients with stenosis in a native coronary artery. N Engl J Med 349:1315-1323
2. Suttorp MJ, Laarman GJ, Rahel BM et al (2006) Primary Stenting of Totally Occluded Native Coronary Arteries II (PRISON II): a randomized comparison of bare metal stent implantation with sirolimus-eluting stent implantation for the treatment of total coronary occlusions. Circulation 114:921-928
3. Grewe PH, Deneke T, Machraoui A et al (2000) Acute and chronic tissue response to coronary stent implantation: pathologic findings in human specimen. J Am Coll Cardiol 35:157-163
4. Stettler C, Wandel S, Allemann S et al (2007) Outcomes associated with drug-eluting and bare-metal stents: a collaborative network meta-analysis. Lancet 370:937-948
5. Adams DF, Abrams HL (1979) Complications of coronary arteriography: a follow-up report. Cardiovasc Radiol 2:89-96
6. Adams DF, Fraser DB, Abrams HL (1973) The complications of coronary arteriography. Circulation 48:609-618
7. Manning WJ, Nezafat R, Appelbaum E et al (2007) Coronary magnetic resonance imaging. Cardiol Clin 25:141-170, vi
8. Dewey M, Teige F, Schnapauff D et al (2006) Combination of free-breathing and breathhold steady-state free precession magnetic resonance angiography for detection of coronary artery stenoses. J Magn Reson Imaging 23:674-681
9. Sakuma H, Ichikawa Y, Suzawa N et al (2005) Assessment of coronary arteries with total study time of less than 30 minutes by using whole-heart coronary MR angiography. Radiology 237:316-321
10. Knollmann FD, Moller J, Gebert A et al (2004) Assessment of coronary artery stent patency by electron-beam CT. Eur Radiol 14:1341-1347
11. Pump H, Mohlenkamp S, Sehnert CA et al (2000) Coronary arterial stent patency: assessment with electron-beam CT. Radiology 214:447-452
12. Mazzarotto P, Di Renzi P, Paluello GM et al (2006) Comparison between four-slice computed tomography and coronary angiography for the assessment of coronary stents. J Cardiovasc Med (Hagerstown) 7:328-334
13. Schuijf JD, Bax JJ, Jukema JW et al (2004) Feasibility of assessment of coronary stent patency using 16-slice computed tomography. Am J Cardiol 94:427-430
14. Seifarth H, Ozgun M, Raupach R et al (2006) 64-Versus 16-slice CT angiography for coronary artery stent assessment: in vitro experience. Invest Radiol 41:22-27
15. Wolf F, Feuchtner GM, Homolka P et al (2007) In vitro imaging of coronary artery stents: Are there differences between 16- and 64-slice CT scanners? Eur J Radiol (Epub ahead of print)
16. Cademartiri F, Schuijf JD, Pugliese F et al (2007) Usefulness of 64-slice multislice computed tomography coronary angiography to assess in-stent restenosis. J Am Coll Cardiol 49:2204-2210
17. Jerrold T, Bushberg EML, Boone JM (1994) Essential physics of medical imaging. Lippincott Williams & Wilkins, Baltimore
18. Lell MM, Panknin C, Saleh R et al (2007) Evaluation of coronary stents and stenoses at different heart rates with dual source spiral CT (DSCT). Invest Radiol 42:536-541
19. Barrett JF, Keat N (2004) Artifacts in CT: recognition and avoidance. Radiographics 24:1679-1691
20. Sirineni GK, Kalra MK, Pottala K et al (2006) Effect of contrast concentration, tube potential and reconstruction kernels on MDCT evaluation of coronary stents: an in vitro study. Int J Cardiovasc Imaging 23:253-263
21. Suzuki S, Furui S, Kuwahara S et al (2007) Assessment of coronary stent in vitro on multislice computed tomography angiography: improved in-stent visibility by the use of 140-kV tube voltage. J Comput Assist Tomogr 31:414-421
22. Maintz D, Seifarth H, Raupach R et al (2006) 64-slice

multidetector coronary CT angiography: in vitro evaluation of 68 different stents. Eur Radiol 16:818-826

23. Alles J, Mudde RF (2007) Beam hardening: analytical considerations of the effective attenuation coefficient of X-ray tomography. Med Phys 34:2882-2889

24. Hsieh J, Molthen RC, Dawson CA et al (2000) An iterative approach to the beam hardening correction in cone beam CT. Med Phys 27:23-29

25. Shikhaliev PM (2005) Beam hardening artefacts in computed tomography with photon counting, charge integrating and energy weighting detectors: a simulation study. Phys Med Biol 50:5813-5827

26. Yan CH, Whalen RT, Beaupre GS et al (2000) Reconstruction algorithm for polychromatic CT imaging: application to beam hardening correction. IEEE Trans Med Imaging 19:1-11

27. Shim SS, Kim Y, Lim SM (2005) Improvement of image quality with beta-blocker premedication on ECG-gated 16-MDCT coronary angiography. AJR Am J Roentgenol 184:649-654

28. Herzog C, Arning-Erb M, Zangos S et al (2006) Multi-detector row CT coronary angiography: influence of reconstruction technique and heart rate on image quality. Radiology 238:75-86

29. Matt D, Scheffel H, Leschka S et al (2007) Dual-source CT coronary angiography: image quality, mean heart rate, and heart rate variability. AJR Am J Roentgenol 189:567-573

30. Scheffel H, Alkadhi H, Plass A et al (2006) Accuracy of dual-source CT coronary angiography: First experience in a high pre-test probability population without heart rate control. Eur Radiol 16:2739-2747

31. Nieman K, Cademartiri F, Raaijmakers R et al (2003) Noninvasive angiographic evaluation of coronary stents with multi-slice spiral computed tomography. Herz 28:136-142

32. Maintz D, Seifarth H, Flohr T et al (2003) Improved coronary artery stent visualization and in-stent stenosis detection using 16-slice computed-tomography and dedicated image reconstruction technique. Invest Radiol 38:790-795

33. Seifarth H, Raupach R, Schaller S et al (2005) Assessment of coronary artery stents using 16-slice MDCT angiography: evaluation of a dedicated reconstruction kernel and a noise reduction filter. Eur Radiol 15:721-726

34. Utsunomiya D, Awai K, Sakamoto T et al (2007) In vitro evaluation of metallic coronary artery stents with sub-millimeter multi-slice computed tomography using an ECG-gated cardiac phantom: relationship between in-stent visualization and stent type. Cardiology 107:254-260

35. Suzuki S, Furui S, Kaminaga T et al (2005) Evaluation of coronary stents in vitro with CT angiography: effect of stent diameter, convolution kernel, and vessel orientation to the z-axis. Circ J 69:1124-1131

36. Schepis T, Koepfli P, Leschka S et al (2007) Coronary artery stent geometry and in-stent contrast attenuation with 64-slice computed tomography. Eur Radiol 17:1464-1473

37. Ehara M, Kawai M, Surmely JF et al (2007) Diagnostic accuracy of coronary in-stent restenosis using 64-slice computed tomography: comparison with invasive coronary angiography. J Am Coll Cardiol 49:951-959

38. Gaspar T, Halon DA, Lewis BS et al (2005) Diagnosis of coronary in-stent restenosis with multidetector row spiral computed tomography. J Am Coll Cardiol 46:1573-1579

SECTION IV

MDCT of Head and Neck

22

CT Angiography of the Neck and Brain

David S. Enterline

Introduction

The evolution of multidetector computed tomography (MDCT) has allowed the development and advancement of CT angiography (CTA). While the concept of carotid artery evaluation by CT was introduced by Heinz and others in 1984 [1, 2], it has taken recent technological advances to bring the current methods into practice. CTA of the neck is used primarily to assess the carotid vessels. As CTA slice thickness and rendering methods have improved, so has the accuracy of stenosis determination. More recently, CTA of the neck has become the standard for traumatic injury. Routine utilization of CTA for the evaluation of carotid and vertebral arteries is now the norm. The technique also has been successfully applied to the intracranial vasculature. Detection of cerebral aneurysms and other vascular diseases are readily identified.

This chapter will discuss CT techniques and contrast optimization of MDCT for CTA of the neck and brain and discuss the interpretation of the diseases commonly evaluated by this technique.

CT Technique

Obtaining great quality CTA of the neck and brain requires optimizing CT technique and acquisition. Thin-slice CT attained while the contrast bolus is present is the fundamental doctrine. While some CT parameters are vendor specific, there are general principles that apply [3]. The scan for neck CTA is set up from the aortic arch to the skull base or to 1 cm above the top of the dorsum sella if additional information is desired about intracranial circulation. Alternatively, the scan can extend to the vertex of the skull. From a practical standpoint, this combined approach is most often used. For CTA of the brain, the scan starts at the C2 level and goes to 1 cm above the dorsum sella or to the vertex. In or-

der to evaluate a suspected vascular lesion more cephalad, such as in the case of an arteriovenous malformation (AVM), the volume covered needs to include this region, too. In most cases, a 20-cm field of view is used. This can be adjusted up or down as the situation warrants; however, use of a smaller field of view improves resolution. Patient chin position is adjusted to a neutral position since the scan is obtained at no gantry tilt, otherwise, the vasculature of the anterior head may be missed. Scanning from caudal to cephalad minimizes the contrast volume needed and venous opacification; however, it does risk producing a nondiagnostic scan if there is not sufficient contrast present.

Slice thickness directly determines resolution in the Z-axis. For neck CTA, use of slices in the 0.5- to 1.5-mm range provides adequate resolution and coverage. In general, for four- and eight-slice scanners, a thickness of 1 mm is used while in 16- and 64-slice scanners, the thinnest option is selected. This is due in large part to the overall detector configuration and length. Gantry rotation times have also decreased with newer scanner iterations. For neck CTA on a 4- or 8-slice scanner, a time of 0.7 s is typically used. For a 16-slice CT, 0.5 or 0.6 s is used while 0.4 s is used for 64-slice CT. This may be manufacturer specific. One interesting variant is a hybrid method. Since imaging a small vessel, such as the 3-mm in-plane middle cerebral artery (MCA), is different than the 5-mm transversely oriented proximal internal carotid artery (ICA), one can scan faster through the neck and then slow down for the circle of Willis where more resolution is needed. An example is to use 0.5-s scans through the neck with 1.0-s scans through the head. Pitch also has a significant impact on image quality. In general, keeping the pitch at about 1 provides a balance between coverage and resolution.

Historically, a tube voltage of 140 kVp was used for CT to minimize tube heating and maximize

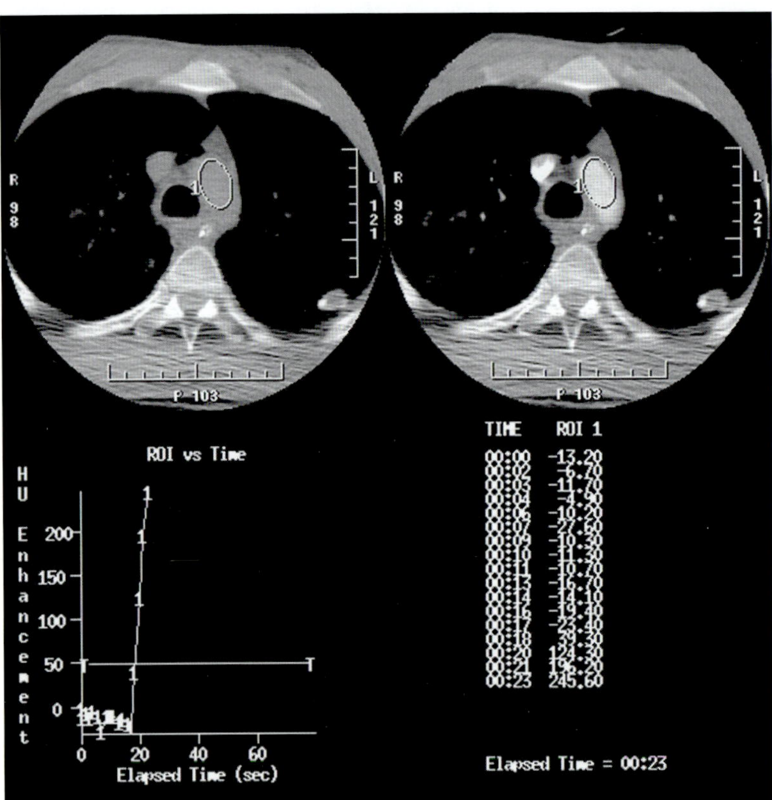

Fig. 1. Automatic triggering for computed tomography angiography (CTA). The cursor is placed in the aorta, and sequential images are obtained during dynamic contrast injection. Scan commences when contrast density in Hounsfield units (HU) reaches a preset value of 50–100 or when the technologist visually sees sufficient opacity in the arteries. Note contrast enhancement versus time curve

tube life. However, one of the key advances of MDCT has been tube technology that improves heat unit dissipation and reliability. This has allowed the use of 120 kVp, which may improve relative opacification of contrast media. The tube load used depends on gantry speed, patient weight and size, and region scanned. In general, the milliampere second (mAs) used should be in the 220–260 range for an average adult patient. For a gantry rotation of 0.7 s, a 380-mA tube load is an acceptable starting point. The newer 16- and 64-slice scanners offer automatic mA adjustments based on in-plane and Z-axis attenuation. A range of mA is set, along with an image quality desired. For CTA of the brain, image quality needs to be set higher with lower noise. Neck studies permit a slightly higher noise setting.

In CT venography (CTV), the basic premise is that the contrast bolus needs to fill the major veins. CT parameters are adapted from CTA protocols. The field of view needs to include the entire head; 22 cm is suggested. For the 4-slice scanner, 2.5 mm slices may be used to provide coverage. Slice thickness of 1.25 mm is used in eight-slice scanners, which may be reduced to thinner slices on the 16- and 64-slice MDCT. Pitch may be increased to about 1.5. Less radiation is needed since the vessels are larger. Tube load and gantry rotation is adjusted for mAs of about 220, with gantry rotation of 0.7–0.8 s.

Contrast Optimization

Contrast timing is a key determinant of CTA image quality. Peak contrast opacification should occur at the time of the scan for each region evaluated. For the neck and brain, the use of high-concentration contrast optimizes visualization of small vessels and defines vessel boundaries for improved accuracy. It permits high iodine flux at an acceptable IV injection rate. Higher IV injection rates provide high iodine flux but at a greater risk of extravasation from the IV site. We typically use 4 ml/s in our patients. Ideally, the bolus of contrast only needs to be present for the length of time that is needed to scan the area of concern, offset by the time it takes to get to the artery of interest. In practice, it is difficult to always reliably time the contrast bolus. An arbitrary injection time of 15 s for the neck or 18 s for the brain might be in error due to poor cardiac output or arterial or venous stenosis. Anxious individuals or trauma patients may have a very rapid transit time due to increased cardiac output.

Bolus tracking and automatic triggering methods have improved with MDCT technology. For neck CTA, the aortic arch with a 500 HU trigger provides a good basis for beginning to scan (Fig. 1). Volume of contrast needed reflects the speed of the scanner, with 100 ml of contrast media needed for four- and eight-slice scanners and

75 ml needed for 16-slice scanners. For brain CTA, ideally, a 100 HU trigger at the distal cervical ICA is used. However, identification of this vessel can prove elusive in some patients, so the aortic arch trigger point can be used with an additional 2–3 s delay added. Contrast requirements for brain CTA is 50 ml for 16-slice and 75 ml for 4- and 8-slice scanners.

Image Processing

The acquired images are checked for adequacy at the scanner and then postprocessed. In the case of 16-slice scanners, the very thin slices are usually reconstructed at a thicker slice thickness of 1 mm. This reduces image noise and number of slices to review while permitting improved three-dimensional (3-D) images and reformation of the thinner slices due to isotropic pixel acquisition. There can be a substantial reduction in radiation exposure to the patient using this technique. The thin-slice data set is sent to the 3-D workstation while the reformatted axial images are sent to the picture archive and communication system (PACS).

The exception to automated processing is the acute stroke patient who is a candidate for thrombolysis intervention. This scenario makes evaluation of the ICA, the basilar artery, the proximal MCA, the anterior cerebral artery (ACA), and the posterior cerebral artery (PCA) immediately at the scanner imperative. This is easy to accomplish by reviewing the data dynamically. If these vessels are not opacified while the other head vessels are and the symptomatic patient is in the therapeutic time window, then immediate intervention is indicated. CT perfusion scans can add value; however, their processing time at this point precludes their routine clinical use.

The CTA data set is best evaluated at the workstation. This workstation may be from a third-party vendor or the scanner vendor. The data set is initially selected, and then a rendering technique selected. Each major vessel may be isolated for review using trimming of the data, isolation of the vessel by selecting an area of interest, or use of a curved multiplanar reconstruction (MPR) technique. In neck CTA, each carotid artery is traced entirely for completeness, with emphasis on the carotid bifurcation. Usually, this is done using both volume-rendered and maximal intensity projection (MIP) methods. For vessels that have little calcification, the 3-D views work best. However, with calcification, the reformatted MIP projections are more accurate. Vertebral arteries are also evaluated from their origins to the basilar artery. Attention to vertebral origins with MIP projections identifies well any areas of stenosis. The raw data set is also evaluated for incidental findings.

For brain CTA, often a different rendering setting is used that optimizes smaller vessel assessment. Again, systematic evaluation of the vessels is needed, as well as an overview of the images for ancillary findings. This may be done by averaging slices and adjusting window and level settings to see brain parenchyma or bone detail. In the case of the circle of Willis, the vital viewing regions include the vertebrobasilar area, the basilar tip, the PCAs, the ACA, the MCA, and their proximal trifurcation vessels; the supraclinoid and cavernous ICAs; and the pericallosal arteries. The 3-D surface-shaded volume-rendered views see these areas best. Reformatted MIP views provide additional and complementary information in the case of vessel calcification, vasculopathy, and aneurysms. Reformatted and source images are used primarily at the skull nase where the clinoids and adjacent bones obscure volume-rendered 3-D views. CTV coverage is of the entire head. Review of the axial data set is supplemented by reformatted MIP images. The 3-D-rendered images are less helpful. In all cases, selected images of important findings are captured and saved. These are then sent to be added to the PACS data set.

CTA of the Neck

Carotid Vascular Disease

Several multicenter trials have established the need to differentiate medical versus surgical therapy on the basis of degree of carotid stenosis. The North America Symptomatic Carotid Artery Trial (NASCET) established that carotid endarterectomy provides an improved outcome over medical therapy in cases where the stenosis measures greater than 70% [4]. Measurement is by diameter of the maximal stenosis divided by diameter of the more distal internal carotid artery beyond any poststenotic dilatation. At 2 years, the stroke risk was reduced from 26% to 9% in the surgical arm while major stroke risk was reduced from 13% to 2.5%. In the 50–69% stenosis group, a modest improvement in outcome was present at 5 years with surgery. Surgical skill was an important determinant in outcome, and the results were better in men than in women [5]. The European Carotid Surgery Trial (ECST) found significant improvement in the surgical endarterectomy group, reducing stroke from 21.9% to 12.3% in stenosis of 70–90% [6]. This trial measured stenosis as the diameter of the stenosis divided by the diameter of the expected vessel wall.

In the asymptomatic patient, there are a few large studies worthy of mention. The Carotid Artery Stenosis with Asymptomatic Narrowing Operation Versus Aspirin (CASANOVA) study and

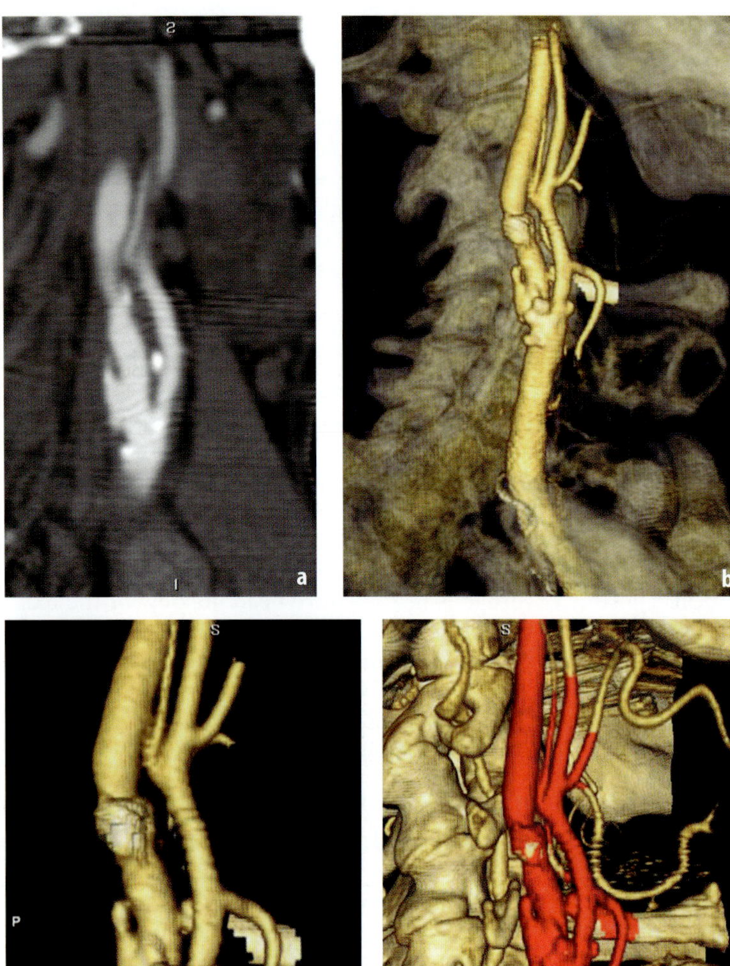

Fig. 2a-d. Carotid vascular disease on computed tomography angiography (CTA). **a** Sagittal reformatted maximum intensity projection (MIP) demonstrates undermined, ulcerated plaque with moderate stenosis. **b** Volume-rendered surface-shaded three-dimensional (3-D) image of moderate stenosis and ulcerated plaque shows calcified plaque. **c** Magnified image with deleted background better exhibits carotid bifurcation region. The calcified plaque is lighter in this scheme, and the ulceration is well depicted posteriorly. **d** Automated vessel definition using a red color scheme example. Note the calcifications are not differentiated in this particular method

the Veterans Administration Asymptomatic Carotid Study (VAACS) are two of the earlier studies that have been overshadowed by the more recent Asymptomatic Carotid Atherosclerosis Study (ACAS) and Asymptomatic Carotid Surgery Trial (ACST) studies [7, 8]. The ACAS trial of 1,662 patients in 39 centers studied patients with greater than 60% stenosis. The 5-year stroke risk was 10.6% in the medical group versus 4.8% in the surgical group, resulting in an effective risk reduction of 1% per year with surgery. The benefit in women was much less with, relative risk reduction of 16% versus 69% in men [9]. The risk of surgery was less than 3%, and angiography constituted 1.2% of the total stroke risk. This often-cited statistic has helped to dramatically reduce the use of diagnostic angiography. The ACST study [10] involving 126 hospital trials in 30 countries followed 3,120 patients with greater than 70% stenosis. It demonstrated a 5-year stroke risk of 11.7% with medical therapy versus 6.4% with surgery. While there is criticism of the methods used in all of these trials, they all have clearly established the need for carotid artery evaluation.

Consequently, the most common indication for CTA of the neck is to assess vascular disease, most commonly carotid stenosis (Figs. 2–4). Its role in noninvasive testing is that of a secondary test along with magnetic resonance angiography (MRA). Ultrasound is a common noninvasive screening test for carotid assessment, and over two thirds of carotid cases are evaluated this way. If this test suggests only mild stenosis, then additional testing is not necessary. However, a moderate or severe degree of stenosis is worthy of further action. In many regions, ultrasound screening alone

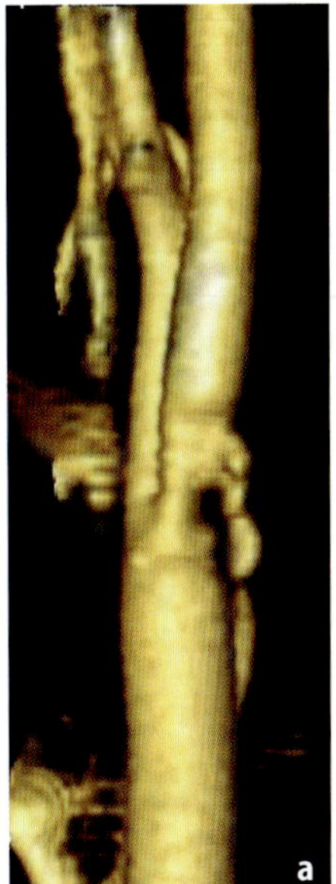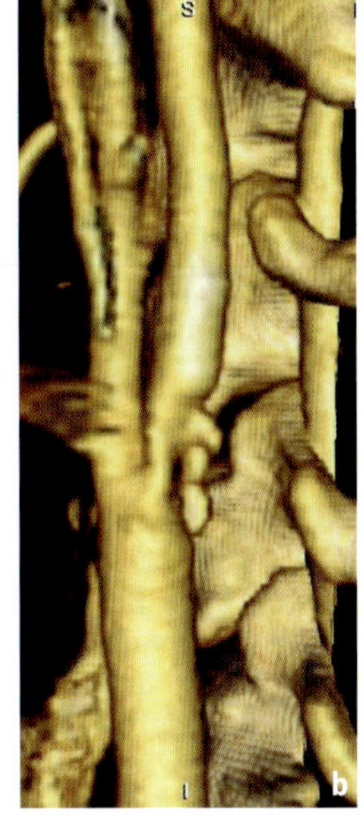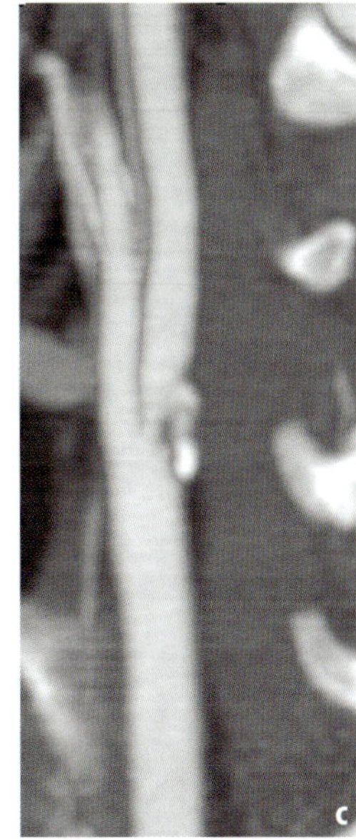

Fig. 3. Carotid vascular disease on computed tomography angiography (CTA). **a** Coronal three-dimensional (3-D) image with eccentric plaque and approximately 70% stenosis. **b** Sagittal 3-D image with minimal calcification posteriorly. **c** Sagittal maximum intensity projection (MIP) reformatted image permits accurate viewing of severe stenosis and minimal calcification. Slice thickness and window/level settings affect visualized narrowing

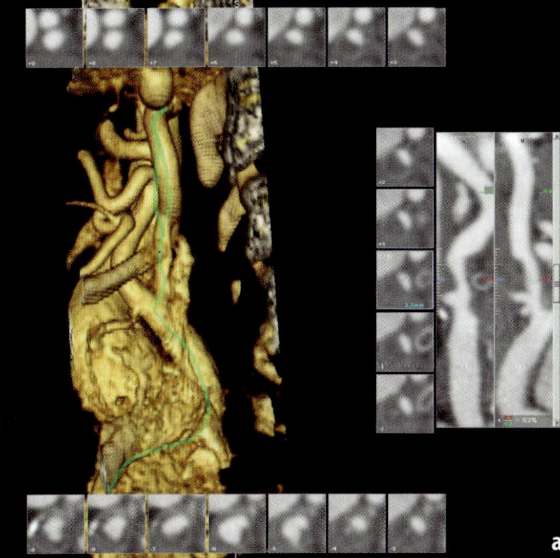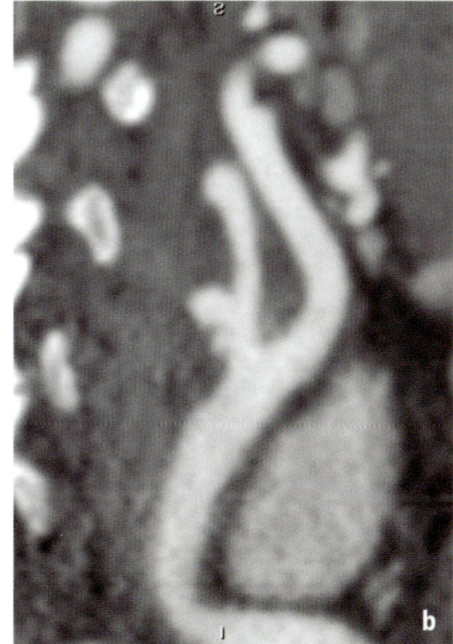

Fig. 4a, b. Carotid vascular disease on computed tomography angiography (CTA). **a** Automated, curved, multiplanar reformation of carotid bifurcation. Multiple images are displayed perpendicular to the vessel long axis. Curved reformatted images to the *right* depict multiple ulcerations. The axial diameters are readily measured. **b** Manually trimmed sagittal maximum intensity projection (MIP) reformation also shows the multiple ulcerations with 50–55% stenosis

is seen as a clear surgical indication. However, the method does tend to exaggerate the degree of stenosis, so in cases of moderate or severe velocities, a correlative test may significantly improve accuracy and minimize false positives, thereby preventing unnecessary interventions. Also, this exam only evaluates a small window around the carotid bifurcation, not the entire vessel. The study by Johnston and Goldstein found a severe stenosis surgery misclassification rate of 28% on ultrasound results alone compared with conventional angiography [11]. While duplex ultrasound alone had a misclassification rate of 18%, the study illus-

trates the value of improved accuracy with multiple tests, reducing the miss rate to 7.9% with concordant exams. Consequently, if ultrasound is used as the screening modality, then MRA or CTA have value to confirm findings and provide additional information useful in patient assessment. This study has been confirmed by others.

MRA is also used widely for carotid evaluation. Most times, MRA is coupled with MR imaging (MRI) of the brain to evaluate the brain for stroke or other conditions and the vessels as a cause of the dysfunction. This "one-stop-shopping" method provides a useful clinical diagnostic procedure that is favored by neurologists. MRA can be obtained using time-of-flight (TOF) methods or with gadolinium enhancement [contrast-enhanced MRA (CEMRA)]. Improvements in MRI scanner gradient coils and slew rates have permitted more rapid data acquisition. Imaging methods such as elliptic-centric data ordering using 3-D fast-gradient-echo sequences or their equivalent allows the more important components of data to be captured when the contrast bolus is highest and for the scan time to be dramatically decreased. MRA is highly accurate. CEMRA tends to mildly overestimate degree of stenosis in the patient with severe stenosis. The two-dimensional (2-D) TOF method overestimates severe stenosis and may result in a "flow gap" due to intravoxel dephasing due to turbulent flow. Calcium is not evaluated since it does not have free hydrogen protons to give signal. The position of the carotid bifurcation is also difficult to assess. In cases of very severe stenosis, slow flow within a patent carotid may not be detected due to saturation effects inherent with MRA methods.

CTA of the neck provides many advantages and a few disadvantages compared with MRA and ultrasound. The entire vessel is evaluated, and the level of the bifurcation is clearly noted relative to the mandible. There is a small risk of allergic reaction due to iodinated contrast media. Radiation risk is difficult to quantify as to its significance but is of lesser importance in the typical older patient. Claustrophobia is certainly less of an issue than in MRI. The detection of calcification is a mixed advantage. This is an important feature to the surgeon and the interventionalist; however, it makes accurate stenosis analysis more difficult. While 3-D surface-shaded volume-rendered images are readily evaluated, in the case of calcification, the MIP reformatted images become the primary image of interpretation. In severe cases, the calcification must be windowed such that the calcium does not visually bloom and yet the vessel is well seen. Correlating the degree of stenosis in multiple planes improves the confidence level for an accurate reading.

Several papers have compared the accuracy of CTA, MRA, ultrasound, and conventional angiography [12, 13]. However, as the technology for each modality improves, the criteria by which they are judged is limited. One of the principal papers was written by Patel and colleagues in 2002 [12]. The sensitivity and specificity of ultrasound were 85% and 71%, of MRA 100% and 57%, and of CTA 65% and 100%, respectively. While the trend of MRA to overestimate and of CTA to underestimating stenosis but be more specific seems to hold, currently, MRA and CTA are considered to both be highly accurate with specificity and sensitivity in the 90–95% range. In our institution, neurologists

favor MRA while vascular surgeons and interventionalists prefer CTA.

Stenosis alone does not fully predict who will present with neurologic events. The character of the carotid plaque is also important. Soft plaque and calcification are well depicted by CTA. Thrombus typically projects as a smooth intraluminal low-density image extending from an area of plaque. The detection of vulnerable plaque is more challenging to identify. The lipid-laden macrophages that are characteristic of vulnerable plaque are less focally defined than they are in the coronary circulation. Stratification of plaque by density is a potential way to suggest vulnerable plaque. Plaque with density below 60 HU is considered to be soft plaque that may be vulnerable while fibrous plaque may extend up to 150 HU. Ulceration is another plaque morphology that is hard to define, even by conventional angiography or direct inspection. A plaque that is undermined with a shelf-like appearance is suggestive of ulceration, but this is not definitive.

Carotid Occlusion

The diagnosis of carotid occlusion is clearly a forte of CTA (Fig. 5). The importance of this distinction lies in the potential for revascularization of a very severe stenosis, or "string sign" and the contraindication of surgery for occlusion. In actuality, it is important to distinguish between a small vessel with a focal severe narrowing that would be amenable to surgery and a diffusely irregular severely narrowed vessel that would preclude surgery. CTA is more of a volume technique than MRA, which is more flow sensitive. Consequently, CTA can provide this important information. With CTA, one can trace the lumen of the carotid artery and see if any contrast is visualized within it. If not, the diagnosis of occlusion is straightforward. Occlusion is also readily seen in the horizontal segment of the ICA. A pitfall is if imaging takes place too soon since slow flow may not be seen in this situation. Also of note is that collaterals from the external carotid artery can reconstitute the distal ICA, including the ophthalmic artery from ethmoidal internal maxillary artery branches, the artery of the foramen rotundum, and the Vidian artery.

Fibromuscular Disease

In addition to vascular stenosis, there are several other disorders that affect the carotid or vertebral arteries in the neck, including many of the collagen vascular disorders. One of these is fibromuscular dysplasia (FMD). This common disorder in-

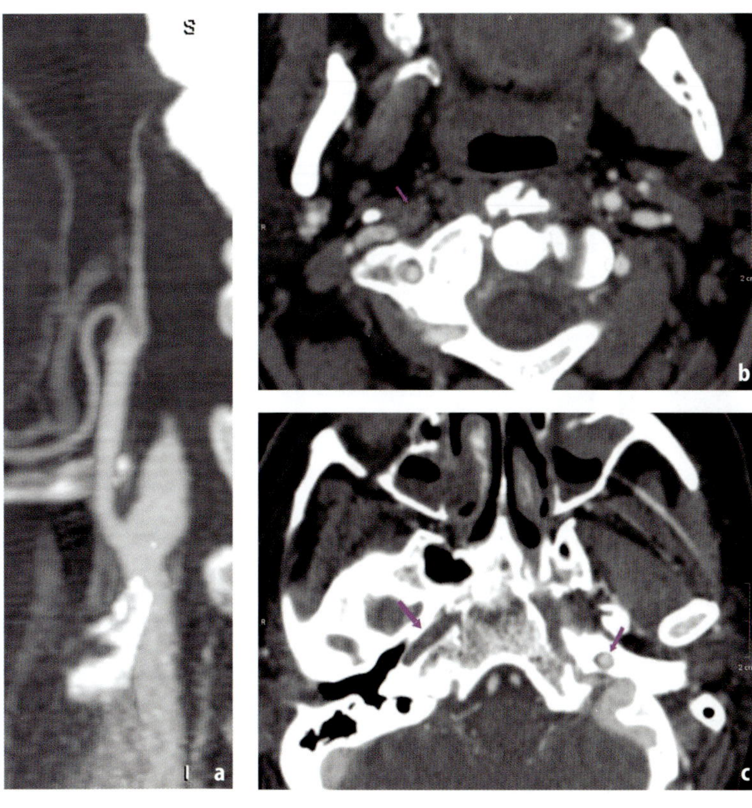

Fig. 5a-c. Carotid occlusion. **a** Sagittal reformatted maximum intensity projection (MIP) demonstrates carotid occlusion. **b** The occluded right internal carotid artery can be well seen on the axial image of the neck (*arrow*). No contrast is present within the lumen. **c** At the skull base, the right carotid occlusion is diagnosed by lack of contrast within the lumen

volves the mid- and distal cervical ICA and the distal vertebral artery. Involvement of the neck vessels is present in 30% of cases; there is a strong female predilection. Irregular beading with small outpouchings and multiple small septations is the characteristic appearance. Areas of more focal dilatations or smooth stenosis are also variants that may be seen. Dissection and pseudoaneurysms are common, and FMD should be considered when these entities present. Intracranial aneurysms are also associated with FMD.

CTA of FMD can be difficult to diagnose (Fig. 6). This is due to the relative smoothing that is inherent to the CTA method. Careful assessment of the mid- and distal ICA and the V3 and V4 vertebral artery segments can demonstrate small irregular undulations or a more irregular enlargement.

Dissection and Pseudoaneurysm

The diagnosis of dissection should be considered in any younger patient who presents with headache or acute neck pain in association with a neurologic complaint. Minimal trauma may be associated. Horner's syndrome of miotic pupil, ptosis, and anhydrosis are frequently seen. The intimal disruption of the vessel results in an expanded vessel and compromised, smoothly narrowed lumen.

Both CTA and MRA are useful in the diagnosis and treatment of dissection (Fig. 7). The expanded vessel can be seen compared with the contralateral vessel, and the intimal flap is typically depicted. If there is flow on both sides of the flap, this is well seen, particularly on the source images. If one lumen is occluded, then thrombus may be evident with flow in the other compromised lumen. By MRA, fat saturation T1 sequences may show methemoglobin in the vessel wall. CTA depicts well vessel expansion and compromised lumen of the vessel. The characteristic involvement of the distal cervical ICA is well seen.

Pseudoaneurysms are often associated with dissections. These represent the focal vessel wall expansion with flow. CTA and MRA are both useful, but CTA demonstrates the location relative to the skull base and the exact dimensions.

The diagnosis of dissection and pseudoaneurysm is readily made by CTA and MRA. These are treated by anticoagulation or antiplatelet therapy in most cases. Consequently, having a noninvasive test to follow therapy is also helpful. Both CTA and MRA can be used for this purpose.

Vertebral Artery Evaluation

The vertebral arteries are well seen by CTA (Fig. 8). However, the adjacent vertebral bodies may overlay the vessel, particularly on the 3-D images. The

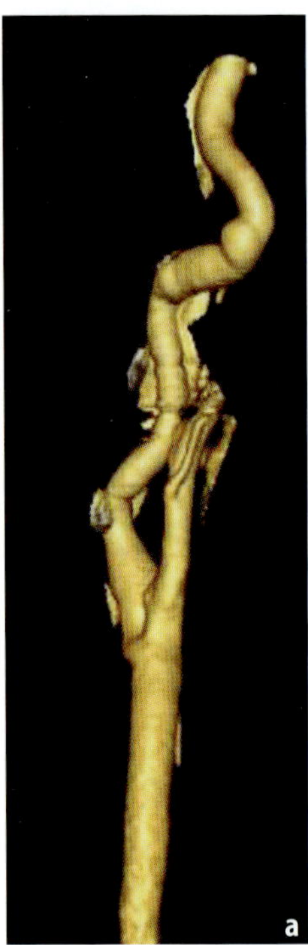
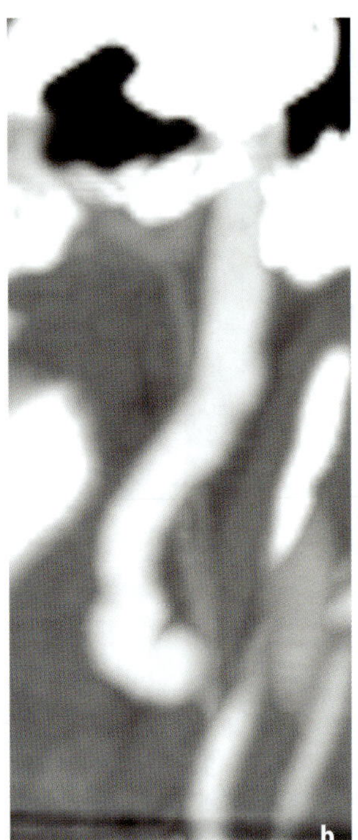
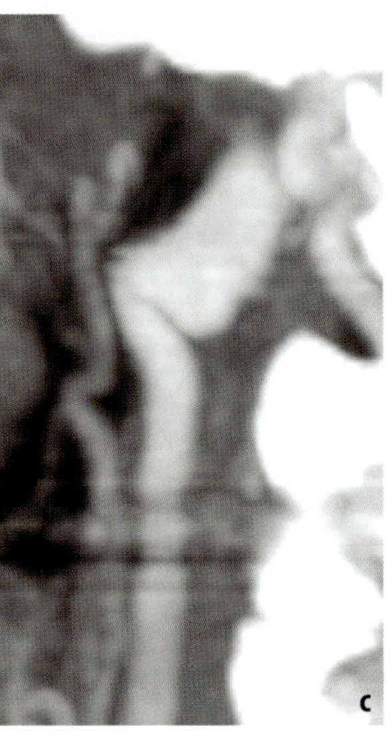

Fig. 6a-c. Fibromuscular dysplasia (FMD). **a** Irregular mid- and distal internal carotid artery (ICA) indicating FMD. **b** Maximum intensity projection (MIP) demonstrates the irregular vessel contour. **c** MIP on a different patient with FMD who also has pseudoaneurysm. Note the enlarged, tortuous vessel

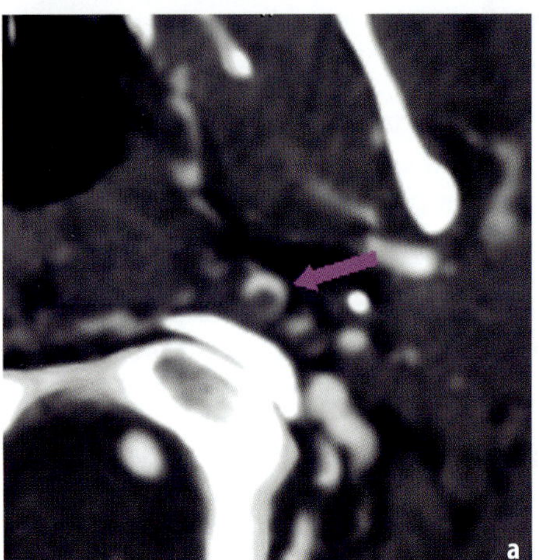
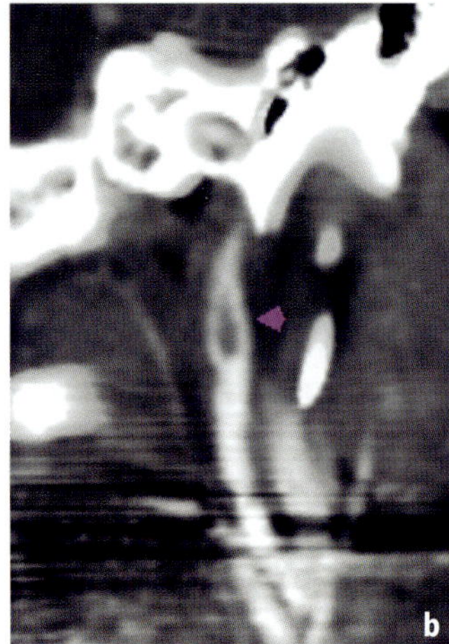

Fig. 7a, b. Carotid dissection. **a** Dissection of the left internal carotid artery (ICA) is diagnosed by enlarged vessel and compromised vessel lumen. Sometimes, a dissection flap is evident. Here, contrast is seen in the false lumen (*arrow*). **b** Reformatted image of dissection in a woman who was thrown from a horse. Note the dissection flap (*arrow*)

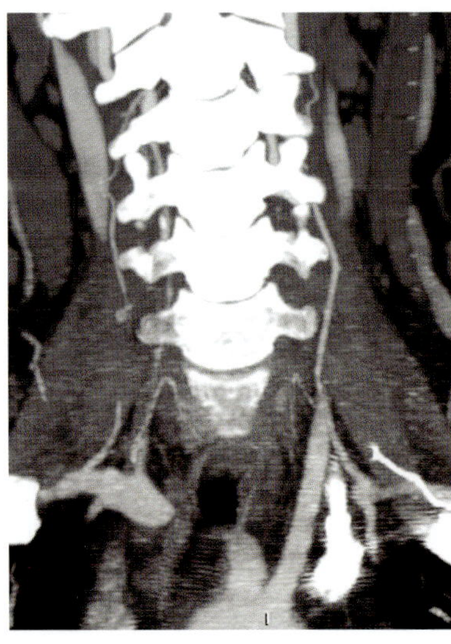

Fig. 8. Vertebral artery occlusion. Origins of the vertebral arteries can usually be well seen using thicker-slab maximum intensity projection (MIP) coronal images. Here, the left vertebral origin is occluded, and the ascending cervical artery reconstitutes the left vertebral artery in the transverse foramen at the C4 level. The right vertebral artery is hypoplastic

reformatted MIP images are useful to identify the vessel along with acquisition data. Normal variations of a dominant left vertebral artery or a vertebral artery ending in the posterior inferior cerebellar artery (PICA) are common. The origins of the vertebral arteries may be obscured by streak artifacts, superimposed contrast from the venous bolus, or calcification related to atherosclerotic disease. By magnifying the area of interest and adjusting the window/level of the image and adjusting the MIP slice thickness, one can usually resolve the vertebral artery well. In the case of atherosclerosis, measuring the maximal stenosis divided by the size of the normal vessel is used. Tortuosity of the vessel is often visualized in the mid-cervical spine region. Dissection of the vessel is more common distally.

Trauma

CTA has become the new standard in evaluating the patient with significant trauma to the neck or head [14]. The thin-slice CT technique provides evaluation of vessels in addition to surrounding soft tissue injury and evidence of fracture. Reformatted images also permit assessment of the cervical spine. Sensitivity for blunt cerebrovascular injury is quoted as 100%, with 94% specificity in a recent study by Berne [14]. Vertebral artery injury was more frequent than carotid injury, and there was a 21% mortality rate with vessel injury. Carotid canal fracture or transverse foramen fracture should alert one to the possibility of major vessel injury, specifically vessel dissection or occlusion (Fig. 9).

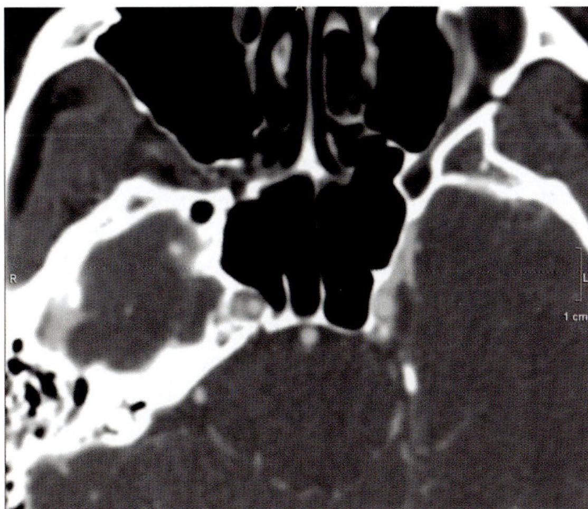

Fig. 9. Carotid traumatic dissection. Computed tomography angiography (CTA) is used extensively to evaluate patients with significant trauma. Here, the right distal petrous internal carotid artery (ICA) is dissected in a patient post motor-vehicle collision. The compromised lumen is seen medial to the dissection laterally

CTA of the Brain

In the past, the evaluation of intracranial vasculature required conventional angiography. However, the development of MRA and CTA provides a noninvasive method of assessing these vessels. A major challenge is the small vessel size. The horizontal segment of the MCA (M1 branch) and the basilar artery are typically 3 mm and the distal ICA is about 4 mm. The more distal branches get progressively smaller. Consequently, voxel resolution is an issue. Small fields of view and thin slices combined with slow table speed and low pitch provide the ability to see most major vessels. Systematic evaluation of intracranial CTA minimizes omissions. While there are many ways to do this, one easy and quick way is outlined as follows:

- Trim the data set to see the back of the foramen magnum and above the top of the basilar artery. Also, trim from the sides to see the MCA branches, excluding most of the calvarium.
- Look at the 3-D view posteriorly to view the vertebral arteries and proximal basilar artery. Rotate along the basilar to see the basilar tip.
- Look from the top of the data set to see the circle of Willis, following the vessels with slight rotations. This will view the posterior and anterior communicating arteries.
- Look from anteriorly to see the ophthalmic artery origins and distal ICAs. The anterior communicating artery and MCAs are also seen from this view with some additional rotation of data.
- Trim data to see just between the ICAs to evaluate the ACA territory branches. Then shift to the right and then to the left to see the MCA territory branches.
- View the coronal and sagittal reformats using MIP, and vary the slab thickness to see vessels of interest, particularly in the cavernous sinus region.
- View the entire data set to look for incidental and related findings, such as stroke, tumor, or AVMs. This may be done by averaging data to 5-mm thickness. Also look at venous drainage for thrombosis.
- Document findings of images of interest.

Stenosis and Occlusion

The major intracranial vessels are usually well seen by CTA [15]. Stenosis represents an area of narrowing in the vessel caliber (Figs. 10, 11). This is calculated as the diameter of the narrowing relative to the normal vessel caliber. Due to the small size of these vessels, it can be difficult to measure this exactly; however, magnification of the image helps to improve accuracy.

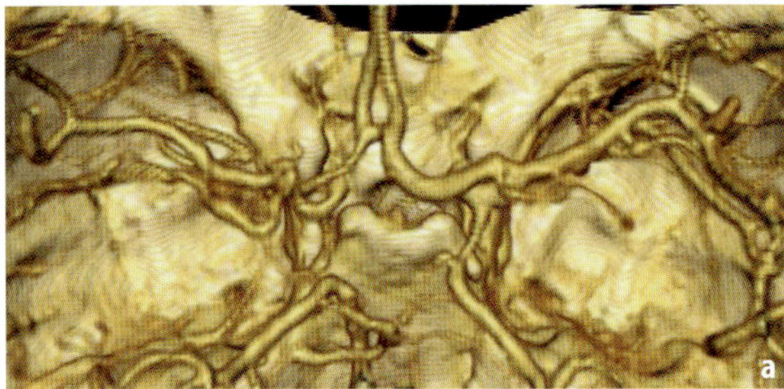

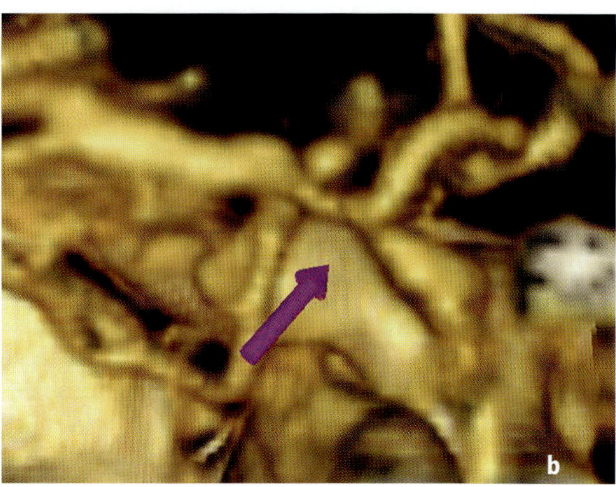

Fig. 10a, b. Intracranial stenosis. **a** Severe distal left internal carotid artery (ICA) and proximal middle cerebral artery (MCA) stenosis in this elderly patient with atherosclerotic disease causes reduced caliber of intracranial vessels. **b** By rotating and cropping the image, the severe stenosis at the ICA–MCA junction is well seen (*arrow*)

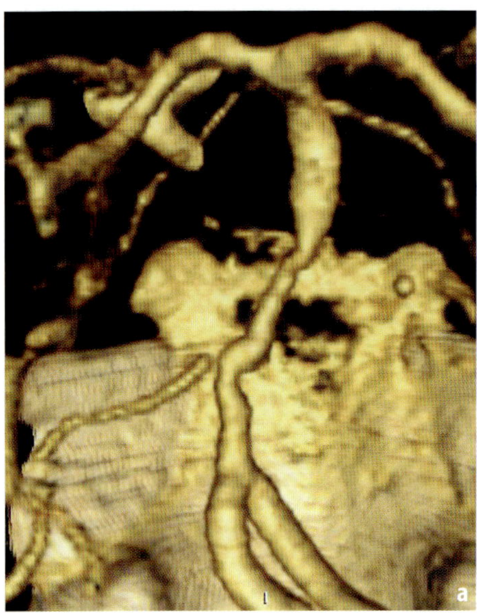

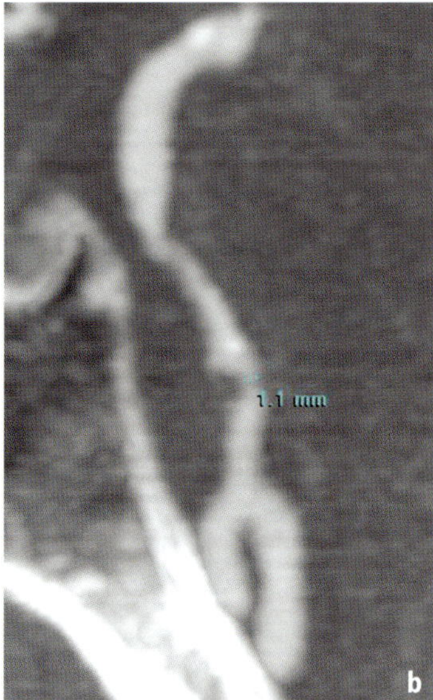

Fig. 11a, b. Intracranial stenosis. **a** Severe stenosis of the proximal and midbasilar artery due to atherosclerotic disease. **b** Sagittal maximum intensity projection (MIP) shows the irregularity of the basilar artery. Measurement of the vessel stenosis is demonstrated

Anomalies of the cerebral vasculature need to be considered as well. The left vertebral artery is equal or dominant in about 75% of patients, so asymmetry of the vertebral arteries is the rule. Frequently, a vertebral artery will diminish in size after the PICA origin. Also, hypoplastic P1 and A1 segments are frequently seen in about 25% of patients. These congenital narrowings should not be interpreted as acquired stenosis. The increased flow in the resultant compensatory feeding vessels makes aneurysms somewhat more likely, so these variations should be noted.

Stenosis of vessels is well seen on the 3-D images when the vessel is not calcified. However, in the setting of calcification, more reliance on MIP reformation is needed. The 3-D images will show a bump along the vessel wall, usually of a different color, but it can be complicated to differentiate the lumen from the calcified plaque. MIP reformation is more accurate to define the percentage stenosis.

In addition, CTA is very useful in the case of anticipated endovascular intervention. Measuring the vessel size, stenosis diameter and length, and landing zones of a stent permit more accurate and, presumptively, safer angioplasty and stent placement.

Occlusion of a branch vessel may be straightforward to detect if one knows the cerebral anatomy to realize that a vessel is missing (Figs. 12, 13). Often, there is a small tail of contrast at the origin or an abrupt caliber change that defines the occlusion site. One pitfall of occlusion in major vessels is due to collateral flow. This reconstitutes the more distal vessel but at a smaller caliber due to reduced pressure and flow. The diagnosis of occlusion is made by tracing the pathway of the vessel and noting that no flow is present in a segment. To be sure of this finding, the image level should be increased using a narrow window to eliminate the possibility of a high-grade stenosis rather than an occlusion.

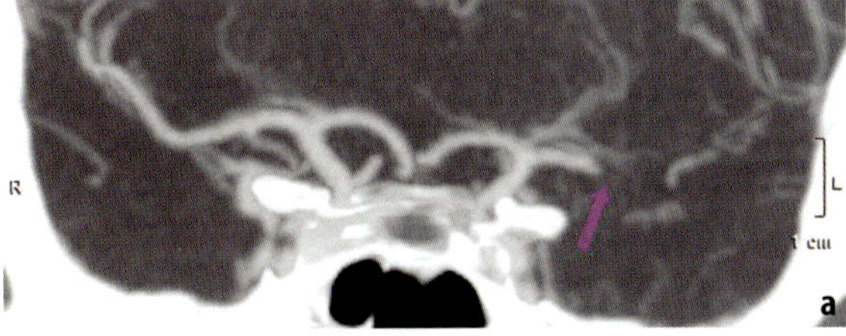

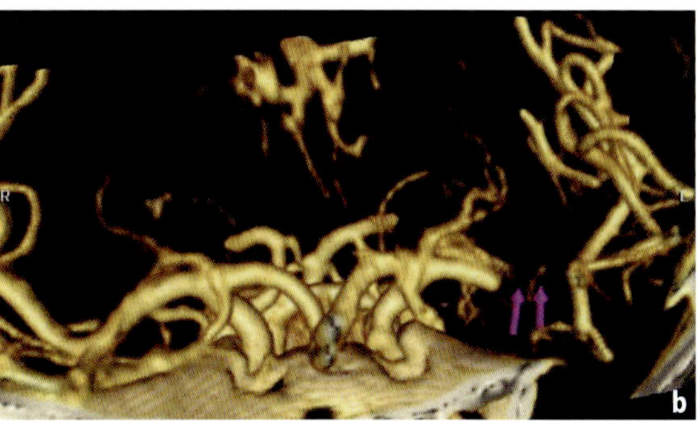

Fig. 12a, b. Acute thrombosis of the left middle cerebral artery (MCA). **a** Patient presents with acute right hemiplegia and aphasia. Thrombosis of the distal MCA is present, with occlusion of the distal M1 MCA segment and proximal M2 branches (*arrow*). **b** Three-dimensional (3-D) image of the acute thrombosis (*arrows*) demonstrates filling defect in contrasted vessels. Note reconstitution of distal collateral MCA branches

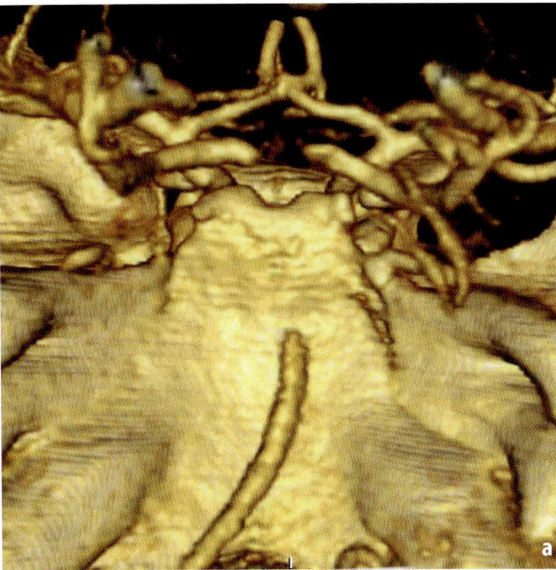

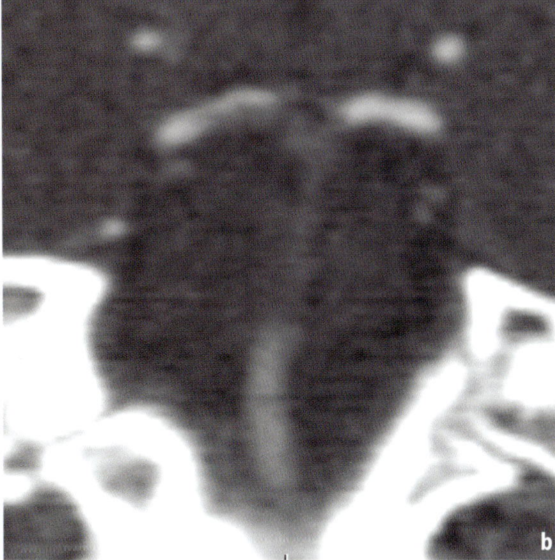

Fig. 13a, b. Acute basilar artery thrombosis. **a** Occlusion of the mid- and distal basilar artery is demonstrated in this patient who suddenly became comatose. **b** Coronal maximum intensity projection (MIP) image shows contrast opacification of the proximal basilar and posterior cerebral arteries with basilar artery thrombosis

Vasculopathy

Vasculopathy is a generalized term referring to any pathologic condition of the blood vessels. As such, it includes stenosis and occlusion and also includes vasospasm and vasculitis.

The detection of vasospasm by CTA has permitted a noninvasive method that complements transcranial Doppler [16]. Vasospasm typically arises in the 4–14 days following subarachnoid hemorrhage and is most common in the 7- to 10-day window. Standard clinical treatment includes "triple H" therapy consisting of hypertension, hypervolemia, and hemodilution in combination with the calcium channel blocker, nimodipine. This is effective in most patients, but in severe cases, endovascular angioplasty or arterial infusion is warranted. CT of the brain to evaluate for hydro-cephalus and infarction is performed prior to intervention. In this situation, CTA can be added to the evaluation although in many cases the decision to proceed to conventional angiography has already been made, negating the value of CTA. The appearance of vasospasm on CTA is that of regions of smooth narrowing of vessels, including the major intracranial vessels.

Vasculitis is an inflammatory infiltration of the blood-vessel wall (Fig. 14). There are many etiologies that can be grouped by the size of the vessel involved. Takayasu's arteritis has large-vessel involvement of the great vessels up to the carotid bifurcation. It shows smooth vessel narrowing and a thickened vessel wall. Giant-cell or temporal arteritis may involve the larger cerebral vessels, including the classic superficial temporal artery. Most of these cases show areas of smooth narrow-

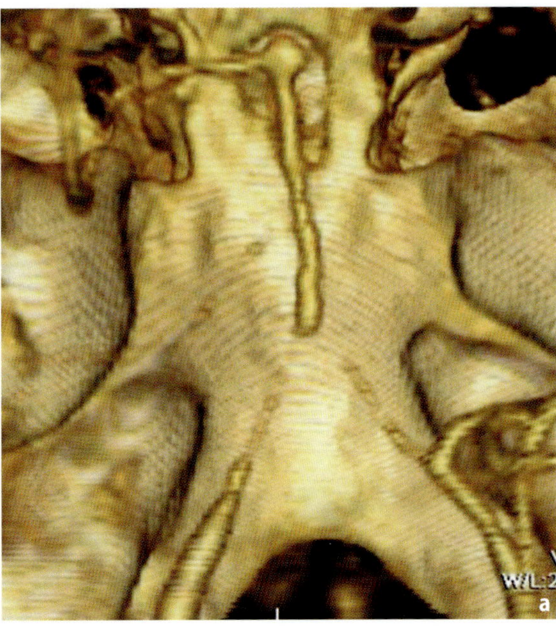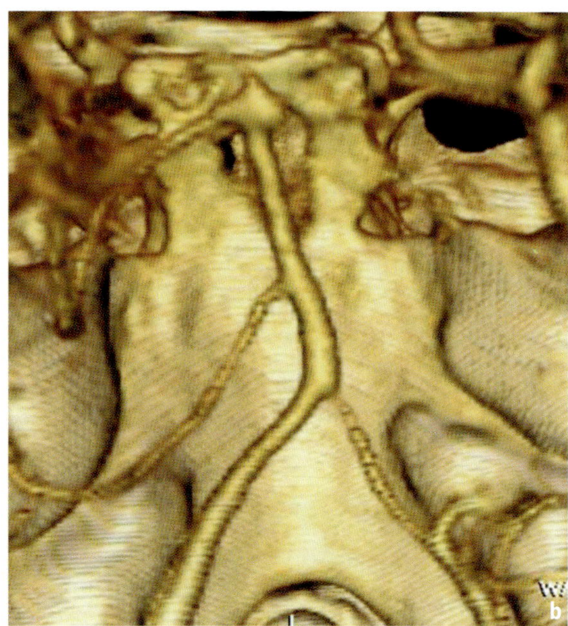

Fig. 14a, b. Vasculopathy. **a** Patient with sarcoid causing intracranial vasculopathy. Note narrowing of the basilar artery, distal vertebral arteries, and anterior inferior cerebellar artery. **b** Same patient after therapy demonstrates marked improvement in vessel caliber

ing of the vessel followed by a return to normal caliber – the so-called "beaded" appearance. There are also multiple autoimmune diseases and even primary CNS vasculitis with involvement of medium- to small-vessel beading. By CTA, involvement of the more proximal vessels is readily detected; however, medium- and small-vessel vasculitis is not able to be reliably found. Consequently, conventional angiography remains the standard diagnostic test.

Aneurysms

The detection of cerebral aneurysms by CTA has dramatically improved in the past few years. In many centers, it has moved to the forefront of evaluating patients with cerebral aneurysms [17–21]. There are two basic scenarios – the evaluation of the patient with subarachnoid hemorrhage (SAH) and the patient being screened or followed for cerebral aneurysm (Figs. 15–17).

SAH in the nontrauma patient without coagulopathy has a high likelihood of being due to a ruptured aneurysm. CT of the brain without contrast provides the diagnosis of SAH in most patients who present with the classical history of severe headache. Rarely, false negative cases may result from delayed presentation of the patient or from minimal amounts of blood in the spinal fluid. A compelling history warrants lumbar puncture (LP) for cerebral spinal fluid (CSF) analysis although the LP may also result in a traumatic tap.

CTA provides a highly sensitive and specific method for detection and evaluation of cerebral aneurysms in all cases. A recent study by Karamessini and colleagues quotes a 93–100% sensitivity and 100% specificity for aneurysms 3 mm or larger. These values are comparable with conventional angiography [20]. In particular, anterior communicating artery aneurysms are seen equivalently or superiorly by CTA since both ACAs are visualized simultaneously.

MCA aneurysms, particularly complex aneurysms, are also seen equally as well or better by digital subtraction angiography (DSA). The basilar tip and artery and distal vertebral arteries are also evaluated equivalently or better by CTA. The posterior communicating artery is seen equivalently to DSA. Aneurysms that are seen better by DSA include those arising from the ICAs proximal to the ophthalmic arteries since adjacent bone can obscure the vessel on CTA. Also, mycotic aneurysms may be missed by CTA if they are not included in the imaging volume or involve small branches.

One advantage of CTA is that the aneurysm neck size and configuration can be accurately measured. Thus, the decision to surgically clip or endovascularly coil can be made in most situations. The need to reconstruct the parent vessel in the case of a broad-necked aneurysm is also suggested. CTA depicts calcified or partially thrombosed aneurysms. Calcification can be difficult to treat surgically. Thrombus within an aneurysm increases the risk of stroke or coil settling resulting

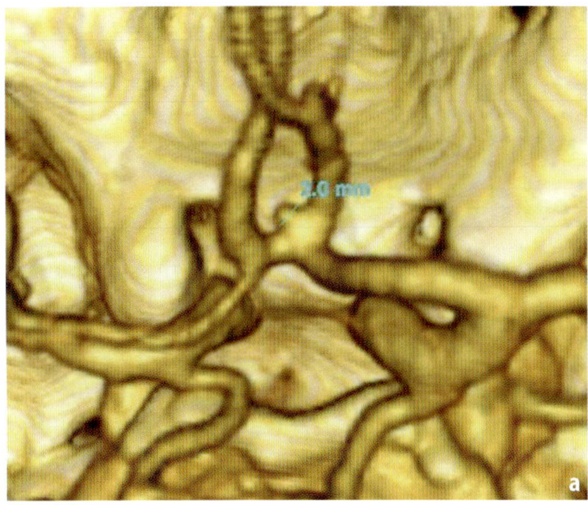

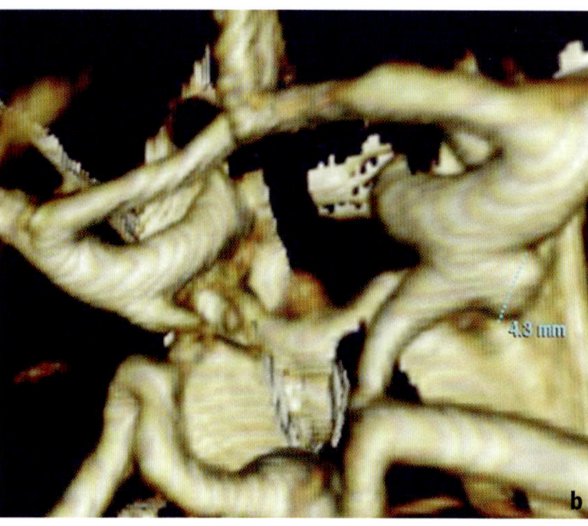

Fig. 15. Anterior communicating artery aneurysm. A small, 2-mm anterior communicating artery aneurysm is well visualized in this patient with prior subarachnoid hemorrhage (SAH) and "negative" cerebral angiography. By opacifying both anterior cerebral arteries simultaneously, the anterior communicating artery is typically seen better than by conventional angiography. Size and contours of the aneurysm are also well depicted

Fig. 16. Posterior communicating artery aneurysm. There is a 4-mm posterior communicating artery aneurysm in this patient who has a prominent associated posterior communicating artery. Note that the aneurysm neck is well seen, as is the contralateral infundibulum

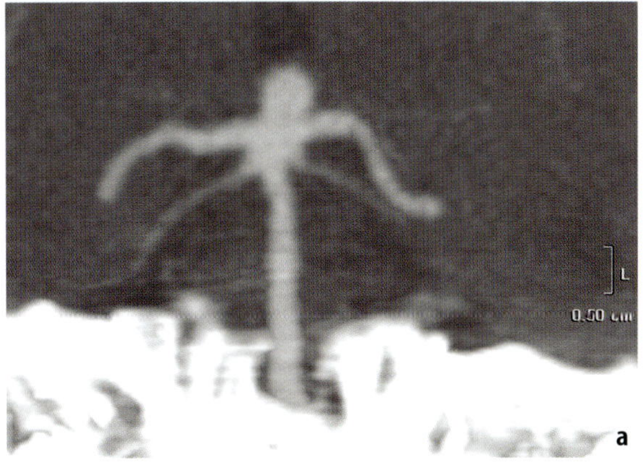

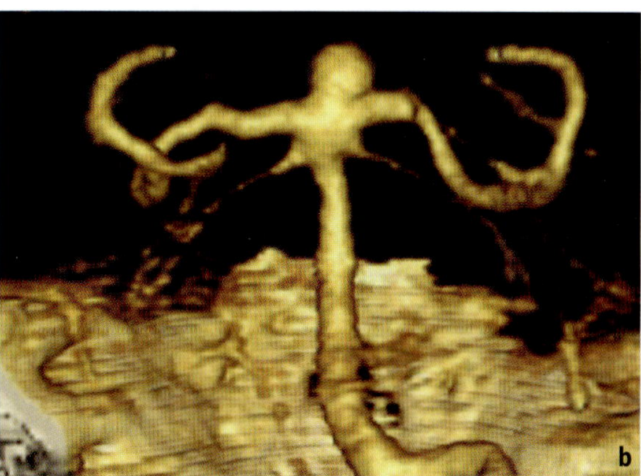

Fig. 17a, b. Basilar artery aneurysm. **a** Coronal maximum intensity projection (MIP) demonstrates the basilar tip aneurysm and relation to the posterior cerebral arteries with relatively broad neck configuration. **b** The three-dimensional (3-D) image gives better perspective of the aneurysm configuration

in incomplete treatment. Cases of endovascular stenting as an adjunct to coiling are also suggested.

An aneurysm may be detected incidentally in many cases where neuroimaging is performed. In the patient without SAH, finding an aneurysm presents a dilemma. Are the risks of rupture high enough to indicate treatment or should the aneurysm be followed medically? The International Study of Unruptured Intracranial Aneurysms (ISUIA) suggested that the risk of rupturing an aneurysm less than 10 mm is very low [22]. Many patients with incidental aneurysms are followed noninvasively to assess for interval change since a growing aneurysm is at higher risk for rupture.

CTA provides an accurate means to measure and compare sequential exams.

Arteriovenous malformations (AVM)

The detection of AVMs is usually made by means other than CTA. In the case of ruptured AVM, brain CT without contrast demonstrates SAH, usually with parenchymal hematoma around the AVM. If the AVM is not ruptured, increased density or calcification at the AVM site is common and may be seen on noncontrasted CT. MRI shows flow voids, mixed signal intensity, and possibly hemo-

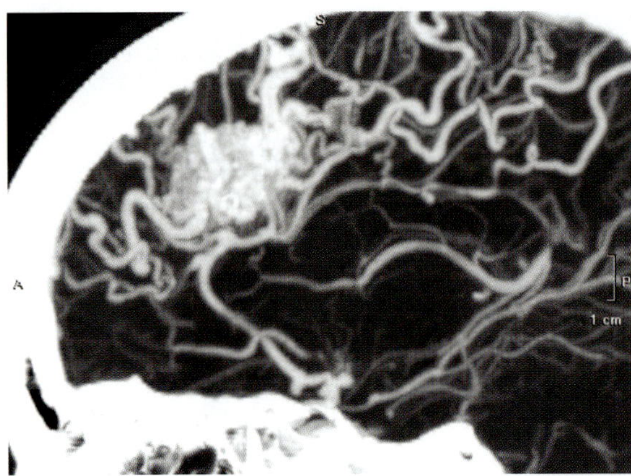

Fig. 18. Arteriovenous malformation (AVM). Sagittal maximum intensity projection (MIP) image demonstrates a 30 cm AVM in the frontal lobe. Note the complex superficial venous drainage pattern. Aneurysms are also present in the distal internal carotid artery (ICA) posteriorly and the anterior communicating artery

siderin at the AVM. Conventional angiography is the procedure of choice for diagnosis since it demonstrates the relative flow in the feeding arteries, including dominant and lesser branches, and the nidus configuration. Most importantly, the venous drainage, including any venous constriction, is seen. CTA can be used to evaluate AVMs; however, the scan volume obviously needs to include the AVM and its feeding and draining vessels. The nidus is well depicted, which may be of benefit for radiosurgery planning. Associated flow-related aneurysms are well seen. However, it is difficult to see all the feeding arteries and to represent the relative flow in each branch (Fig. 18).

CT Venography of the Brain

CTV is a variation of CTA whereby the area of interest is the venous drainage rather than the arterial supply to the brain. As such, the timing reflects the transit time of blood to fill the venous system.

CTV Protocol

The entire head is included, using a 22-cm field of view with craniocaudal scanning using thin slices. For a 16-slice scanner, a pitch over 1 can be used with rotation time of 0.7 s. Tube load in the 320-mA range for 120 kVp with noise index of 5 provides excellent image quality. Image reconstruction at 2.5 mm or 1.25 mm is suggested. At the workstation, CTV is evaluated somewhat differently than CTA. The axial images provide the most in-

formation while reformatted data depicts the venous sinuses well. The 3-D images are sliced to look at the vertex and then the posterior head as an adjunct to the 2-D images.

Congenital Variants

The right transverse and sigmoid sinus are dominant in 50–75% of patients. Consequently, seeing a small left-venous sinus is common. Typically, the transverse sinus is smaller, and the sigmoid is a little larger due to inflow from the vein of Labbe and posterior fossa veins. The true size of the sigmoid sinus is easy to determine since the bony defect of the vein coincides with the vein on the CT source images.

The ability of CTV to show a hypoplastic sinus is one of its principal advantages over MR venography (MRV). Frequently, small low-density defects are visualized in the major venous sinuses. These represent arachnoid granulations where CSF is resorbed. MRV may mistakenly portray these defects as nonobstructive thrombus.

The significance of sinus stenosis is uncertain. If the sinuses connect, then compromise of one sinus is not of consequence. However, sometimes the sagittal sinus or straight sinus drains via only one transverse sinus. In these circumstances, severe sinus stenosis could be symptomatic [23]. Restriction of venous outflow inherently increases intracranial pressure, but the degree and nature of compensation is unknown. It has been postulated that there is an association with pseudotumor cerebri; however, the nature of this link and the contribution of other factors, such as the demographic association of an obese woman of childbearing age, is unknown.

Venous Thrombosis

Contrast-filled venous sinuses are commonly seen in almost every CTA and contrast-enhanced brain CT. By adjusting the window and level to see the contrast-filled veins, the entire venous system can be readily traced. Thrombosis represents a filling defect within the sinus and is readily evaluated [24] (Fig. 19). As a consequence of the venous obstruction, collateral veins along the sinus may be seen. As the thrombosis matures, the clot becomes adherent and synechia are seen. While thrombosis is demonstrated superiorly by CTV over MRV, MRI is better than CT at looking at the sequelae of the thrombosis. This includes venous infarction and cerebral edema. Hemorrhage, which is common with venous infarction, can be seen with both modalities.

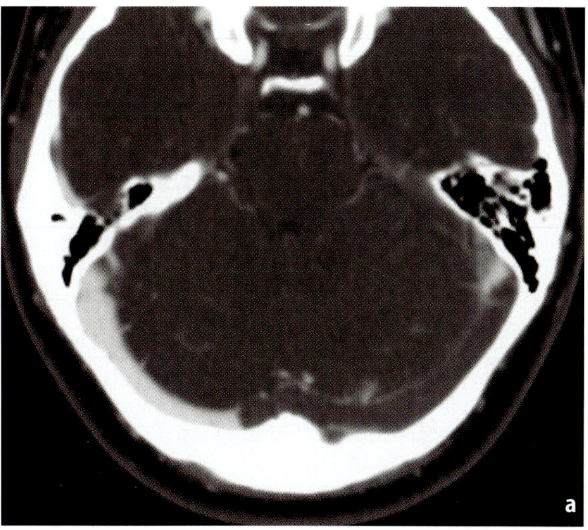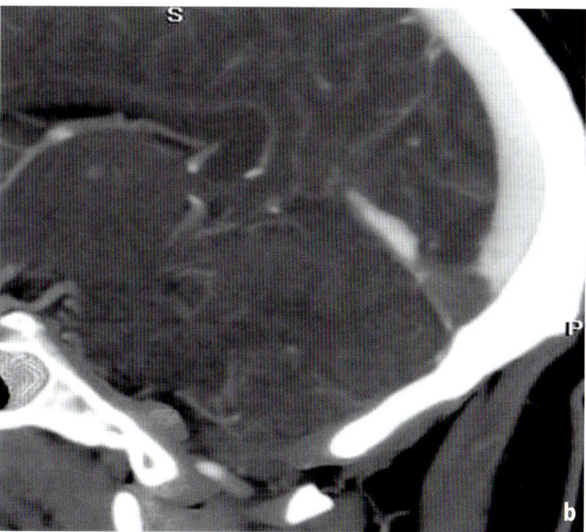

Fig. 19a, b. Venous thrombosis. **a** Axial image demonstrates a large filling defect of the left transverse sinus involving the torcula. This indicates acute thrombosis. **b** Sagittal maximum intensity projection (MIP) image demonstrates thrombus within the torcula. The posterior superior sagittal sinus and the straight sinus are widely patent and opacify with contrast

Summary

CTA provides an excellent method of evaluating the vasculature of the neck and brain. Technical improvements in MDCT and the improvement in workstation software provide for accurate diagnosis in a timely manner. In many cases, this currently replaces conventional angiography. The evaluation of carotid stenosis; trauma to the neck; and detection of cerebral stenosis, aneurysm, and thrombosis are but some of the growing indications for the routine utilization of CTA.

References

1. Heinz ER, Fuchs J, Osborne D et al (1984) Examination of the extracranial carotid bifurcation by thin-section dynamic CT: direct visualization of intimal atheroma in man (Part 2). AJNR Am J Neuroradiol 5(4):361-366
2. Heinz ER, Pizer SM, Fuchs H et al (1984) Examination of the extracranial carotid bifurcation by thin-section dynamic CT: direct visualization of intimal atheroma in man (Part 1). AJNR Am J Neuroradiol 5(4):355-359
3. Enterline D, Lowry CR, Tanenbaum LN (2005) Brain, and head and neck applications. In: Multidetector CT protocols developed for GE scanners. BDI, Princeton, pp E1-57
4. North American Symptomatic Carotid Endarterectomy Trial Collaborators (1991) Beneficial effect of carotid endarterectomy in symptomatic patients with high-grade carotid stenosis. N Engl J Med 325:445-453
5. Barnett HJ, Taylor DW, Eliasziw M et al for the North American Symptomatic Carotid Endarterectomy Trial Collaborators (1998) Benefit of carotid endarterectomy in patients with symptomatic moderate or severe stenosis. N Engl J Med 12:339(20):1415-1425
6. European Carotid Surgery Trialists' Collaborative Group (1991) MRC European carotid surgery trial: interim results for symptomatic patients with severe (70–99%) or with mild (0–29%) carotid stenosis. Lancet 337:1235-1243
7. Hobson RW 2nd, Weiss DG, Fields WS et al (1993) The Veterans Affairs Cooperative Study Group. Efficacy of carotid endarterectomy for asymptomatic carotid stenosis. N Engl J Med 28:328(4):221-227
8. CASANOVA Study Group (1991) Carotid surgery versus medical therapy in asymptomatic carotid stenosis. Stroke 22(10):1229 1235
9. Executive Committee for the Asymptomatic Carotid Atherosclerosis Study (1995) Endarterectomy for asymptomatic carotid artery stenosis. JAMA 273:1421-1428
10. Halliday A, Mansfield A, Marro J et al for the MRC asymptomatic carotid surgery trial (ACST) collaborative group (2004) Prevention of disabling and fatal strokes by successful carotid endarterectomy in patients without recent neurological symptoms: randomized controlled trial. Lancet 363:1491-1502
11. Johnston DCC, Goldstein LB (2001) Clinical carotid endarterectomy decision making: Noninvasive vascular imaging versus angiography. Neurology 56:1009-1015
12. Patel SG, Collie DA, Wardlaw JM et al (2002) Outcome, observer reliability, and patient preferences if CTA, MRA, or Doppler ultrasound were used, individually or together, instead of digital subtraction angiography before carotid endarterectomy. J Neurol Neurosurg Psychiatry 73(1):21-28
13. Randoux B, Marro B, Koskas F et al (2001) Carotid artery stenosis: prospective comparison of CT, three-dimensional gadolinium-enhanced MR, and conventional angiography. Radiology 220(1):179-185
14. Berne JD, Norwood SH, McAuley CE, Villareal DH (2004) Helical computed tomographic angiography: an excellent screening test for blunt cerebrovascular

injury. J Trauma 57(1):11-17

15. Bash S, Villablanca JP, Jahan R et al (2005) Intracranial vascular stenosis and occlusive disease: evaluation with CT angiography, MR angiography, and digital subtraction angiography. AJNR Am J Neuroradiol 26(5):1012-1021

16. Goldsher D, Shreiber R, Shik V (2004) Role of multisection CT angiography in the evaluation of vertebrobasilar vasospasm in patients with subarachnoid hemorrhage. AJNR Am J Neuroradiol 25(9):1493-1498

17. Dammert S, Krings T, Moller-Hartmann W (2004) Detection of intracranial aneurysms with multislice CT: comparison with conventional angiography. Neuroradiology 46(6):427-434

18. Hoh BL, Cheung AC, Rabinov JD (2004) Results of a prospective protocol of computed tomographic angiography in place of catheter angiography as the only diagnostic and pretreatment planning study for cerebral aneurysms by a combined neurovascular team. Neurosurgery 54(6):1329-1340

19. Kangasniemi M, Makela T, Koskinen S et al (2004) Detection of intracranial aneurysms with two-dimensional and three-dimensional multislice helical computed tomographic angiography. Neurosurgery 54(2):336-340

20. Karamessini MT, Kagadis GC, Petsas T et al (2004) CT angiography with three-dimensional techniques for the early diagnosis of intracranial aneurysms. Comparison with intra-arterial DSA and the surgical findings. Eur J Radiol 49(3):212-223

21. White PM, Teasdale EM, Wardlaw JM, Easton V (2001) Intracranial aneurysms: CT angiography and MR angiography for detection prospective blinded comparison in a large patient cohort. Radiology 219(3):739-749

22. International Study of Unruptured Intracranial Aneurysms Investigators (1998) Unruptured intracranial aneurysms: risk of rupture and risks of surgical intervention. N Engl J Med 339:1725–1733

23. Rajpal S, Niemann DB, Turk AS (2005) Transverse venous sinus stent placement as treatment for benign intracranial hypertension in a young male: case report and review of the literature. J Neurosurg 102 [Suppl 3]:342-346

24. Casey SO, Alberico RA, Patel M et al (1996) Cerebral CT venography. Radiology 198:163-170

MDCT Perfusion in Acute Stroke

Sanjay K. Shetty, Michael H. Lev

Introduction

Acute cerebrovascular stroke ranks amongst the foremost causes of morbidity and mortality in the world [1]. In acute settings, the rapid evaluation of acute stroke is invaluable due to the ability to treat patients with thrombolytics. In addition to anatomic information about the acute stroke, state-of-the-art radiologic techniques can also provide critical information about capillary-level hemodynamics and the brain parenchyma. Computed tomography perfusion (CTP) provides this information and can help in understanding the pathophysiology of stroke [2–5]. CTP helps the physician to identify critically ischemic or irreversibly infarcted tissue ("core") and to identify severely ischemic but potentially salvageable tissue ("penumbra"). This information can guide triage and management in acute stroke.

Overall application of CT and magnetic resonance (MR) perfusion techniques and estimation of cerebral perfusion parameters such as cerebral blood flow (CBF), cerebral blood volume (CBV), and mean transit time (MTT) are similar for both MR imaging (MRI) and CT. However, faster imaging time, affordability, and wider availability of CT technology in the acute setting makes the combination of CT angiography (CTA) and CTP a potential surrogate marker of stroke severity, likely exceeding the National Institutes of Health Stroke Scale (NIHSS) or the Alberta Stroke Program Early CT Score (ASPECTS) as a predictor of outcome [6–14].

CTP: Scanning Technique

Scanning protocol for acute stroke must facilitate patient triage. At Massachusetts General Hospital, the scanning protocol for acute stroke has the following three parts: the noncontrast CT; CTA from aortic arch to vertex; and dynamic, first-pass, cine CTP (Table 1). The noncontrast CT excludes hemorrhage prior to thrombolysis [15] and can reveal a large territory infarction [such as a hypodensity occupying greater than one third of the middle cerebral artery (MCA) territory], which is also considered to be a contraindication to thrombolysis [16].

The CTA component of acute stroke protocol provides information about important vessels of the head and neck and generates source images (CTA-SI), which serve as relevant data for tissue level perfusion. According to theoretical perfusion models, the CTA-SI data are predominantly blood-volume rather than blood-flow weighted [17–19]. As this perfused blood volume technique requires the assumption of an approximately steady-state level of contrast media during the period of image acquisition [18], our CTA protocols use a biphasic contrast injection to attain a better approximation of the steady state [20, 21].

Finally, for dynamic, quantitative CTP, an additional bolus of contrast is administered (at a rate of 4–7 ml/s) during continuous cine imaging over a single region of the brain. In order to track the "first pass" of the contrast bolus through the intracranial vasculature without recirculation effects, images over 45–60 s are acquired. The coverage volume of each acquisition depends on the vendor and type of the multidetector CT (MDCT) scanner. We use two contrast boluses to acquire two slabs of CTP data at different locations to increase overall Z-axis coverage [22]. Appropriate scanning planes allow multiple vascular territories to be assessed [3, 23, 24]. It is important to include a major intracranial artery in at least one image slice in each acquisition for CTP map reconstruction (Fig. 1). In this respect, the previously acquired CTA data allows one to target the tissue of interest with the CTP, which is important given the relatively restricted Z-axis coverage obtained even

Table 1. Sample acute stroke computed tomography (CT) protocol employed at the authors' institution, incorporating CT angiography (CTA) and CT perfusion (CTP). The protocol is designed to answer the four basic questions necessary for stroke triage described. Note the alteration in the kilovolt peak (kVp) for perfusion acquisition. Parameters are presented for illustrative purposes and have been optimized for the scanner currently employed (General Electric Healthcare Lightspeed 16) in our emergency department. Parameters should be optimized for each scanner

Scan series	Unenhanced	CTA head	CTA neck	Cine perfusion ×2
Contrast		Biphasic contrast injection: 2.5 cc/s for 50 cc, then 1.0 cc/s for 20 cc		7 cc/sec for 40 cc for each CTP acquisition
Scan delay		Delay: 25 s (35 s if poor cardiac output, including atrial fibrillation)		Delay: 5 s (each series is a 60-s cine acquisition)
Range	C1 to vertex	C1 to vertex	Arch to C1	Two CTP slabs
Slice thickness	5 mm	2.5 mm	2.5 mm	5 mm
Image spacing	5 mm	2.5 mm	2.5 mm	N/A
Table feed	5.62 mm	5.62 mm	5.62 mm	N/A
Detectors configuration (mm)	16×0.625	16×0.625	16×0.625	16×1.25
Pitch	0.562:1	0.562:1	0.562:1	N/A
Mode	Helical	Helical	Helical	Cine 4i
kVp	140	140	140	80
mA	220	200	250	200
Rotation time	0.5 s	0.5 s	0.5 s	1 s
Scan FOV	Head	Head	Large	Head
Retrospective slice thickness/interval	None	1.25/0.625 mm	1.25/1.0 mm	None

Standard reconstruction algorithm is used for all image reconstruction
CTA computed tomography angiography, *CTP* computed tomography perfusion, *kVp* kilovolt peak, *mA* milliampere, *FOV* field of view

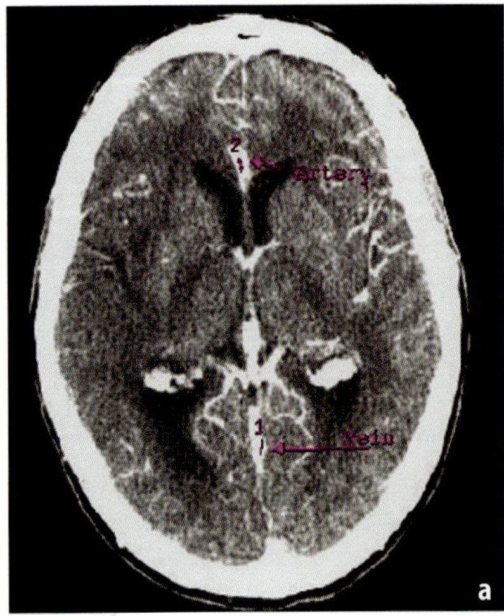
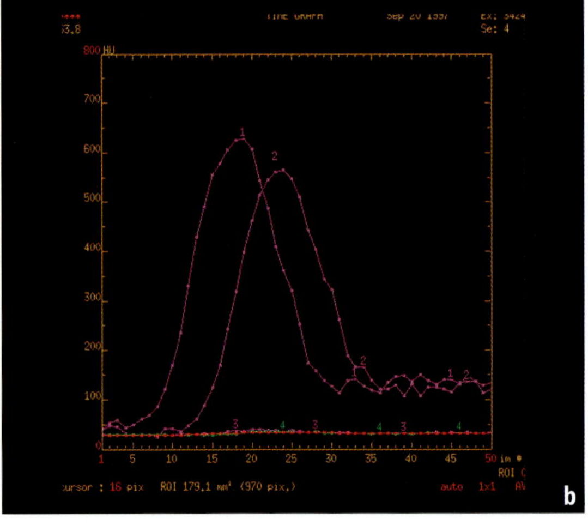

Fig. 1a, b. Computed tomography perfusion (CTP) postprocessing. Appropriate region of interest (ROI) placement on an artery (a major vessel running perpendicular to the plane of section to avoid volume averaging) and on a vein (also running perpendicular to the plane of section and placed to avoid the inner table of the skull) (**a**). The time density curves (TDC) generated from this artery (*A*) and vein (*V*) show the arrival, peak, and passage of the contrast bolus over time (**b**). These TDCs serve as the arterial input function (AIF) and the venous output for the subsequent deconvolution step with two CTP acquisitions. To keep the total iodine dose for acute stroke protocol within reasonable limits, the contrast bolus for the CTA is restricted to allow two 40-cc boluses for the CTP acquisition.

It is also important to bear in mind that there is considerable variability in CTP scanning protocols, as this technique has only recently gained acceptance as a clinical tool and because construction of perfusion maps depends on the particular mathematical model used to analyze the dynamic, contrast-enhanced data. Algorithm-dependent differences in contrast injection rates exist, and, regardless of injection rate, higher contrast concentrations are likely to produce maps with improved signal-to-noise ratios [25].

CTP: Comparison with Perfusion-Weighted MR (MR-PWI)

CTP has several advantages and disadvantages compared with perfusion-weighted MR (MR-PWI). Wider availability and easy, rapid scanning in seriously ill patients with monitors or ventilators make CTP a feasible option. Furthermore, in patients with absolute contraindication to MR, CT may be the only option. Although capillary-level hemodynamics can be assessed with both MR-PWI and CTP, there are several important distinctions between these two techniques (Table 2, Fig. 2). Dynamic susceptibility contrast MR-PWI techniques depend on induction of the indirect T2* effect in adjacent tissues by high concentrations of gadolinium. Thus, MR-PWI may have more "contamination" from large vascular structures and is also limited in certain regions of brain because of susceptibility effects from adjacent structures. On the other hand, CTP depends on direct visualization of the contrast medium. As there is a linear relationship between attenuation and contrast concentration in CT, CTP readily allows quantitation. This is not possible with MR-PWI.

Another advantage of CTP is that CT has greater spatial resolution than MRI. Thus, visual evaluation of core/penumbra mismatch may be more reliable with CTP than with MR-PWI [26, 27].

Conversely, there are notable disadvantages of CTP when compared with MR-PWI. These include limited Z-axis coverage and more labor-intensive postprocessing of CTA and CTP data sets. Another limitation of our CTP protocol is the use of a large amount of contrast material, which may be particularly problematic in older patients, who are most likely to be undergoing evaluation for acute stroke. Several studies have highlighted the issue of radiation risk inherent to CT [3, 28].

CTP: Fundamentals

CTP and MR-PWI evaluate capillary, tissue-level circulation, which is beyond the resolution of traditional anatomic imaging and provides valuable information about blood flow to the brain parenchyma [29]. Cerebral blood flow can be assessed using various parameters, which include CBF, CBV, and MTT. For accurate analysis of CTP maps, it is important to understand associations between these perfusion parameters, as cerebral perfusion pressure drops in acute stroke. CBV is the total blood volume in a given unit volume of the brain, which includes blood in the tissues and blood in the larger vessels such as arteries, arterioles, capillaries, venules, and veins. CBV is measured as units of milliliters of blood per 100 g of cerebral tissue (ml/100 g). CBF is the blood volume moving through a given unit volume of brain per unit time. CBF is measured in units of milliliters of blood per 100 g of brain tissue per minute. MTT is the mean of the transit time of blood through a given region of the brain, which depends on the distance traveled between arterial inflow and venous outflow. MTT is related to both CBV and CBF according to the central volume principle, which

Table 2. Advantages and disadvantages of computed tomography perfusion (CTP) relative to magnetic resonance (MR) perfusion-weighted imaging (PWI)

Advantages	Disadvantages
• Wider availability of CT with lower cost	• Associated radiation dose
• Improved resolution with quantitative perfusion information	• Risks and complications of iodine-based contrast
• Rapid acquisition	• Limited scan coverage
• Easier monitoring and intervention in critical patients	• More complex data postprocessing
• Possible in patients with pacemakers or other contraindications to MR or in patients who cannot be screened for MR safety	

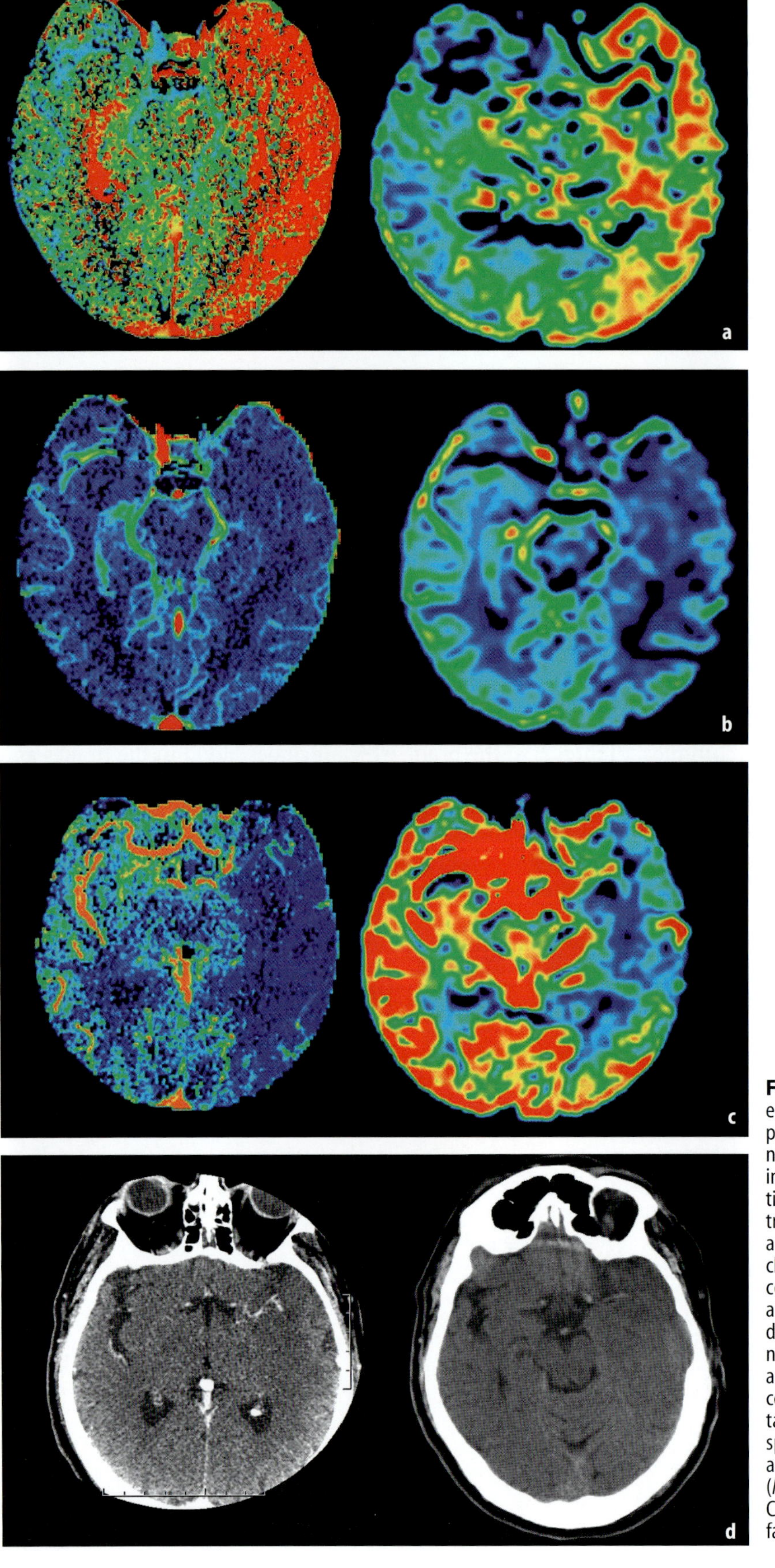

Fig. 2a-d. Correlation of computed tomography perfusion (CTP) and perfusion-weighted magnetic resonance (MR-PWI) images. Perfusion images obtained 1 h apart in a patient presenting with left lower extremity weakness. CTP images (*left*) and MR perfusion images (*right*), including mean transit time (MTT) (**a**), cerebral blood volume (CBV) (**b**), and cerebral blood flow (CBF) (**c**), demonstrate a large perfusion abnormality in the left middle cerebral artery (MCA) distribution. Note the concordance between the data obtained with each modality. Corresponding computed tomography angiography source images (CTA-SI) (*left*) and subsequent unenhanced CT are also shown, revealing an infarct in the left MCA distribution (**d**)

states that MTT=CBV/CBF [30, 31].

The CTP parameters of CBV, CBF, and MTT can be difficult to quantify in practice. The dynamic, first-pass, CTP approach is performed with the dynamic intravenous administration of contrast agent, which is tracked with serial scanning during its first-pass circulation through the capillary bed of brain tissue. Depending on the assumptions regarding the arterial inflow and the venous outflow of the contrast agent, CBV, CBF, and MTT can then be calculated. Dynamic, first-pass CTP models assume that the agent used for perfusion measurement is *nondiffusible* (neither absorbed nor metabolized) in the tissue bed through which it traverses. Therefore, "contrast leakage" outside of the intravascular space in cases of blood brain barrier breakdown associated with tumor, infection, or inflammation, requires a more complex model for calculations. The two major mathematical models used for calculating CTP parameters include deconvolution based and nondeconvolution-based methods.

Nondeconvolution-based CTP models depend on the application of the *Fick principle* to a given region of interest (ROI) within the cerebral parenchyma. A time-density curve (TDC) is derived for each pixel, and CBF is calculated based on the concept of conservation of flow. This calculation is dependent on the assumptions made regarding blood inflow and outflow to the brain region. Although common models simplify the calculations by assuming that there is no venous outflow, these models necessitate high injection rates. CBV can be estimated as the area under the "fitted" tissue TDC divided by the area under the fitted arterial TDC [17]. This equation forms the basis for the quantitative estimation of CBV using the "whole-brain perfused blood volume" when it is assumed that there is a steady state of contrast concentration in the arteries and capillaries [18, 19]: CBV is a function of the density of tissue contrast, normalized by the density of arterial contrast, after soft tissue components have been removed by coregistration and subtraction of the noncontrast scan.

Deconvolution models to estimate CTP parameters have also been validated in a number of studies [32–40]. These methods allow direct computation of CBF, which is applicable for even relatively slow injection rates [41] and compensates for inability to deliver a complete, instantaneous contrast bolus into the artery supplying a given region of brain. Indeed, a contrast bolus (especially one that is given via a peripheral vein) does undergo delay and dispersion before arriving in the cerebral circulation. With the deconvolution model, correct CBV and CBF are estimated by calculating the *residue function*. CBF is calculated directly as proportional to the maximum *height* of the scaled residue function curve. CBV is represented as the *area* under the scaled residue function curve. Once CBF and CBV are estimated, MTT is calculated using the central volume principle.

Potential imaging pitfalls in the calculation of CBF with the deconvolution model include partial volume averaging as well as patient motion, which can lead to underestimation of the arterial input function (AIF). To minimize errors in CTP parameters due to these pitfalls, image coregistration software programs can be used to correct for patient motion and to carefully select ROIs for the AIF. Comparison with the contralateral (normal) side to establish a percentage change from normal can also be a useful adjunctive technique, particularly since the reliability of quantitative CTP parameters is in the range of 20–25%.

In general, nondeconvolution models are more sensitive to changes in underlying vascular anatomy than the deconvolution models. The reason is that nondeconvolution cerebral CTP models assume that a single feeding artery and a single draining vein supports blood circulation in a given area, and that the precise arterial, venous, and tissue TDC can be uniquely identified by imaging. This assumption is an oversimplification of cerebral circulation. In fact, a delay correction is present in most available CTP processing software, so that this oversimplification is less of a concern in CTP.

CTP: Data Postprocessing

In emergent cases, CTP can allow immediate detection of perfusion changes by direct visual inspection of the axial source images at the user interface. Review of CTP data set at an image workstation using a "movie" or cine mode can provide information about relative perfusion changes over time. However, detection of subtle perfusion changes requires advanced postprocessing and quantification. To accomplish this, source CTP images are usually networked to a freestanding workstation for computation of quantitative, first-pass, cine cerebral perfusion maps. Users are generally required to input some information for quantification purposes (Fig. 1), which include:

- *Arterial Input ROI*: A small ROI is placed over the central portion of a large intracranial artery (with maximal peak contrast intensity), preferably orthogonal to the image acquisition plane so that partial volume averaging can be minimized. It is critical to ensure that the image acquisition slab for CTP contains a major intracranial artery to generate the AIF. Some programs allow ROI selection in a semiautomated manner.
- *Venous Outflow ROI*: In addition to an arterial

ROI, a small venous ROI with similar attributes is also selected, most commonly at the superior sagittal sinus. For certain programs, appropriate venous ROI are crucial for accurate CTP maps [42].

Major variations in the aforementioned input values may cause variation in the image quality of CTP maps as well as variation in the CBF, CBV, and MTT.

CTP: Clinical Indications and Applications

Advanced "functional" imaging of acute stroke in the first 12 h can include the following [42]:
- Inclusion of cases most likely to benefit from thrombolysis
- Exclusion of cases most likely to hemorrhage
- Extension of the time window beyond 3 h for intravenous thrombolysis and 6 h for anterior circulation intra-arterial thrombolysis
- Triage to other available therapies, such as hypertension or hyperoxia
- Appropriate treatment of "wake-up" strokes, for which precise time of onset is unknown
- Management decisions regarding admission to neurological intensive care unit or discharge from emergency department

The Desmoteplase in Acute Ischemic Stroke (DIAS) trial suggests that intravenous desmoteplase can be used in an extended therapeutic window of 3–9 h postictus, with substantial improvements in reperfusion rates and clinical outcomes achieved in patients with a diffusion/perfusion mismatch on MRI [43]. On the basis of this study and other ongoing studies, some investigators have cautiously proposed the use of either MR-PWI or CTP for extending the traditional therapeutic time window [44, 45]. These authors cite evidence of a relevant volume of salvageable cerebral tissue present in the 3- to 6-h time frame in more than 80% of acute stroke patients [43, 46, 47].

CTP: Infarct Detection

Several studies have opined that CTA-SI, like diffusion-weighted MRI, can detect tissue destined to infarct despite successful recanalization [11, 48, 49]. In theory, if an approximately steady state of contrast in the cerebral arteries and parenchyma during image acquisition is assumed, CTA-SI are predominantly blood-volume rather than blood-flow weighted [17–19, 50]. An early report suggested that CTA-SI can be used to delineate minimal final infarct size and to identify "infarct core" in an acute stroke [48]. CTA-SI subtraction maps, ob-

tained by commercially available platforms for coregistration and subtraction of the noncontrast head CT from the CTA source images, can provide information about quantitative blood-volume maps of the entire brain [3, 18, 19]. As these maps cover the entire brain, they are especially appealing for clinical use. An exploratory study in patients with MCA stem occlusion who underwent intra-arterial thrombolysis after imaging revealed that CTA-SI and CTA-SI subtraction maps improve conspicuity of cerebral infarct when compared with nonenhanced CT in hyperacute stroke.

In another study, CTA-SI preceding diffusion-weighted MRI was performed in patients with clinically suspected acute stroke presenting within 12 h of symptom onset (42 patients were scanned within 6 h) [11]. The authors reported that CTA-SI and diffusion-weighted imaging (DWI) lesion volumes were independent predictors of final infarct volume, and overall sensitivity and specificity for parenchymal stroke detection were 76% and 90% for CTA-SI, and 100% and 100% for diffusion-weighted imaging, respectively. Although diffusion-weighted imaging is more sensitive than CTA-SI for detection of small lacunar and distal infarcts, both diffusion-weighted imaging techniques are highly accurate predictors of final infarct volume. It is important to remember that, like diffusion-weighted imaging, not every acute hypodense ischemic lesion seen with CTA-SI is destined to infarct [51, 52] (Fig. 3). In the presence of early complete recanalization, CTA-SI can show occasional dramatic sparing of regions with reduced blood pool.

CTP maps can also improve detection of acute infarct, improving both sensitivity (MTT maps) and specificity (relative CBF and relative CBV maps) for the detection of infarct relative to noncontrast CT images [53] (Fig. 4). These maps are also more accurate for determining the extent of infarct, especially for the percentage of MCA territory infarct [53]. A prior study has shown that the relative CBV (rCBV) map correlated better with final infarct volume than admission diffusion-weighted imaging [54].

CTP: Interpretation of Penumbra and Core

Advanced stroke imaging in acute settings must allow for evaluation of the viability of ischemic tissue that transcends an arbitrary "clock time" [55–57]. Two thresholds from prior experimental studies gave rise to the original theory of penumbra [58, 59]. One threshold defined a specific CBF value below which there was no cortical function, without extracellular potassium increment or pH

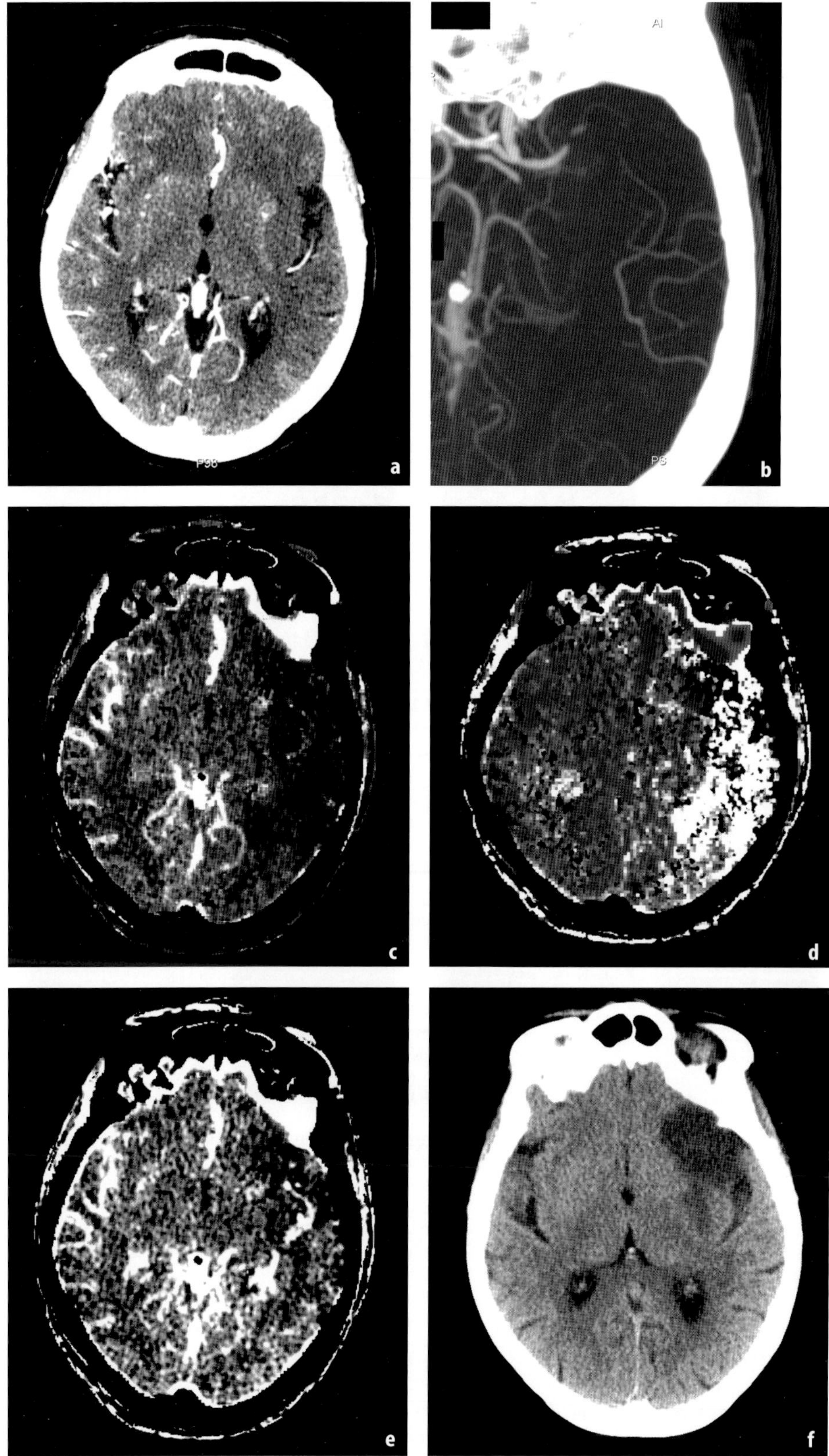

Fig. 3a-f. Reversal of computed tomography angiography source images (CTA-SI) abnormality. An 80-year-old woman presented with a devastating exam. CTA-SI initially demonstrated a large area of hypodensity in the left middle cerebral artery (MCA) distribution (**a**). CTA shows occlusion of the distal left internal carotid artery (ICA) and the entire left middle cerebral artery (MCA) (**b**). CT perfusion (CTP) images obtained at the same time, including cerebral blood flow (CBF) (**c**), mean transit time (MTT) (**d**), and cerebral blood volume (CBV) (**e**), show a large CBF/MTT abnormality involving nearly the entire left MCA territory while the CBV shows only a small area of abnormality anteriorly. After successful intra-arterial thrombolysis, subsequent unenhanced CT shows that the infarct is confined to the initial CBV abnormality (**f**). Although the CTA-SI abnormality characteristically predicts infarct, this case demonstrates the unusual possibility of a reversal of the CTA-SI abnormality. The final infarct volume was better predicted by the initial CBV map

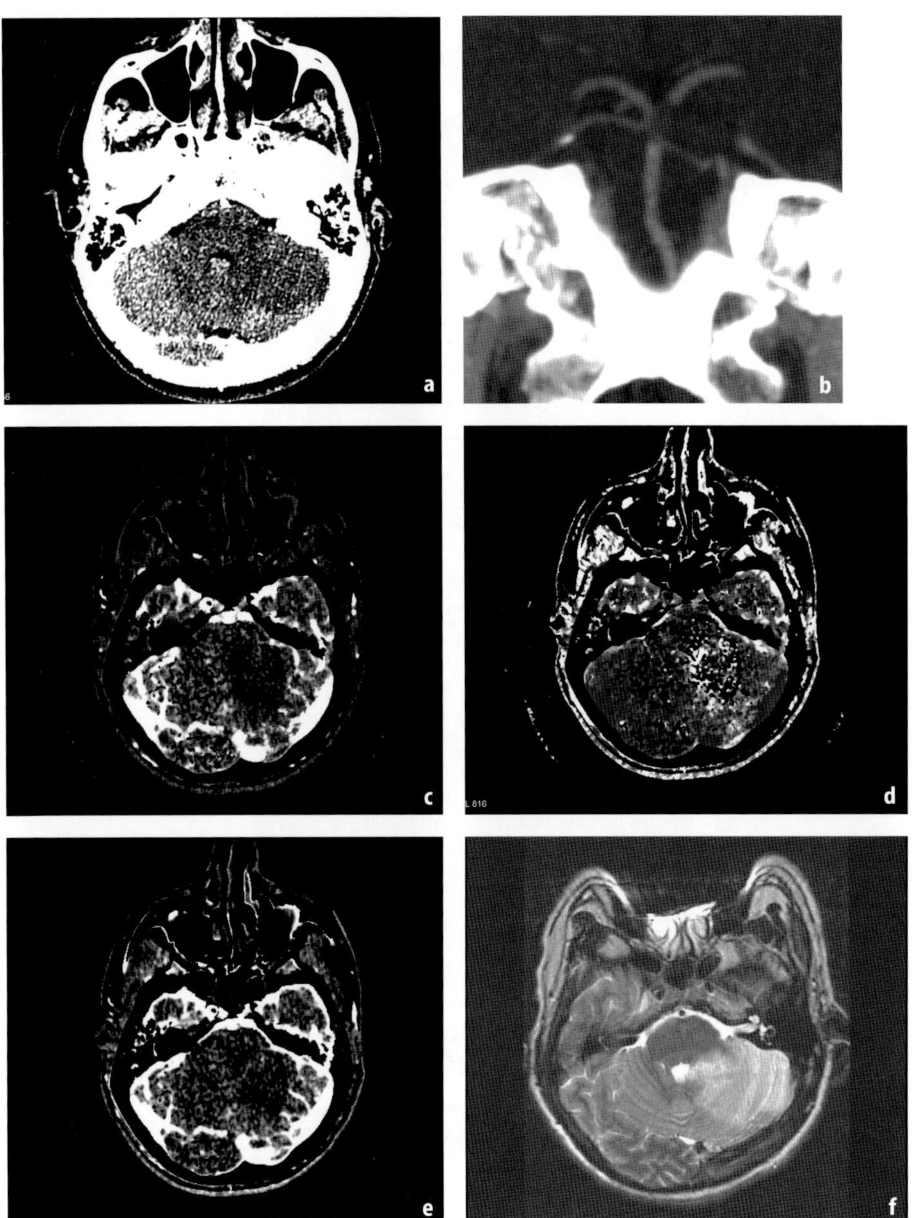

Fig. 4a-f. Matched-perfusion defects. A 36-year-old man presented with acute onset ataxia. Computed tomography angiography source images (CTA-SI) demonstrates an infarct in the left cerebellar hemisphere (**a**). CTA reformat shows thrombus at the basilar tip (**b**). Concurrent CT perfusion (CTP) images, including cerebral blood flow (CBF) (**c**), mean transit time (MTT) (**d**), and cerebral blood volume (CBV) (**e**), show no evidence of a perfusion mismatch to suggest additional territory at risk. T2-weighted magnetic resonance (MR) image obtained 5 days later show an infarct in the left superior cerebellar artery distribution, with no interval expansion of the infarct territory as predicted by the matched perfusion defect initially (**f**). Note that MR perfusion is typically limited in the posterior fossa due to susceptibility artifact

reduction. The second threshold defined a CBF value below which cellular integrity was disrupted. Subsequently, a clinically relevant "operationally defined penumbra," which defines hypoperfused but potentially salvageable tissue, has gained acceptance with emergence of advanced cross-sectional imaging techniques and modern stroke therapy protocols [55, 59–61].

"Ischemic penumbra" can be defined as ischemic but still viable tissue. The operationally defined penumbra may be described as the volume of tissue in the region of CBF/CBV mismatch on CTP maps, where the region of CBV abnormality represents the infarct tissue core and the CBF/CBV mismatch identifies the surrounding region of hypoperfused tissue that is potentially salvageable (Figs. 5 and 6). Dynamic, single-slab CTP with quantitative maps of CBF, CBV, and MTT can describe regions of ischemic penumbra.

Prior human and animal studies with MRI, positron emission tomography (PET), single photon emission tomography (SPECT), and xenon,

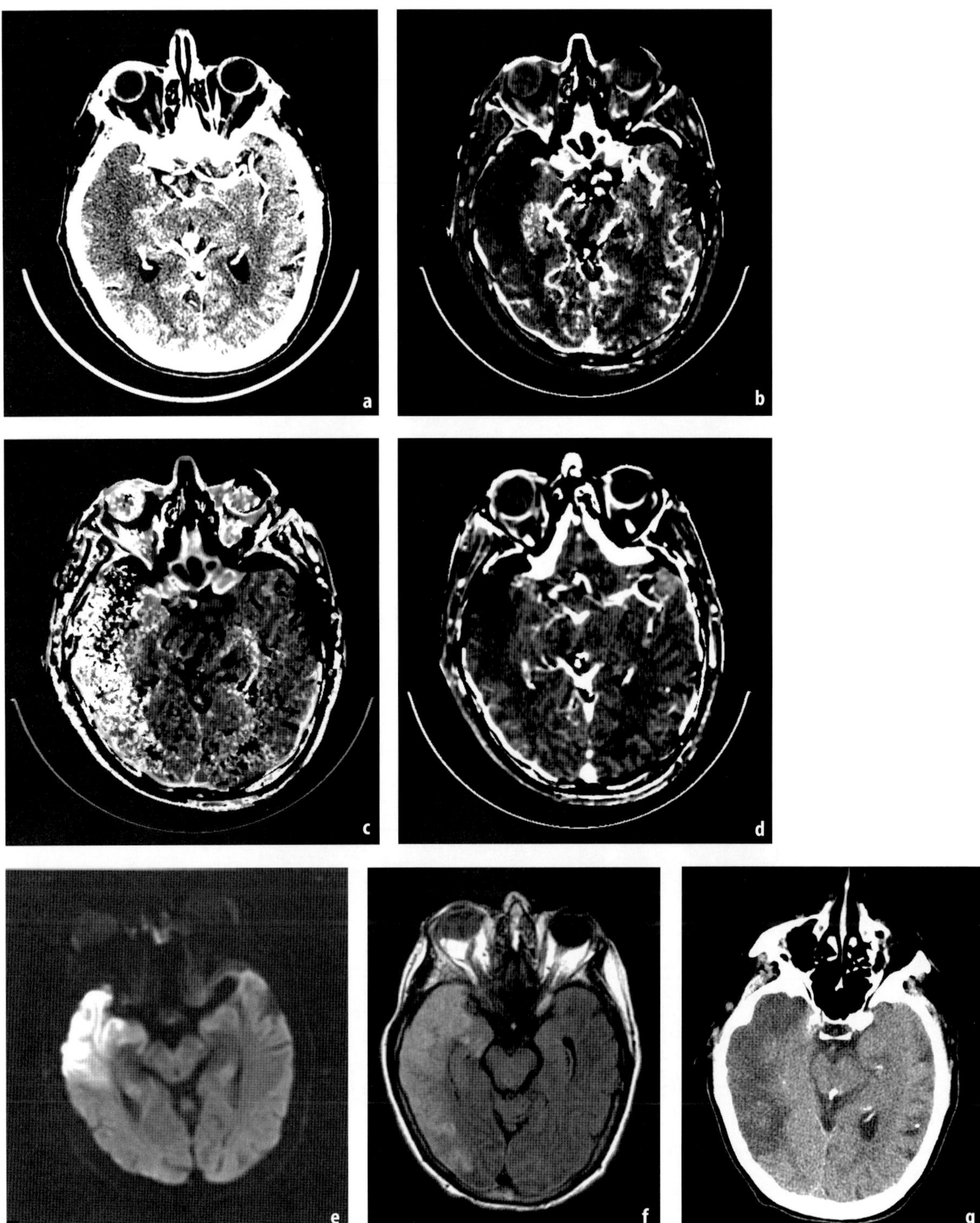

Fig. 5a-g. Expansion of infarct into territory at risk. A 77-year-old woman presented with acute left-sided weakness. Initial computed tomography angiography source images (CTA-SI) performed several hours postictus demonstrates an area of infarct in the anterior right temporal lobe (**a**). CT perfusion (CTP) images obtained concurrently, including cerebral blood flow (CBF) (**b**), mean transit time (MTT) (**c**), and cerebral blood volume (CBV) (**d**) show an area of mismatch posteriorly within the right temporal lobe. Note that the initial infarct corresponds to the CBV abnormality. Diffusion-weighted image (DWI) obtained 30 min later confirms that the infarct is limited to the area seen on CTA-SI and CBV (**e**). Therapy was withheld because of suspected hemorrhage in the cerebellum (not shown). Subsequent magnetic resonance MR (2 days later) (**f**) and CT (5 days later) (**g**) reveal expansion of the infarct into the region at risk as predicted on the initial CTP

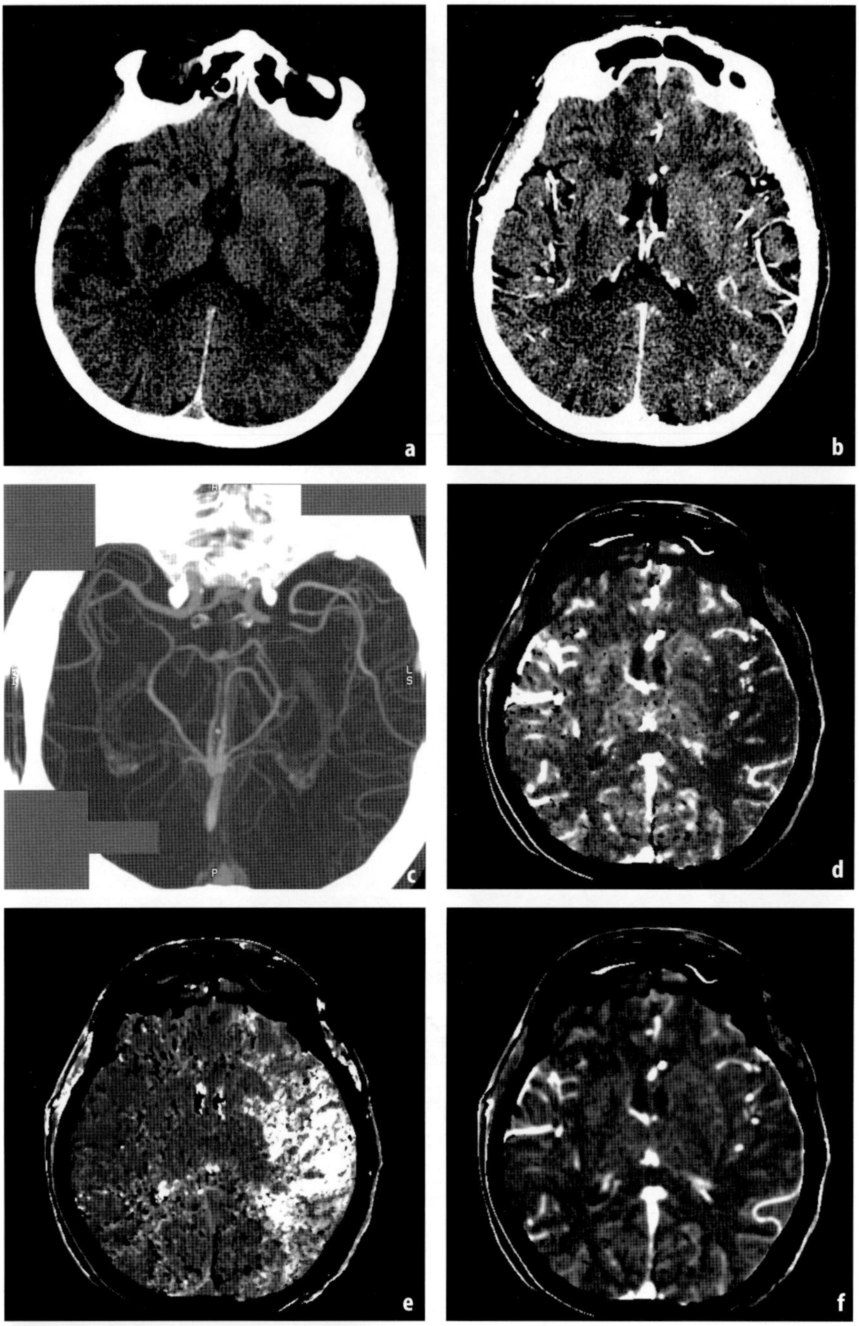

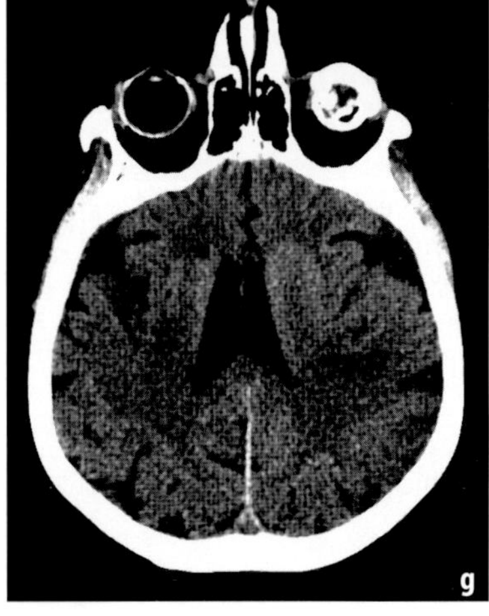

Fig. 6a-g. Successful therapy to preserve territory at risk. A 76-year-old woman presented with acute onset weakness and dysphasia. Computed tomography (CT) (**a**) and CT angiography source images (CTA-SI) (**b**) show no evidence of infarct while CTA reformat shows nonocclusive thrombus in the proximal M1 segment (**c**). Concurrent CT perfusion (CTP), including cerebral blood flow (CBF) (**d**), mean transit time (MTT) (**e**), and cerebral blood volume (CBV) (**f**) show a large area of CBF/CBV mismatch, suggesting territory at risk. The patient underwent intravenous (IV) thrombolysis and an attempt at intra-arterial (IA) mechanical thrombolysis. Unenhanced CT 2 day later shows only small areas of infarct in the posterior left temporal lobe and inferior parietal lobe, in a region much smaller than the territory at risk (**g**). The patient was unable to have a magnetic resonance (MR) image because of a pacemaker

Table 3. Normal values for perfusion parameters in brain tissue. Adapted from [80]

CTP	CBF	CBV	MTT
Gray matter	60 ml/100 g per minute	4 ml/100 g	4 s
White matter	25 ml/100 g per minute	2 ml/100 g	4.8 s

CTP computed tomography perfusion, *CBF* cerebral blood flow, *CBV* cerebral blood volume, *MTT* mean transit time

Table 4. Summary of computed tomography perfusion (CTP) interpretation

Small CBV, larger CBF
- Ideal for therapy
- Perfusion mismatch identifies territory at risk
- Consider no treatment if prolonged time postictus

CBV/CBF match
- No territory at risk
- No therapy regardless of lesion size

Large CBV, larger CBF
- Possible therapy based on time postictus, size
- Perfusion mismatch suggests territory at risk
- Consider no therapy if CBV is greater than 100 ml

CBV cerebral blood volume, *CBF* cerebral blood flow

which investigated the role of CTP in acute stroke triage, have assumed predefined threshold values for infarct core and ischemic penumbra and determined the accuracy of these modalities in predicting stroke outcome [22]. An excellent correlation ($r=0.946$) was noted between diffusion-weighted imaging and CTP-CBV infarct core and the MR-MTT and CT-CBF ischemic penumbra with assumed cutoff values of $\geq34\%$ reduction from baseline CTP-CBF for ischemic penumbra and ≤2.5 ml/100 g CTP-CBV for infarct core [22] (refer to Table 3 for normal values).

The interpretation of CTP in acute stroke is summarized in Table 4. CTP-CBF/CBV mismatch correlates significantly with increase in lesion size. Acute stroke patients who are not treated or are unsuccessfully treated and have a large CBF/CBV mismatch exhibit substantial increase in lesion size on follow-up imaging (Fig. 5). However, in patients without substantial mismatch or with early, complete recanalization, progression of their initial CTA-SI lesion volume is not exhibited (Fig. 6). Hence, CBF/CBV mismatch might serve as a marker of salvageable tissue, which can be useful in triaging patients for thrombolysis [62].

Interpretation of CTP-CBV maps can benefit from a semiautomated thresholding approach to segmentation for a more precise definition of the infarct size [27]. More sophisticated probability maps, synthesizing information derived from different CTP parameters, as well as other imaging series may eventually provide a means to facilitate interpretation of CTP, particularly in the acute setting (Fig. 7).

Prior studies with MR perfusion have shown that CBF maps are superior to MTT maps for distinguishing viable from nonviable penumbra, as MTT maps depict circulatory derangements that are not necessarily ischemic changes (such as large-vessel occlusions with compensatory collateralization and reperfusion hyperemia following revascularization) [63–65].

There have been several improvements in the traditional penumbra model. As not all tissue within the operationally defined penumbra is destined to infarct, the operationally defined penumbra is an oversimplified term. Indeed, there is an area of "benign oligemia" in the region of the CTP-CBV/CBF mismatch that is not expected to infarct even in the absence of reperfusion. Thus, refinement of the traditional penumbra model is important from a clinical standpoint, as therapies based on an overestimated "at-risk" tissue volume can be overaggressive and result in higher risks and complications of treatment for tissue that may not have progressed to infarct even without these therapies. Very few studies have addressed this problem using CTP. Prior studies have reported a significant difference between the MR-CBF thresholds for ischemic penumbra likely to infarct and penumbra likely to remain viable [63, 65]. They also suggested a good correlation between MR perfusion and CTP parameters [50, 66–69]. We reported that normalized, or relative, CBF (rCBF) is the most robust

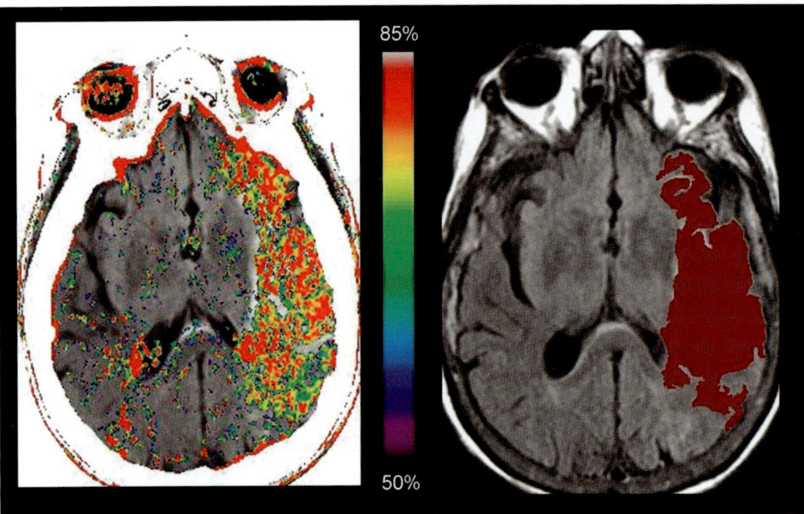

Fig. 7. Probability maps. Scans from a patient who presented to the emergency department with acute stroke symptoms of aphasia and right hemiparesis. The image on the *left* is a probability map constructed from the admission computed tomography angiography source images (CTA-SI) and CT perfusion (CTP) data, with brain regions likely to be irreversibly injured despite successful treatment shown in color. On the *right* is a follow-up magnetic resonance (MR) scan, with the region of the final stroke shown in red. This portends improved methods for visualizing perfusion defects and synthesizing several imaging parameters into a single set of images, facilitating interpretation. Figure courtesy of Ona Wu, Ph.D.

CTP parameter for differentiating viable from nonviable penumbra. In general, CTP-CBF penumbra with less than 50% reduction from baseline values has a high probability of survival. Conversely, CTP-CBF penumbra with a greater than two-thirds reduction from baseline values has a high probability of infarction. Furthermore, no region with an average rCBV less than 0.68, absolute CBF less than 12.7 ml/100 g per minute, or absolute CBV less than 2.2 ml/100 g survived. Due to differences in CBV and CBF between gray matter (GM) and white matter (WM) (Table 3), it is important that the contralateral ROI used for normalization have the same GM/WM ratio as the ipsilateral ischemic area under study.

CTP: Relationship with Clinical Outcome

As stated in the prior section, estimation of the penumbra is technically challenging. Depending on the applied techniques, there is substantial variation in CBF thresholds for various states of tissue perfusion among different studies [70]. However, several studies, evaluating heterogeneous cohorts of patients receiving different therapies, have consistently reported that there is a strong correlation between clinical outcome and initial infarct core lesion volume, regardless of the technique used for measuring it (DWI, CT-CBV, subthreshold xenon CT-CBF, or noncontrast CT) [71–75]. One of these studies reported that clinical outcome was influenced by two factors: recanalization at 24 h (p=0.0001) and day-0 lesion volume on diffusion-weighted imaging (p=0.03) [76]. Likewise, a CTP study in patients with MCA stem occlusions and patients with admission whole-brain CTP lesions volumes greater than 100 ml (about a third of the

volume of the MCA territory) had poor clinical outcomes, irrespective of degree of recanalization [49]. Furthermore, final infarct volume was closely approximated by the lesion size of the initial whole-brain CTP in patients from the same cohort who had early complete MCA recanalization.

In addition to the prediction of clinical outcome from identification of infarct core, CTP, particularly the extent of early CBF reduction in patients with acute stroke, may also help in predicting risk of hemorrhage. Our initial studies indicate that severe hypoperfusion relative to normal cerebral tissue on whole-brain CTP images may also help to localize ischemic regions more likely to have hemorrhage after intra-arterial thrombolysis [77]. Our results are also supported by a recent SPECT study in patients with complete recanalization within 12 h of stoke onset [78]. This study demonstrated that patients with less than 35% of normal blood flow at infarct core had substantially higher risk for hemorrhage [79]. Supportive evidence suggests that cerebral parenchyma with severe ischemia with early reperfusion have the highest risk for hemorrhage [73, 78].

Conclusion

Technologic revolution in MDCT hardware and software has enhanced speed, coverage, and resolution of CTP. CTP has the potential to decrease morbidity of acute stroke. Incorporation of CTP as part of a "one-stop" acute stroke imaging examination is possible with the current MDCT scanners to rapidly and accurately answer the crucial questions related to acute stroke triage. As new treatments are developed for stroke, the potential clinical applications of CTP in the diagnosis, triage, and therapeutic monitoring of these diseases will increase.

References

1. Heart disease and stroke statistics – 2004 update (2003) American Heart Association, 2003, Dallas
2. Lev MH, Farkas J, Rodriguez VR et al (2001) CT angiography in the rapid triage of patients with hyperacute stroke to intraarterial thrombolysis: accuracy in the detection of large vessel thrombus. J Comput Assist Tomogr 25(4):520–528
3. Lev MH, Gonzalez RG (2002) CT Angiography and CT Perfusion Imaging. In: Toga AW, Mazziotta JC (eds) Brain mapping: the methods, 2nd edn. Academic Press, San Diego, pp 427–484
4. Wildermuth S, Knauth M, Brandt T et al (1998) Role of CT angiography in patient selection for thrombolytic therapy in acute hemispheric stroke. Stroke 29(5):935–938
5. Knauth M, vonKummer R, Jansen O et al (1997) Potential of CT angiography in acute ischemic stroke. AJNR Am J Neuroradiol18(6):1001–1010
6. Albers GW (1999) Expanding the window for thrombolytic therapy in acute stroke. The potential role of acute MRI for patient selection. Stroke 30(10):2230–2237
7. Barber PA, Demchuk AM, Zhang J, Buchan AM (2000) Validity and reliability of a quantitative computed tomography score in predicting outcome of hyperacute stroke before thrombolytic therapy. ASPECTS Study Group. Alberta Stroke Programme Early CT Score. Lancet 355(9216):1670–1674
8. Broderick JP, Lu M, Kothari R et al (2000) Finding the most powerful measures of the effectiveness of tissue plasminogen activator in the NINDS tPA stroke trial. Stroke 31(10):2335–2341
9. Schellinger PD, Jansen O, Fiebach JB et al (2000) Monitoring intravenous recombinant tissue plasminogen activator thrombolysis for acute ischemic stroke with diffusion and perfusion MRI. Stroke 31(6):1318–1328
10. Tong D, Yenari M, Albers G et al (1998) Correlation of perfusion- and diffusion-weighted MRI with NIHSS Score in acute (<6.5 hour) ischemic stroke. Neurology 50(4):864–870
11. Berzin T, Lev M, Goodman D et al (2001) CT perfusion imaging versus MR diffusion-weighted imaging: prediction of final infarct size in hyperacute stroke [abstract]. Stroke 32:317
12. Warach S (2001) New imaging strategies for patient selection for thrombolytic and neuroprotective therapies. Neurology 57 [Suppl 2]:48–52
13. Von Kummer R, Holle R, Grzyska U, Hofmann E et al (1996) Interobserver agreement in assessing early CT signs of middle cerebral artery infarction. AJNR Am J Neuroradiol 17:1743–1748
14. Grotta JC, Chiu D, Lu M et al (1999) Agreement and variability in the interpretation of early CT changes in stroke patients qualifying for intravenous rtPA therapy. Stroke 30(8):1528–1533
15. Von Kummer R, Allen KL, Holle R et al (1997) Acute stroke: usefulness of early CT findings before thrombolytic therapy. Radiology 205(2):327–333
16. Von Kummer R (2003) Early major ischemic changes on computed tomography should preclude use of tissue plasminogen activator. Stroke 34(3):820–821
17. Axel L (1980) Cerebral blood flow determination by rapid-sequence computed tomography. Radiology 137:679–686
18. Hunter GJ, Hamberg LM, Ponzo JA et al (1998) Assessment of cerebral perfusion and arterial anatomy in hyperacute stroke with three-dimensional functional CT: Early clinical results. AJNR Am J Neuroradiol 19:29–37
19. Hamberg LM, Hunter GJ, Kierstead D et al (1996) Measurement of cerebral blood volume with subtraction three-dimensional functional CT. AJNR Am J Neuroradiol 17(10):1861–1869
20. Bae KT, Tran HQ, Heiken JP (2000) Multiphasic injection method for uniform prolonged vascular enhancement at CT angiography: pharmacokinetic analysis and experimental porcine model. Radiology 216(3):872–880
21. Fleischmann D, Rubin GD, Bankier AA, Hittmair K (2000) Improved uniformity of aortic enhancement with customized contrast medium injection protocols at CT angiography. Radiology 214(2):363–371
22. Wintermark M, Reichhart M, Thiran JP et al (2002) Prognostic accuracy of cerebral blood flow measurement by perfusion computed tomography, at the time of emergency room admission, in acute stroke patients. Ann Neurol 51(4):417–432
23. Aksoy FG, Lev MH (2000) Dynamic contrast-enhanced brain perfusion imaging: technique and clinical applications. Semin Ultrasound CT MR 21(6):462–477
24. Eastwood JD, Lev MH, Provenzale JM (2003) Perfusion CT with iodinated contrast material. AJR Am J Roentgenol 180(1):3–12
25. Lev MH, Kulke SF, Weisskoff RM et al (1997) Dose dependence of signal to noise ratio in functional MRI of cerebral blood volume mapping with sprodiamide. J Magn Reson Imaging 7:523–527
26. Coutts SB, Simon JE, Tomanek AI et al (2003) Reliability of assessing percentage of diffusion-perfusion mismatch. Stroke 34(7):1681 1683
27. Roccatagliata L, Lev MH, Mehta N et al (2003) Estimating the size of ischemic regions on CT perfusion maps in acute stroke: is freehand visual segmentation sufficient? In: Proceedings of the 89th Scientific Assembly and Annual Meeting of the Radiological Society of North America, 2003, Chicago, p. 1292
28. Mullins ME, Lev MH, Bove P et al (2004) Comparison of image quality between conventional and low-dose nonenhanced head CT. AJNR Am J Neuroradiol 25(4):533–538
29. Villringer A, Rosen BR, Belliveau JW et al (1988) Dynamic imaging with lanthanide chelates in normal brain: Contrast due to magnetic susceptibility effects. Magn Reson Med 6:164–174
30. Meier P, Zieler K (1954) On the theory of the indicator-dilution method for measurement of blood flow and volume. J Appl Physiol 6:731–744
31. Roberts G, Larson K (1973) The interpretation of mean transit time measurements for multi-phase tissue systems. J Theor Biol 39:447–475
32. Cenic A, Nabavi DG, Craen RA et al (1999) Dynamic CT measurement of cerebral blood flow: a validation study. AJNR Am J Neuroradiol 20(1):63–73
33. Cenic A, Nabavi DG, Craen RA et al (2000) A CT method to measure hemodynamics in brain tumors: validation and application of cerebral blood flow maps. AJNR Am J Neuroradiol 21(3):462–470

34. Nabavi DG, Cenic A, Dool J et al (1999) Quantitative assessment of cerebral hemodynamics using CT: stability, accuracy, and precision studies in dogs. J Comput Assist Tomogr 23(4):506–515
35. Nabavi DG, Cenic A, Craen RA et al (1999) CT assessment of cerebral perfusion: experimental validation and initial clinical experience. Radiology 213(1):141–149
36. Nabavi DG, Cenic A, Henderson S et al (2001) Perfusion mapping using computed tomography allows accurate prediction of cerebral infarction in experimental brain ischemia. Stroke 32(1):175–183
37. Ostergaard L, Weisskoff RM, Chesler DA et al (1996) High resolution of cerebral blood flow using intravascular tracer bolus passages. Part I: Mathematical Approach ad Statistical Analysis. Magnetic Resonance Imaging in Medicine 36(5):715–725
38. Ostergaard L, Chesler DA, Weisskoff RM et al (1999) Modeling cerebral blood flow and flow heterogeneity from magnetic resonance residue data. J Cereb Blood Flow Metab 19(6):690–699
39. Wintermark M, Thiran JP, Maeder P et al (2001) Simultaneous measurement of regional cerebral blood flow by perfusion CT and stable xenon CT: a validation study. AJNR Am J Neuroradiol 22(5):905–914
40. Wirestam R, Andersson L, Ostergaard L et al (2000) Assessment of regional cerebral blood flow by dynamic susceptibility contrast MRI using different deconvolution techniques. Magn Reson Med 43(5):691–700
41. Wintermark M, Maeder P, Thiran JP (2001) Quantitative assessment of regional cerebral blood flows by perfusion CT studies at low injection rates: a critical review of the underlying theoretical models. Eur Radiol 11(7):1220–1230
42. Sanelli PC, Lev MH, Eastwood JD et al (2004) The effect of varying user-selected input parameters on quantitative values in CT perfusion maps. Academic Radiology 11(10):1085–1092
43. Hacke W, Albers G, Al-Rawi Y et al (2005) The Desmoteplase in Acute Ischemic Stroke Trial (DIAS): a phase II MRI-based 9-hour window acute stroke thrombolysis trial with intravenous desmoteplase. Stroke 36(1):66–73
44. Schellinger PD, Fiebach JB, Hacke W (2003) Imaging-based decision making in thrombolytic therapy for ischemic stroke: present status. Stroke 34(2):575–583
45. Rother J (2003) Imaging-guided extension of the time window: ready for application in experienced stroke centers? Stroke 34(2):575–583
46. Rother J, Schellinger PD, Gass A et al (2002) Effect of intravenous thrombolysis on MRI parameters and functional outcome in acute stroke <6 hours. Stroke 33(10):2438–2445
47. Parsons MW, Barber PA, Chalk J et al (2002) Diffusion- and perfusion-weighted MRI response to thrombolysis in stroke. Ann Neurol 51(1):28–37
48. Lev MH, Segal AZ, Farkas J et al (2001) Utility of perfusion-weighted CT imaging in acute middle cerebral artery stroke treated with intra-arterial thrombolysis: prediction of final infarct volume and clinical outcome. Stroke 32(9):2021–2028
49. Schramm P, Schellinger PD, Fiebach JB et al (2002). Comparison of CT and CT angiography source images with diffusion-weighted imaging in patients with acute stroke within 6 hours after onset. Stroke 33(10):2426–2432
50. Schramm P, Schellinger PD, Klotz E et al (2004) Comparison of perfusion computed tomography and computed tomography angiography source images with perfusion-weighted imaging and diffusion-weighted imaging in patients with acute stroke of less than 6 hours' duration. Stroke 35:1652–1658
51. Kidwell CS, Saver JL, Mattiello J et al (2000) Thrombolytic reversal of acute human cerebral ischemic injury shown by diffusion/perfusion magnetic resonance imaging. Ann Neurol 47(4):462–469
52. Kidwell CS, Saver JL, Starkman S et al (2002) Late secondary ischemic injury in patients receiving intraarterial thrombolysis. Ann Neurol 52(6):698–703
53. Wintermark M, Fischbein NJ, Smith WS et al (2005) Accuracy of dynamic perfusion CT with deconvolution in detecting acute hemispheric stroke. AJNR Am J Neuroradiol 26(1):104–112
54. Bisdas S, Donnerstag F, Ahl B (2004) Comparison of perfusion computed tomography with diffusion-weighted magnetic resonance imaging in hyperacute ischemic stroke. J Comput Assist Tomogr 28(6):747–755
55. Warach S (2003) Measurement of the ischemic penumbra with MRI: it's about time. Stroke 34(10):2533–2534
56. Wu O, Koroshetz WJ, Ostergaard L et al (2001) Predicting tissue outcome in acute human cerebral ischemia using combined diffusion- and perfusion-weighted MR imaging. Stroke 32(4):933–942
57. Barber PA, Darby DG, Desmond PM et al (1998) Prediction of stroke outcome with echoplanar perfusion- and diffusion-weighted MRI. Neurology 51(2):418–426
58. Astrup J, Siesjo BK, Symon L (1981) Thresholds in cerebral ischemia – the ischemic penumbra. Stroke 12(6):723–725
59. Sorensen AG, Buonanno FS, Gonzalez RG et al (1996) Hyperacute stroke: evaluation with combined multisection diffusion- weighted and hemodynamically weighted echo-planar MR imaging. Radiology 199(2):391–401
60. Sunshine JL, Tarr RW, Lanzieri CF et al (1999) Hyperacute stroke: ultrafast MR imaging to triage patients prior to therapy. Radiology 212:325–332
61. Schlaug G, Benfield A, Baird AE et al (1999) The ischemic penumbra: operationally defined by diffusion and perfusion MRI. Neurology 53(7):1528–1537
62. Mehta N, Lev MH, Mullins ME et al (2003) Prediction of final infarct size in acute stroke using cerebral blood flow/cerebral blood volume mismatch: added value of quantitative first pass CT perfusion imaging in successfully treated versus unsuccessfully treated/untreated patients. In: Proceedings of the 41st Annual Meeting of the American Society of Neuroradiology, 2003, Washington
63. Rohl L, Ostergaard L, Simonsen CZ et al (2001) Viability thresholds of ischemic penumbra of hyperacute stroke defined by perfusion-weighted MRI and apparent diffusion coefficient. Stroke 32(5):1140–1146
64. Grandin CB, Duprez TP, Smith AM et al (2001) Usefulness of magnetic resonance-derived quantitative measurements of cerebral blood flow and volume in prediction of infarct growth in hyperacute stroke. Stroke 32(5):1147–1153

65. Schaefer PW, Ozsunar Y, He J et al (2003) Assessing tissue viability with MR diffusion and perfusion imaging. AJNR Am J Neuroradiol 24(3):436–443
66. Eastwood JD, Lev MH, Wintermark M et al (2003) Correlation of early dynamic CT perfusion imaging with whole-brain MR diffusion and perfusion imaging in acute hemispheric stroke. AJNR Am J Neuroradiol 24(9):1869–1875
67. Wintermark M, Reichhart M, Cuisenaire O et al (2002) Comparison of admission perfusion computed tomography and qualitative diffusion- and perfusion-weighted magnetic resonance imaging in acute stroke patients. Stroke 33(8):2025–2031
68. Lev MH, Hunter GJ, Hamberg LM et al (2002) CT versus MR imaging in acute stroke: comparison of perfusion abnormalities at the infarct core. In: Proceedings of the 40th Annual Meeting of the American Society of Neuroradiology, 2002, Vancouver
69. Lev MH (2003) CT versus MR for acute stroke imaging: is the "obvious" choice necessarily the correct one? AJNR Am J Neuroradiol 24(10):1930–1931
70. Heiss WD (2000) Ischemic penumbra: evidence from functional imaging in man. J Cereb Blood Flow Metab 20(9):1276–1293
71. Jovin TG, Yonas H, Gebel JM et al (2003) The cortical ischemic core and not the consistently present penumbra is a determinant of clinical outcome in acute middle cerebral artery occlusion. Stroke 34(10):2426–2433
72. Lev MH, Roccatagliata L, Murphy EK et al (2004) A CTA based, multivariable, "benefit of recanalization" model for acute stroke triage: core infarct size on CTA source images independently predicts outcome. In: Proceedings of the 42nd Annual Meeting of the American Society of Neuroradiology, 2004, Seattle
73. Suarez J, Sunshine J, Tarr R et al (1999) Predictors of clinical improvement, angiographic recanalization, and intracranial hemorrhage after intra-arterial thrombolysis for acute ischemic stroke. Stroke 30:2094–2100
74. Molina CA, Alexandrov AV, Demchuk AM et al (2004) Improving the predictive accuracy of recanalization on stroke outcome in patients treated with tissue plasminogen activator. Stroke 35(1):151–156
75. Baird AE, Dambrosia J, Janket S et al (2001) A three-item scale for the early prediction of stroke recovery. Lancet 357(9274):2095–2099
76. Nighoghossian N, Hermier M, Adeleine P et al (2003) Baseline magnetic resonance imaging parameters and stroke outcome in patients treated by intravenous tissue plasminogen activator. Stroke 34(2):458–463
77. Swap C, Lev M, McDonald C et al (2002) Degree of oligemia by perfusion-weighted CT and risk of hemorrhage after IA thrombolysis. In: Stroke – Proceedings of the 27th International Conference on Stroke and Cerebral Circulation, 2002, San Antonio
78. Ogasawara K, Ogawa A, Ezura M et al (2001) Brain single-photon emission CT studies using 99mTc-HMPAO and 99mTc-ECD early after recanalization by local intraarterial thrombolysis in patients with acute embolic middle cerebral artery occlusion. AJNR Am J Neuroradiol 22(1):48–53
79. Ueda T, Sakaki S, Yuh W (1999) Outcome in acute stroke with successful intra- arterial thrombolysis procedure and predictive value of initial single-photon emission-computed tomography. J Cereb Blood Flow Metab 19:99–108
80. Calamante F, Gadian DG, Connelly A (2000) Delay and dispersion effects in dynamic susceptibility contrast MRI: simulatinos using singular value decomposition. Magn Reson Med 44(3):466–473

SECTION IV

MDCT of Trauma

24

MDCT of Abdominal Trauma

Robert A. Halvorsen

Introduction

Trauma is a significant public health problem, representing the third leading cause of death in the United States. Trauma is also the leading cause of mortality in Americans under the age of 40. With the widespread availability of multidetector-row computed tomography (MDCT) in trauma centers, the traditional workup of trauma patients has changed. Blunt chest injuries are now frequently studied with MDCT to evaluate the aorta, and workup of the blunt trauma victim with abdominal injury is evolving with MDCT. MDCT now allows not only the detection of injuries but provides new information on the severity of injuries with improved detection of vascular injury manifested by "active extravasation." Until recently, patients with a history of penetrating trauma went directly to the operating room for surgical therapy without preoperative imaging. Today, MDCT is often performed in patients with penetrating trauma in order to best identify vascular injuries prior to surgical intervention.

This chapter reviews the technique of MDCT and discusses major findings in abdominal MDCT in the trauma patient. The varied manifestations of bleeding are emphasized. Common mistakes and pitfalls in interpretation are described along with a step-by-step technique for interpretation.

MDCT Utilization in the Trauma Patient

Workup of the blunt trauma patient has evolved with the advent of MDCT. In the past, a large number of patients with deceleration injuries had abdominal CT in the search for solid-organ or hollow viscus injury, but few had a chest CT. With the installation of MDCT scanners in major trauma centers, the frequency of chest CT in the trauma pa-

tient has increased dramatically. MDCT provides the capability to perform high-definition multiplanar reconstruction (MPR) based upon thin sections reconstructed from MDCT raw data. Chest MDCT with MPR effectively produces CT angiograms, probably equal in quality to angiography (Fig. 1). A trauma surgeon can be provided definitive information concerning aortic injuries almost immediately with MDCT without the additional contrast load and invasiveness of traditional angiography. At many institutions, MDCT of the chest has almost completely replaced angiography in the initial workup of patients with possible aortic injuries. Angiography is often relegated to the role of a problem-solving tool. An MDCT of the chest not only provides diagnostic information concerning potential aortic injuries but also evaluates lungs, pleura, and bones. MPRs of the thorax

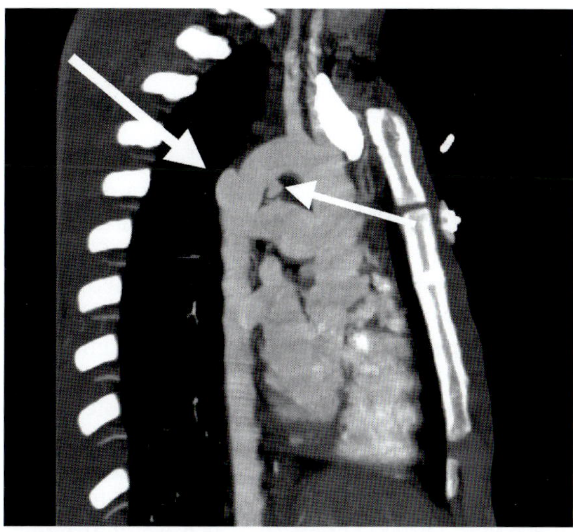

Fig. 1. Computed tomography angiogram (CTA) of motor vehicle accident victim demonstrating two pseudoaneurysms of the aorta (*arrows*), the smaller located on the anterior surface at the bottom of the aortic arch and the second located on the posterior proximal descending thoracic aorta

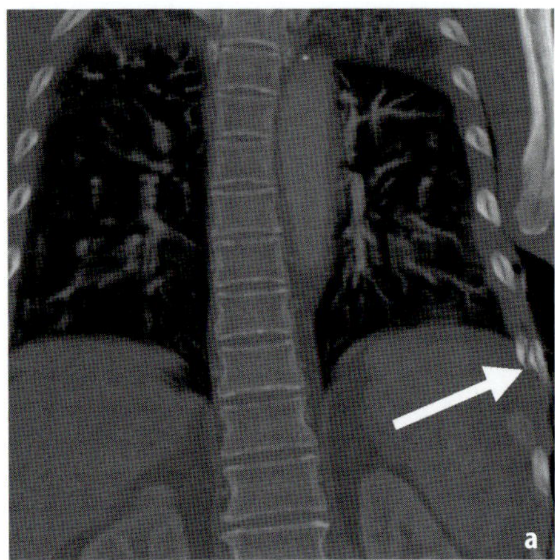
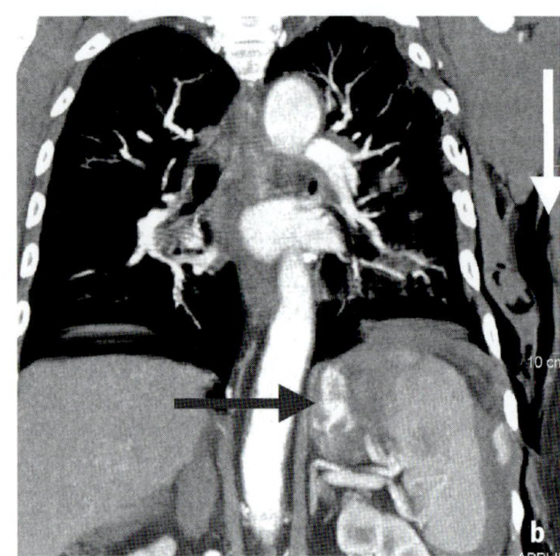
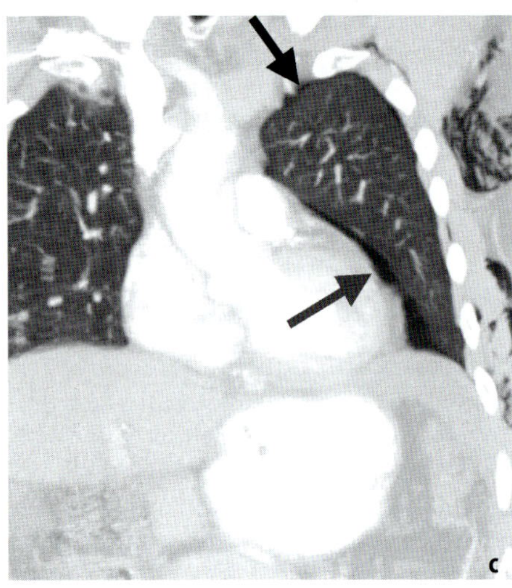

Fig. 2a-c. Computed tomography (CT) of high-speed motor vehicle accident victim. **a** Coronal CT with bone windows readily identifies rib fracture (*arrow*). **b** Soft tissue coronal view demonstrates large amount of subcutaneous emphysema (*white arrow*) and active extravasation in upper abdomen medial to spleen (*black arrow*). **c** Lung window in coronal projection demonstrates medial and small apical pneumothorax (*black arrows*)

facilitate detection of rib and spine fractures (Fig. 2a)

Alternative Strategies in MDCT Acquisitions

While the introduction of MDCT has dramatically changed the way many thoracic injuries are evaluated, it has had a lesser impact on evaluation of the abdomen and pelvis. Optimal use of MDCT below the diaphragm has not yet been established. Evaluation of the abdomen and pelvis with MDCT is currently performed differently in different institutions. Some centers, such as Massachusetts General Hospital, advocate the use of a "whole-body" CT in the trauma patient [1]. They utilize a continuous scanning technique through the areas to be scanned, such as cervical spine, chest, abdomen, and pelvis. Other centers, such as ours, continue to perform separate MDCT data acquisitions for each type of CT. For instance, a patient who has multiple types of CT studies in our Emergency Department will have them performed sequentially but

not continuously, facilitating the optimization of contrast enhancement timing and radiation dose. Sequential rather than continuous scanning makes possible the use of different types of reconstruction algorithms for different anatomical segments.

Alternative Means of MDCT Interpretation

Another variable is the availability of freestanding image processing workstations. Workstations linked to CT scanners allow the interpreting radiologist to take raw data at the workstation and make customized MPRs. Off-line reconstruction has the added benefit of allowing the technologist to move on to the next patient without waiting for the CT computers to perform the MPRs. Alternatively, technologists can produce routine MPRs using standard imaging planes, such as sagittal or coronal planes. Our technologists obtain routine coronal and sagittal MPRs in chest trauma patients and also reconstruct an oblique sagittal MPR along the plane of the aortic arch (Fig. 1). When obtaining MPRs using the 16-detector-row MDCT scanner computer, time costs are of interest. An MDCT of the chest requires a 20/second scan time. Initial reconstruction at 3 mm is performed, and axial images are sent to our PACS system for interpretation. This initial reconstruction requires 3 min 20 s. Then, to obtain MPRs, the raw data is reconstructed at thinner intervals and MPRs are constructed, requiring 7 min 10 s. Therefore, in order to prepare data obtained from an MDCT of the chest for interpretation, scan time (data acquisition) is only 20 s, but total reconstruction time is 10 min 30 s.

Changes in Interpretation Strategies with MDCT

Interpretation of MDCT in trauma patients requires attention to detail. The use of a rigorous routine in the interpretation of these studies significantly diminishes missed traumatic lesions [2]. We routinely review all trauma CTs with five settings:
- Lung window
- Soft tissue window
- Liver window
- Bone window
- MPR: sagittal and coronal multiplanar reconstructions

Interpretation: Routine Approach

Following is a detailed routine for interpretation of abdominal and pelvic MDCT in trauma patients:

Lung Windows
In our experience, the most frequently overlooked finding in trauma CT is a pneumothorax. We use lung windows to search for pneumothorax as well as pneumoperitoneum (Figs. 2c, 3, and 4). Not only the entire chest, but also the abdomen and pelvis are scanned from top to bottom using lung windows for the detection of free intraperitoneal air, intraperitoneal air adjacent to bowel loops, and retroperitoneal air.

Soft Tissue Windows
After scanning from top to bottom using lung windows, we switch to soft tissue windows and scroll from bottom back to top. This primary initial soft tissue survey is performed to search for free intraperitoneal fluid consistent with blood in a trauma patient (Fig. 5) Intraperitoneal fluid in a trauma patient is most likely due to either solid-organ or bowel injury and is a good indicator of injury severity. Careful attention is paid to the presence or absence of free fluid in the pelvis, where small amounts of fluid are easily overlooked. After the initial survey of the abdomen for blood, individual organs are scrutinized. When intraabdominal fluid is encountered on an MDCT of a trauma patient, an analysis of fluid density is extremely helpful. Clotted blood next to or adjacent to a bleeding site is called a sentinel clot [4] (Fig. 6). This clotted blood will be of higher density than the more serous blood further away from the site of bleeding. Identification of the sentinel clot is helpful in identifying the site of bleeding.

Spleen Survey
We evaluate the spleen twice. First, we look within the splenic parenchyma for areas of low or high density. Low density can represent splenic laceration or fracture. Fracture of a solid organ is defined as a laceration that extends from one capsular surface to the other. Splenic lacerations are usually identified because of the hematoma within the splenic parenchyma (Fig. 6). Whenever a

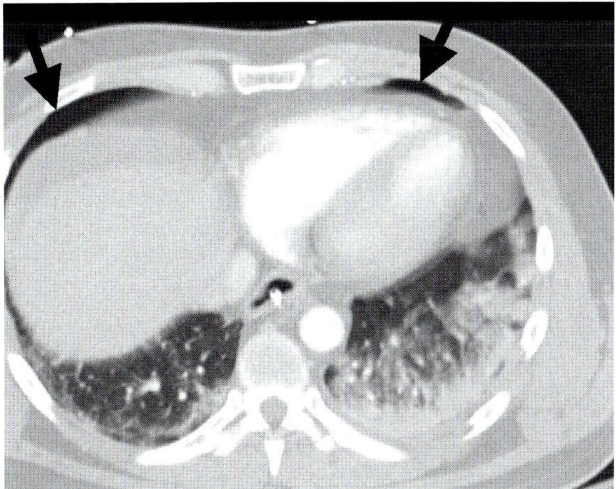

Fig. 3. Computed tomography (CT) of motor vehicle accident victim. Demonstrates bilateral pneumothoraces

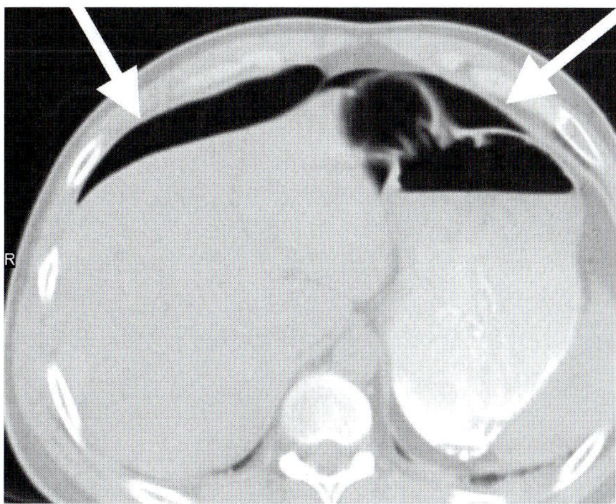

Fig. 4. Motor vehicle accident victim with pneumoperitoneum. Demonstrates subphrenic air (*arrows*)

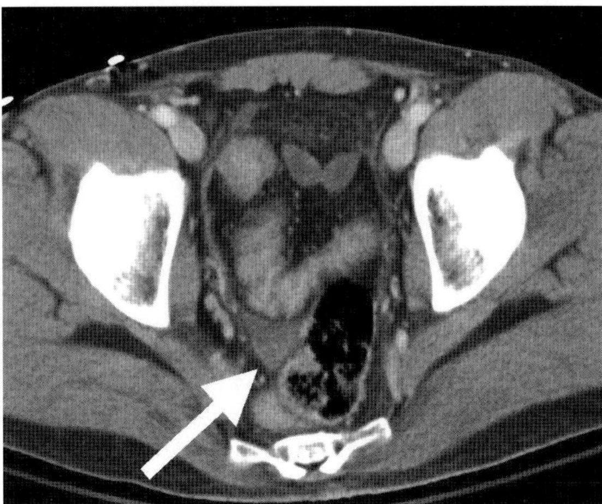

Fig. 5. Free intraperitoneal blood (*arrow*) in pelvis in blunt-trauma victim

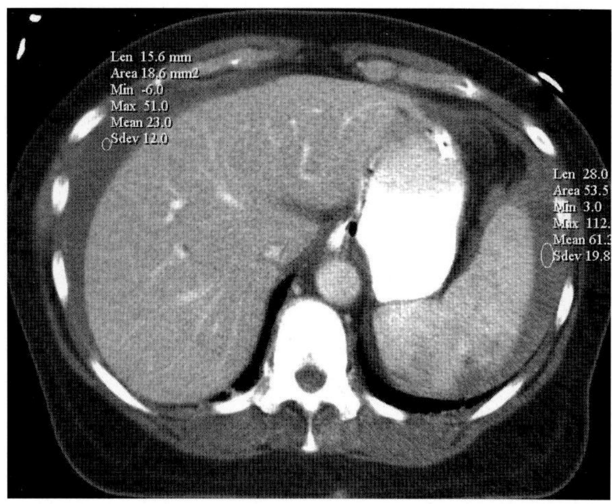

Fig. 6. Sentinel clot. Motor vehicle accident victim with splenic laceration. Perisplenic blood has higher density [61 Hounsfield units (HU)] compared with perihepatic blood (23 HU). Higher-density blood adjacent to the spleen is the "sentinel clot," helping to identify the source of bleeding. Lower-density blood adjacent to the liver is more serous in nature

hematoma is identified in the spleen or in any portion of an abdominal and pelvic CT, one should always search for active extravasation. Active extravasation of contrast material signifies arterial bleeding. Recognition of arterial bleeding or active extravasation has dramatically increased with the introduction of MDCT with rapid administration of high-concentration contrast media (Fig. 7). In 1989, Sivit et al. [5] reported the first demonstration of active intraabdominal arterial bleeding in a patient with splenic rupture from blunt trauma. Gavant et al. were among the first to describe the usefulness of detecting active bleeding in predicting the need for surgical intervention [3]. Jeffrey et al. [6] and later Federle et al. [7] further characterized and clarified the importance of active extravasation in helical CT. Detection of active extravasation on CT implies arterial bleeding and is usually considered an indication for splenic arteriography with possible embolization as alternative to surgery.

Traditionally, splenic injuries have been classified using a CT-based scoring or grading system [8]. Such grading systems may be misleading, as a minor injury may go on to a devastating delayed bleed:

- Grade 1: Subcapsular hematoma or laceration <1 cm
- Grade II: Larger subcapsular hematoma or laceration 1–3 cm
- Grade III: Capsular disruption or laceration >3 cm
- Grade IVA: Shattered spleen or active extravasation into spleen or subcapsular hematoma or pseudo aneurysm or arteriovenous fistula (Fig. 7)

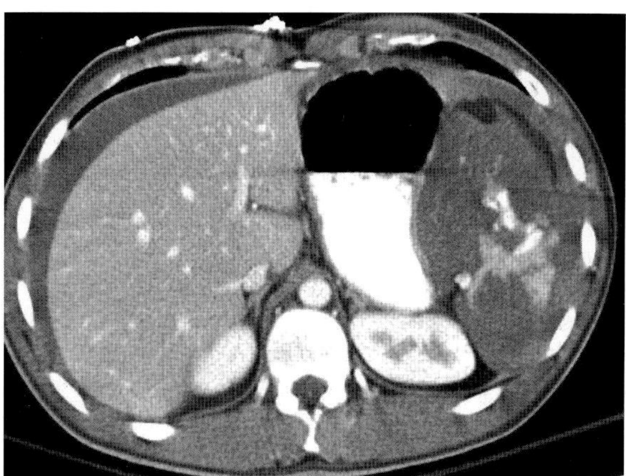

Fig. 7. Motor vehicle accident victim with splenic injury demonstrating active intrasplenic arterial bleeding

- Grade IVB: Active intraperitoneal bleeding (Fig. 8)

The severity predicted by traditional CT scoring systems for solid-organ injury using the American Association for the Surgery of Trauma (AAST) scoring system is controversial, with a number of authors finding them unhelpful [8–11], while others find them of use in patients with massive splenic injury, as most patients with Grades IVA or IVB splenic injury will require catheter embolization or surgery [12].

Liver Survey
The liver is the most frequently injured organ in trauma patients in general when both blunt and penetrating trauma is considered, while in blunt trauma patients, the spleen is the most commonly

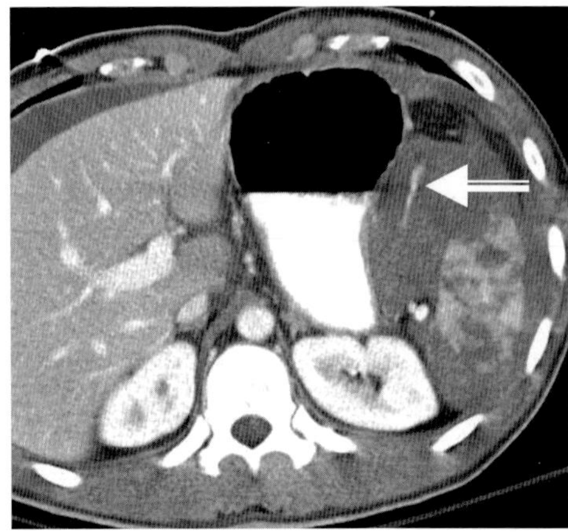

Fig. 8. Motor vehicle accident victim with severely injured spleen with active intraperitoneal bleeding (*arrow*) and evidence of a shattered spleen

injured organ. Survey of the liver is similar to that of the spleen, with an initial review of the deep hepatic parenchyma in the search for laceration or hematoma. A second review of each slice containing liver is performed to evaluate the margin of the liver in the search for subtle lacerations and perihepatic blood. Finally, one should evaluate the right paracolic gutter for small amounts of fluid. Occasionally in a patient with extensive respiratory motion, subtle hepatic injuries will not be detectable, but perihepatic blood, especially in the upper right paracolic gutter, will point to the site of injury.

With hepatic injuries, as with any solid organ injury, it is important to look for signs of active extravasation manifested as high-density contrast equivalent to arterial structures on the same slice (Fig. 9). But besides arterial injury, venous injury is of extreme importance in hepatic trauma. With liver injuries, it is essential to look for signs of he-

patic vein damage. Traumatic avulsion of the hapatic vein occurs in approximately 13% of liver injuries, often as a result of avulsion of the right hepatic vein from the inferior vena cava. Such vein damage is suggested on CT when lacerations extend around the inferior vena cava or into the porta hepatis (Fig. 10). With venous injuries, active extravasation is usually not detected. As the liver parenchyma itself compresses the laceration of the vein, no large hematomas are encountered. However, if the patient goes to the operating room and the surgeon elevates the liver, the tamponading effect of the liver parenchyma against the bleeding site is removed, and patients frequently exsanguinate on the operating room table. Therefore, if there is a detectable deep injury in the liver near the hepatic veins or the inferior vena cava (Fig. 11), the surgeon should be alerted to the finding prior to any operative intervention. With venous injuries, control of the inferior vena cava is obtained prior to elevating the liver in order to prevent exsanguination.

Pancreatic and Duodenal Injury

Duodenal hematomas may be subtle, with only mild thickening of the duodenal wall. Paraduodenal fluids often have a triangular, pointed shape and suggest a tear of the serosal surface of the duodenum (Fig. 12).

Pancreatic lacerations are often associated with duodenal injuries but can occur without CT-detectable duodenal hematoma. Pancreatic lacerations are often difficult to diagnose on the immediate trauma MDCT. Traumatic pancreatic injuries require time to produce edema within the pancreas. The initial CT may fail to show pancreatic injury unless a laceration within the pancreas is large enough to be visualized or there is peripancreatic

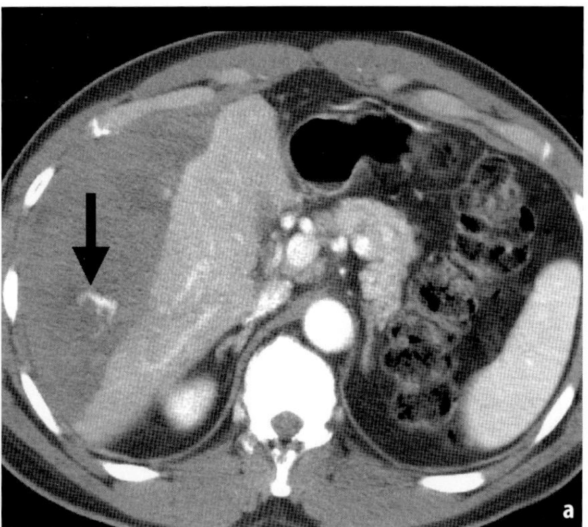

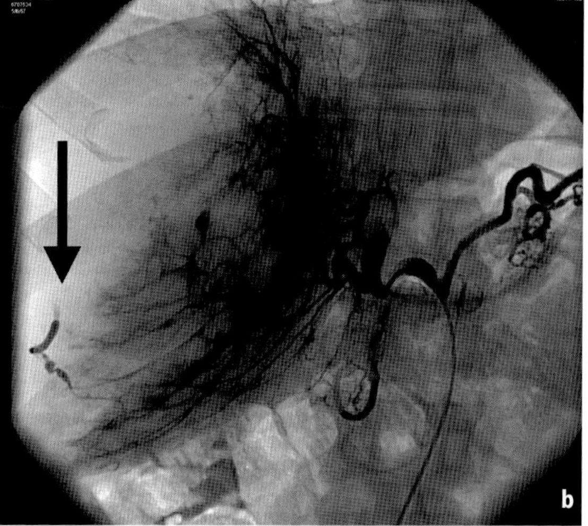

Fig. 9a, b. Large subcapsular hematoma with active arterial bleeding from hepatic injury. **a** Linear area of active extravasation (*arrow*) lateral to liver within subcapsular hematoma on axial computed tomography (CT). **b** Celiac artery angiogram demonstrates active extravasation (*arrow*) in subcapsular hematoma mimicking vessel

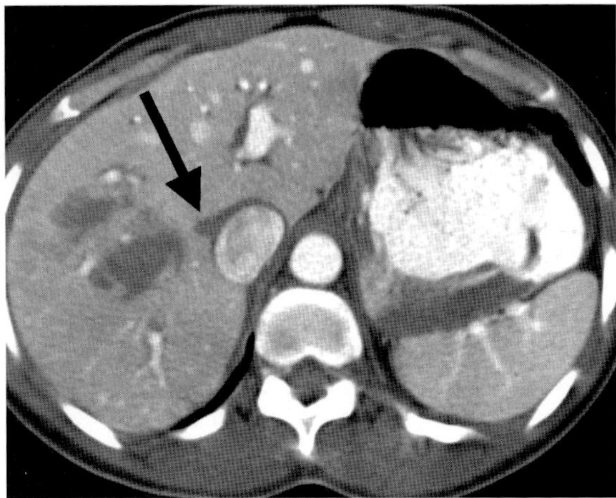

Fig. 10. Hepatic laceration with extension to inferior vena cava (*arrow*)

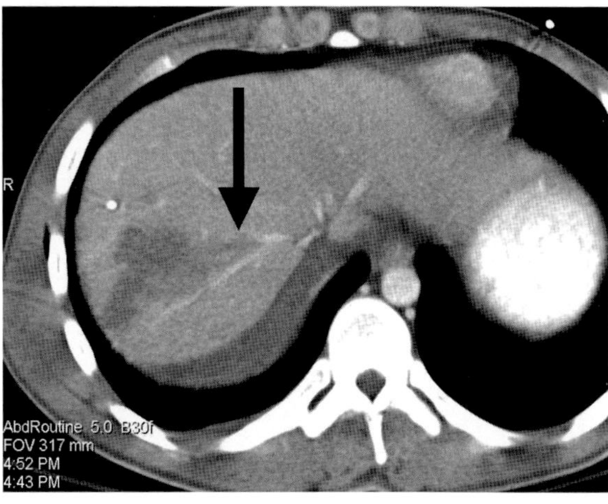

Fig. 11. Hepatic laceration extends along right hepatic vein and its branches (*arrow*)

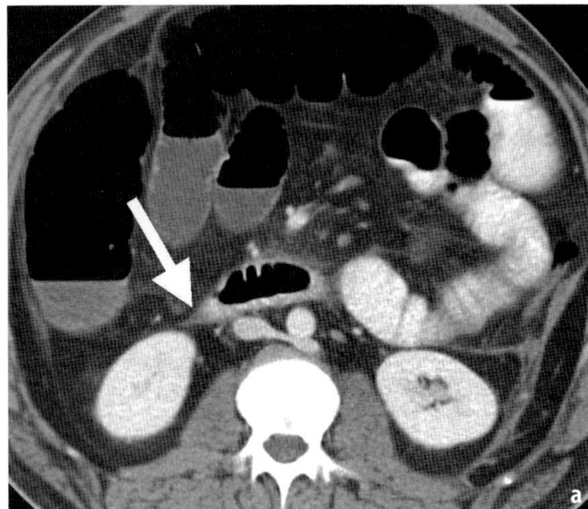

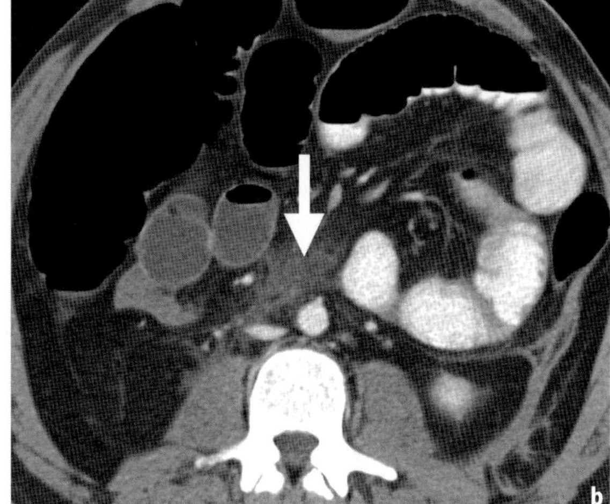

Fig. 12a, b. Periduodenal hematoma (*arrow*) with triangular shape (**a**). Retroperitoneal hematoma (*arrow*) (**b**)

bleeding. Always look for fluid density between the pancreas and the splenic vein (Fig. 13) Normally, only fat is found between the pancreas and the splenic vein. If fluid is visible, then either traumatic pancreatitis or actual bleeding on the posterior pancreatic surface is present. More obvious pancreatic injuries will be detected as a linear laceration extending through the tissue of the pancreas. Pancreatic injuries often occur slightly to the right or left of midline in locations where the pancreas is sheered against the side of the vertebral body. Therefore, lacerations typically occur either at the junction of the head and body of the pancreas to the right of the spine or within the body just to the left of midline (Fig. 14). The severity of a pancreatic injury is predominantly dependent upon the status of the main pancreatic duct. Bruises to the pancreas can often be treated conservatively. However,

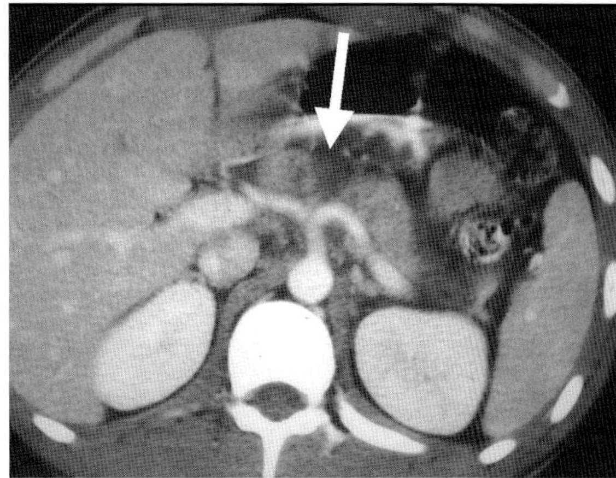

Fig. 13. Motor vehicle accident victim with pancreatic laceration (*white arrow*) through body of pancreas. This is a typical location for a deceleration injury due to shearing of the pancreas along side the vertebral body

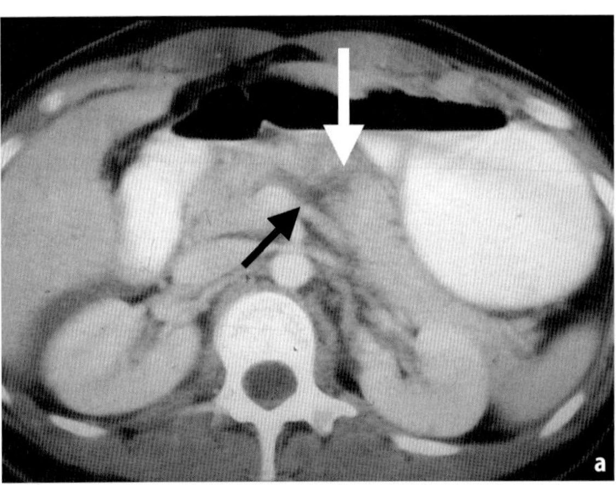
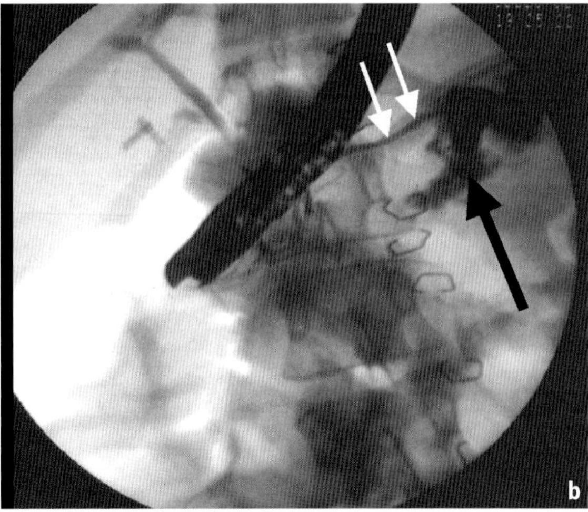

Fig. 14a, b. Motor vehicle accident victim with shearing injury of pancreatic body. **a** Laceration of posterior aspect of pancreas (*white arrow*) with blood separating pancreas from splenic vein (*black arrow*). **b** Endoscopic retrograde cholangiopancreatography (ERCP) demonstrates large area of extravasation (*black arrow*) from pancreatic duct (*white arrows*)

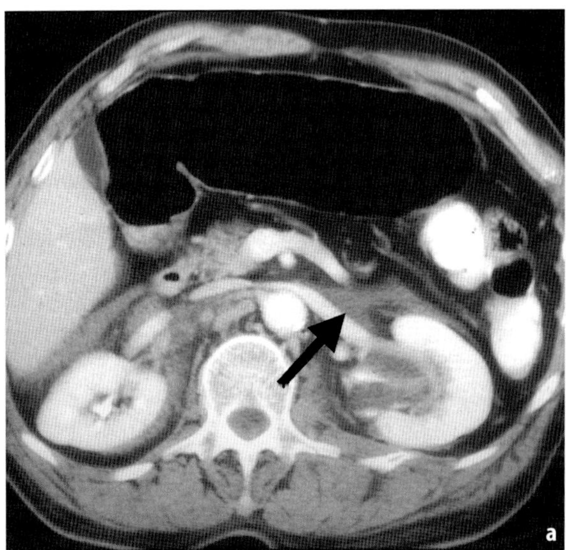
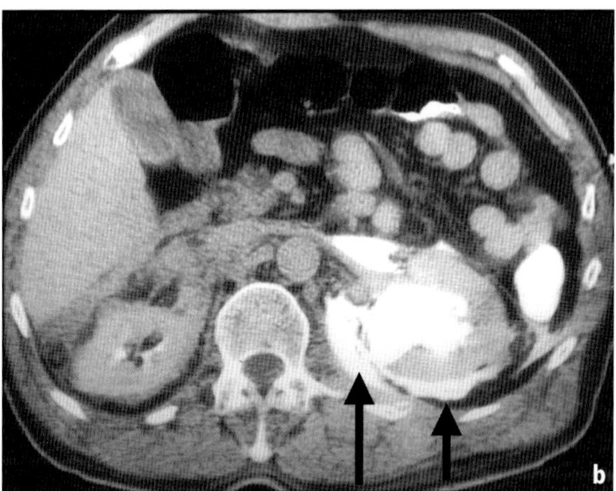

Fig. 15a, b. Left renal injury: patient status post motor vehicle accident. **a** Initial computed tomography (CT) study demonstrated fluid anterior to left kidney (*arrow*) and unusual fullness of renal pelvis. **b** Five-minute delayed image demonstrates urinoma (*arrows*). Fluid adjacent to the kidney and in the renal pelvis is extravasated urine, not blood

a laceration or transection of the main pancreatic duct usually requires a surgical repair.

Patients with duodenal or pancreatic injury should be monitored carefully for significant pancreatic injuries. Even if a patient has only mild swelling of the pancreas or inhomogeneity in blunt trauma, a follow-up CT is often warranted. Serum amylase may be used to detect change in amylase level suggesting traumatic pancreatitis, although the initial amylase obtained in the Emergency Room may be misleading. For instance, patients who have been subjected to head and neck injury may have an elevated amylase because of salivary gland injury. And the initial amylase in a pancreatic trauma patient may be normal while it may rise later.

In patients with questionable pancreatic in-juries, especially with an elevating amylase on serial lab tests, a magnetic resonance cholangiopancreatography (MRCP) or occasionally an endoscopic retrograde cholangiopancreatography (ERCP) may be useful to better assess continuity of the main pancreatic duct (Fig. 14).

Kidneys

With renal trauma, CT findings include laceration, fracture, and perirenal blood or urine. Kidney analysis in the trauma patient is different from that of the liver or spleen. While perihepatic or perisplenic fluid is usually due to blood, perinephric fluid may represent either urine or blood. Therefore, when renal trauma is suspected, it is essential to obtain delayed CT images (Fig. 15) Generally, such delayed images should be obtained after a sufficient length of time for contrast to have been excreted into the renal collecting system, allowing for the detection of urinomas. Typically, a 3-min delay is adequate. Our routine includes initial evaluation of the abdominal CT prior to removing the patient from the CT table. If the patient demonstrates any abnormality in the kidney region, delayed imaging is obtained. If the patient is known to have hematuria prior to CT, then delayed images are protocoled in prior to initiation of the CT examination.

Retroperitoneal Structures

While adrenal injuries are often associated with renal injuries, solitary adrenal hematomas can occur without detectable renal injury. Adrenal injuries usually manifest as simple adrenal masses.

It is important to image the inferior vena cava in the detection of shock. Shock is identified on CT as a flat or slit-like inferior vena cava on at least three slices in the infrahepatic inferior vena cava. We typically look at the inferior vena cava at the level of the left renal vein (Fig. 16). Please note that a flat or slit-like inferior vena cava seen on one or two sections only may be simply due to a rapid inspiration of the patient, sucking blood out of the abdomen into the thorax if the patient gasps during CT examination. Therefore, one should see a narrowed inferior vena cava on three slices to increase specificity of this finding.

We recently reviewed our experience of shocked or hypotensive patients studied with CT in our Emergency Department and identified that a small spleen is an additional finding of hypotension (Fig. 17). In a series of patients who were hypotensive either in the ambulance during transportation to or on arrival in the Emergency Room, we found that mean spleen volume in hypotensive patients was 142 cc. Following fluid resuscitation, the spleen in the same patients was noted to increase to a mean volume of 227 cc.

Hollow Viscus Injury

Identification of bowel injury in a blunt trauma patient is difficult. Bowel injury is often not detectable on clinical examination and can easily be overlooked on a CT study. Findings suggestive of bowel injury include free intraperitoneal air, free intraperitoneal fluid, and wall thickening of the bowel. Unfortunately, extraluminal gas has been reported to be detectable on CT, with a range of 46–63% [13–15]. When a loop of bowel that is fluid filled and does not contain air is ruptured, there will be no initial release of gas into the peritoneum. Therefore, a CT obtained soon after a bowel injury will often fail to detect extraluminal gas. Extraluminal contrast has been reported as a helpful finding in abdominal trauma CT. However, in one study, extraluminal contrast was detected in only 19% of cases [16]. In our experience, extraluminal contrast is infrequently identified. As CT scans are obtained more rapidly following abdominal trauma, the incidence of detectable extraluminal contrast has declined. Patients are scanned so quickly after arrival in the Emergency Room that administered contrast, either given orally or via nasogastric tube, often has not had time to reach the site of bowel injury. Reports from the radiology literature suggest an overall sensitivity for bowel injury ranging between 88% and 93% [16]. However, in the nonradiology literature there have been reports of significantly lower accuracy rates. In a 1998 study from a large trauma center in Texas involving 19,621 patients, CT missed hollow viscus injuries in 43% of children and 21% of adults [17].

Bowel injury has been studied in an experimental model by a group of English surgeons [18].

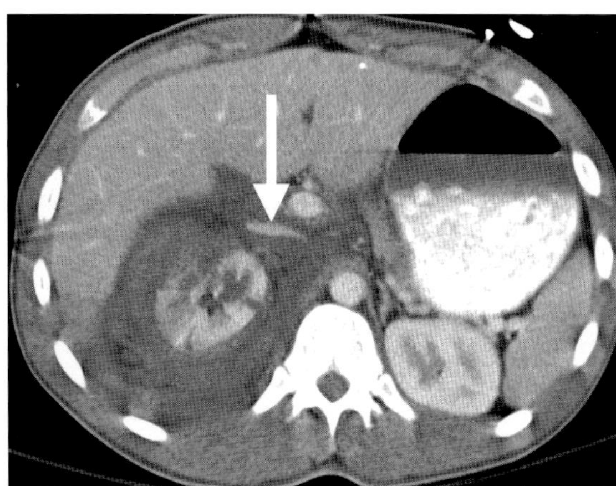

Fig. 16. Motor vehicle accident victim with hepatic and renal injuries and hypotension demonstrating slit-like inferior vena cava (*arrow*)

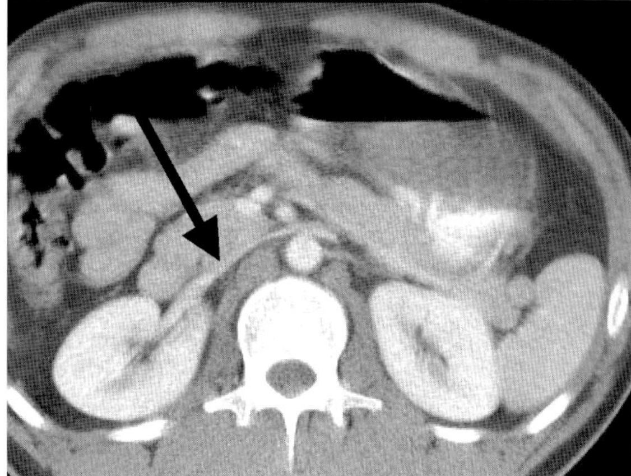

Fig. 17. Motor vehicle accident victim with bleeding into thigh from femoral fracture demonstrates slit-like inferior vena cava (*black arrow*) and small spleen due to hypotension

Their model used the pig and studied deceleration injuries. Their experiment consisted of anesthetized pigs thrown by a mechanical device into a solid object. They found that bowel injury occurred in 100% of the pigs when the speed at impact was 100 mph (161 kph) or greater. In a similar fashion to that of humans, they found that small-bowel injuries were twice as frequent as colonic injuries. Small-bowel injuries consisted of perforation or mesenteric avulsions while colonic injuries were usually serosal tears. The authors hypothesized that the increased frequency of small-bowel injuries was due to the fact that the small bowel is mobile and the colon is relatively fixed in the retroperitoneum.

Detection of intraperitoneal fluid is critical in the identification of bowel injury [19]. However, peritoneal fluid seen in the trauma patient can be either from traumatic or nontraumatic origin. Traumatic causes of intraperitoneal fluid include blood from a solid organ injury, blood from a bowel injury, bowel contents, and blood from a mesenteric injury but also can be due to bile from a ruptured gallbladder or biliary tree or urine from a ruptured bladder. Peritoneal fluid seen in the trauma patient can also arise from a combination of more than one injury. There are also nontraumatic causes of intraperitoneal fluid, which can be quite problematic. The most difficult cause is encountered in women of childbearing age who have a small amount of what is termed "physiologic fluid in the pelvis." In an ongoing study at our institution, we reviewed 175 CTs of women of childbearing age who were referred for evaluation of blunt trauma. Of those patients who had no evidence of injury on CT and required no operative management of abdominal injury, approximately 50% were identified to have at least a small amount of intraperitoneal fluid. In order to better characterize this fluid, density, volume, and location were analyzed. Using CT reconstruction at a 5-mm interval, of the 175 patients, only one had fluid seen on more than three slices in the pelvis with no evidence of injury. Therefore, identification of a "trace" amount of fluid seen on less than three slices seems likely to be an adequate predictor of a nontraumatic, physiologic fluid collection.

Fluid location is also extremely helpful in identifying the site of bleeding. As discussed above, the concept of a sentinal clot is quite useful. Since blood clots adjacent to the site of bleeding, when a higher density blood collection is encountered with a density that approaches that of adjacent muscles, the site of bleeding is likely to be adjacent to this clotted blood. More serous blood is seen further away from the bleeding site.

With solid-organ injuries initial bleeding occurs adjacent to the injured organ then extends down the pericolic gutters and into the pelvis. Only after readily accessible potential spaces are filled, fluid will extend between the leaves of the mesentery. With a large amount of intraperitoneal blood from a solid organ injury "interloop" fluid will be detected. However, if bleeding occurs due to a bowel injury, the initial bleeding initially occurs into the interloop space. Therefore, if a patient has blood caught between the leaves of the mesentery and does not have blood in the pericolic gutters or pelvis, then bleeding is likely to be from a bowel injury.

Mesenteric or interloop fluid can be differentiated from the bowel by its shape [20], often manifesting as V- or triangular-shaped fluid collections between the leaves of the mesentery that are easily discerned from the more rounded shape of fluid within bowel loops (Fig. 18). The etiology of the V or triangular shape is simply that the mesentery leaves converge at the root of the mesentery, and any fluid caught between the leaves tends to have a point or apex of a triangle that points toward the mesentery root (Figs. 18 and 19).

Another sign of possible bowel injury on abdominal and pelvic MDCT is a group of "matted-together" bowel loops (Fig. 20). This matted-together appearance is due to blood extending between loops of unopacified bowel. This is a relatively nonspecific appearance and can occasionally be seen in normal unopacified bowel but should be considered a warning sign for possible bowel injury.

Bowel-wall thickening is an important finding in bowel injury. Since most small- and large-bowel loops are not opacified with contrast on a CT obtained in a trauma patient, one must be able to identify bowel-wall thickening without contrast. One useful trick is to remember that bowel-wall thickening is almost always circumferential in a trauma patient. Therefore, look at the anterior portion of a

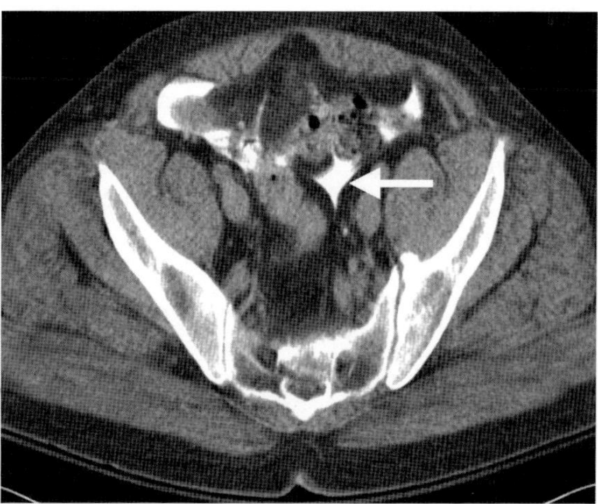

Fig. 18. Motor vehicle accident victim with extravasated urine from a bladder rupture: iodinated contrast caught between leaves of mesentery produces "V" shape (*arrow*) in upper pelvis

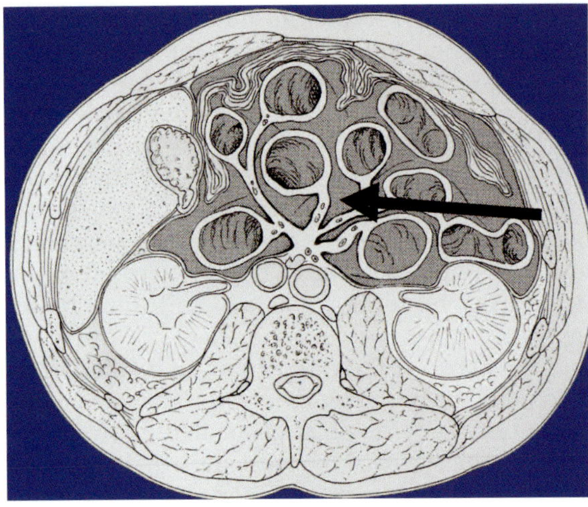

Fig. 19. Fluid caught between the leaves of the mesentery on this diagram demonstrates triangular shape (*arrow*)

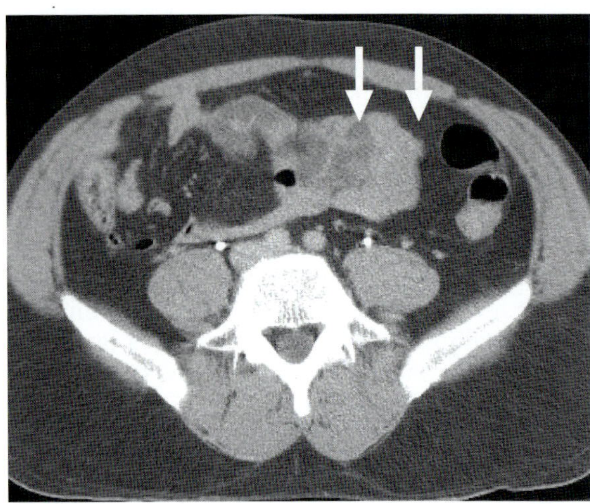

Fig. 20. Motor vehicle accident victim with bowel injury demonstrating "matted-together loop" appearance (*arrows*)

bowel loop. While bowel contents may make the bowel wall look thickened posteriorly, often, there is enough air or fluid in the lumen to identify whether or not there is anterior-wall thickening due to circumferential injury. An additional trick is to call bowel-wall thickening only when it is seen in the same bowel loop on two contiguous slices.

Identification of bowel injury is important. In our experience at San Francisco General Hospital, 46 patients with bowel injury had a delay in diagnosis resulting in more than 6 h from the time of injury to operative intervention [13]. There was a mortality rate of 4.3%, which corresponds to reports of mortality from bowel injury in the literature, which is up to 5.9%. One of the two deaths that occurred in our series was due to delayed diagnosis of a single jejunal perforation. Delay in diagnosis often occurred when the radiologist had identified an abnormality on the CT but the significance of the CT findings was not appreciated. For instance, a radiology report described colonic wall thickening with pericolonic soft tissue stranding, but the impression failed to mention "possible" or "probably colonic injury." In trauma patients with multiple problems, it is quite useful to be specific in reporting possible bowel injury. While the findings on CT may be subtle, the consequence of a delay in diagnosis can be severe.

Conclusion

Since almost any portion of the abdomen and pelvis can be injured in a trauma patient, it is quite useful to use a routine interpretation technique that ensures that the radiologist reviews all appropriate structures.

References

1. Novelline RA, Rhea JT, Rao PM, Stuk JL (1999) State-of-the-art. Helical CT in emergency radiology. Radiology 213(2):321–339
2. Halvorsen RA Jr, McCormick VD, Evans SJ (1994) Computed tomography of abdominal trauma; a step by step approach. Emerg Radiol 1:283–291
3. Gavant ML, Schurr M, Flick PA et al (1997) Predicting clinical outcome of nonsurgical management of blunt splenic injury: using CT to reveal abnormalities of splenic vasculature. AJR Am J Roentgenol 168(1):207–212
4. Orwig D, Federle MP (1989) Localized clotted blood as evidence of visceral trauma on CT: the sentinel clot sign. AJR Am J Roentgenol 153(4):747–749
5. Sivit CJ, Peclet MH, Taylor GA (1989) Life-threatening intraperitoneal bleeding: demonstration with CT. Radiology 171:430
6. Jeffrey RB Jr, Cardoza JD, Olcott EW (1991) Detection of active intraabdominal hemorrhage: value of dynamic contrast-enhanced CT. AJR Am J Roentgenol 156:725–729
7. Federle MP, Courcoulas AP, Powell M et al (1998) Blunt splenic injury in adults: clinical and CT criteria for management, with emphasis on active extravasation. Radiology 206:137–142
8. Mirvis SE, Whitley NO, Gens DR (1989) Blunt splenic trauma in adults: CT-based classification and correlation with prognosis and treatment. Radiology 171:33–39
9. Umlas SL, Cronan JJ (1991) Splenic trauma: can CT grading systems enable prediction of successful nonsurgical treatment? Radiology 178:481–487
10. Kohn JS, Clark DE, Isler RJ et al (1994) Is computed tomographic grading of splenic injury useful in the nonsurgical management of blunt trauma? J Trauma Mar 36(3):385–389; discussion 390
11. Becker CD, Spring P, Glattli A, Schweizer W (1994) Blunt splenic trauma in adults: can CT findings be used to determine the need for surgery? AJR Am J Roentgenol 162:343–347

12. Federle MP (2004) Splenic trauma. In: Federle, Jeffrey, Desser, Anne, Eraso (eds) Diagnostic Imaging: Abdomen. Amirsys, Salt Lake City, pp I:6:20–21

13. Harris HW, Morabito DJ, Mackersie RC et al (1999) Leukocytosis and free fluid are important indicators of isolated intestinal injury after blunt trauma. J Trauma 46:656–659

14. Mirvis SE, Gens DR, Shanmuganathan K (1992) Rupture of the bowel after blunt abdominal trauma: diagnosis with CT. AJR Am J Roentgenol 159:1217–1221

15. Sherck J, Shatney C (1996) Significance of intraabdominal extraluminal air detected by CT scan in blunt abdominal trauma. J Trauma 40:674–675

16. West OC (2000) Intraperitoneal abdominal injuries. In: West OC, Novelline RA, Wilson AJ (eds) Emergency and trauma radiology. American Roentgen Ray Society, Washington, pp 87–98

17. Allen GS, Moore FA, Cox CSJ et al (1998) Hollow viscus injury and blunt trauma. J Trauma 45:69–77

18. Cripps N, Cooper G (1997) Intestinal injury mechanisms after blunt abdominal impact. Ann R Coll Surg Engl 79:115–120

19. Dowe MF, Shanmuganathan K, Mirvis SE et al (1997) CT findings of mesenteric injury after blunt trauma: implications for surgical intervention. AJR Am J Roentgenol 168:425–428

20. Halvorsen RA Jr, McKenney K (2002) Blunt trauma to the gastrointestinal tract: CT findings with small bowel and colonic injuries. Emerg Radiol 9(3): 141–145

25

Role of MDCT in the Evaluation of Musculoskeletal Trauma

Sunit Sebastian, Hamid Salamipour

Introduction

Technical advances in the past decade have made computed tomography (CT) increasingly valuable in the early clinical management of patients with polytrauma. The development of multidetector CT (MDCT) has transformed CT from a simple, cross-sectional imaging technique to an advanced, three-dimensional (3-D) imaging modality, enabling excellent 3-D displays [1]. Multislice CT scanning is associated with a substantial gain in performance, decreased scan times, reduced section collimation, and reduction in scan length. The combined value of MDCT and 3-D reformations in assessment of the musculoskeletal system has been documented in the literature. The high contrast interface between bone and adjacent tissues in the musculoskeletal system makes it ideal for 3-D evaluation. The increased acquisition speed of MDCT with superior image resolution enables rapid diagnostic work up and institution of therapy in the setting of musculoskeletal trauma. This chapter will discuss the various techniques and applications of MDCT in orthopedic trauma. The use of 3-D reformations in the evaluation of musculoskeletal trauma will also be emphasized. The use of minimally invasive techniques such as CT angiography in the work up of a patient with skeletal trauma in appropriate indications will also be highlighted.

MDCT: Technical Considerations

MDCT significantly increases body coverage and thus reduces scanning time in most instances. Innovative detector arrays allow the acquisition of 0.5-mm-thick slices, with isotropic voxels [2]. This enables multiplanar reconstruction (MPR) images to be created in any plane with the same spatial resolution as the original sections without degradation of image quality.

MDCT in the Setting of Musculoskeletal Trauma

Extensive anatomic coverage is necessary in the evaluation of a patient with musculoskeletal trauma. MDCT is capable of acquiring multiple data sets simultaneously in each slice, leading to larger areas of scan coverage without correspondingly increasing the pitch and slice thickness [3]. This leads to longer scan ranges, near-isotropic imaging, better multiplanar reformatting, and 3-D rendering. Reduced scan times and motion artifacts are valuable in the evaluation of musculoskeletal trauma, especially in pediatric patients. MDCT can decrease artifacts related to metallic implant devices. Recently, automatic tube current modulation has been used to allow scanning of the musculoskeletal system with significantly less radiation [4].

MDCT Scanning Protocols

Technological advances in MDCT have led to the newer strategies to evaluate patients with orthopedic trauma. Radiation dose reduction is a significant issue that must be addressed in the evaluation of trauma patients in an emergent setting. Tables 1 and 2 present scanning protocols for facial and cervical trauma and extremity trauma, respectively, for a 16-slice MDCT scanner.

Table 1. Scanning protocol for facial and cervical trauma with AutomA technique on a 16-slice MDCT scanner (GE Healthcare)

Noise index	15–20
Tube current range:	
• Face	10–180 mA
• Cervical spine	10–270 mA
Gantry rotation time	0.5 s
Voltage	120 kVp
Beam pitch	0.938:1
Table speed	18.75 mm/rotation
Detector configuration	16×1.25 mm
Reconstructed slice thickness:	
• Face	1.25 mm
• Cervical spine	2.5 mm

Table 2. Scanning protocol for extremity trauma with AutomA technique on a 16-slice MDCT scanner (GE Healthcare)

Noise index	15–20
Tube current range	75–440
Gantry rotation time	0.5 s
Voltage	120 kVp
Beam pitch	0.938:1
Table speed	18.75 mm/rotation
Detector configuration	16×1.25 mm
Reconstructed slice thickness	1.25-2.5 mm (soft tissue & bone algorithm)

Indications for MDCT in Musculoskeletal Trauma

MDCT can be used to evaluate fractures of the spine, pelvis, and extremities. It has almost replaced plane radiography in the evaluation of skeletal trauma and is the standard of care in modern-day radiology practices. MDCT can also be used for the evaluation of soft tissue, tendons, and articular cartilage in conjunction with arthrography. Additional indications include postoperative evaluation of metallic implants. Complex intra-articular fractures of the extremities can also be evaluated thoroughly. Multiplanar reformatted images provide additional information regarding complex musculoskeletal injuries. Three-dimensional or volume-rendered images can play a crucial role in the further management of the patient.

Spinal Trauma

Traumatic injuries to the spine can cause permanent damage and are associated with high morbidity and mortality [5]. Spinal cord injuries are more common in males (75–85%), with the majority of the patients being younger than 30 years of age. The faster speed of acquisition and superior image resolution without significant patient manipulation has made MDCT the imaging method of choice for evaluation of a patients with of musculoskeletal trauma. Cervical spine injuries are associated with higher morbidity and mortality. Subtle fractures of the cervical spine may be difficult to diagnose on axial images alone. MPR images generated immediately after the scan in the sagittal and coronal planes can depict these fractures more precisely (Fig. 1). This serves as a roadmap for the surgeon and can prove to be a valuable guide for management of the patient.

The major mechanisms of spinal injury include hyperflexion, hyperextension, rotation, and vertical compression. Anterior wedge fractures of the thoracolumbar spine can be caused by flexion or compression injuries. These fractures can also cause posterior ligament injury with dislocation of facet joints.

The "seat belt" type injury is the most common type of injury associated with flexion distraction forces. Three patterns of seat belt injury described include:
- Type 1, or chance fracture: caused by disruption of posterior bony elements
- Type 2, or Smith fracture: caused by rupture of posterior ligaments
- Type 3: tear in annulus fibrosus causes subluxation injury

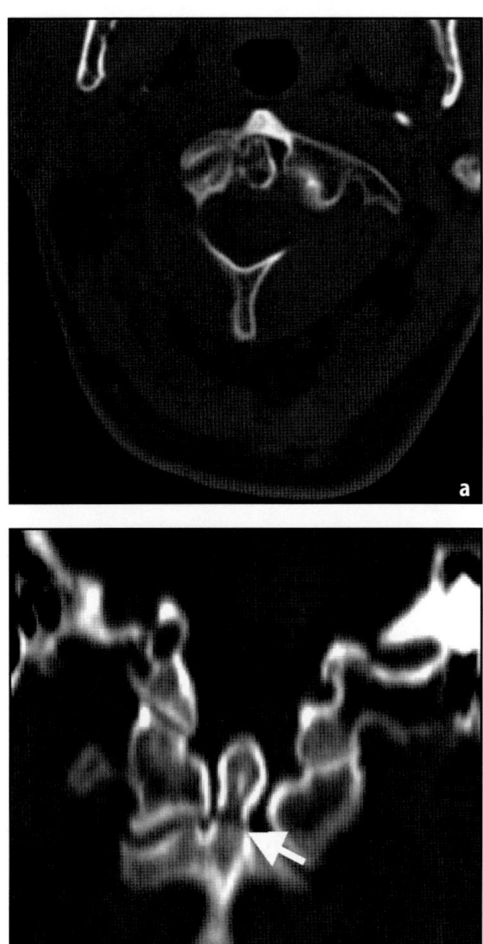

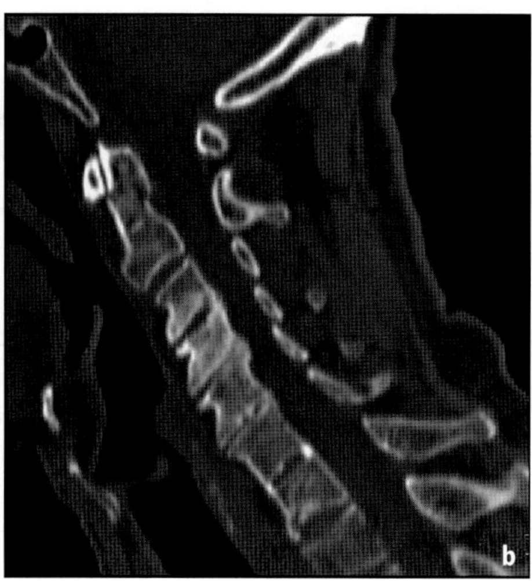

Fig. 1a–c. A 67-year-old man with history of motor vehicle crash. Axial CT scan shows subtle lucency at the base of the dens (**a**). Axial CT scan does not reveal the extent of the injury, which is perpendicular to the imaging plane. **b** Sagittal reformatted CT scan shows lucency through the dens just above the body of C2. **c** Coronal reformatted CT scan shows type II dens fracture in greater detail

The second cervical vertebra is the most common level of injury, involving the odontoid in 30% of the cases. The vertebral body is the most frequent site of fracture [6]. Spinal stability is crucial in determining the nature of injury and deciding the course of treatment. The most important determinant of spinal stability is the integrity of the middle column [7]. Instability of the spine is associated with inability to maintain normal alignment under normal physiological forces. The early detection of neurological injury associated with spinal instability is vital in preventing long-term disability.

Whiplash injuries result from a collision that includes sudden acceleration or deceleration. The person is often involved in a rear-end automobile collision or injured as a result of contact sports. The head swings backward, followed by a forward flexion, causing injuries to the cervical spine due to the relative weakness of the anterior longitudinal ligament. Tears or thrombotic obstruction of the vertebral artery and traumatic dissection of the extracranial part of the internal carotid arteries may occur even after moderate injury [8] .Whiplash injuries can cause significant morbidity

and impairment. A detailed history of the mechanism of trauma and thorough clinical examination can help make a diagnosis of whiplash injury. MD-CT is useful to determine subtle fractures and facet lesions, which can be missed on plain radiography. MDCT is more sensitive than MRI in the detection of fractures of the posterior elements of the spine and to injuries of the craniocervical junction [9].

Screening helical CT has a sensitivity of 98.3%, a specificity of 100%, and an accuracy of 99.9% in the detection of clinically important fractures of the cervical spine [10]. Intravenous contrast should be administered to evaluate soft tissue and vascular structures in the region of trauma. Volume-rendered images can help detect subtle or hidden fractures that may have been missed on routine axial images. The 3-D images provide exact orientation of the fracture fragments and possible compression of the spinal cord by the displaced fracture fragments. This information is invaluable in planning treatment of the patient. MD-CT allows improved imaging of orthopedic hardware by minimizing streak artifacts that traditionally plague CT in this setting.

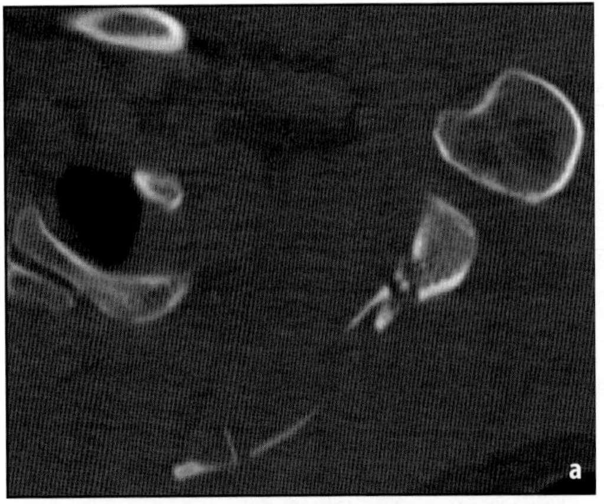
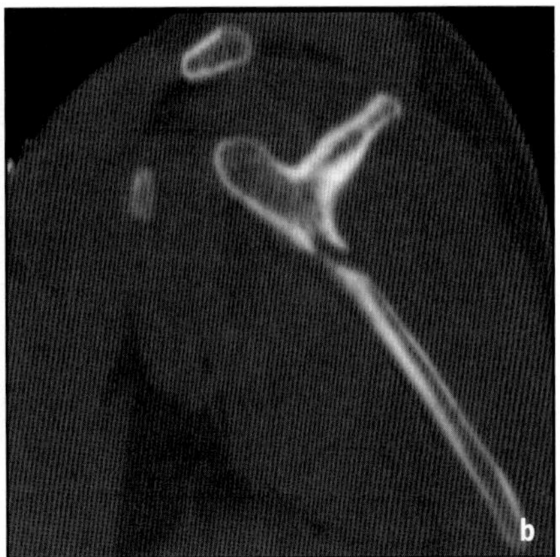
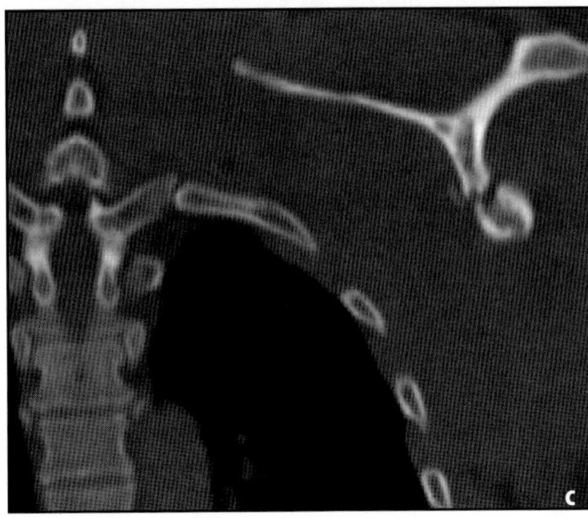

Fig. 2a-c. A 40-year-old man involved in a motor vehicle accident. Axial images show comminuted fracture of the body of the scapula (**a**). Sagittal (**b**) and coronal (**c**) reformatted images show the relationship of the fracture fragments to better advantage. There is minimal displacement of the fracture fragments

Upper Extremity Trauma

Sternoclavicular Joint

Blunt chest trauma, such as can occur in motor vehicle accidents, is usually associated with injuries to the sternoclavicular joint. Fractures of the ribs or shoulder joint are commonly associated with sternoclavicular joint trauma. Injury to the thoracic aorta and mediastinal vessels can occur with posterior displacement of the fracture fragments. CT angiography (CTA) must be performed if vascular injury is suspected. Complete obstruction of the brachiocephalic vein and impingement of the aorta can present with no clinical evidence of complication. A high index of suspicion is needed to prevent serious complications, which may appear insidiously in these injuries [11].

Shoulder Joint

MDCT has high sensitivity in the detection and evaluation of fractures of the shoulder with complex anatomical relationships. Scapular fractures can be difficult to detect on plain radiographs, but MDCT can demonstrate scapular fractures with a high degree of accuracy (Fig. 2). Fractures of the lesser tubercle and coracoid process are difficult to diagnose on plain radiographs and can present as occult fractures. MDCT in conjunction with MPR is proven to be useful in the evaluation of complex proximal humerus fractures where the extent of the fractures and alignment of fracture fragments is not adequately depicted on radiography [12] Additional information regarding injury to the lung, chest wall, clavicle, and axillary artery can also be attained. The number and relative rotation of fracture fragments can be accurately determined, especially with the use of 3-D reformatted images, thus proving valuable information when planning open reduction and internal fixation [13].

Elbow Joint

Acute elbow trauma is common in both adult and pediatric age groups. Plain radiographs can be equivocal, especially in children, and inadequate characterization may warrant the use of MDCT, with fractures being the most common finding.

Volume-rendered images can provide detailed information regarding the alignment of fracture fragments. Automatic tube-current modulation has been demonstrated to effectively minimize radiation from the MDCT examination of the elbow in pediatric patients [14].

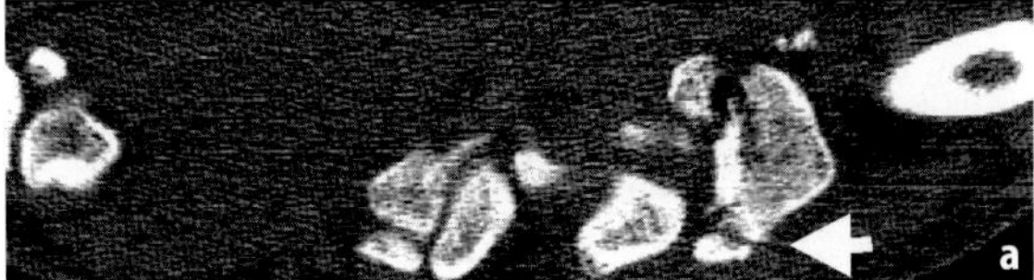

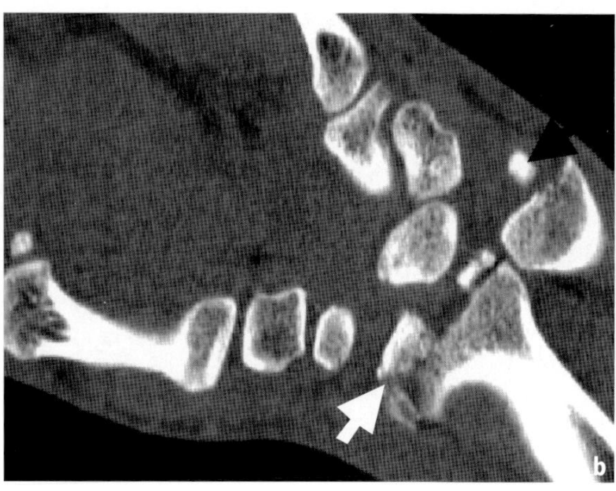

Fig. 3a, b. A 38-year-old man with history of fall on outstretched hand. Axial image shows comminuted fracture of the distal radius (**a**). Coronal reformatted images better demonstrate comminuted fractures of the distal radius involving the articular surface and fracture of the ulnar styloid process (*black arrowhead*) (**b**)

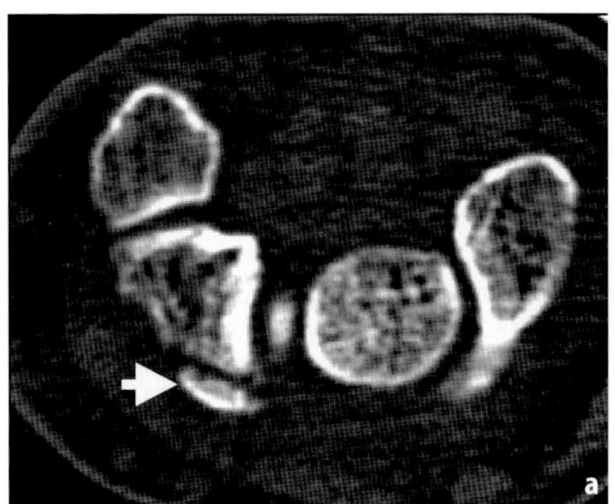

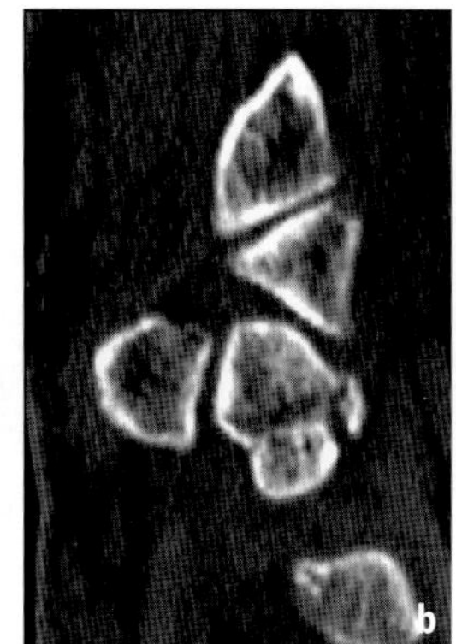

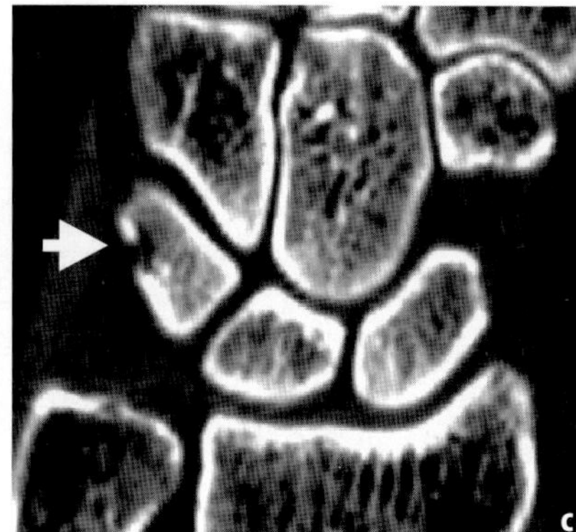

Fig. 4a-c. A 51-year-old man with history of industrial accident to the wrist joint. Triquetral avulsion fracture (*arrow*) on axial image (**a**) is better demonstrated on sagittal (**b**) and coronal (**c**) reformatted images

Wrist Joint

MDCT examinations are not dependent on the wrist position in the CT gantry due to its ability to generate 3-D reformatted images. Distal radio-ulnar joint injuries can occur independently or in unison with distal radius fractures and Galeazzi fractures. Diagnosis of stable, partially unstable (subluxation), and unstable (dislocation) patterns of injury can be based on MDCT evaluation. The early diagnosis and suitable treatment of an acute distal radioulnar joint injury is crucial to prevent development of a chronic disorder [15]. Complex fractures involving the distal radius and ulna can be accurately assessed with multiplanar reformats using MDCT (Fig. 3). Also, 3-D CT imaging is useful in evaluating extensor tendons proximal to the metacarpophalangeal joint. This method increases the accuracy of diagnosis and is useful in surgical planning and patient education [16]. Volume-rendered CT can be performed with cast material without significantly decreasing image quality. MDCT provides quick and accurate information in assessing complex wrist fractures [17]. Arthrography is superior to diagnose scapholunate ligament tears and ulnolunate and ulnotriquetral ligament defects [18]. Carpal bone avulsion injuries can be clearly assessed in the sagittal and coronal planes (Fig. 4).

Pelvis

Plain radiography has low sensitivity in determining if the pelvic injury is stable or not. Tile classification describes pelvic injuries as stable, rotationally unstable, or rotationally and vertically unstable [19]. MDCT with MPRs and 3-D reformats has greater sensitivity in detection of complex pelvic and acetabular traumatic injuries and is preferred as the imaging of choice in severe trauma in the emergency department [20]. Comminuted acetabular fractures can be better visualized on the multiplanar reformat images (Fig. 5). A vascular map of the abdominal aorta, iliac, and femoral vessels can be obtained after contrast administration, especially in the setting of penetrating trauma.

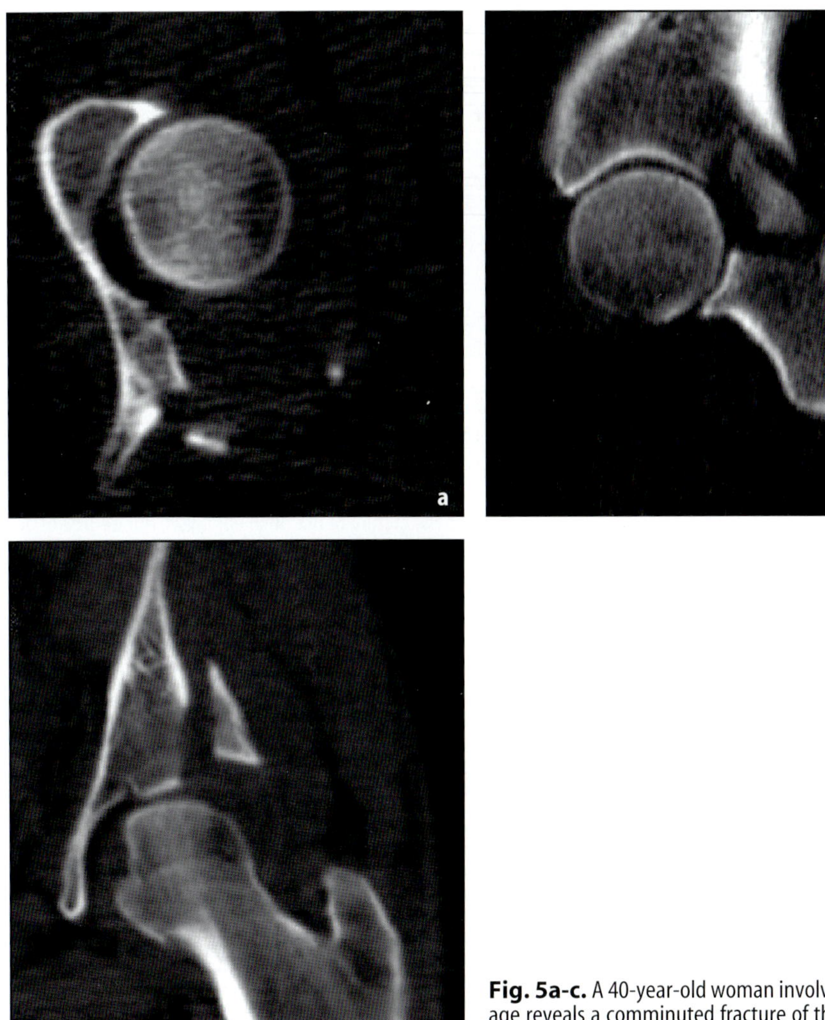

Fig. 5a-c. A 40-year-old woman involved in a motor vehicle accident. Axial image reveals a comminuted fracture of the posterior acetabulum (**a**). Sagittal (**b**) and coronal (**c**) images depict the fracture without dislocation of the hip joint

Lower Extremity Trauma

Knee Joint
Subtle fractures can be missed on plain radiography. Intra-articular extension of the fracture line can be depicted clearly using sagittal and coronal reformats (Fig. 6). This is critical in determining appropriate therapy. CT arthrography and virtual arthroscopy have shown good diagnostic accuracy in detecting anterior cruciate ligament and meniscal abnormalities [21]. Patellofemoral joint evaluation after arthroscopic stabilization can be assessed in various degrees of knee flexion [22].

Ankle Joint
On axial CT images alone, it can be difficult to interpret the complex anatomy of the ankle and foot. Comminuted fractures of the distal tibia and fibula can be accurately assessed using MDCT (Fig. 7). Articular facets of the subtalar joints may not be seen clearly depicted on routine axial scans. MPR images can significantly improve visualization of the subtalar joint anatomy. Talar and calcaneal injuries can also be easily assessed (Fig. 8). Volume rendering is useful for determining anatomic relationships between ankle tendons and underlying bones. Surface shaded display is valuable when fractures extend to the articular cortex and a disarticulated view is needed [23].

Summary

MDCT enables rapid and thorough evaluation of the musculoskeletal system. It has transformed an axial imaging modality to a multiplanar one in which reformations and 3-D reconstructions can be obtained routinely and at will [24]. Evolving techniques such as automatic exposure control have led to lower radiation doses in MDCT evalua-

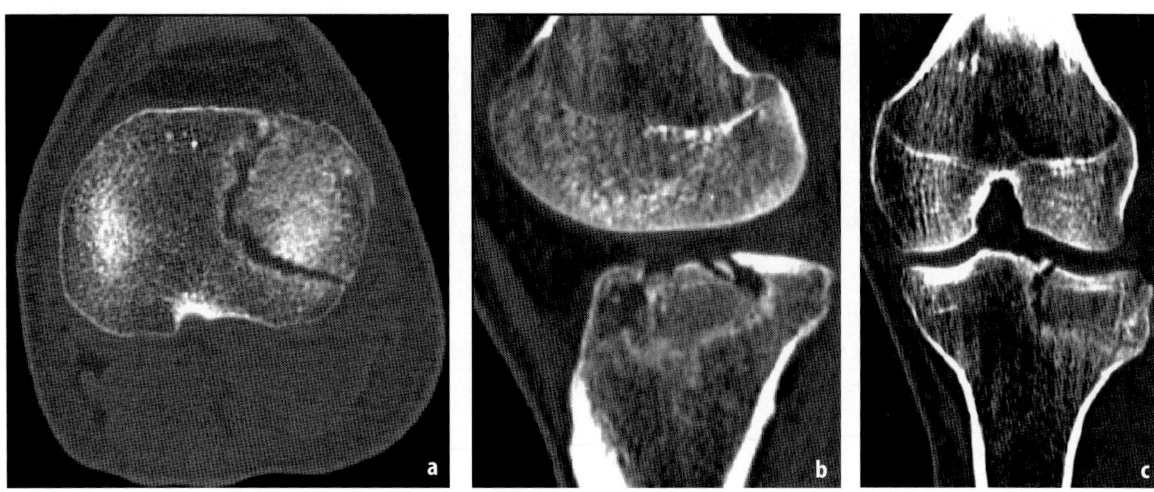

Fig. 6a-c. A 39-year-old man with history of fall from a motorcycle. Axial image shows fracture of the tibial epiphysis, but degree of depression is difficult to assess (**a**). Sagittal (**b**) and coronal (**c**) images reveal fracture involving the tibial plateau with extension to the articular surface of the knee joint. Degree of depression can be accurately determined

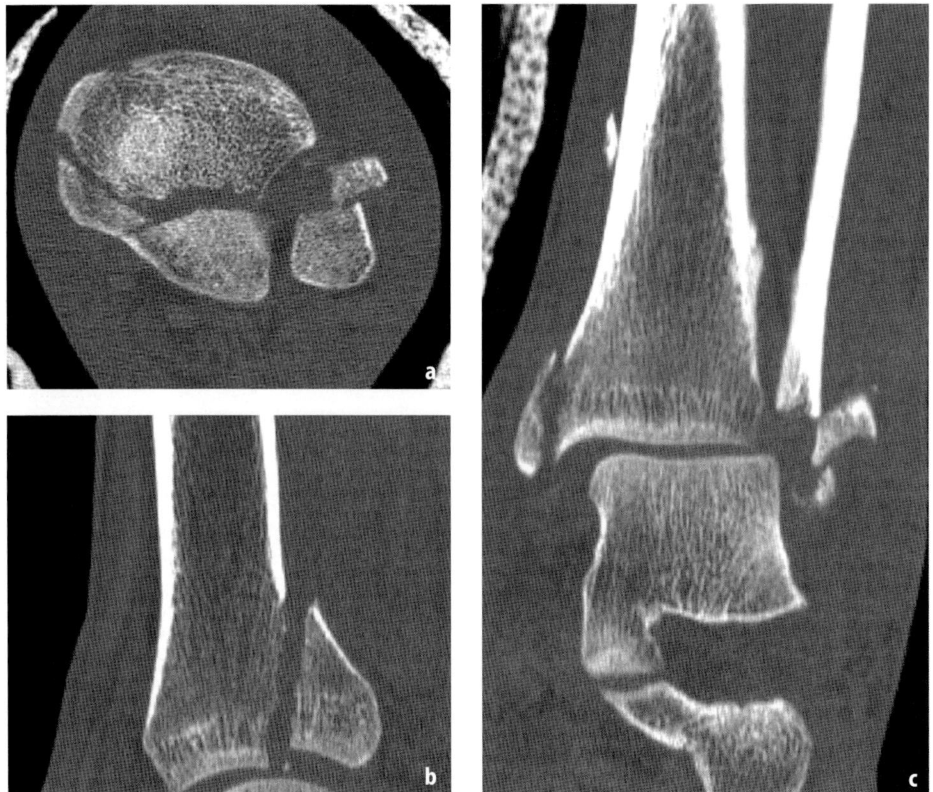

Fig. 7a-c. A 31-year-old man with fracture due to a motor vehicle accident. Fracture involves the distal tibia, as well as the fibula. Alignment is difficult to assess (**a**). Sagittal reformats demonstrate pilon fracture with displacement (**b**). Coronal reconstructions show complexity of fracture, with involvement of distal fibula (**c**)

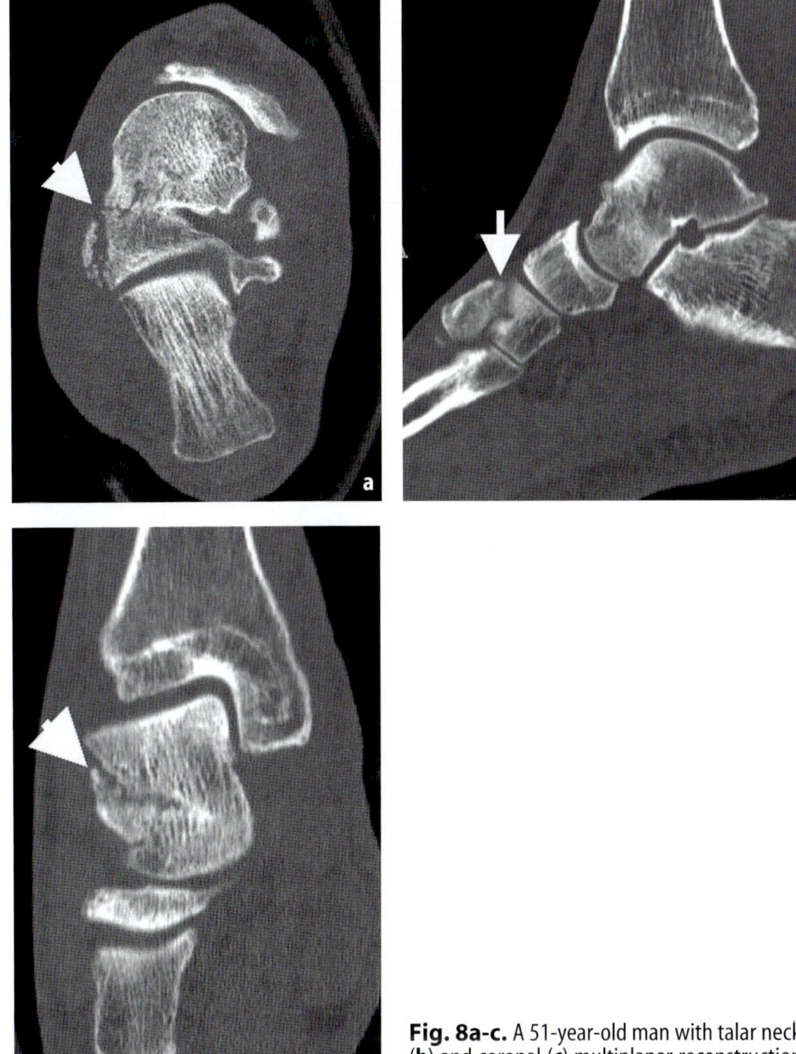

Fig. 8a-c. A 51-year-old man with talar neck fracture due to fall from height (**a**). Sagittal (**b**) and coronal (**c**) multiplanar reconstructions from MDCT images show that joint alignment is still maintained

tion of the musculoskeletal system. Appropriate scanning protocols should be tailored to incorporate these advances.

Acknowledge

We would like to acknowlege Jay Curtin for his valuable assistance in preparing the figures.

References

1. Prokop M (2003) General principles of MDCT. Eur J Radiol 45[Suppl 1]:S4–10
2. El-Khoury GY, Bennett L, Ondr GJ (2004) Multidetector-row computed tomography. J Am Acad Orthop Surg 12(1):1–5
3. Rydberg J, Buckwalter KA, Caldemeyer KS et al (2000) Multisection CT: scanning techniques and clinical applications. Radiographics 20:1787–1806
4. Dalal T, Kalra MK, Rizzo SM et al (2005) Metallic prosthesis: technique to avoid increase in CT radiation dose with automatic tube current modulation in a phantom and patients. Radiology 236(2):671–675
5. Harris JH Jr (2000) Spine, including soft tissues of the pharynx and neck. In: Harris JH Jr, Harris WH (eds) The radiology of emergency medicine. Lippincott Williams and Wilkins, Philadelphia, pp 137–298
6. Goldberg W, Mueller C, Panacek E et al (2001) Distribution and patterns of blunt traumatic cervical spine injury. Ann Emerg Med 38:17–21
7. El-Khoury GY, Moore TE, Kathol MH (1992) Radiology of the thoracic spine. Clin Neurosurg 38:261–295
8. Viktrup L, Knudsen GM, Hansen SH (1995) Delayed onset of fatal basilar thrombotic embolus after whiplash injury. Stroke 26: 2194–2196
9. Crim JR., Moore K, Brodke D (2001) Clearance of the cervical spine in multitrauma patients: the role of advanced imaging. Semin Ultrasound CT MRI 22(4):283–305

10. Ptak T, Kihiczak D, Lawrason JN et al (2001) Screening for cervical spine trauma with helical CT: Experience with 676 cases. Emerg Radiol 8:315–319
11. Mirza AH, Alam K, Ali A (2005) Posterior sternoclavicular dislocation in a rugby player as a cause of silent vascular compromise: a case report. Br J Sports Med 39(5):28
12. Haapamaki VV, Kiuru MJ, Koskinen SK (2004) Multidetector CT in shoulder fractures. Emerg Radiol 11(2):89–94
13. Jurik AG, Albrechtsen J (1994)The use of computed tomography with two- and three-dimensional reconstructions in the diagnosis of three- and four-part fractures of the proximal humerus. Clin Radiol 49(11):800–804
14. Chapman VM, Kalra M, Halpern E et al (2005)16-MDCT of the posttraumatic pediatric elbow: optimum parameters and associated radiation dose AJR Am J Roentgenol 185(2):516–521
15. Nicolaidis SC, Hildreth DH, Lichtman DM (2000) Acute injuries of the distal radioulnar joint. Hand Clin 16(3):449–359
16. J Sunagawa T, Ishida O, Ishiburo M et al (2005) Three-dimensional computed tomography imaging: its applicability in the evaluation of extensor tendons in the hand and wrist. Comput Assist Tomogr 29(1):94–98
17. Kiuru MJ, Haapamaki VV, Koivikko MP, Koskinen SK (2004).Wrist injuries; diagnosis with multidetector CT. Radiol 10(4):182–185
18. Klein HM, Vrsalovic V, Balas R, Neugebauer F (2002). Imaging diagnostics of the wrist: MRI and arthrography/arthro-CT. Rofo 174(2):177–182
19. Pennal GF, Tile M, Waddell JP, Garside H (1980) Pelvic disruption: assessment and classification. Clin Orthop 151:12–21
20. Their ME, Bensch FV, Koskinen SK et al (2005) Diagnostic value of pelvic radiography in the initial trauma series in blunt trauma. Eur Radiol 15(8):1533–1537
21. Lee W, Kim HS, Kim SJ et al (2004) CT arthrography and virtual arthroscopy in the diagnosis of the anterior cruciate ligament and meniscal abnormalities of the knee joint. Korean J Radiol 5(1):47–54
22. Schroder RJ, Weiler A, Hoher J et al (2003) Computed tomography of the patellofemoral alignment after arthroscopic reconstruction following patella dislocation. Rofo 175(4):547–555
23. Choplin RH, Buckwalter KA, Rydberg J, Farber JM (2004) CT with 3D rendering of the tendons of the foot and ankle: technique, normal anatomy, and disease. Radiographics 24(2):343–356
24. Salamipour H, Jimenez RM, Brec SL et al (2005) Multidetector row CT in pediatric musculoskeletal imaging. Pediatr Radiol 35(6):555–564

26

MDCT in Children: Scan Techniques and Contrast Issues

Donald P. Frush

Introduction

Computed tomography (CT) is an essential imaging modality in the evaluation of infants and children [1]. Technical advances, especially with multi-detector-array CT (MDCT) have provided increased opportunities for established uses as well as for new applications, such as evaluation of possible appendicitis, renal colic, and cardiovascular abnormalities. However, these technical advances are often complex and can be confusing. This complexity arises from the equipment, with increasing numbers of channels or arrays, and from the scan technique, consisting of multiple options for scan settings and intravenous (IV) contrast medium administration. Only with a solid understanding of these technical considerations will diagnostic MDCT in children be optimized. Therefore, this chapter focuses on the technical aspects of MDCT rather than on its applications. In addition to this technical discussion, issues in patient safety related to MDCT are addressed, including radiation management as a fundamental responsibility of the radiologist and radiology personnel [2].

MDCT in Children: General Considerations

While scan technique, including CT parameters and IV contrast administration, are certainly pivotal in a successful CT examination in an infant or child, several other responsibilities must be recognized. First, the radiology team needs to determine that CT is the correct examination. It may be that delaying the CT examination or using other modalities, such as sonography or magnetic resonance (MR), in which there is no ionizing radiation, are better options. Once it is decided that a CT examination is appropriate, the correct examination should be ordered. For example, an abdomen scan including the pelvis is not required for an evaluation of some upper abdominal abnormalities, such as localized or follow-up hepatic or renal disease. Following this determination, the technical aspects of CT examination should be addressed. These can be divided into the pre-scan (or patient preparation) and the scanning components. The scanning components consist of IV contrast medium administration and CT parameters, which are emphasized in the subsequent discussion. However, a brief discussion of patient preparation, which subsumes patient safety issues, is warranted here.

Without adequate patient preparation, even the optimal IV contrast administration technique and other aspects of the CT scanning protocol may not be sufficient to yield a diagnostic examination. The radiology team, including the technologist, must assess the need for patient sedation prior to patient arrival. With the faster scanners, in general, sedation is only required in children between 1 and 2 years of age. This will depend on the type of scan, as non-contrast examinations probably have a smaller window of age in children for which the use of sedation is necessary. In addition, it is important to know the specific clinical question. This will help the radiologist to tailor the examination–thus preventing overscanning–and optimize the technique. For example, a lower tube current [milliampere (mA)] setting or peak kilovoltage (kVp) could be used when looking for large abnormalities, high-contrast regions (i.e., lung or musculoskeletal evaluation), or in follow-up examinations. In addition, the presence of potential material causing artifacts (Fig. 1), including surgical clips, stents, or caval contrast (Fig. 2) for cardiovascular assessment, is particularly important. Designing CT suites that maximize the comfort of the child while creating an environment that is both child friendly and efficient will reduce both child and parent anxiety, providing for a higher scan success rate.

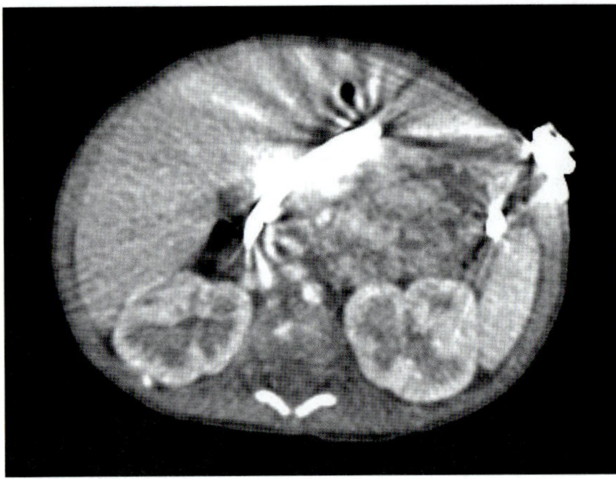

Fig. 1. A 10-week-old girl with multiple anomalies and hemody-namically significant gastrointestinal bleeding. Axial, contrast-enhanced computed tomography (CT) image through the upper abdomen demonstrates marked streak artifact from the enteric feeding tube, substantially limiting scan quality

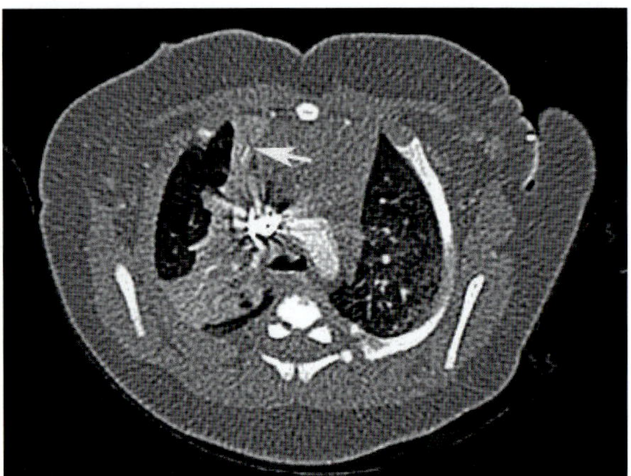

Fig. 2. In this infant with sequestration, suboptimal CT angiography technique potentially obscured critical information. A single axial image from a CT angiogram demonstrates marked streak artifact from caval contrast. This compromised the ability to see the tiny systemic artery (*arrow*) that likely originated from the right internal mammary artery to supply the sequestration, evident in the right posterior lung. In addition, a relatively high noise (bone vs. soft) algorithm was incorrectly used for image reconstruction, further compromising detail

Table 1. Percent of pediatric radiologists routinely using gastrointestinal high-density contrast material. Reproduced from [24], with permission from the American Journal of Roentgenology

Esophageal contrast for chest CT	3/89 (3%)
Oral contrast for abdomen CT (non-trauma)	86/92 (93%)
Oral contrast for abdomen CT (trauma)	31/92 (34%)
Rectal contrast for abdomen CT	0/92 (0%)

Patient preparation considerations may also include enteric contrast material (Tables 1 and 2). Because there is usually less intra-abdominal and pelvic fat in the pediatric age group, oral high-density contrast and IV contrast media are recommended for abdomen/pelvis CT. Recently, for scanning of the abdomen and pelvis in the pediatric population, there has been decreasing reliance on enteric contrast material, particularly in the setting of trauma but also for the evaluation of inflammatory processes (Table 2). If a high-density contrast material (e.g., barium or water-soluble iodinated material in some other liquid medium, such as apple juice or a soft drink) is not tolerated by the child, it is helpful to have the child drink any preferred liquid to provide some potential for discrimination of bowel lumen from the wall and adjacent structures [3] (Fig. 4). The use of routine rectal contrast in children is also decreasing. This had been most commonly used for assessment of appendicitis, but major pediatric institutions are now using either anterograde passage of enteric contrast or no contrast material at all.

The safety issues for MDCT in children are

Table 2. Oral contrast for abdominal and pelvic computed tomography (CT) in infants and children[a]. Reproduced from [5], with permission from Elsevier

Age	Amount[b] (1.5–3.0% solution)
1–6 months	60–120 ml (2–4 oz)
6–12 months	120–180 ml (4–6 oz)
1–4 years	180–270 ml (6–9 oz)
4–8 years	270–360 ml (9–12 oz)
8–12 years	360–480 ml (12–16 oz)
12–16 years	480–600 ml (16–20 oz)

> 16 years adult volume
[a]45 min 0–1.5 h prior to examination.
[b]An additional volume 1/2 of the original volume can be given about 15 min before the examination phase

those related to sedation, IV contrast medium administration, and radiation exposure. As sedation is becoming more often performed by non-radiology specialists, this will not be addressed here further [4] other than to say it is still the responsibility of the radiology team (1) to provide appropriate pediatric-sized support, including resuscitation

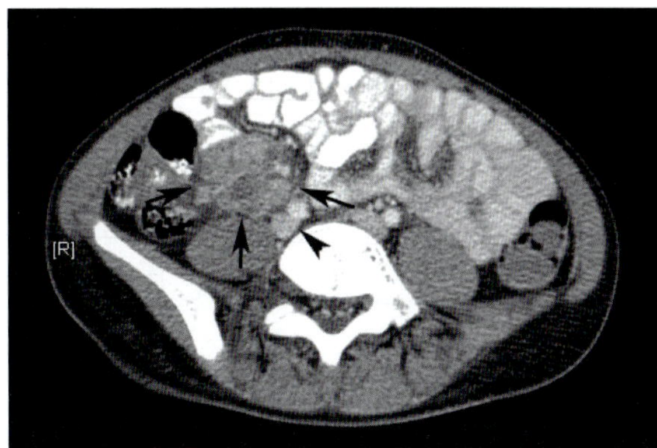

Fig. 3. Approximately 10-year-old girl with mesenteric adenitis as a solitary mass. Both oral- and IV-contrast-enhanced CT examination shows a nodal mass (*arrows*) in the right lower quadrant. The mass is readily seen despite little abdominal fat due to opacification of the adjacent bowel and vessels (*arrowhead*). Reproduced from [5], with permission from Elsevier

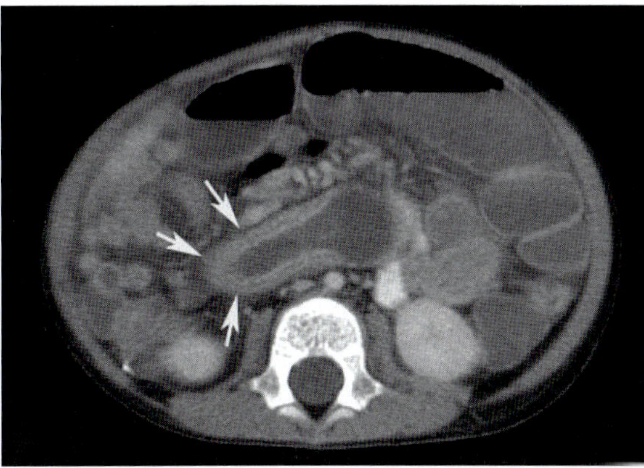

Fig. 4. Young immunocompromised (bone marrow transplant) boy with bowel obstruction who was at risk for post-transplant lymphoproliferative disorder. Axial, IV-contrast-enhanced CT at the mid-abdominal level shows thickening and mucosal enhancement of a proximal jejunal segment (*arrows*). Mucosal enhancement could have been obscured with high-density oral contrast. At resection, only inflammatory changes were present. Reproduced from [5], with permission from Elsevier

equipment, when children are part of the CT practice; (2) to help in designing the program in regards to the imaging needs for sedation (e.g., how long will the child have to hold still, what "still" means, and if inspiratory or expiratory pause is needed). In general, low-osmolarity contrast media are recommended for use in children [6]. The occurrence of adverse affects in children is extremely low. In one recent investigation of contrast-enhanced CT in just under 11,000 patients under 19 years of age, there were no severe reactions. Mild and moderate reactions were seen in 0.144 and 0.009% of this group, respectively [7].

That said, life-threatening reactions still do occur in children, and IV contrast material, for this and other reasons, is considered a "medication." Appropriate response to life-threatening reactions (i.e., anaphylactic reactions) in children is something that is very unfamiliar to radiologists. For that reason, facilities should adhere to regulatory guidelines regarding appropriate support equipment for children and to make use of available expertise. In a recent investigation, Gaca et al. demonstrated that access to a resuscitation tool and familiarity with the algorithm to use this tool may improve the outcome of children who experience anaphylactic reactions while in the radiology department [8].

The final safety consideration for children is radiation exposure. Optimization of the radiation dose in pediatric CT cannot be under-emphasized [9-13]. An in-depth discussion of the issues related to radiation biology is beyond the intent of this chapter, but can be found in a recent review [14]. In short, the actual risks are debatable. However, the radiologists and radiology team should adhere to the ALARA (as low as reasonably achievable) principle. To that end, CT should only be performed when appropriate, and, when appropriate, the technique should be adjusted based on the size of the child and clinical indication. To this end, technical guidelines for CT settings in the subsequent portion of this chapter should provide an adequate and appropriate balance of image quality in radiation dose [15]. Pediatric MDCT radiation dose estimations and practical methods for dose estimations for radiologists can be found in several recent sources [16-18].

Scan Technique and Contrast Issues

Contrast Issues

There are unique considerations with respect to children and IV contrast administration for MDCT. These primarily relate to the great range of sizes in pediatric imaging, from less than 1 kg to more than 100 kg. The overall amount of contrast may range from as small as a few milliliters up to an adult dose of 150 ml. The scan onset related to contrast administration, given the large range of sizes in children, is not standard. For an infant, the onset of scanning for a CT angiogram may be as short as 10 s following the initiation of contrast. The same exam in an adult-sized teenager may have a delay that approaches 60 s. In addition, the angiocatheter gauge will differ. Perfectly acceptable contrast-enhanced scanning including CT angiography can be performed through a 24-gauge angiocatheter in infants and small children. This is generally not acceptable for adult patients. The location of the angiocatheters may also differ in children; access sites such as the feet and hands are more common, particularly in small and ill children in whom standard IV access is limited. Given these challenges, however, attention to IV contrast administration details will translate to excellent diagnostic IV contrast MDCT scanning even in the most complex case [19]. These details consist of type, dose, and rate of contrast medium administration; route of administration; method of injection; and timing of scan initiation.

Type of IV Contrast Media

Low-osmolarity, non-ionic contrast material is recommended for pediatric CT. In general, the concentration is about 300 mgI/ml. While the benefits of high-concentration IV contrast media (e.g., 370 mgI/ml) [20] are increasingly advocated for adult-body imaging, including CT angiography, there has been no systematic review of scan quality and safety in children. It is likely that applications for high-concentration contrast media in adults will eventually find their way to some applications in children. For CT angiography, especially if there is fluid restriction, higher concentrations of contrast (i.e., 370 mgI/ml) can be considered.

Dose of IV Contrast Medium

The amount of contrast material in pediatric-body MDCT depends on the examination being performed. In general, 2.0 ml/kg is recommended for abdomen and pelvis (or combined chest, abdomen, and pelvis or neck scanning with either chest and/or abdomen and pelvis) imaging. For CT angiographic evaluation and isolated contrast-enhanced examination of the chest, a dose of 1.5 ml/kg is usually sufficient. For higher concentrations, the amount can be scaled back relative to the increase in iodine concentration. There are few, if any, published data in the diagnostic radiology literature about the maximum amount of contrast that can be administered. This would obviously depend somewhat on renal function, but in patients in whom renal function is relatively normal, 3.0 ml/kg is a reasonable ceiling. This gives one the opportunity to increase the overall doses noted above if extensive coverage is required in complicated cases. For example, neck scanning may require both venous and arterial information that is not optimized if the neck is scanned early in a combined neck, chest, abdomen, and pelvis MDCT examination. In this situation, a split bolus of 60%/40% (1.8/1.2 ml/kg) with a total dose of 3.0 ml/kg can be used, scanning the neck after completion of a chest, abdomen, and pelvis sequence. This dose of contrast medium in a patient

with normal renal function is reasonable, since concern is not raised until the contrast amount in small children reaches 5-6 ml/kg in conventional angiographic evaluation of the heart and great vessels [21].

For specialized examinations, consideration can be given to a biphasic administration, in which a portion of the bolus, i.e., two thirds, is given at the usual rate (approximately 2.0 ml/s), with a delay before beginning diagnostic scanning of 25–35 s from onset of contrast administration; just before scanning is initiated, the final one third is given (Fig. 5). This will provide both adequate venous enhancement, such as portal-vein opacification, and increasing arterial enhancement. This can be done if both arterial and venous information needs to be maximized (e.g., in cases of vascular malformations).

Rate of Administration of IV Contrast Medium

The rate of administration will depend on individual practice preferences. Basically, there are two general ways to administer a contrast agent to children for MDCT. One is to use one or relatively few fixed durations of injection. Thus, the rate will vary depending on the size of the child to get all the contrast administered within the fixed window of time. However, an increasingly common method of administration is a millimeter per second (ml/s) rate. This preference is probably due to the increasing number of detector rows and progressively shorter scan durations (e.g., less than 1 s for neonatal chest imaging with 64-slice MDCT). The ml/s contrast administration technique optimizes arterial opacification and provides for a higher peak enhancement than obtained with the slower rate of administration. The ml/s technique depends on the size of the angiocatheter (Table 3), but a target of 2.0 ml/s is adequate for almost all pediatric-body MDCT in younger children (< 12 years of age).

Route of Administration for IV Contrast Medium

The administration of IV contrast medium for pediatric MDCT depends on both the type and location of the IV catheter. For example, an umbilical venous catheter in a newborn is an excellent option for administration of contrast medium, including for CT angiography. Children are more likely to have smaller (i.e., 24- and 22-gauge) angiocatheters than adults. In particular, even a 24-gauge angiocatheter can provide excellent cardiovascular CT angiographic evaluations [19]. Most

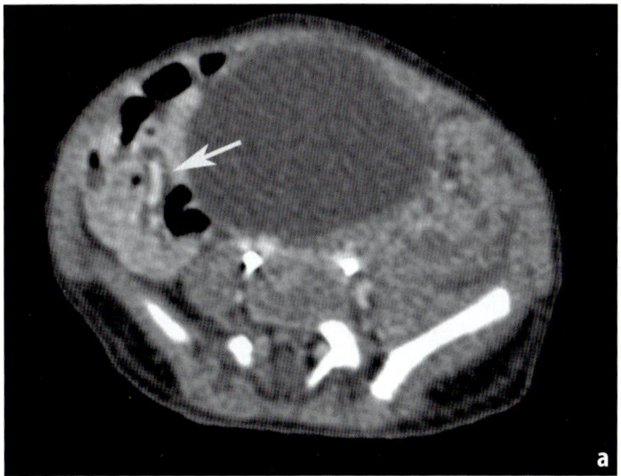

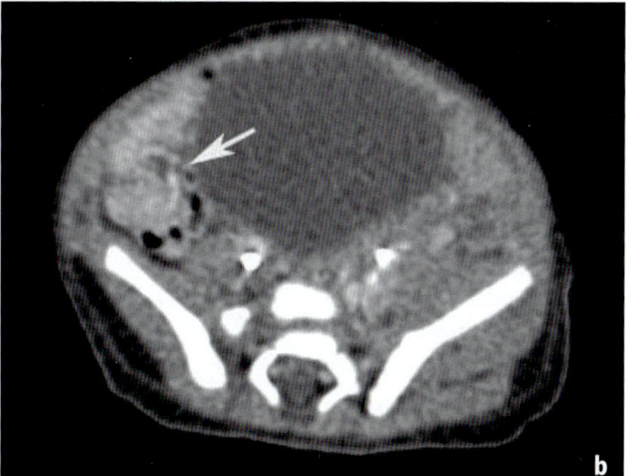

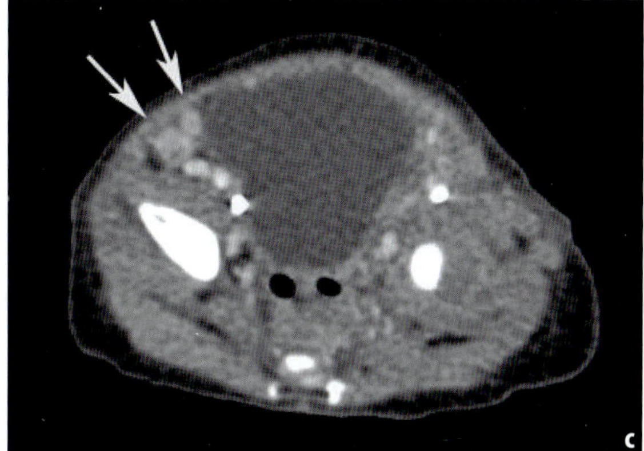

Fig. 5a-c. A 10-week-old girl (same child as in Fig. 1) with hemodynamically significant gastrointestinal bleeding. Technique: 120 kVp, 80 mA, 0.5 s (40 mAs), 0.938 pitch, 3.75-mm-thick. A dual-injection technique was used in which 60% of the 370 mgI/ml contrast medium was administered initially with a standard 25-s delay. Near the end of this delay, the remaining 40% of a total dose of 2.0 ml/kg was administered to provide additional arterial information. No oral contrast was given. **a** Axial image at the upper iliac crest shows prominent vascularity asymmetrically distributed to the right lower quadrant. There is also slightly more enhancement of bowel in this region. **b** Image slightly lower shows two vessels (*arrow*) that are again prominent and bowel that is enhancing more than bowel on the left side of the abdomen. **c** At the level of the lower pelvis, the mucosal or mural enhancement (*arrows*) is more clearly defined. Note the good opacification of the iliac arteries and veins. These changes were felt to be responsible for gastrointestinal bleeding, likely due to increased perfusion from non-specific inflammation. No obvious mass or vascular malformation was present. The child responded to conservative therapy

Table 3. Angiocatheter size and suggested rates of administration for pediatric computed tomography (CT) angiography

Catheter gauge	Administration rate (ml/s)
24	1.5–2.0
22	2.0–4.0
18, 20	3.0–7.0

central venous accesses, including ports, are also amenable to IV contrast administration, if the rate of administration is not excessive (> 2.5 ml/s). Generally, rates of administration of up to 2.5 ml/s will cover the majority of contrast-enhanced pediatric-body MDCT applications. The lumen diameter of peripherally inserted central catheters (PICCs) has been traditionally too small, but investigational work supports their potential use together with a power injector [23]. Newer large-lumen PICCs have yet to be evaluated for dynamic IV contrast administration in children.

Method of Administration for IV Contrast Medium

Either manual- or power-injector administration is available for pediatric contrast-enhanced MDCT. In general, with angiocatheters that withdraw and flush easily and are lumen caliber ≥22-gauge, power injection gives a more consistent enhancement, with a predictable time course of administration than manual technique. The use of power injectors with central venous catheters is acceptable, but the practice is not universal [24]. This decision should be based on individual practice standards. For catheters in which the blood return is absent or the catheter flushes poorly (but there is no swelling), or with a 24-gauge catheter in a peripheral site (hand or foot), manual injection should generally be considered.

Scan Timing for IV Contrast Medium

The timing of scan onset with respect to contrast administration is critical. For most abdomen and

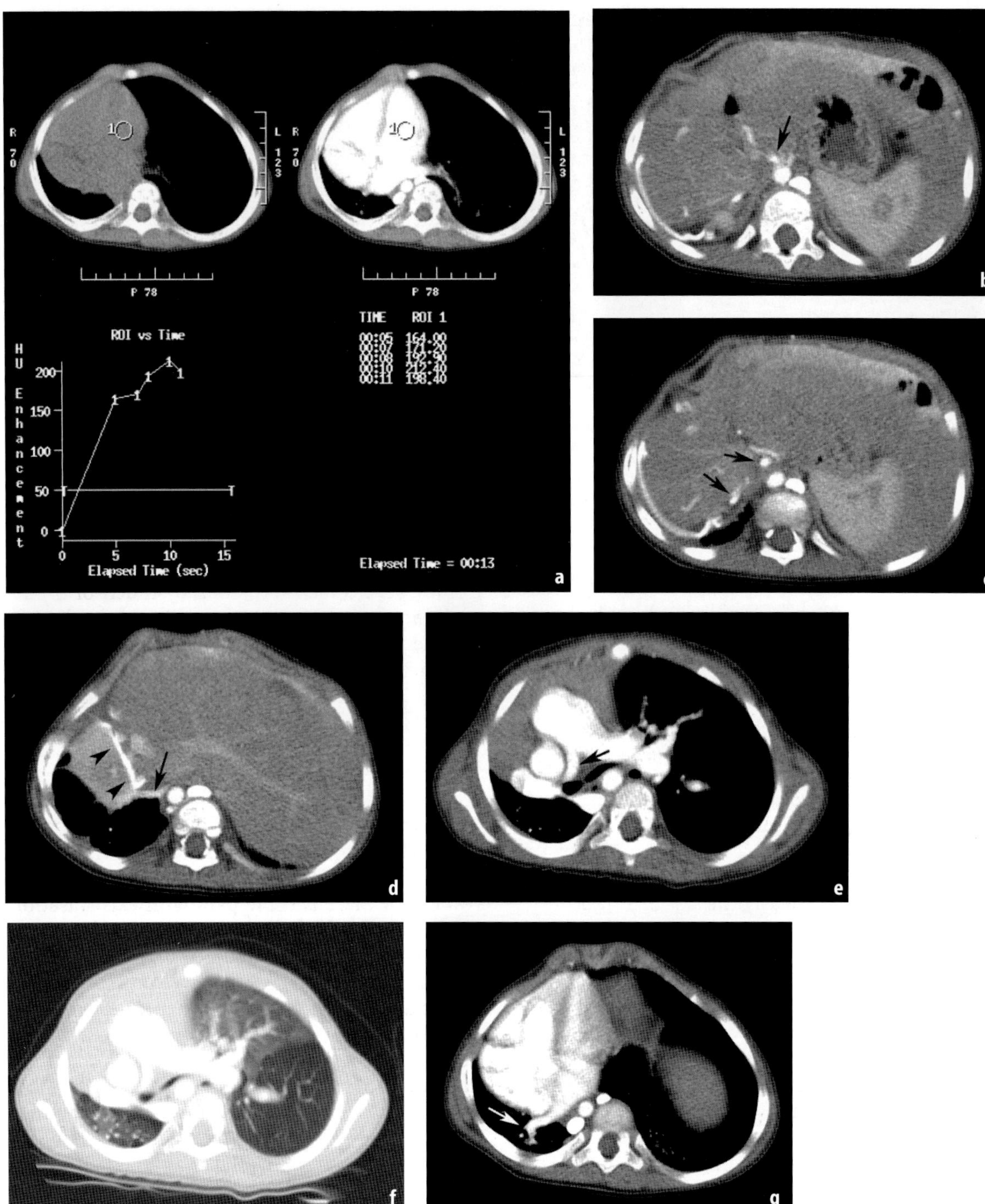

Fig. 6a-g. A 2-year-old boy with a complex history, including right congenital diaphragmatic hernia, pulmonary sequestration, right lung hypoplasia, and left lung congenital lobar emphysema in addition to structural cardiac disease. Technique: 120 kVp, 65 mA, 0.5 s (33 mAs), 0.938 pitch, 3.75-mm-thick, computed tomography (CT) angiogram was performed to define the congenital disorders of the lung. A total of 20 ml of 370 mgI/ml contrast medium was delivered by hand bolus. Bolus tracking was performed: **a** sequential enhancement of the aorta is depicted in the table. **b** Axial image at the level of the celiac axis demonstrates the origin of the systemic arterial supply (*arrow*). **c** Slightly more superiorly, the course of this artery (*arrows*) is seen at the level of the diaphragm. **d** More superiorly, the artery (*arrow*) extends above the diaphragm. Note the surgical changes following congenital diaphragmatic hernia repair (*arrowheads*). **e** Axial image at the level of the pulmonary artery shows the hypoplastic right pulmonary artery (*arrow*). **f** Lung window and level at the same level show hyperinflation of the left lower lobe due to congenital lobar emphysema. **g** Slightly inferior, the sequestered lung drained normally but into a single right lung vein (*arrow*)

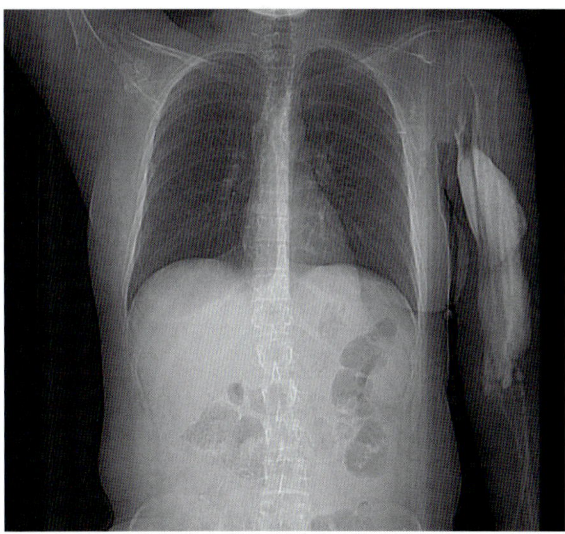

Fig. 7. Extravasation of non-ionic contrast material into the left arm in a teenager. There were no long-term sequelae from this extravasation

pelvis scanning, the desired scanning phase is the portovenous phase. For 4- to 16-detector scanners, a delay of 20–30 s after *completion* of contrast administration is suggested [25]. For 64-slice scanners, a delay of about 35 s after completion of contrast administration is recommended. For arterial-phase imaging, either an empirical delay or bolus tracking can be used. An empirical delay can be problematic given the great variation in size of children. Thus, an empirical delay is most useful in children who are nearly the size of adults.

When systemic arterial enhancement is indicated, the scan initiation time will depend on the scan duration. For shorter regions of coverage (e.g., in a small child) or for faster scanning (higher number of detector arrays), peak arterial opacification occurs at the end of or just after all contrast is administered and the scan should thus begin at that time point. For longer duration scans, the duration of the scan will need to span more of the injection period and scanning may have to begin slightly earlier than at the end of contrast injection. As this can be somewhat difficult to compute and may be unpredictable, especially if manual administration is the technique used, bolus-tracking software is extremely helpful [26] (Fig. 6), virtually eliminating the uncertainties with pediatric CT angiography [19, 21, 26, 27].

There are two methods for using bolus tracking. The first is to watch a region of interest (ROI) over the desired vessel to see when enhancement is going to be optimal. This can be determined based on the triggering of some predetermined attenuation of the ROI, or be visually triggered when the enhancement is deemed adequate. Scanning can

then be initiated at this point. The second is to use a test bolus [21]. Even for small children, a test bolus of 10% of the total amount of contrast used for the diagnostic scan can give information about when opacification of either the right ventricle, used for pulmonary arterial opacification, or left ventricle, for systemic arterial opacification, has been achieved. This method is less successful with a foot vein due to the mixing of a larger portion of venous blood from the lower torso than from the upper torso. With this method, tracking images start just before or during the onset of injection and the time to reach the desired region is recorded [21]. This technique is useful for neonates and for infants up to about 6 months of age to optimize timing for contrast enhancement. In general, a few (2–5) seconds are added to the time it takes the test bolus to reach the desired structure, since that initial time recorded for the test bolus simply represents the front end of the larger diagnostic scan bolus. By using the delay of arrival of the test bolus, one would not be taking advantage of the additional enhancement provided by much of the remaining contrast dose for the diagnostic phase of the examination.

One comment on the use of extravasation detectors is important. Unless the amount injected is going to be greater than the minimum level for threshold detection by the detector (such as 35 ml), these devices are not useful in children. It is recommended that for all children, but particularly for younger ones, the IV site be directly monitored during injection. This is particularly important if the child is sedated and may not be able to respond if there is some pain with extravasation. With the use of non-ionic agents, the chances of long-term sequelae from extravasation are extremely low (Fig. 7). While, thus far, there are no published reports in children, our experience over the last 15 years, consisting of the exclusive use of non-ionic contrast media in children, is that there have been no long-term adverse effects.

MDCT Scan Techniques

The discussion here includes general scan techniques (Tables 4–18) followed by considerations for more specialized, organ- or region-based scanning for pediatric-body MDCT.

Multi-phase scanning is not as routine in pediatric-body imaging as it is in adults. Usually, sufficient information can be obtained with a single phase during contrast administration or from a non-contrast-enhanced examination [28]. In general, multi-phase imaging in children should be less than 5% of all IV contrast-enhanced body MDCT protocols. When multi-phase imaging is indicated, then individual parameters such as tube

Table 4. Pediatric routine chest. GE LightSpeed 16 slice

Protocol	Pediatric routine chest
Vendor and detector rows	GE LightSpeed 16 slice
Phase (pre, arterial, venous, etc.)	Consider arterial for all chest
Scan range	Apex through sulcus
Detector configuration	16×0.625 if reformations anticipated
	16×1.25 for other
Rotation time (s)	0.5
Pitch	0.938 or 1.375 (see Table 11)
Table speed (mm/rotation)	18.75 (lower pitch, 16×1.25) or
	27.5 (higher pitch, 16×1.25)
kVp	Size adjusted (Table 11)
mA	Size adjusted (Table 11)
AEC	Optional (Table 13)
Reconstruction algorithm	Soft tissue
Prospective slice thickness (mm)	3.75–5.0 (Table 11)
Reconstruction interval (mm)	2.5 (favored)–5.0
Oral contrast (pos or neg)	None
IV contrast concentration (mg/ml)	300
IV contrast volume (ml)	1.5 ml/kg to adult dose as maximum
IV contrast dose (g)	Based on weight
IV contrast injection rate (ml/s)	1.5–3.0 injector; manual: fast as possible
Scan delay (fixed or bolus tracking)	At end of injection (minimal delay) or CTA technique (Table 10)
Saline chaser (ml)	Optional
Other	5-mm-thick/2.5 spacing coronals for trauma, assessment, congenital malformations, airway depiction

current (mA) and kVp can be adjusted. For example, for assessment of possible enhancement of a renal cyst vs. a solid lesion, a relatively low-dose pre-contrast examination can be performed of the region of the kidneys alone for baseline attenuation, followed by routine size-based technical parameters for the nephrographic phase (Fig. 8). When an excretory phase is necessary, such as for CT urography, then a lower kVp and lower mA are usually sufficient, given the excellent contrast in the collecting system. There are a number of selectable CT parameters that are principle determinants of scan quality and dose. These consists of tube current, peak kilovoltage, gantry cycle time (in seconds) and table speed, and the effective collimation (i.e., beam width) or pitch.

While detector configuration, consisting of the number of detector rows and the detector thickness, also are determinants of scan quality, these are becoming more limited as options as the number of detector rows increase. However, a few points are worthy of discussion. For multi-planar or three-dimensional reconstructions, it is recommended that the thinnest detector configuration is used (sub-mm if available). In addition, one should be familiar with effective collimation and radiation dose for pediatric MDCT related to over-beaming and over-ranging. For over-ranging, there is a portion of the beam beyond the desired scan range at the beginning and end of the region scanned that is necessary for image formation within the scan extent. This can be several centimeters for 16-slice MDCT [29]. With a larger beam width (effective collimation) such as 64×0.625 mm (40 mm) vs. 32×0.625 mm (20 mm), there is more over-ranging with the larger effective collimation when a smaller range is scanned (e.g., an infant's chest) with all other factors stable. Therefore, if a small range is going to be imaged, then a smaller effective collimation will reduce the dose. However, there is also a dose penalty per rotation, since there is an unused portion of the beam for each rotation outside of the detectors. This means that the more rotations per region scanned, the higher the dose. Thus, there is a dose penalty for the narrower beam width. There is a balance between the dose penalties for over-beaming and for over-ranging. This is complex and will depend on the pitch and collimation, as well as other factors that may vary between manufactur-

Table 5. Pediatric routine abdomen and pelvis. GE LightSpeed 16

Protocol	Pediatric routine abdomen and pelvis
Vendor and detector rows	GE LightSpeed 16
Phase (pre; arterial, venous, etc.)	Portal venous*
Scan range	Diaphragm to symphysis pubis
Detector configuration	64×0.625 if reformations anticipated; otherwise 16×1.25
Rotation time (s)	0.5
Pitch	0.938 or 1.375 (Table 12)
Table speed (mm/rotation)	18.75 (lower pitch, 16×1.25) or 27.5 (higher pitch, 16×1.25)
kVp	Size adjusted (Table 12)
mA	Size adjusted (Table 12)
AEC	Optional (Table 13)
Reconstruction algorithm	Soft tissue
Prospective slice thickness (mm)	3.75–5.0 (Table 12)
Reconstruction interval (mm)	2.5 (favored)–5.0
Oral contrast (pos or neg)	Positive
IV contrast concentration (mg/ml)	300
IV contrast volume (ml)	2.0 ml/kg to adult dose as maximum
IV contrast dose (g)	Based on weight
IV contrast injection rate (ml/s)	1.5–3.0 injector; manual: fast as possible
Scan delay (fixed or bolus tracking)	25–30 s following *completion of injection*
Saline chaser (ml)	Optional
Other	*Delays for liver lesions, evaluation of renal collecting system 5-mm-thick/2.5 spacing coronals for acute abdomen (e.g., appendicitis, obstruction), complex disorder including masses, trauma

Table 6. Pediatric routine chest. GE VCT 64 slice

Protocol	Pediatric routine chest
Vendor and detector rows	GE VCT 64 slice
Phase (pre, arterial, venous, etc.)	Consider arterial for all chest
Scan range	Apex through sulcus
Detector configuration	64×0.625
Rotation time (s)	0.4
Pitch	0.984 or 1.375 (Table 14)
Table speed (mm/rotation)	39.37 (for lower pitch) or 55 (for highes pitch) (Table 14)
kVp	Size adjusted (Table 14)
mA	Size adjusted (Table 14)
AEC	Optional (Table 13)
Reconstruction algorithm	Soft tissue
Prospective slice thickness (mm)	3.75–5.0 (Table 14)
Reconstruction interval (mm)	2.5 (favored)–5.0
Oral contrast (pos or neg)	None
IV contrast concentration (mg/ml)	300
IV contrast volume (ml)	1.5 ml/kg to adult dose as maximum
IV contrast dose (g)	Based on weight
IV contrast injection rate (ml/s)	1.5–3.0 injector; manual: fast as possible
Scan delay (fixed or bolus tracking)	At end of injection (minimal delay) or CTA technique (Table 10)
Saline chaser (ml)	Optional
Other	5-mm-thick/2.5 spacing coronals for trauma, assessment, congenital malformations, airway depiction

Table 7. Pediatric routine abdominal and pelvis. GE VCT 64 slice

Name of the protocol	Pediatric routine abd/pelvis
Vendor and detector rows	GE VCT 64 slice
Phase (pre; arterial, venous, etc)	Portal venous
Scan range	Diaphragm to symphysis pubis
Detector configuration	64×0.625
Rotation time (sec)	0.4
Pitch	0.984 or 1.375 (Table 15)
Table speed (mm/rotation)	39.37 (lower) or 55 (higher); pitch (Table 15)
kVp	Size adjusted (Table 15)
mA	Size adjusted (Table 15)
AEC	Optional (Table 13)
Reconstruction algorithm	Soft tissue
Prospective slice thickness (mm)	3.75 – 5.0 (Table 15)
Reconstruction interval (mm)	2.5 (favored) – 5.0
Oral contrast (pos or neg)	None
IV contrast concentration (mg/ml)	300
IV contrast volume (cc)	2.0 ml/kg to adult dose as max
IV contrast dose (grams)	Based on weight
IV contrast injection rate (cc/sec)	1.5-3.0 injector; manual: fast as possible
Scan delay (fixed or bolus tracking)	35 s following completion of injection
Saline chaser (cc)	NA
Other	5-mm thick/2.5 spacing coronals for acute abdomen (e.g., appendicitis, obstruction), complex disorders including masses, trauma

Table 8. Pediatric routine chest. Siemens Definition

Protocol	Pediatric routine chest
Vendor and detector rows	Siemens definition
Phase (pre, arterial, venous, etc.)	Consider arterial for all chest
Scan range	Apex through sulcus
Detector configuration	64×0.6
Rotation time (s)	0.5
Pitch	1.0 or 1.4 (Table 16)
Table speed (mm/rotation)	NA
kVp	Size adjusted (Table 16)
Note: mAs_{eff} not mA	Size adjusted (Table 16)
AEC	(insufficient experience at this point)
Reconstruction algorithm	Soft tissue (kernel B31f)
Prospective slice thickness (mm)	3.0–5.0 (Table 16)
Reconstruction interval (mm)	2.5 (favored)–5.0
Oral contrast (pos or neg)	None
IV contrast concentration (mg/ml)	300
IV contrast volume (ml)	1.5 ml/kg to adult dose as maximum
IV contrast dose (g)	Based on weight
IV contrast injection rate (ml/s)	1.5–3.0 injector; manual: fast as possible
Scan delay (fixed or bolus tracking)	At end of injection (minimal delay) or CTA technique (Table 10)
Saline chaser (ml)	Optional
Other	5-mm-thick/2.5 spacing coronals for trauma, assessment, congenital malformations, airway depiction

Table 9. Pediatric routine abdomen and pelvis. Siemens Definition

Protocol	Pediatric routine abdomen and pelvis
Vendor and detector rows	Siemens definition
Phase (pre, arterial, venous, etc.)	Portal venous*
Scan range	Diaphragm to symphysis pubis
Detector configuration	64×0.6
Rotation time (s)	0.5
Pitch	1.0 or 1.4 (Table 17)
Table speed (mm/rotation)	NA
kVp	Size adjusted (Table 17)
Note: mAs_{eff} not mA	Size adjusted (Table 17)
AEC	(insufficient experience at this point)
Reconstruction algorithm	Soft tissue (kernel B31f)
Prospective slice thickness (mm)	3.0–5.0 (Table 17)
Reconstruction interval (mm)	2.5 (favored)–5.0
Oral contrast (pos or neg)	Positive
IV contrast concentration (mg/ml)	300
IV contrast volume (cc)	2.0 ml/kg to adult dose as maximum
IV contrast dose (g)	Based on weight
IV contrast injection rate (ml/s)	1.5–3.0 injector; manual: fast as possible
Scan delay (fixed or bolus tracking)	35 s following *completion of injection*
Saline chaser (ml)	Optional
Other	*Delays for liver lesions, evaluation of renal collecting system 5-mm-thick/2.5 spacing coronals for acute abdomen (e.g., appendicitis, obstruction), complex disorders including masses, trauma

Table 10. Pediatric routine CTA. GE VCT 64 and LightSpeed 16

Protocol	Pediatric routine CTA
Vendor and detector rows	GE VCT 64 and LightSpeed 16
Phase (pre, arterial, venous, etc.)	Arterial
Scan range	Varies for indication
Detector configuration	16×0.625, 64×0.625
Rotation time (s)	0.4, 0.5
Pitch	1.375
Table speed (mm/rotation)	55
kVp	Size adjusted (Table 18)
mA	Size adjusted (Table 18)
AEC	No recommendations
Reconstruction algorithm	Soft
Display slice thickness (mm)	1.25–5.0 (Table 18)
Reconstruction thickness (mm)	0.625
Reconstruction interval (mm)	0.5–1.0
Oral contrast (pos or neg)	None
IV contrast concentration (mg/ml)	300–370
IV contrast volume (ml)	1.5 ml/kg to adult dose as maximum
IV contrast dose (g)	Based on weight
IV contrast injection rate (ml/s)	1.5–5.0 injector; manual: fast as possible
Scan delay (fixed or bolus tracking)	Bolus tracking (SmartPrep); usual visual trigger for $\leq$ 7 years; adult HU trigger in older children
Saline chaser (ml)	Optional
Other	In small (e.g., < 1 year) children, begin bolus tracking (start contrast when first image displayed) *before starting contrast* so that peak of bolus not missed; can use test bolus (10% of total dose) even in infants

Table 11. Pediatric chest 16-slice GE LightSpeed multi-detector computed tomography (MDCT)

Zone	Weight	Length	Age	mA	kVp	Pitch	Thick
Pink	5.5–7.4 kg	60–67 cm	2.5–5.5 months	55	100	.938	3.75
Red	7.5–9.4 kg	67–75 cm	5.5–11.5 months	60	100	.938	3.75
Purple	9.5–11.4 kg	75–85 cm	11.5–22 months	65	120	.938	3.75
Yellow	11.5–14.4 kg	85–97 cm	22 months–3 years, 2 months	50	120	.938	5
White	14.5–18.4 kg	97–109 cm	3 years, 2 months–5 years, 2 months	55	120	1.38	5
Blue	18.5–23.4 kg	109–121 cm	5 years, 2 months–7 years, 4 mo	65	120	1.38	5
Orange	23.5–29.4 kg	121–133 cm	7 years, 4 months–9 years, 2 mo	70	120	1.38	5
Green	29.5–36.4 kg	133–147 cm	9 years, 2 months–13 years, 6 months	75	120	1.38	5
Black	36.5–55 kg	>147 cm	>13 years, 6 months	90	120	1.38	5

Table 12. Pediatric abdomen/pelvis 16-slice GE LightSpeed multi-detector computed tomography (MDCT)

Zone	Weight	Length	Age	mA	kVp	Pitch	Thick
Pink	5.5–7.4 kg	60–67 cm	2.5–5.5 months	70	120	.938	3.75
Red	7.5–9.4 kg	67–75 cm	5.5–11.5 months	85	120	.938	3.75
Purple	9.5–11.4 kg	75–85 cm	11.5–22 months	90	120	.938	3.75
Yellow	11.5–14.4 kg	85–97 cm	22 months–3 years, 2 months	65	120	.938	5
White	14.5–18.4 kg	97–109 cm	3 years, 2 months–5 years, 2 months	70	120	1.38	5
Blue	18.5–23.4 kg	109–121 cm	5 years, 2 months–7 years, 4 months	80	120	1.38	5
Orange	23.5–29.4 kg	121–133 cm	7 years, 4 months–9 years, 2 months	90	120	1.38	5
Green	29.5–36.4 kg	133–147 cm	9 years, 2 months–13 years, 6 months	100	140	1.38	5
Black	36.5–55 kg	>147 cm	>13 years, 6 months	105	140	1.38	5

Table 13. AEC guidelines for pediatric GE multi-detector computed tomography (MDCT)

				Noise Index	
Zone	Weight	Length	Age	Chest	Abd Pelvis
Pink	5.5–7.4 kg	60–67 cm	2.5–5.5 months	9.5	6.5
Red	7.5–9.4 kg	67–75 cm	5.5–11.5 months	10.0	7.5
Purple	9.5–11.4 kg	75–85 cm	11.5–22 months	10.5	8.5
Yellow	11.5–14.4 kg	85–97 cm	22 months–3 years, 2 months	11	9.5
White	14.5–18.4 kg	97–109 cm	3 years, 2 months–5 years, 2 months	12	10.5
Blue	18.5–23.4 kg	109–121 cm	5 years, 2 months–7 years, 4 months	13	11.5
Orange	23.5–29.4 kg	121–133 cm	7 years, 4 months–9 years, 2 months	14	12.5
Green	29.5–36.4 kg	133–147 cm	9 years, 2 months–13 years, 6 months	15	13.5
Black	36.5–55 kg	>147 cm	>13 years, 6 months	16	14

Note: Max (ceiling) should be set to mA in tables depending on region and scanner so that routine mA *is not exceeded*

Table 14. Pediatric chest 64-slice GE multi-detector computed tomograhy (MDCT)

Zone	Weight	Length	Age	mA	kVp	Pitch	Thick
Pink	5.5–7.4 kg	60–67 cm	2.5–5.5 months	70	100	.98	3.75
Red	7.5–9.4 kg	67–75 cm	5.5–11.5 months	80	100	.98	3.75
Purple	9.5–11.4 kg	75–85 cm	11.5–22 months	90	100	.98	3.75
Yellow	11.5–14.4 kg	85–97 cm	22 months–3 years, 2 months	70	120	1.38	5
White	14.5–18.4 kg	97–109 cm	3 years, 2 months–5 years, 2 months	75	120	1.38	5
Blue	18.5–23.4 kg	109–121 cm	5 years, 2 months–7 years, 4 months	80	120	1.38	5
Orange	23.5–29.4 kg	121–133 cm	7 years, 4 months–9 years, 2 months	90	120	1.38	5
Green	29.5–36.4 kg	133–147 cm	9 years, 2 months–13 years, 6 months	95	120	1.38	5
Black	36.5–55 kg	> 147 cm	>13 years, 6 months	110	120	1.38	5

Table 15. Pediatric abdomen/pelvis 64-slice GE multi-detector computed tomography (MDCT)

Zone	Weight	Length	Age	mA	kVp	Pitch	Thick
Pink	5.5–7.4 kg	60–67 cm	2.5–5.5 months	85	120	.98	3.75
Red	7.5–9.4 kg	67–75 cm	5.5–11.5 months	100	120	.98	3.75
Purple	9.5–11.4 kg	75–85 cm	11.5–22 months	110	120	.98	3.75
Yellow	11.5–14.4 kg	85–97 cm	22 months–3 years, 2 months	85	120	1.38	5
White	14.5–18.4 kg	97–109 cm	3 years, 2 months–5 years, 2 months	90	120	1.38	5
Blue	18.5–23.4 kg	109–121 cm	5 years, 2 months–7 years, 4 months	100	120	1.38	5
Orange	23.5–29.4 kg	121–133 cm	7 yr, 4 months–9 years, 2 months	110	120	1.38	5
Green	29.5–36.4 kg	133–147 cm	9 years, 2 months–13 years, 6 months	115	140	1.38	5
Black	36.5–55 kg	>147 cm	>13 years, 6 months	130	140	1.38	5

Table 16. Pediatric chest Siemens Definition multi-detector computed tomography (MDCT)

Zone	Weight	Length	Age	mAseff	kVp	Pitch	Thick
Pink	5.5–7.4 kg	60–67 cm	2.5–5.5 months	60	100	1.0	3.75
Red	7.5–9.4 kg	67–75 cm	5.5–11.5 months	65	100	1.0	3.75
Purple	9.5–11.4 kg	75–85 cm	11.5–22 months	75	120	1.0	3.75
Yellow	11.5–14.4 kg	85–97 cm	22 months–3 years, 2 months	45	120	1.4	5
White	14.5–18.4 kg	97–109 cm	3 years, 2 months–5 years, 2 months	50	120	1.4	5
Blue	18.5–23.4 kg	109–121 cm	5 years, 2 months–7 years, 4 months	50	120	1.4	5
Orange	23.5–29.4 kg	121–133 cm	7 years, 4 months–9 years, 2 months	55	120	1.4	5
Green	29.5–36.4 kg	133–147 cm	9 years, 2 months–13 years, 6 mo	60	120	1.4	5
Black	36.5–55 kg	>147 cm	>13 years, 6 months	65	120	1.4	5

Table 17. Pediatric abdomen/pelvis Siemens Definition multi-detector computed tomography (MDCT)

Zone	Weight	Length	Age	mAseff	kVp	Pitch	Thick
Pink	5.5–7.4 kg	60–67 cm	2.5–5.5 months	70	120	1.0	3.75
Red	7.5–9.4 kg	67–75 cm	5.5–11.5 months	80	120	1.0	3.75
Purple	9.5–11.4 kg	75–85 cm	11.5–22 months	90	120	1.0	3.75
Yellow	11.5–14.4 kg	85–97 cm	22 months–3 years, 2 months	55	120	1.4	5
White	14.5–18.4 kg	97–109 cm	3 years, 2 months–5 years, 2 months	60	120	1.4	5
Blue	18.5–23.4 kg	109–121 cm	5 years, 2 months–7 years, 4 months	60	120	1.4	5
Orange	23.5–29.4 kg	121–133 cm	7 years, 4 months–9 years, 2 months	65	120	1.4	5
Green	29.5–36.4 kg	133–147 cm	9 years, 2 months–13 years, 6 months	70	140	1.4	5
Black	36.5–55 kg	>147 cm	>13 years, 6 months	80	140	1.4	5

Table 18. Pediatric computed tomography angiography (CTA) 16-and 64-slice GE multi-detector computed tomography (MDCT)

Zone	Weight	Length	Age	mA[a]	kVp	Pitch	Thick[b]
Pink	5.5–7.4 kg	60–67 cm	2.5–5.5 months	100	80	1.375	1.25–5.0
Red	7.5–9.4 kg	67–75 cm	5.5–11.5 months	110	80	1.375	1.25–5.0
Purple	9.5–11.4 kg	75–85 cm	11.5–22 months	120	80	1.375	1.25–5.0
Yellow	11.5–14.4 kg	85–97 cm	22 months–3 years, 2 months	130	100	1.375	1.25–5.0
White	14.5–18.4 kg	97–109 cm	3 years, 2 months–5 years, 2 months	140	100	1.375	1.25–5.0
Blue	18.5–23.4 kg	109–121 cm	5 years, 2 months–7 years, 4 months	150	100	1.375	1.25–5.0
Orange	23.5–29.4 kg	121–133 cm	7 years, 4 months–9 years, 2 months	160	120	1.375	1.25–5.0
Green	29.5–36.4 kg	133–147 cm	9 years, 2 monthso–13 years, 6 months	180	120	1.375	1.25–5.0
Black	36.5–55 kg	>147 cm	>13 years, 6 months	200+	120	1.375	1.25–5.0

[a]mA can be about 10–20% lower for chest CTA
[b]Display
For coronal and sagittal reformats and 3-D, reconstruct axial data set at 0.625 mm at 0.5- to 1.0-mm intervals. Multi-planar thickness and interval should be similar to axial

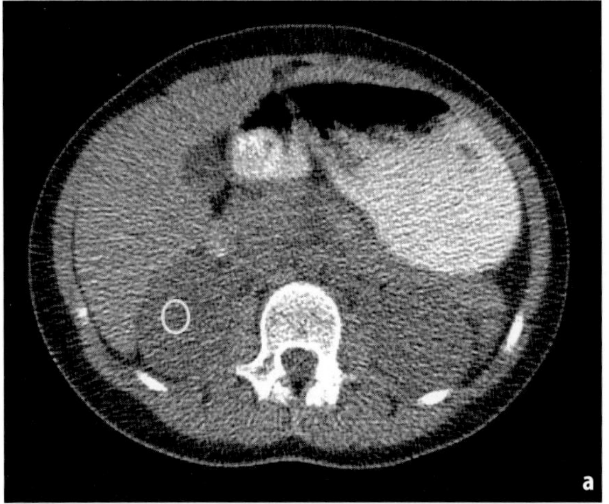
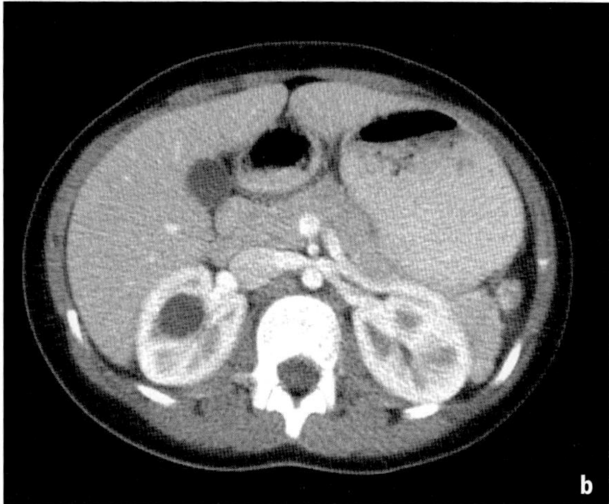
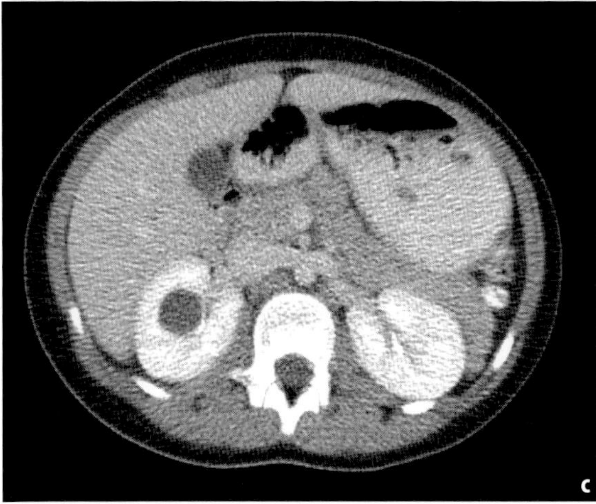

Fig. 8a-c. An 8 year-old girl in whom a complex cyst was detected on sonography (not shown). **a** Initial non-contrast low-dose examination was performed at 10 mAs for renal localization. The cyst (in region of oval ROI) measured 10 HU, lower than adjacent kidney. **b** Arterial and lower-dose nephrographic (**c**) phases showed no enhancement. Reproduced from [5], with permission from Elsevier

ers [29]. For the GE scanner, the threshold for overall dose savings for changing to the larger effective collimation of the 64-slice scanner (40 mm) is at a scan range of just over 20 cm. This means that if the scan distance is less than about 20 cm, then the 32 × 0.625-mm configuration should be used for dose savings.

Tube current is a primary modulator of image noise. Increasing tube current decreases noise, or mottle (Fig. 9). There are guidelines for tube-current settings for pediatric-body MDCT [1, 5, 30]. As a rule, tube current should be adjusted based on the size of the child (smaller cross-sectional areas do not require as high an mA as larger cross-sectional areas), in addition to other considerations such as clinical indication and body region scanned (these are addressed below).

Gantry cycle time should be as fast as possible. This will decrease image artifacts and result in the scanning being completed quicker, an advantage with children. The product of tube current and gantry cycle time, or milliampere second (mAs), therefore should have the fastest cycle time as the second factor.

Peak kilovoltage contributes to both image noise and contrast. A decrease in kVp will increase contrast but also increase noise. As with tube current, guidelines for kVp in pediatric MDCT have been published [1, 5]. In general, over the past few years, increased efforts have been directed toward decreasing kVp [31]. For high-contrast examinations (e.g., chest, skeletal assessment, and CT angiography) in small children, a low kVp (80–120 kVp) will increase contrast sufficiently that there is a relative improvement in the contrast-to-noise ratio even though noise also increases. Even for abdomen and pelvis MDCT in small children, 120 kVp is recommended.

Despite the increasing number of detector rows, scan pitches in the range of 1.0–1.75 for pediatric-body MDCT, as for single slice- and 4-slice helical CT, are still recommended [32, 33]. Based on empirical observations of image artifacts, protocols (16-24 slice MDCT) generally call for pitches of approximately 1.0 in the youngest children, increasing to approximately 1.375 in older children.

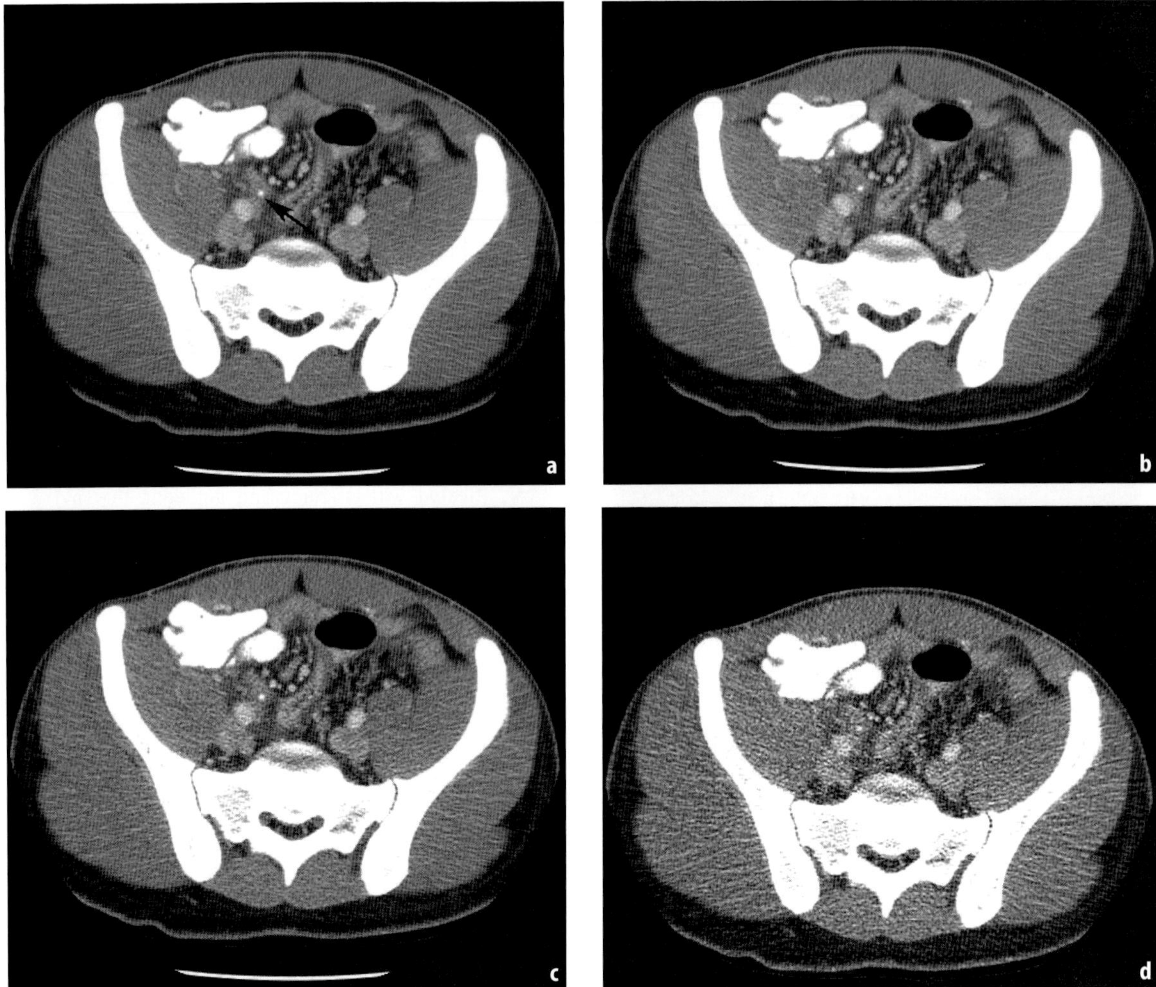

Fig. 9a-d. A 20-year-old man with acute appendicitis. Axial, oral, and IV-contrast-enhanced CT image in the lower pelvis was performed at 340 mA (**a**) and shows the thickened appendix with a small appendicolith (*arrow*). Simulated tube current (noise addition) reductions to 240 mA (**b**), 140 mA (**c**), and 40 mA (**d**) demonstrate progressive loss in image quality. Diagnostic quality is still evident at least as low as 240 mA but is limited at 40 mA. Reproduced from [5], with permission from Elsevier

Specialized MDCT Techniques

There are certain organ systems or regions for which MDCT of children have unique technical considerations. The following addresses these special technical considerations, which are aimed at maximizing diagnostic yield while minimizing radiation dose. While not exhaustive, this discussion covers the majority of specialized examinations in children, i.e., chest MDCT, skeletal evaluation, CT angiography, and evaluation of the urinary tract.

Pediatric Chest MDCT

Because of the intrinsically high contrast resolution between parenchyma, consisting predominantly of vessels, and aerated lung, lower settings for kVp and mA should be considered in children.

In addition, children (routinely at about 6 years of age) should be encouraged to hold their breath. With faster scanning, scan durations of just a few seconds are possible in children with limited (<10 s) breath-holding capability, typical of those younger than about 8 years of age. Coaching for this maneuver is sometimes helpful. In the evaluation of interstitial lung disease, a lower dose is achieved when a single axial thin (1–1.25 mm) slice is obtained at intervals yielding 6-10 to slices. An alternate to this technique is to extract thin sections from a helically performed examination. Again, breath-holding is recommended, as movement artifacts have a substantial impact in interstitial lung disease evaluation. When breath-holding is not possible, either intubation (Fig. 10) with suspended respiration or control-assisted ventilation is useful [34]. Without breath-holding, only a few salvageable high-resolution (thin slices) images of

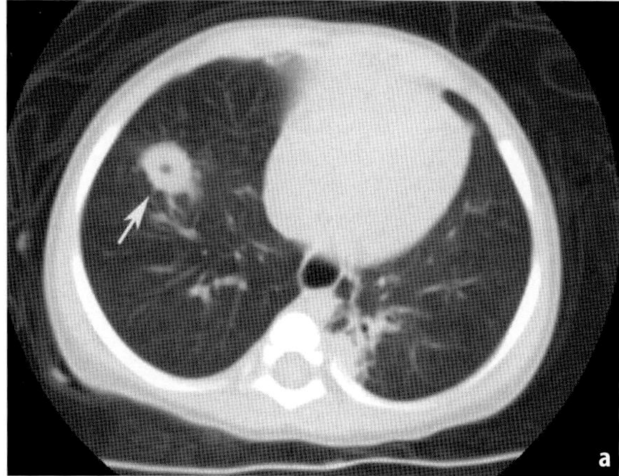
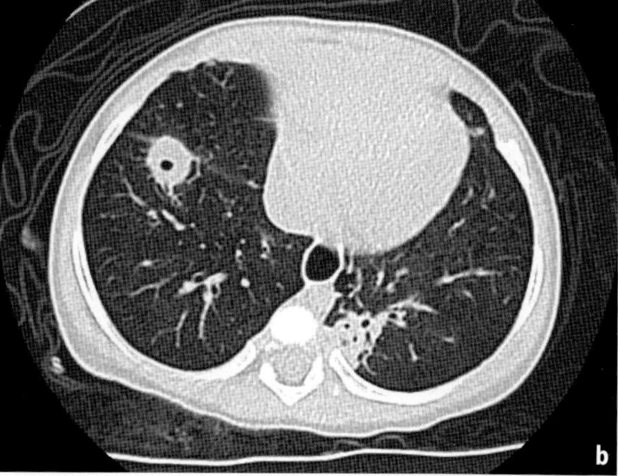
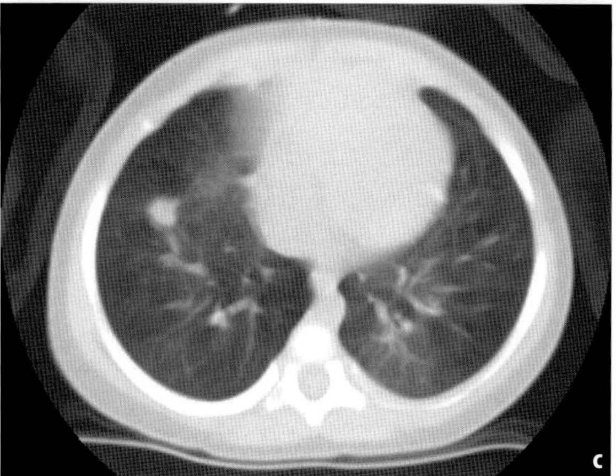

Fig. 10a-c. A 13-month-old girl with sickle cell disease and cystic fibrosis (treated with steroids and antibiotic therapy) with parenchymal opacities, as seen on chest X-ray. Technique: 120 kVp, 65 mA, 0.5 s (33 mAs), pitch 0.938, 3.75-mm-thick images of the chest performed, with the patient under general anesthesia, for assessment of possible fibrosis and parenchymal opacities using high-resolution CT. **a** Thicker image demonstrates the cavitary lesion (*arrow*) in the right middle lobe as well as consolidation medially on the left. **b** Axial 1.25-mm-thick image extracted from the helical dataset better demonstrates these changes, including the airways in the consolidation on the left. No fibrosis was present. **c** Follow-up CT 1 month later was limited to the lower chest and shows substantial resolution of previous opacities. This was performed at 60 mA, 0.5 s (30 mAs), 0.938 pitch, 3.75-mm-thick. The dose-length product for the follow-up examination was 21.54 mGy·cm, with a conversion factor of 0.016 mSv (mGy.cm)$^{-1}$ [16], yielding an estimated dose equivalent of about 10-15 chest X-rays. Note in **c** the movement artifact since the patient was not intubated for this examination and image quality is therefore degraded compared with **a**

natural pauses in lung movement at end inspiration or end expiration are available.

In general, especially in younger children, in whom there is limited amount of mediastinal fat, IV contrast medium is recommended. This is not as standard as in adult chest CT. In an evaluation of the skeletal system, such as pectus abnormalities, or for isolated lung parenchyma abnormalities, such as interstitial lung disease or metastatic disease in the setting of Wilms tumor or extrathoracic sarcomas, a non-contrast examination is adequate.

When reconstructions are anticipated, i.e., cardiovascular abnormalities, potential congenital lung malformations, or for major airway depiction, the thinnest detector configuration should be selected so that high-quality reconstruction can be performed.

Pediatric Urinary Tract CT

This is one of the few organ systems in which multi-phase CT should be considered. In the assessment of cystic abnormalities (i.e., enhancement), a pre-contrast evaluation is obligatory (Fig. 8). To examine the renal or subjacent arterial vascula-

ture, an arterial phase is helpful in addition to the nephrographic phase. In settings of possible abnormalities of the collecting system (i.e., calyceal diverticulum, renal trauma with extravasation of contrast medium, or assessment of the urinary collecting system anatomy such as a ureteropelvic junction obstruction or in a setting of duplication), an excretory phase is necessary (Fig. 11). For these applications, however, there can be individual adjustments in technique to minimize the additional radiation dose. For example, for excretory-phase imaging, the kVp, mA, or both can be reduced due to the excellent contrast differentiation between the collecting system and adjacent soft tissues. In general, a delay of about 10-15 min following the administration of contrast is adequate for depicting the ureters and to provide up to moderate bladder filling. A longer delay may be necessary to adequately distend the bladder if this is the region that needs assessment.

In the evaluation of renal stones, IV contrast is not indicated unless there is an abnormality that may be mimicking renal colic, such as appendicitis. For these examinations, a lower tube current of 40 mAs (Fig. 11) is acceptable for stone detection even in adult-sized teenagers (personal communication, Dr. B. Karmazyn, Indianapolis, IN, USA).

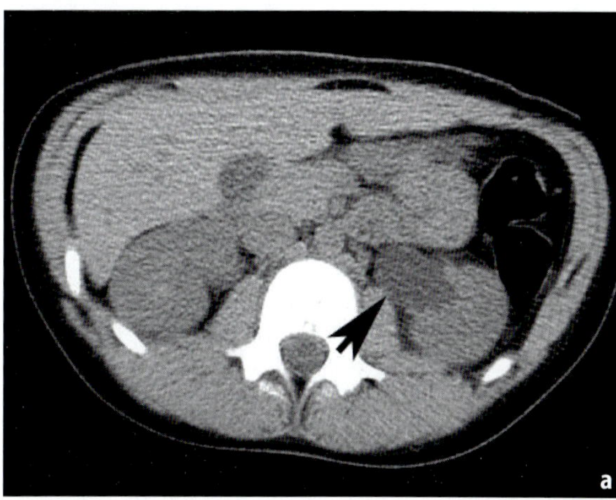
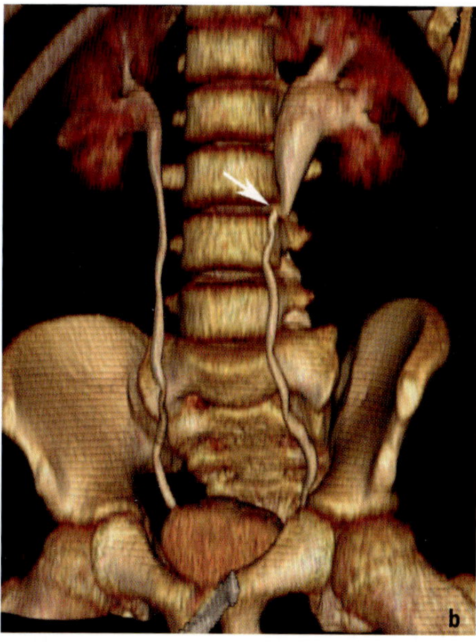

Fig. 11a, b. A 9 year-old-boy with right flank pain. Renal stone protocol was initially performed. Technique: 120 kVp, 100 mA, 0.4 s (40 mAs), 1.375 pitch, 5.0-mm-thick. No stones were seen but there was dilation of the collecting system (*short arrow*) in (**a**), associated with left perinephric stranding. To assess for possible other causes, such as appendicitis, a subsequent examination was performed using 36 mAs. Some delayed images were obtained 15 min after contrast administration, as it was felt that the patient may have had a ureteropelvic junction (UPJ) obstruction. (**b**) Volume-rendered 3D reconstruction shows the UPJ obstruction (*arrow*), which was due to a focal nondistensible collecting system at surgery. An alternative imaging strategy, if appendicitis was not in the differential diagnosis, would be to have obtained an ultrasound following the non-contrast computed tomography (CT)

Pediatric Skeletal CT

As with chest and CT angiography, lower kVp and mA can be considered for skeletal evaluation. Since multi-planar and volume reconstructions are typically performed, the thinnest detector configuration (preferably sub-mm) should be selected (Figs. 12, 13).

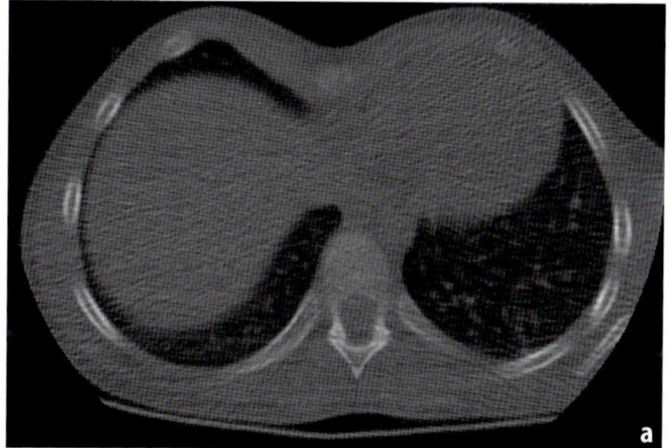
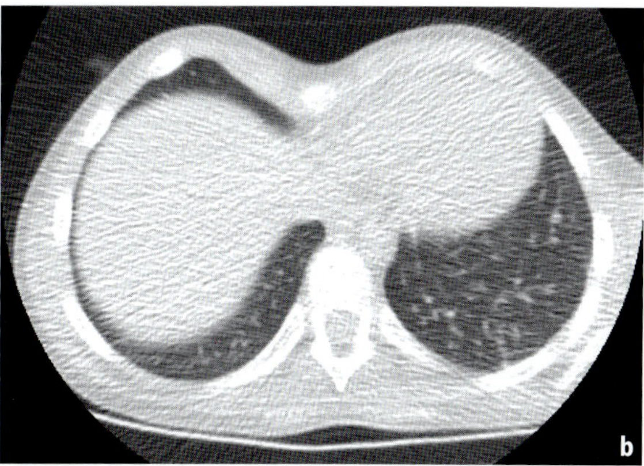
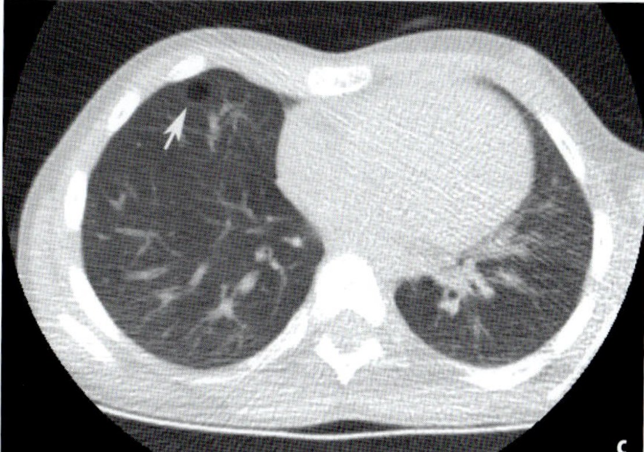

Fig. 12a-c. An 8 year-old-girl assessed for pectus excavatum deformity. Technique: 80 kVp, 20 mA, 0.5 s (10 mAs), pitch 1.375, 5-mm slice thickness, yielding a dose-length product of 4.78 mGy.cm. With this dose-length product and a conversion factor of 0.013 mSv (mGy cm)$^{-1}$ [15], this is the equivalent of less than five chest X-rays. **a** Bone window and level in lower chest demonstrates the pectus deformity well (Haller index 4:1). With lung window and level note preservation of parenchymal detail. **c** Image slightly higher shows a well-defined cystic area that was present on a prior CT and unchanged in appearance. Prior CT was done at approximately 10 times the dose (image not shown)

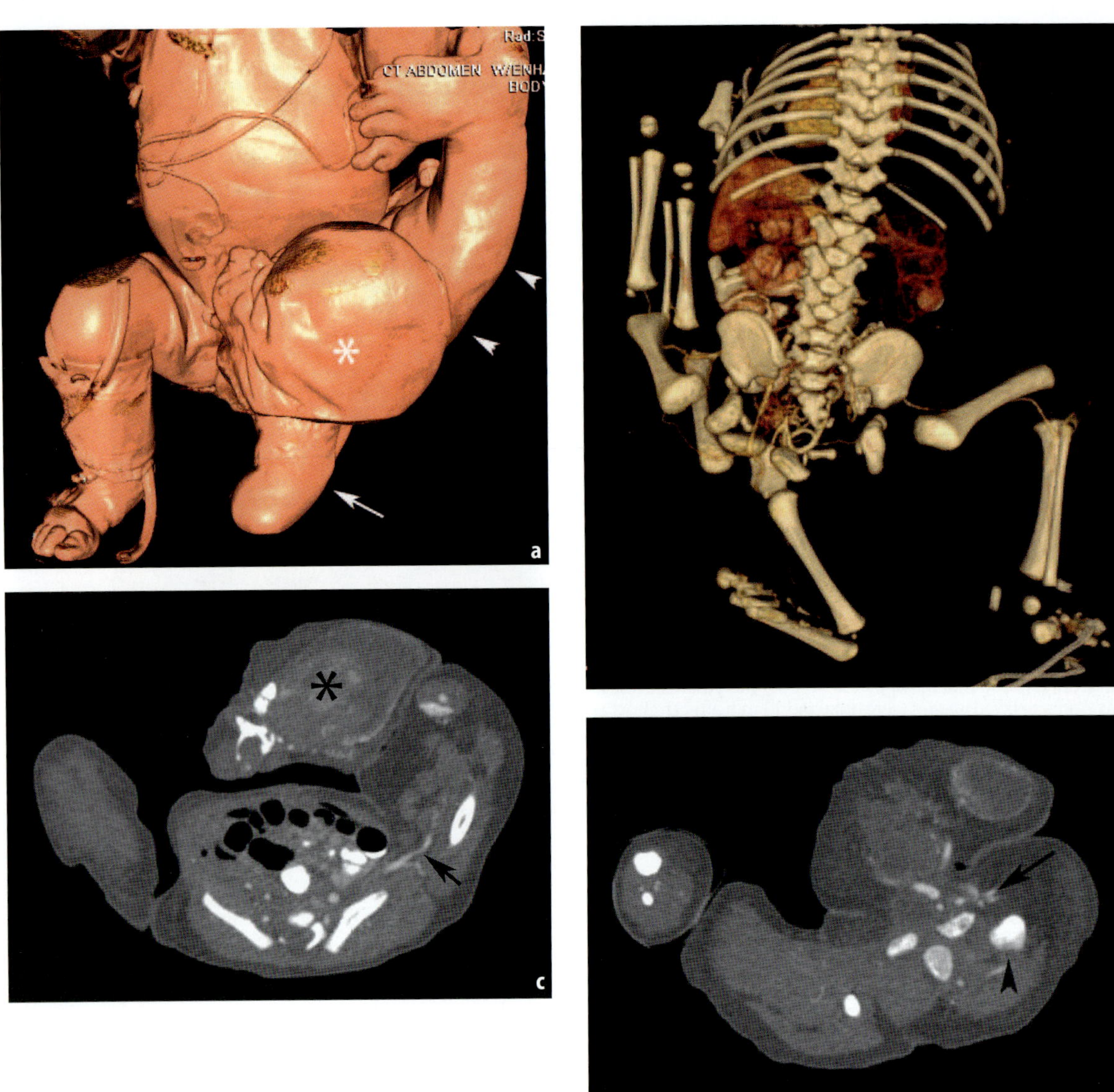

Fig. 13a-d. Newborn, heteropagus (incomplete conjoint) twin, consisting of a partial twin arising from the pelvic region. Technique: 100 kVp, 160 mA, 0.4 s (64 mAs), 0.984 pitch, 2.5-mm-thick images. **a** 3-D surface display shows the incomplete twin (*) arising from the left hemipelvis region. The infant's normal lower extremity is inferior to this tissue (*arrow*), with the lower extremity of the more well-developed portion of the incomplete twin seen extending superiorly (*arrowheads*). Computed tomography (CT) angiographic technique was performed to help define the relationship of the vasculature and osseous structures for operative planning. Information from the CT angiogram obviated conventional angiography. **b** Volume-rendered 3-D image for bone detail, viewed posteriorly, demonstrates the native lower extremity inferiorly with two lower extremities from the incomplete twin arising from the hemipelvis and extending superiorly. **c** Axial image from level of the iliac crest demonstrates the course of a common iliac vessel supplying both the full twin's lower extremity and the incomplete twin's (*) lower extremity. **d** *Arrow* demonstrates the origin of the vascularity for the incomplete twin's lower extremities. The acetabulum and subjacent proximal femur (*arrowhead*) of the complete twin are seen

Pediatric CT Angiography

The technique for assessing the cardiovascular system was discussed above, in the context of IV contrast administration. While the kVp can be decreased for CT angiographic evaluation, a slightly higher tube current (up to 50% above that used for general body CT (see Table 18) is generally used (Fig. 14). Because images as thin as 0.625–1.25 mm may also be reviewed for small vessel detail, a higher mA will reduce the noise in these data sets. It is important to realize that pediatric CT angiography comprises more than simply arterial enhancement. CT angiographic technical considerations may need to be modified in any examination in which vascular enhancement is important, including venous opacification (in this case, delayed images after an arterial phase should be obtained)

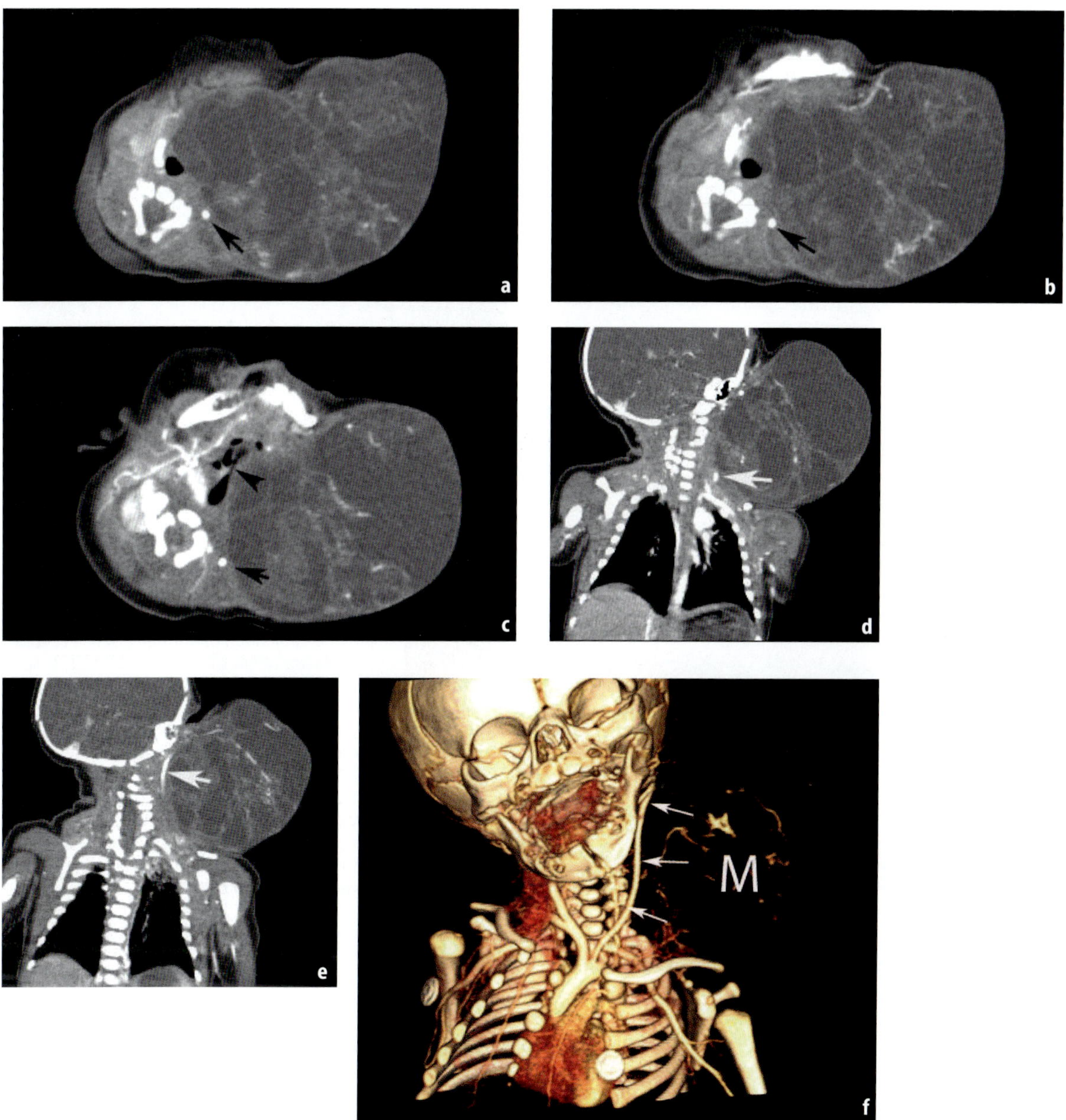

Fig. 14a-f. Newborn girl with left neck lymphatic malformation. Computed tomography (CT) angiogram for pre-operative planning. Technique: 100 kVp, 160 mA, 0.5 s (80 mAs), 0.984 pitch, 2.5-mm-thick. Axial images from just above the thoracic inlet (**a**) level of the mandible (**b**) and, more superiorly, in the mandible (**c**) demonstrate the large multi-cystic mass and its relationship to the mandible and deeper structures within the neck, as well as the densely opacified left carotid artery (*arrows* in **a-c**), which is displaced posteriorly and laterally. Note narrowing of the airway (*arrow*) in (**c**) just at the level of the larynx due to the mass. Coronal reformations show the course of the displaced left, carotid artery (*arrow*) at the level of the aortic arch (**d**), and at a slightly more posterior location (**e**). The course of the common carotid artery (*arrows*) is best demonstrated in the volume-rendered 3D image (**f**). Note the relationship of the common carotid artery (*arrows*) medial to the mass (*M*). There is also some superior positioning and a deformation of the left mandible due to chronic mass effect. Because airway and bone information was necessary for surgical planning, and sedation would have likely been necessary, magnetic resonance angiography was not performed

(Fig. 15) or a simultaneous depiction of artery and veins requiring a biphasic-type administration (Fig. 5), as discussed regarding IV contrast administration. There are several reviews of the recommended techniques for thoracic and body MDCT angiography in children [21, 22, 27, 35].

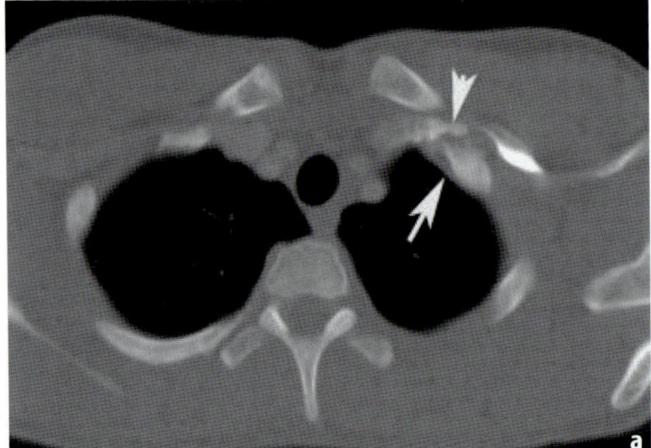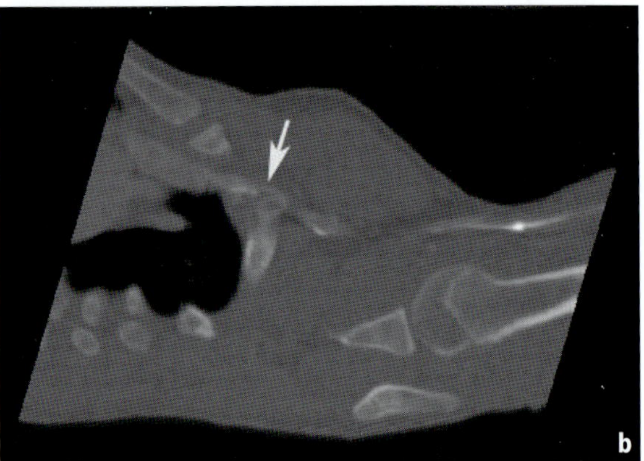

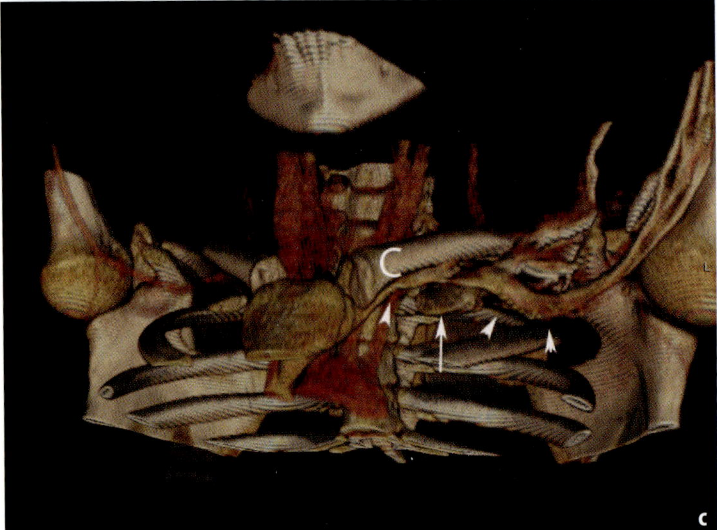

Fig. 15a-c. A 15-year-old-boy with left upper extremity numbness and swelling due to thoracic inlet compression. **a** Axial image from an MDCT examination performed elsewhere (technical factors unavailable) shows the course of the subclavian vein (*arrowhead*) adjacent to the left first rib with a slightly thickened end (*arrow*). **b** Curved reformat reconstruction demonstrates narrowing of the vein at the *arrow* at the level of the first rib (*arrow*). **c** Volume-rendered reconstruction shows the course of the vein (*arrowheads*) with narrowing between the left first rib (*arrow*) and inferior clavicle. CT examination was performed only through the upper chest, thereby limiting the radiation dose

Additional Technical Considerations

Recommendations for region- or organ-specific lower dose scanning in children address chest [36-38], airway [39], brain [40], sinuses [41, 42], skeletal evaluation [43, 44], and CT colonography [45]. Two other methods for dose management include tube-current modulation and in-plane shielding (using dose-attenuating material within the scan range to shield relatively radiosensitive organs or regions). For tube-current modulation, two excellent reviews are available [46, 47]. The dose-saving benefits of this technology in children have been reported [48-50], with one investigation finding dose savings of up to 43% compared with non-modulated examinations [50]. Although its value is debated [51], breast shielding in pediatric chest MDCT has also been shown to reduce the dose in children, with savings of up to 53% if used in conjunction with tube-current modulation [52, 53]. These authors noted that not all types of tube-current modulation technology are amenable to use with breast shields, since the dose may be increased through the shielded region to compensate for the higher-attenuation shields [53].

Conclusion

In the pediatric population, IV contrast-enhanced MDCT can be challenging. However, with attention to issues of scan preparation, and the use of a scan technique that takes into account the administration of IV contrast medium and individual CT settings, these challenges can be minimized. In addition, adequate attention to technique should address safety considerations, particularly radiation dose, in children. By subscribing to the principle that adequate diagnostic information and the child's welfare are the responsibilities of radiologists and the radiology team, the benefit to the child of MDCT examinations is optimized.

References

1. Donnelly LF, Frush DP (2003) Pediatric multidetector body CT. Radiol Clin North Am 41:637-655
2. Frush DP, Frush KS (2006) In a new kind of light: patient safety in pediatric radiology. Clin Ped Emerg Med 7:255-260
3. Donnelly LF (1997) Commentary: oral contrast medium administration for abdominal CT–reevalu-

ating the benefits and disadvantages in the pediatric patient. Pediatr Radiol 27:770

4. Kaste S, Laningham F, Stazzone M et al (2007) Safety in pediatric MR and cardiac CT. Pediatr Radiol 37:409-412

5. Frush DP (2005) Multislice CT–Pediatric Principles and Protocols. In: Knollman F, Coakley FV, eds. Elsevier Inc., Philadelphia, PA, 179-201

6. Cohen MD, Smith JA (1994) Intravenous use of ionic and nonionic contrast agents in children. Radiology 191:793

7. Dillman JR, Strouse PJ, Ellis JH et al (2007) Incidence and severity of acute allergic-like reactions to i.v. nonionic iodinated contrast material in children. AJR Am J Roentgenol 188(6):1643-1647. Erratum in: AJR Am J Roentgenol 2007 Sep;189(3):512

8. Gaca AM, Frush DP, Hohenhaus S et al (2007) Enhancing pediatric safety: using simulation to assess radiology resident preparedness for anaphylaxis from intravenous contrast media. Radiology 245:236-44

9. UNSCEAR (2000) Medical radiation exposures, annex D. United Nations Scientific Committee on the Effects of Atomic Radiation Report to the General Assembly; New York

10. Frush DP, Applegate K (2004) Computed tomography and radiation: Understanding the issues. J Am Coll of Radiol 1:113-119

11. Brenner DJ, Hall EJ (2007) Computed Tomography – An Increasing Source of Radiation Exposure. NEJM 357:2277-2284

12. Frush DP, Donnelly LF, Rosen N (2003) CT and radiation risks: What pediatric health care providers should know. Pediatrics 112:951-957

13. Amis ES Jr, Butler PF, Applegate KE et al (2007) American College of Radiology white paper on radiation dose in medicine. J Am Coll Radiol 4:272-84

14. Slovis TL, Frush DP, Berdon WE et al (2007) Biological Effects of Diagnostic Radiation on Children. In: Slovis T (ed) Caffey's Pediatric Diagnostic Imaging. 11th Edition. Elsevier 3-12

15. Frush DP (2006) Categorical Course in Physics: Ra diation Dose and Image Quality for Pediatric CT: clinical considerations. Radiological Society of North American 167-182

16. Thomas KE, Wang BB (2008) Age-specific effective doses for Pediatric MSCT examinations at a large children's hospital using DLP conversion coefficients; a simple estimation method. Pediatr Radiol (In press)

17. Huda W, Vance A (2007) Patient radiation doses from adult and pediatric CT. AJR Am J Roentgenol 188:540-6

18. Huda W (2008) Computing effective doses to pediatric patients undergoing body CT examinations. Pediatr Radiol (In press)

19. Cohen RA, Frush DP, Donnelly LF (2000) Data acquisition for pediatric CT angiography: problems and solutions. Pediatr Radiol 30:813-822

20. Fleischmann D (2003) Use of high-concentration contrast media in multiple-detector-row CT: principles and rationale. Eur Radiol 13(Suppl 5):M14-20

21. Frush DP, Herlong RJ (2005) Pediatric thoracic CT angiography. Pediatr Radiol 35:11-25

22. Chan FP, Rubin GD (2005) MDCT angiography of pediatric vascular diseases of the abdomen, pelvis, and extremities. Pediatr Radiol 35:40-53

23. Salis AI, Eclavea A, Johnson MS et al (2004) Maximal flow rates possible during power injection through currently available PICCs: an in vitro study. J Vasc Interv Radiol 15:275-281

24. Hollingsworth CL, Frush DP, Cross M et al (2003) Helical CT of the body: A survey of techniques used for pediatric patients. AJR Am J Roentgenol 180:401-406

25. Frush DP, Donnelly LF, Bisset GS (2001) Technical innovation: Effect of scan delay on hepatic enhancement for pediatric abdominal multislice helical CT. AJR Am J Roentgenol 176:1559-1561

26. Frush DP, Spencer EB, Donnelly LF et al (1999) Optimizing contrast-enhanced abdominal CT in infants and children using bolus tracking. AJR Am J Roentgenol 172:1007

27. Frush DP (2005) Technique of pediatric thoracic CT angiography. Radiol Clin North Am 43(2):419-433

28. da Costa e Silva EJ, da Silva GA (2007) Eliminating unenhanced CT when evaluating abdominal neoplasms in children. AJR Am J Roentgenol 189:1211-1214

29. van der Molen AJ, Geleijns J (2007) Overranging in multisection CT: quantification and relative contribution to dose–comparison of four 16-section CT scanners. Radiology 242:208-216

30. Donnelly LF, Emery KH, Brody AS et al (2001) Minimizing radiation dose for pediatric body applications of single-detector helical CT: Strategies at a large children's hospital. AJR Am J Roentgenol 176(2):303-306

31. Arch ME, Frush DP (2008) Pediatric Body MDCT: A Five-Year Follow-Up Survey of Scan Parameters Used by Pediatric Radiologists. AJR Am J Roentgenol February 2008 (In press)

32. Vade A, Demos TC, Olson MC et al (1996) Evaluation of image quality using 1:1 pitch and 1.5:1 pitch helical CT in children: a comparative study Pediatr Radiol 26:891-893

33. Vade A, Olson MC, Vittore CP et al (1999) Hepatic enhancement analysis in children using Smart Prep monitoring for 2:1 pitch helical scanning. Pediatr Radiol 29:689-693

34. Long FR, Castile RG, Brody AS et al (1999) Lungs in infants and young children: improved thin-section computed tomography with a noninvasive controlled-ventilation technique: initial experience. Radiology 212:588-593

35. Siegel MS (2003) Multiplanar and three-dimensional multidetector row CT of thoracic vessels and airways in the pediatric population. Radiology 229:641-650

36. Lucaya J, Piqueras J, García-Peña P et al (2000) Low-dose high-resolution CT of the chest in children and young adults: dose, cooperation, artifact incidence, and image quality. AJR Am J Roentgenol 175:985-992

37. Rogalla P, Stover B, Scheer I et al (1999) Low-dose spiral CT; applicability to paediatric chest imaging. Pediatr Radiol 29:565-569

38. Ambrosino MM, Genieser NB, Roche KJ et al (1994) Feasibility of high-resolution, low-dose chest CT in evaluating the pediatric chest. Pediatr Radiol 24:6-10

39. Pacharn P, Poe SA, Donnelly LF (2002) Low-tube-current multidetector CT for children with suspected extrinsic airway compression. AJR Am J Roentgenol 179:1523-1527

40. Cohnen M, Fischer H, Hamacher J et al (2000) CT of the head by reduced current and kilovoltage: relationship between image quality and dose reduction. Am J Neuroradiol 21:1654-1660

41. Hein E, Rogalla P, Klingebiel R et al (2002) Low-dose CT of the paranasal sinuses with eye lens protection: effect on image quality and radiation dose. Eur Radiol 12:1693-1696

42. Mulkens TH, Broers C, Fieuws S (2005) Comparison

of effective doses for low-dose MDCT and radiographic examination of sinuses in children. AJR Am J Roentgenol 184:1611-1618

43. Salamipour H, Jimenez RM, Brec SL et al (2005) Multidetector row CT in pediatric musculoskeletal imaging. Pediatr Radiol 35:555-564

44. Chapman VM, Kalra M, Halpern E et al (2004) 16-MDCT of the posttraumatic pediatric elbow: optimum parameters and associated radiation dose. AJR Am J Roentgenol 185:516-521

45. Anupindi S, Perumpillichira J, Jaramillo D et al (2005) Low-dose CT colonography in children: initial experience, technical feasibility, and utility. Pediatr Radiol 35:518-524

46 Kalra MK, Maher MM, Toth TL et al (2004) Techniques and applications of automatic tube current modulation for CT. Radiology 233:649-657

47. McCollough CH, Bruesewitz MR, Kofler JM Jr (2006) CT dose reduction and dose management tools: overview of available options. Radiographics 26:503-512

48. Greess H, Nömayr A, Wolf H et al (2002) Dose reduction in CT examination of children by an attenuation-based on-line modulation of tube current (CARE Dose). Eur Radiol 12:1571-1576

49. Greess H, Wolf H, Baum U et al (2000) Dose reduction in computed tomography by attenuation-based on-line modulation of tube current: evaluation of six anatomical regions. Eur Radiol 10:391-394

50. Greess H, Lutze J, Nomayr A et al (2004) Dose reduction in subsecond multislice spiral CT examination of children by online tube current modulation. Eur Radiol 14:995-999

51. Geleijns J, Salvadó Artells M, Veldkamp WJ et al (2006) Quantitative assessment of selective in-plane shielding of tissues in computed tomography through evaluation of absorbed dose and image quality. Eur Radio 16:2334-40

52. Fricke BL, Donnelly LF, Frush DP et al (2003) In-Plane bismuth breast shields for pediatric CT: effects on dose and imaging quality using experimental and clinical data. AJR Am J Roentgenol 180:407-411

53. Coursey C, Frush D, Yoshizumi T et al (2008) Pediatric chest MDCT and tube current modulation: effect on radiation dose with breast shielding. Pediatric chest MDCT using tube current modulation: effect on radiation dose with breast shielding. AJR Am J Roentgenol 190: 54-61

APPENDIX

MDCT Protocols

Authors

Lincoln L. Berland
Department of Radiology
University of Alabama at Birmingham
Birmingham, AL, USA

W. Dennis Foley
Medical College of Wisconsin
Milwaukee, WI, USA

Donald P. Frush
Department of Radiology
Duke University Medical Center
Durham, NC, USA

Jay P. Heiken
Mallinckrodt Institute of Radiology
Washington University School of Medicine
St. Louis, MO, USA

Vassilios Raptopoulos
Department of Radiology
Beth Israel Deaconess Medical Center
Boston, MA, USA

Dushyant V. Sahani
Department of Radiology
Massachusetts General Hospital
Harvard Medical School
Boston, MA, USA

Note to the readers:
Protocols described in this section and elsewhere in this textbook may need adjustments for type of CT equipment, scanning protocols, type and concentration of contrast agent, patients' size and condition, and clinical indication for CT scanning.

MDCT Protocols - Chest CT

Name of the protocol	Chest
Vendor and detector rows	Philips 16
Phase	Portal venous
Scan range	Apex to costophrenic recess
Detector configuration	16 × 0.75
Rotation time (s)	0.5
Pitch	0.95
Table speed (mm/rotation)	11.4
kVp	120
mA	250 (average patient) with DoseRight™
Reconstruction algorithm	Filter kernel C
Prospective slice thickness (mm)	5
Reconstruction interval (mm)	5
Oral contrast	None
IV contrast concentration (mg/ml)	370
IV contrast volume (cc)	80
IV contrast injection rate (cc/s)	3
Scan delay (fixed or bolus tracking)	Fixed @ 40 s
Saline chaser (cc)	40
Other	3-mm coronal MIP recon from 2.5-mm slices

Name of the protocol	Chest
Vendor and detector rows	Philips 40 and 64
Phase	Portal venous
Scan range	Apex to costophrenic recess
Detector configuration	40 × 0.625 or 64 × 0.625
Rotation time (s)	0.5
Pitch	1.17
Table speed (mm/rotation)	29.2 (40-slice), 46.8 (64-slice)
kVp	120
mA	250 (average patient) with DoseRight™
Reconstruction algorithm	Filter kernel C
Prospective slice thickness (mm)	5
Reconstruction interval (mm)	5
Oral contrast	None
IV contrast concentration (mg/ml)	370
IV contrast volume (cc)	80
IV contrast injection rate (cc/s)	3
Scan delay (fixed or bolus tracking)	Fixed @ 45 s
Saline chaser (cc)	40
Other	3-mm coronal MIP recon from 2.5-mm slices

Name of the protocol	Chest
Vendor and detector rows	GE 16
Phase	Arterial
Scan range	Inferior neck through adrenal glands
Detector configuration	16 × 1.25
Rotation time (s)	0.5
Pitch	1.375
Table speed (mm/rotation)	27.5
kVp	120
mA	AutomA 3-D Noise index 15.8
Reconstruction algorithm	Standard
Prospective slice thickness (mm)	2.5
Reconstruction interval (mm)	2.5
Oral contrast	None
IV contrast concentration (mg/ml)	350–370
IV contrast volume (cc)	75
IV contrast injection rate (cc/s)	3
Scan delay (fixed or bolus tracking)	25
Saline chaser (cc)	
Comment (1)	Routine sagittal and coronal reformations from 1.25-mm axial data with 50% overlap. Reformations 2.5-mm thick

Name of the protocol	Chest
Vendor and detector rows	GE 64
Phase	Arterial
Scan range	Inferior neck through adrenal glands
Detector configuration	64 × 0.625
Rotation time (s)	0.5
Pitch	1.375
Table speed (mm/rotation)	55
kVp	120
mA	AutomA 3-D Noise index 15.8
Reconstruction algorithm	Standard
Prospective slice thickness (mm)	2.5
Reconstruction interval (mm)	2.5
Oral contrast	None
IV contrast concentration (mg/ml)	350–370
IV contrast volume (cc)	75
IV contrast injection rate (cc/s)	3
Scan delay (fixed or bolus tracking)	25
Saline chaser (cc)	
Comment	Routine sagittal and coronal reformations from 0.625-mm axial data. Reformations 2.5-mm thick

Name of the protocol	Chest
Vendor and detector rows	Siemens 16
Phase	
Scan range	Above apex of lungs to below adrenal glands
Detector configuration	16 × 0.75
Rotation time (s)	0.5*
Pitch	1
Table speed (mm/rotation)	12
kVp	120
Effective mAs	140*
Reconstruction algorithm	Soft tissue (B20f); lung (B60f)
Prospective slice thickness (mm)	5
Reconstruction interval (mm)	5
Oral contrast	None
IV contrast concentration (mg/ml)	370
IV contrast volume (cc)	75
IV contrast injection rate (cc/s)	3*
Scan delay (fixed or bolus tracking)	25 s
Saline chaser (cc)	30 (optional)
Other	* For very large patients (>250 lbs), increase rotation time to 1.0 s and injection rate to 4ml/s. Increase effective mAs as needed

Name of the protocol	Chest
Vendor and detector rows	Siemens 64
Phase	
Scan range	Above apex of lungs to below adrenal glands
Detector configuration	64 × 0.6
Rotation time (s)	0.5*
Pitch	1
Table speed (mm/rotation)	19.2
kVp	120
Effective mAs	180**; ***
Reconstruction algorithm	Soft tissue (B20f); lung (B60f)
Prospective slice thickness (mm)	5
Reconstruction interval (mm)	5
Oral contrast	None
IV contrast concentration (mg/ml)	370
IV contrast volume (cc)	75
IV contrast injection rate (cc/s)	3***
Scan delay (fixed or bolus tracking)	25
Saline chaser (cc)	30 (optional)
Other	* Increase rotation time for very large patients ** Use CARE Dose 4-D *** For very large patients (>250 lbs), increase injection rate to 4 ml/s in addition to increasing volume to 125 ml. Increase effective mAs as needed

Name of the protocol	Chest (Chest Pain)
Vendor and detector rows	GE 16 Pro
Phase	Arterial*
Scan range	Above the arch to base of heart**
Detector configuration	16 × 0.625
Rotation time (s)	0.5
Pitch	0.938
Table speed (mm/rotation)	9.37
kVp	120***
mA	AEC (NI 11.57; range 150 – 500)***
Reconstruction algorithm	Standard
Prospective slice thickness (mm)	5****
Reconstruction interval (mm)	5
Oral contrast	None
IV contrast concentration (mg/ml)	350
IV contrast volume (cc)	90 (100 if CT venography)
IV contrast injection rate (cc/s)	4
Scan delay (fixed or bolus tracking)	200 HU at pulmonary artery
Saline chaser (cc)	30
Other	* Combined phase PA & aorta ** CT venography: pelvis to below knees: 3 min later (controversial) *** Pregnancy: 100 kVp; 200 mA **** 5 × 5-mm Coronal and sagittal slices routinely

Name of the protocol	Chest (Chest Pain)
Vendor and detector rows	GE 64 VCT
Phase	Arterial*
Scan range	Above the arch to base of heart**
Detector configuration	64 × 0.625
Rotation time (s)	0.5
Pitch	1.37
Table speed (mm/rotation)	54
kVp	120***
mA	AEC (NI 11.57; range 150 – 500)***
Reconstruction algorithm	Standard
Prospective slice thickness (mm)	5****
Reconstruction interval (mm)	5
Oral contrast	None
IV contrast concentration (mg/ml)	350
IV contrast volume (cc)	75 (100 if venography)
IV contrast injection rate (cc/s)	4
Scan delay (fixed or bolus tracking)	200 HU at pulmonary artery
Saline chaser (cc)	30
Other	* Combined phase PA & aorta ** CT venography: pelvis to below knees: 3 min later (controversial) *** Pregnancy: 100 kVp; 200 mA **** 5 × 5-mm coronal and sagittal slices routinely

Name of the protocol	Chest (Chest Pain)
Vendor and detector rows	Toshiba 16 Aquilion
Phase	Arterial*
Scan range	Above the arch to base of heart**
Detector configuration	16 × 1
Rotation time (s)	0.5
Pitch	0.937
Table speed (mm/rotation)	14.99
kVp	120***
mA	AEC (SD 12; range 150 – 500)***
Reconstruction algorithm	Standard
Prospective slice thickness (mm)	5****
Reconstruction interval (mm)	5
Oral contrast	None
IV contrast concentration (mg/ml)	350
IV contrast volume (cc)	100
IV contrast injection rate (cc/s)	4
Scan delay (fixed or bolus tracking)	200 HU at pulmonary artery
Saline chaser (cc)	30
Other	* Combined phase PA & aorta ** CT venography: pelvis to below knees: 3 min later (controversial) *** Pregnancy: 100 kVp; 200 mA **** 5 × 5-mm coronal and sagittal slices routinely

Name of the protocol	Chest (Chest Pain)
Vendor and detector rows	Toshiba 64 Aquilion
Phase	Arterial*
Scan range	Above the arch to base of heart**
Detector configuration	64 × 0.5
Rotation time (s)	0.5
Pitch	0.828
Table speed (mm/rotation)	53
kVp	120***
mA	AEC (SD 12; range 150 – 500)***
Reconstruction algorithm	Standard
Prospective slice thickness (mm)	5****
Reconstruction interval (mm)	5
Oral contrast	None
IV contrast concentration (mg/ml)	350
IV contrast volume (cc)	75 (100 if venography)
IV contrast injection rate (cc/s)	4
Scan delay (fixed or bolus tracking)	200 HU at pulmonary artery
Saline chaser (cc)	30
Other	* Combined phase PA & aorta ** CT venography: Pelvis to below knees: 3 min later (controversial) *** Pregnancy: 100 kVp; 200 mA **** 5 × 5-mm coronal and sagittal slices routinely

Name of the protocol	Abdomen-Pelvis
Vendor and detector rows	Philips 16
Phase	Portal venous
Scan range	Diaphragm to ischium
Detector configuration	16 × 0.75
Rotation time (s)	0.75
Pitch	0.95
Table speed (mm/rotation)	11.4
kVp	120
mA	250 (average patient) with DoseRight™
Reconstruction algorithm	Filter kernel C
Prospective slice thickness (mm)	5
Reconstruction interval (mm)	5
Oral contrast	Positive
IV contrast concentration (mg/ml)	370
IV contrast volume (cc)	100-130 lbs: 85 ml, 130-200: 115, 200-240: 140, >240: 175
IV contrast injection rate (cc/s)	Adjust rate to target duration of 30 s
Scan delay (fixed or bolus tracking)	40 s after injection completion
Saline chaser (cc)	40
Other	3-mm coronals recon from 2.5-mm slices

Name of the protocol	Abdomen-Pelvis
Vendor and detector rows	Philips 40 and 64
Phase	Portal venous
Scan range	Diaphragm to ischium
Detector configuration	40 × 0.625 or 64 × 0.625
Rotation time (s)	0.75
Pitch	1.17
Table speed (mm/rotation)	29.2 (40-slice), 46.8 (64-slice)
kVp	120
mA	250 (average patient) with DoseRight™
Reconstruction algorithm	Filter kernel C
Prospective slice thickness (mm)	5
Reconstruction interval (mm)	5
Oral contrast	Positive
IV contrast concentration (mg/ml)	370
IV contrast volume (cc)	100–130 lbs: 85 ml, 130–200: 115, 200–240: 140, >240: 175
IV contrast injection rate (cc/s)	Adjust rate to target duration of 30 s
Scan delay (fixed or bolus tracking)	40 s after injection completion
Saline chaser (cc)	40
Other	3-mm coronals recon from 2.5-mm slices

Name of the protocol	CTA Abdomen-Pelvis
Vendor and detector rows	Philips 16
Phase	Arterial
Scan range	Diaphragm to pubic symphysis
Detector configuration	16 × 0.75
Rotation time (s)	0.75
Pitch	1.25
Table speed (mm/rotation)	15
kVp	120
mA	250 (average patient) with DoseRight™
Reconstruction algorithm	Filter kernel C
Prospective slice thickness (mm)	1.5 (for 3-D, MIP), 5 (for axial review)
Reconstruction interval (mm)	1.0 (for 3-D, MIP), 5 (for axial review)
Oral contrast	None
IV contrast concentration (mg/ml)	370
IV contrast volume (cc)	100–130 lbs: 85 ml, 130–200: 115, 200–240: 140, >240: 175
IV contrast injection rate (cc/s)	4
Scan delay (fixed or bolus tracking)	Tracking: descending aorta @ 100 HU
Saline chaser (cc)	40
Other coronals	Volume-rendered 3-D

Name of the protocol	CTA Abdomen-Pelvis
Vendor and detector rows	Philips 40 and 64
Phase	Arterial
Scan range	Diaphragm to pubic symphysis
Detector Configuration	40 × 0.625 or 64 × 0.625
Rotation Time (s)	0.75
Pitch	1.17
Table Speed (mm/rotation)	29.2 (40-slice), 46.8 (64 slice)
kVp	120
mA	250 (average patient) with DoseRight™
Reconstruction algorithm	Filter kernel C
Prospective slice thickness (mm)	1.5 (for 3-D, MIP), 5 (for axial review)
Reconstruction interval (mm)	1.0 (for 3-D, MIP), 5 (for axial review)
Oral contrast	None
IV contrast concentration (mg/ml)	370
IV contrast volume (cc)	100–130 lbs: 85 ml, 130–200: 115, 200–240: 140, >240: 175
IV contrast injection rate (cc/s)	4
Scan delay (fixed or bolus tracking)	Tracking: descending aorta @ 100 HU
Saline chaser (cc)	40
Other coronals	Volume-rendered 3-D

Name of the protocol	Abdomen-Pelvis
Vendor and detector rows	GE 16
Phase	Hepatic (portal venous)
Scan range	Dome of liver through pubic bones
Detector configuration	16 × 1.25
Rotation time (s)	0.5
Pitch	1.375
Table speed (mm/rotation)	27.5
kVp	120 – 140 (dependent on body habitus)
mA	AutomA 3-D Noise index 15.8
Reconstruction algorithm	Standard
Prospective slice thickness (mm)	2.5
Reconstruction interval (mm)	2.5
Oral contrast	Positive
IV Contrast concentration (mg/ml)	350–370
IV Contrast volume (cc)	150
IV Contrast injection rate (cc/s)	4
Scan Delay (fixed or bolus tracking)	Smart Prep (50 HU Threshold)
Saline chaser (cc)	
Comment (1)	Oral contrast for all IV contrast dependent on renal function Rectal contrast at discretion of radiologist
Comment (2)	Sagittal and coronal reformations for solid mass lesions, fluid collections, bowel obstruction

Name of the protocol	Abdomen-Pelvis
Vendor and detector rows	GE 64
Phase	Hepatic (portal venous)
Scan range	Dome of liver through pubic bones
Detector configuration	64 × 0.625
Rotation time (s)	0.5
Pitch	0.984
Table speed (mm/rotation)	40
kVp	120 – 140 (dependent on body habitus)
mA	AutomA 3-D Noise index 15.8
Reconstruction algorithm	Standard
Prospective slice thickness (mm)	2.5
Reconstruction interval (mm)	2.5
Oral contrast	Positive
IV contrast concentration (mg/ml)	350–370
IV contrast volume (cc)	150
IV contrast injection rate (cc/s)	4
Scan delay (fixed or bolus tracking)	Smart prep (50 HU Threshold)
Saline chaser (cc)	
Comment (1)	Oral contrast for all IV contrast dependent on renal function Rectal contrast at discretion of radiologist
Comment (2)	Sagittal and coronal reformations for mass lesions, fluid collections, bowel obstruction

Name of the protocol	Lower Extremity CTA
Vendor and detector rows	GE 16
Phase	Arterial
Scan range	Supraceliac aorta to feet
Detector configuration	16 × 1.25
Rotation time (s)	0.5
Pitch	1.375
Table speed (mm/rotation)	27.5
kVp	120 – 140 (dependent on body habitus)
mA	AutomA 3-D Noise index 14
Reconstruction algorithm	Standard
Prospective slice thickness (mm)	1.25 (3-D imaging) 2.5 (workstation review)
Reconstruction interval (mm)	1.25 (3-D imaging) 2.5 (workstation review)
Oral contrast	None
IV contrast concentration (mg/ml)	370
IV contrast volume (cc)	110 (standard)
IV contrast injection rate (cc/s)	5
Scan Delay (fixed or bolus tracking)	Time to peak on preliminary minibolus in supraceliac aorta plus 4 s
Saline chaser (cc)	50 ml, 5 ml/s

Name of the protocol	Lower Extremity CTA
Vendor and detector rows	GE 64
Phase	Arterial
Scan range	Supraceliac aorta to feet
Detector configuration	64 × 0.625
Rotation time (s)	0.5 (standard) see comment
Pitch	1.375 (standard) see comment
Table speed (mm/rotation)	55 (standard) see comment
kVp	120 – 140 (dependent on body habitus)
mA	AutomA 3-D Noise index 14
Reconstruction algorithm	Standard
Prospective slice thickness (mm)	0.625 (3-D imaging) 2.5 (workstation review)
Reconstruction interval (mm)	0.625 (3-D imaging) 2.5 (workstation review)
Oral contrast	None
IV contrast concentration (mg/ml)	370
IV contrast volume (cc)	90 (standard) see comment
IV contrast injection rate (cc/s)	6
Scan delay (fixed or bolus tracking)	Time to peak on preliminary mini bolus in supra celiac aorta plus 4 s
Saline chaser (cc)	50 ml, 6 ml/s
Comment	Preliminary determination of arterial flow velocity. Table speed adjusted (by changing rotation time, pitch, and beam width in that order) to equal flow velocity. Contrast injection time equals scan delay of 4 s plus acquisition interval

Name of the protocol	Abdomen/Pelvis
Vendor and detector rows	Siemens 16
Phase	Portal venous
Scan range	Above diaphragm to lesser trochanters
Detector configuration	16 × 1.5
Rotation time (s)	0.5*
Pitch	1
Table speed (mm/rotation)	24
kVp	120
Effective mAs	200*
Reconstruction algorithm	Soft tissue (B20f)
Prospective slice thickness (mm)	5*
Reconstruction interval (mm)	5
Oral contrast	Positive
IV contrast concentration (mg/ml)	370
IV contrast volume (cc)	125 (100<150 lbs; 150>250 lbs)
IV contrast injection rate (cc/s)	3
Scan delay (fixed or bolus tracking)	65
Saline chaser (cc)	30 (optional)
Other	* For very large patients, increase rotation time to 1.0 s, mAs to 380 eff, and slice thickness to 10-mm

Name of the protocol	Abdomen/Pelvis
Vendor and detector rows	Siemens 64
Phase	Portal venous
Scan range	Above diaphragm to lesser trochanters
Detector configuration	64 × 0.6*
Rotation time (s)	0.5*
Pitch	1
Table speed (mm/rotation)	19.2
kVp	120
Effective mAs	240*;**
Reconstruction algorithm	Soft tissue (B20f)
Prospective slice thickness (mm)	5
Reconstruction interval (mm)	5
Oral contrast	Positive
IV contrast concentration (mg/ml)	370
IV contrast volume (cc)	125 (100<150 lbs; 150>250 lbs)
IV contrast injection rate (cc/s)	3
Scan delay (fixed or bolus tracking)	65 s***
Saline chaser (cc)	30 (optional)
Other	* For very large patients, increase detector collimation to 1.2, rotation time to 1.0, and mAs to 380 eff ** Use CARE Dose 4-D *** Increase scan delay by 10 s for every 0.5 ml/s decrease in injection rate

Name of the protocol	Chest-Abd-Pelvis
Vendor and detector rows	Philips 16
Phase	Portal venous
Scan range	Apex to costophrenic recess (chest), then diaphragm to ischium (abd-pelv)
Detector configuration	16 × 0.75
Rotation time (s)	0.75
Pitch	0.95
Table speed (mm/rotation)	11.4
kVp	120
mA	250 (average patient) with DoseRight™
Reconstruction algorithm	Filter kernel C
Prospective slice thickness (mm)	5
Reconstruction interval (mm)	5
Oral contrast	Positive
IV contrast concentration (mg/ml)	370
IV contrast volume (cc)	100–130 lbs: 85 ml, 130–200: 115, 200–240: 140, >240: 175
IV contrast injection rate (cc/s)	Adjust rate to target duration of 30 s
Scan delay (fixed or bolus tracking)	Fixed @ 40 s (chest), 40 s after injection completion (abd-pelv)
Saline chaser (cc)	40
Other	Chest and abd-pelvis split because of timing 3-mm coronal MIP recon from 2.5-mm slices

Name of the protocol	Chest-Abd-Pelvis
Vendor and detector rows	Philips 40 and 64
Phase	Portal venous
Scan range	Apex to costophrenic recess (chest), then diaphragm to ischium (abd-pelv)
Detector configuration	40 × 0.625 or 64 × 0.625
Rotation time (s)	0.75
Pitch	1.17
Table speed (mm/rotation)	29.2 (40-slice), 46.8 (64 slice)
kVp	120
mA	250 (average patient) with DoseRight™
Reconstruction algorithm	Filter kernel C
Prospective slice thickness (mm)	5
Reconstruction interval (mm)	5
Oral contrast	Positive
IV contrast concentration (mg/ml)	370
IV contrast volume (cc)	100–130 lbs: 85 ml, 130–200: 115, 200–240: 140, >240: 175
IV contrast injection rate (cc/s)	Adjust rate to target duration of 30 s
Scan delay (fixed or bolus tracking)	Fixed @ 45 s (chest), 40 s after injection completion (abd-pelv)
Saline chaser (cc)	40
Other	Chest and abd-pelvis split because of timing 3-mm coronal MIP recon from 2.5-mm slices

Name of the protocol	Chest, Abdomen, Pelvis
Vendor and detector rows	GE 16
Phase	Vascular (chest), hepatic (portal venous) (abd, pelvis)
Scan range	Inferior neck through pubic bones
Detector configuration	16×1.25
Rotation time (s)	0.5
Pitch	1.375
Table speed (mm/rotation)	27.5
kVp	120 – 140 (dependent on body habitus)
mA	AutomA 3-D Noise index 15.8
Reconstruction algorithm	Standard
Prospective slice thickness (mm)	2.5
Reconstruction interval (mm)	2.5
Oral contrast	Positive
IV contrast concentration (mg/ml)	350–370
IV contrast volume (cc)	150
IV contrast injection rate (cc/s)	4
Scan delay (fixed or bolus tracking)	60
Saline chaser (cc)	
Comment (1)	Oral contrast for all IV contrast dependent on renal function Rectal contrast at discretion of radiologist
Comment (2)	Sagittal and coronal reformations for abdominal mass lesions, fluid collections, bowel obstruction

Name of the protocol	Chest, Abdomen, Pelvis
Vendor and detector rows	GE 64
Phase	Vascular (chest), hepatic (portal venous) (abd, pelvis)
Scan range	Inferior neck through pubic bones
Detector configuration	64×0.625
Rotation time (s)	0.5 s
Pitch	1.375
Table speed (mm/rotation)	55
kVp	120 – 140 (dependent on body habitus)
mA	AutomA 3-D Noise index 15.8
Reconstruction algorithm	Standard
Prospective slice thickness (mm)	2.5
Reconstruction interval (mm)	2.5
Oral contrast	Positive
IV contrast concentration (mg/ml)	350–370
IV contrast volume (cc)	150
IV contrast injection rate (cc/s)	4
Scan delay (fixed or bolus tracking)	65
Saline chaser (cc)	
Comment (1)	Oral contrast for all IV contrast dependent on renal function Rectal contrast at discretion of radiologist
Comment (2)	Sagittal and coronal reformations for abdominal mass lesions, fluid collections, bowel obstruction

Name of the protocol	Chest, Abdomen, Pelvis
Vendor and detector rows	Siemens 16
Phase	
Scan range	Above lung apex to lesser trochanters
Detector configuration	16 × 1.5*
Rotation time (s)	0.5*
Pitch	1
Table speed (mm/rotation)	24
kVp	120
Effective mAs	180*
Reconstruction algorithm	Soft tissue (B20f); lung (B60f)
Prospective slice thickness (mm)	5
Reconstruction interval (mm)	5
Oral contrast	Positive
IV contrast concentration (mg/ml)	370
IV contrast volume (cc)	125 (100<150 lbs; 150>250 lbs)
IV contrast injection rate (cc/s)	3
Scan delay (fixed or bolus tracking)	55
Saline chaser (cc)	30 (optional)
Other	* For very large patients, increase rotation time to 1.0 s and increase effective mAs as needed. Can also increase slice thickness to 10 mm

Name of the protocol	Chest, Abdomen, Pelvis
Vendor and detector rows	Siemens 64
Phase	
Scan range	Above lung apex to lesser trochanters
Detector configuration	64 × 0.6*
Rotation time (s)	0.5*
Pitch	1
Table speed (mm/rotation)	19.2
kVp	120
Effective mAs	220*; **
Reconstruction algorithm	Soft tissue (B20f); lung (B60f)
Prospective slice thickness (mm)	5
Reconstruction interval (mm)	5
Oral contrast	Positive
IV contrast concentration (mg/ml)	370
IV contrast volume (cc)	125 (100<150 lbs; 150>250 lbs)
IV contrast injection rate (cc/s)	3
Scan delay (fixed or bolus tracking)	60 ***
Saline chaser (cc)	30 (optional)
Other	* For very large patients, increase detector collimation to 1.2, rotation time to 1.0, and mAs to 380 eff. ** Use CARE Dose 4D *** Increase scan delay by 10 s for every 0.5 ml/s decrease in injection rate

MDCT Protocols - Pancreas

Name of the protocol	Pancreas-Staging
Vendor and detector rows	Philips 16
Phase	Noncontrast, pancreatic, portal venous
Scan range	Diaphragm to crest (noncontrast and panc), diaphragm to ischium (PV)
Detector configuration	16 × 0.75
Rotation time (s)	0.75
Pitch	0.95
Table speed (mm/rotation)	11.4
kVp	120
mA	275 (average patient) with DoseRight™
Reconstruction algorithm	Filter kernel C
Prospective slice thickness (mm)	5 (noncontrast), 3 (panc, PV), 5 (pelvis)
Reconstruction interval (mm)	5 (noncontrast), 3 (panc, PV), 5 (pelvis)
Oral contrast	Water or VoLumen™. Give cup water on table to fill duodenum
IV contrast concentration (mg/ml)	370
IV contrast volume (cc)	100–130 lbs: 85 ml, 130–200: 115, 200–240: 140, >240: 175
IV contrast injection rate (cc/s)	Adjust rate to target duration of 30 s
Scan delay (fixed or bolus tracking)	Tracking @ 100 HU+15 s (panc), 50 s after trigger (PV)
Saline chaser (cc)	40
Other	3-mm coronals recon from 2-mm slices 3-D surface from Panc phase Curved planar reformations

Name of the protocol	Pancreas-Staging
Vendor and detector rows	Philips 40 and 60
Phase	Noncontrast, pancreatic, portal venous
Scan range	Diaphragm to crest (noncontrast and panc), diaphragm to ischium (PV)
Detector configuration	40 × 0.625 or 64 × 0.625
Rotation time (s)	0.75
Pitch	1.17
Table speed (mm/rotation)	29.2 (40-slice), 46.8 (64 slice)
kVp	120
mA	275 (average patient) with DoseRight™
Reconstruction algorithm	Filter kernel C
Prospective slice thickness (mm)	5 (noncontrast), 3 (panc, PV), 5 (pelvis)
Reconstruction interval (mm)	5 (noncontrast), 3 (panc, PV), 5 (pelvis)
Oral contrast	Water or VoLumen™. Give cup water on table to fill duodenum
IV contrast concentration (mg/ml)	370
IV contrast volume (cc)	100–130 lbs: 85 ml, 130–200: 115, 200–240: 140, >240: 175
IV contrast injection rate (cc/s)	Adjust rate to target duration of 30 s
Scan delay (fixed or bolus tracking)	Tracking @ 100 HU+20 s (panc), 55 s after trigger (PV)
Saline chaser (cc)	40
Other	3-mm coronals recon from 2-mm slices 3-D surface from panc phase Curved planar reformations

Name of the protocol	Pancreatic
Vendor and detector rows	GE 16
Phase	Late arterial, hepatic (portal venous)
Scan range	Diaphragm through inferior liver (1st pass) Diaphragm through iliac crest (2nd Pass)
Detector configuration	16×1.25
Rotation time (s)	0.5
Pitch	1.375
Table speed (mm/rotation)	27.5
kVp	120 – 140 (dependent on body habitus)
mA	AutomA 3-D Noise index 15.8
Reconstruction algorithm	Standard
Prospective slice thickness (mm)	2.5
Reconstruction interval (mm)	2.5
Oral contrast	Negative
IV contrast concentration (mg/ml)	350–370
IV contrast volume (cc)	150
IV contrast injection rate (cc/s)	6
Scan delay (fixed or bolus tracking)	Time to peak on preliminary mini bolus in supra celiac aorta plus 15 s (late arterial phase) and 45 s (hepatic phase)
Saline chaser (cc)	
Comment (1)	Staging of suspected pancreatic carcinoma
Comment (2)	Initial exam in patient with severe acute pancreatitis
Comment (3)	Sagittal and coronal reformations for all abnormal studies
Comment (4)	CT pancreatography for abnormal pancreas
Comment (5)	CT cholangiography (Min IP) for dilated biliary system

Name of the protocol	Pancreatic
Vendor and detector rows	GE 64
Phase	Late arterial, hepatic (portal venous)
Scan range	Dome diaphragm thru inferior liver (1st Pass) Dome diaphragm thru iliac crest (2nd Pass)
Detector configuration	64×0.625
Rotation time (s)	0.5
Pitch	0.984
Table speed (mm/rotation)	40
kVp	120 – 140 (dependent on body habitus)
mA	AutomA 3-D Noise index 15.8
Reconstruction algorithm	Standard
Prospective slice thickness (mm)	2.5
Reconstruction interval (mm)	2.5
Oral contrast	Negative
IV contrast concentration (mg/ml)	350–370
IV contrast volume (cc)	150
IV contrast injection rate (cc/s)	6
Scan delay (fixed or bolus tracking)	Time to peak on preliminary minibolus in supraceliac aorta plus 15 s (late arterial phase) and 45 s (hepatic phase)
Saline chaser (cc)	
Comment (1)	Staging of suspected pancreatic carcinoma
Comment (2)	Initial exam in patient with severe acute pancreatitis
Comment (3)	Sagittal and coronal reformations for all abnormal studies
Comment (4)	CT pancreatography for abnormal pancreas
Comment (5)	CT cholangiography (Min IP) for dilated biliary system

Name of the protocol	Pancreas - Staging
Vendor and detector rows	Siemens 16
Phase	Noncontrast/pancreatic/portal venous
Scan range	Above diaphragm to iliac crest*
Detector configuration	16 × 1.5/0.75/1.5
Rotation time (s)	0.5
Pitch	0.9
Table speed (mm/rotation)	22/11/22
kVp	120
Effective mAs	180
Reconstruction algorithm	Soft tissue (B20f)
Prospective slice thickness (mm)	5/3 & 1/2 **
Reconstruction interval (mm)	5/3 & 0.8/2 **
Oral contrast	Water or VoLumen
IV contrast concentration (mg/ml)	370
IV contrast volume (cc)	125 (100<150 lbs; 150>250 lbs)
IV contrast injection rate (cc/s)	4
Scan delay (fixed or bolus tracking)	Bolus tracking with 15 s delay after arterial threshold for pancreatic phase ***
Saline chaser (cc)	40 (optional)

Other	* For pancreatic phase: Above top of pancreas to bottom of liver
	** Noncontrast: 5 × 5
	    Pancreatic: 3 × 3 & 1 × 0.8
	    Venous: 2 × 2
	*** Alternatively, can use fixed scan delay (40 s/60 s)

Name of the protocol	Pancreas - Staging
Vendor and detector rows	Siemens 64
Phase	Noncontrast/pancreatic/portal venous
Scan range	Above diaphragm to iliac crest*
Detector configuration	64 × 0.6
Rotation time (s)	0.5
Pitch	0.9
Table speed (mm/rotation)	17.3
kVp	120
Effective mAs	240**
Reconstruction algorithm	Soft tissue (B20f)
Prospective slice thickness (mm)	5 / 3 & 1 / 5&2 ***
Reconstruction interval (mm)	5 / 3 & 0.7 / 5&1 ***
Oral contrast (pos or neg)	Water or VoLumen
IV contrast concentration (mg/ml)	370
IV contrast volume (cc)	125 (100<150 lbs; 150>250 lbs)
IV contrast injection rate (cc/s)	4
Scan delay (fixed or bolus tracking)	Bolus tracking with 20 sec delay after 100 HU arterial threshold for pancreatic phase ***
Saline chaser (cc)	40 (optional)
Other	* For pancreatic phase: Above top of pancreas to bottom of liver ** Use CARE dose 4D *** Alternatively, can use fixed scan delay (45 s/65 s)

MDCT Protocols - Enterography

Name of the protocol	CT Enterography
Vendor and detector rows	Philips 16
Phase	Arterial, portal venous
Scan range	Diaphragm to ischium
Detector configuration	16 × 0.75
Rotation time (s)	0.5
Pitch	1.25
Table speed (mm/rotation)	15
kVp	120
mA	275 (average patient) with DoseRight™
Reconstruction algorithm	Filter kernel C
Prospective slice thickness (mm)	3 (both series)
Reconstruction interval (mm)	2 (both series)
Oral contrast	450 ml VoLumen™ every 20 min × 3. 300 ml water when on table
IV contrast concentration (mg/ml)	370
IV contrast volume (cc)	100–130 lbs: 85 ml, 130–200: 115, 200–240: 140, >240: 175
IV contrast injection rate (cc/s)	Adjust rate to target duration of 30
Scan delay (fixed or bolus tracking)	Bolus tracking (arterial), 40 s after injection completion (PV)
Saline chaser (cc)	40
Other	Coronals recon of both series 3-D surface rendered of arterial phase

Name of the protocol	CT Enterography
Vendor and detector rows	Philips 40 and 64
Phase	Arterial, portal venous
Scan range	Diaphragm to ischium
Detector configuration	40 × 0.625 or 64 × 0.625
Rotation time (s)	0.75
Pitch	1.17
Table speed (mm/rotation)	29.2 (40-slice), 46.8 (64-slice)
kVp	120
mA	275 (average patient) with DoseRight™
Reconstruction algorithm	Filter kernel C
Prospective slice thickness (mm)	3 (both series)
Reconstruction interval (mm)	2 (both series)
Oral contrast	450 ml VoLumen™ every 20 min × 3. 300 ml water when on table
IV contrast concentration (mg/ml)	370
IV contrast volume (cc)	100–130 lbs: 85 ml, 130–200: 115, 200–240: 140, >240: 175
IV contrast injection rate (cc/s)	Adjust rate to target duration of 30 s
Scan delay (fixed or bolus tracking)	Bolus tracking (arterial), 40 s after injection completion (PV)
Saline chaser (cc)	40
Other	Coronals recon of both series 3-D surface rendered of arterial phase

Name of the protocol	CT Enterography
Vendor and detector rows	GE 16
Phase	Hepatic (portal venous)
Scan range	Dome of diaphragm to pubic bones
Detector configuration	16 × 1.25
Rotation time (s)	0.5
Pitch	1.375
Table speed (mm/rotation)	27.5
kVp	120 – 140 (dependent on body habitus)
mA	AutomA 3-D Noise index 15.8
Reconstruction algorithm	Standard
Prospective slice thickness (mm)	2.5
Reconstruction interval (mm)	2.5
Oral contrast	VoLumen™
IV contrast concentration (mg/ml)	350–370
IV contrast volume (cc)	150
IV contrast injection rate (cc/s)	4
Scan delay (fixed or bolus tracking)	Smart Prep (hepatic att threshold 50)
Saline chaser (cc)	
Comment (1)	Volumen 450 ml given at 45, 30, and 15 min prior to scanning. 8 oz of water 1 min prior to scanning
Comment (2)	Coronal and sagittal image reformation routine

Name of the protocol	CT Enterography
Vendor and detector rows	GE 64
Phase	Hepatic (portal venous)
Scan range	Dome of diaphragm to pubic bones
Detector configuration	64 × 0.625
Rotation time (s)	0.5
Pitch	0.984
Table speed (mm/rotation)	40
kVp	120 – 140 (dependent on body habitus)
mA	AutomA 3-D Noise index 15.8
Reconstruction algorithm	Standard
Prospective slice thickness (mm)	2.5
Reconstruction interval (mm)	2.5
Oral contrast	VoLumen™
IV contrast concentration (mg/ml)	350–370
IV contrast volume (cc)	150
IV contrast injection rate (cc/s)	4
Scan delay (fixed or bolus tracking)	Smart Prep (hepatic att threshold 50)
Saline chaser (cc)	
Comment (1)	VoLumen 450 ml given at 45, 30 and 15 min prior to scanning , 8 oz of water 1 min prior to scanning
Comment (2)	Sagittal and coronal reformation routine

Name of the protocol	CTE Enterography
Vendor and detector rows	Siemens 16
Phase	Portal venous (– 5 s)
Scan range	Above diaphragm to lesser trochanters
Detector configuration	16 × 1.5
Rotation time (s)	0.5
Pitch	1
Table speed (mm/rotation)	24
kVp	120
Effective mAs	180
Reconstruction algorithm	Soft tissue (B20f)
Prospective slice thickness (mm)	5 & 2*
Reconstruction interval (mm)	5 & 2*
Oral contrast	VoLumen
IV contrast concentration (mg/ml)	370
IV contrast volume (cc)	125 (100<150 lbs; 150>250 lbs)
IV contrast injection rate (cc/s)	3
Scan delay (fixed or bolus tracking)	60
Saline chaser (cc)	30 (optional)

Other	* Two reconstructions:
	  5 × 5
	  2 × 2

Comment	Also reconstruct coronals (2 × 2)

Name of the protocol	Enterography (CTE)
Vendor and detector rows	Siemens 64
Phase	Portal venous (– 5 s)
Scan range	Above diaphragm to lesser trochanters
Detector configuration	64 × 0.6
Rotation time (s)	0.5
Pitch	1
Table speed (mm/rotation)	19.2
kVp	120
Effective mAs	240*
Reconstruction algorithm	Soft tissue (B20f)
Prospective slice thickness (mm)	5 and 2**
Reconstruction interval (mm)	5 and 2**
Oral contrast (pos or neg)	VoLumen
IV contrast concentration (mg/ml)	370
IV contrast volume (cc)	125 (100<150 lbs; 150>250 lbs)
IV contrast injection rate (cc/s)	3
Scan delay (fixed or bolus tracking)	60
Saline chaser (cc)	30 (optional)

Other	* Use CARE Dose 4D
	** Two reconstructions:
	  5 × 5
	  2 × 2

Comment	Also reconstruct coronals (2 × 2)

MDCT Protocols - Mesenteric

Name of the protocol	CTA Mesenteric
Vendor and detector rows	Philips 16
Phase	Arterial
Scan range	Diaphragm to mid-pelvis (arterial), diaphragm to ischium (PV)
Detector configuration	16 × 0.75
Rotation time (s)	0.5
Pitch	1.25
Table speed (mm/rotation)	15
kVp	120
mA	250 (average patient) with DoseRight™
Reconstruction algorithm	Filter kernel B
Prospective slice thickness (mm)	1.5 (for 3D, MIP), 5 (for axial review and for PV)
Reconstruction interval (mm)	1.0 (for 3D, MIP), 5 (for axial review and for PV)
Oral contrast	None
IV contrast concentration (mg/ml)	370
IV contrast volume (cc)	100–130 lbs: 85 ml, 130–200: 115, 200–240: 140, >240: 175
IV contrast injection rate (cc/s)	4
Scan delay (fixed or bolus tracking)	Tracking: descending aorta @100 HU, 55 s after trigger (PV)
Saline chaser (cc)	40
Other	Coronals – 10-mm MIP slab @ 3-mm Volume rendered 3-D

Name of the protocol	CTA Mesenteric
Vendor and detector rows	Philips 40 and 64
Phase	Arterial
Scan range	Diaphragm to mid-pelvis (arterial), diaphragm to ischium (PV)
Detector configuration	40 × 0.625 or 64 × 0.625
Rotation time (s)	0.5
Pitch	1.17
Table speed (mm/rotation)	29.2 (40-slice), 46.8 (64 slice)
kVp	120
mA	250 (average patient) with DoseRight™
Reconstruction algorithm	Filter kernel B
Prospective slice thickness (mm)	1.5 (for 3-D, MIP), 5 (for axial review and for PV)
Reconstruction interval (mm)	1.0 (for 3-D, MIP), 5 (for axial review and for PV)
Oral contrast	None
IV contrast concentration (mg/ml)	370
IV contrast volume (cc)	100–130 lbs: 85 ml, 130–200: 115, 200–240: 140, >240: 175
IV contrast injection rate (cc/s)	4
Scan delay (fixed or bolus tracking)	Tracking: descending aorta @100 HU, 55 s after trigger (PV)
Saline chaser (cc)	40
Other	Coronals – 10-mm MIP slab @ 3-mm Volume-rendered 3-D

Name of the protocol	Mesenteric
Vendor and detector rows	GE 16
Phase	Arterial, portal venous (double pass)
Scan range	Supra celiac aorta to inferior pubic bones
Detector configuration	16×0.625 (1st pass) 16×1.25 (2nd pass)
Rotation time (s)	0.5
Pitch	1.375
Table speed (mm/rotation)	13.75 (1st Pass) 27.5 (2nd Pass)
kVp	120 – 140 (dependent on body habitus)
mA	AutomA 3-D Noise index 14 (1st pass) Noise index 15.8 (2nd pass)
Reconstruction algorithm	Standard
Prospective slice thickness (mm)	0.625 (for 3-D imaging) 2.5 (workstation review)
Reconstruction interval (mm)	0.625 (for 3-D imaging) 2.5 (workstation review)
Oral contrast	None
IV contrast concentration (mg/ml)	370
IV contrast volume (cc)	100
IV contrast injection rate (cc/s)	6
Scan delay (fixed or bolus tracking)	Time to peak on preliminary minibolus in supraceliac aorta plus 4 s
Saline chaser (cc)	50 ml (at 6 ml/s)
Comment	Double pass examination, 2nd pass begins 15 s after the 1st pass and acquires a mesenteric capillary and early portal venous phase

Name of the protocol	Mesenteric
Vendor and detector rows	GE 64
Phase	Arterial, portal venous (double pass)
Scan range	Supra celiac aorta to inferior pubic bones
Detector configuration	64×0.625
Rotation time (s)	0.5 s
Pitch	0.984
Table speed (mm/rotation)	40
kVp	120 – 140 (dependent on body habitus)
mA	AutomA 3-D Noise index 14 (1st pass) Noise index 15.8 (2nd pass)
Reconstruction algorithm	Standard
Prospective slice thickness (mm)	0.625 (3-D imaging) 2.5 (workstation review)
Reconstruction interval (mm)	0.625 (3-D imaging) 2.5 (workstation review)
Oral contrast	None
IV contrast concentration (mg/ml)	370
IV contrast volume (cc)	100
IV contrast injection rate (cc/s)	6
Scan delay (fixed or bolus tracking)	Time to peak on preliminary minibolus in supraceliac aorta plus 4 s
Saline chaser (cc)	50 ml (at 6 ml/s)
Comment	Double pass examination, 2nd pass begins 15 s after the 1st pass and acquires a mesenteric capillary and early portal venous phase

Name of the protocol	Mesenteric/Ischemic Bowel
Vendor and detector rows	Siemens 16
Phase	Arterial/portal venous
Scan range	Above diaphragm to lesser trochanters
Detector configuration	16 × 1.5
Rotation time (s)	0.5
Pitch	1
Table speed (mm/rotation)	24
kVp	120
Effective mAs	180
Reconstruction algorithm	Soft tissue (B20f)
Prospective slice thickness (mm)	2
Reconstruction interval (mm)	2
Oral contrast	Water or none
IV contrast concentration (mg/ml)	370
IV contrast volume (cc)	100 (75<150 lbs; 125>250 lbs)
IV contrast injection rate (cc/s)	3
Scan delay (fixed or bolus tracking)	CARE Bolus*
Saline chaser (cc)	40 (optional)
Other	* Begin monitoring scans at 15 s Add 4-s delay after threshold (120 HU) is reached

Name of the protocol	Mesenteric/Ischemic Bowel
Vendor and detector rows	Siemens 64
Phase	Arterial/portal venous
Scan range	Above diaphragm to lesser trochanters
Detector configuration	64 × 0.6
Rotation time (s)	0.5
Pitch	1
Table speed (mm/rotation)	19.2
kVp	120
Effective mAs	240*
Reconstruction algorithm	Soft tissue (B20f)
Prospective slice thickness (mm)	2
Reconstruction interval (mm)	2
Oral contrast	Water or none
IV contrast concentration (mg/ml)	370
IV contrast volume (cc)	100 (75<150 lbs; 125>250 lbs)
IV contrast injection rate (cc/s)	4
Scan delay (fixed or bolus tracking)	CARE Bolus for arterial phase**/then 60 s
Saline chaser (cc)	40 (optional)
Other	* Use CARE Dose 4-D ** Begin monitoring scans at 15 s Add 5-s delay after threshold (120 HU) is reached

MDCT Protocols - Kidneys

Name of the protocol	Renal Mass (Preintervention Planning) (Note: Detection protocol similar to CTU)
Vendor and detector rows	Philips 16
Phase	Noncontrast, arterial, nephrographic/excretory
Scan range	Diaphragm to upper pelvis (noncontrast), diaphragm to mid-pelvis (arterial), diaphragm to ischium (neph/excret)
Detector configuration	16×0.75
Rotation time (s)	0.75
Pitch	0.95
Table speed (mm/rotation)	15
kVp	120
mA	275 (average patient) with DoseRight™
Reconstruction algorithm	Filter kernel B
Prospective slice thickness (mm)	5 (noncontrast), 2 (arterial) 3, (neph/excret)
Reconstruction interval (mm)	5 (noncontrast), 2 (arterial and neph/excret)
Oral contrast	Water or VoLumen™
IV contrast concentration (mg/ml)	370
IV contrast volume (cc)	100–130 lbs: 85 ml, 130–200: 115, 200–240: 140, >240: 175
IV contrast injection rate (cc/s)	Adjust rate to target duration of 30 s
Scan delay (fixed or bolus tracking)	Bolus tracking (arterial), 100 s after injection begins (neph/excret)
Saline chaser (cc)	40
Other	Administer 250 ml normal saline IV Administer additional ~1/5 iodine dose by hand, wait 10 min, then do nephrographic/excretory phase with remainder. Administer Lasix, 10 mg IV prior to contrast injection Contraindications: Allergy to Lasix, sulfa drugs, BP < 90 systolic 3-mm coronal MPR recon from 2.5-mm slices Oblique thin-slab MIPs oriented to renal axis 3-D Surface volume rendering

Name of the protocol	Renal Mass (Pre-intervention Planning) (Note: Detection protocol similar to CTU)
Vendor and detector rows	Philips 40 and 64
Phase	Noncontrast, arterial, nephrographic/excretory
Scan range	Diaphragm to upper pelvis (noncontrast), diaphragm to mid-pelvis (arterial), diaphragm to ischium (neph/excret)
Detector configuration	40 × 0.625 or 64 × 0.625
Rotation time (s)	0.75
Pitch	1.17
Table speed (mm/rotation)	34.4–55 (40-64 slice noncontrast), 29.2–46.8 (40-64 slice Arterial and neph/excret)
kVp	120
mA	275 (average patient) with DoseRight™
Reconstruction algorithm	Filter kernel B
Prospective slice thickness (mm)	5 (noncontrast), 2 (arterial) 3, (neph/excret)
Reconstruction interval (mm)	5 (noncontrast), 2 (arterial and neph/excret)
Oral contrast	Water or VoLumen™
IV contrast concentration (mg/ml)	370
IV contrast volume (cc)	100–130 lbs: 85 ml, 130–200: 115, 200–240: 140, >240: 175
IV contrast injection rate (cc/s)	Adjust rate to target duration of 30 s
Scan delay (fixed or bolus tracking)	Bolus tracking (arterial), 100 s after injection begins (neph/excret)
Saline chaser (cc)	40
Other	Administer 250 ml normal saline IV Administer additional ~1/5 Iodine dose by hand, wait 10 min, then do nephrographic/excretory phase with remainder. Administer Lasix, 10 mg IV prior to contrast injection Contraindications: allergy to Lasix, sulfa drugs, BP < 90 systolic 3-mm coronal MPR from 2.5-mm slices Oblique thin-slab MIPs oriented to renal axis 3-D surface volume rendering

Name of the protocol	Renal Mass
Vendor and detector rows	GE 16
Phase	Arterial, nephrogram (double-pass)
Scan range	Diaphragm to mid pelvis (1st pass) Diaphragm to inferior pelvis (2nd Pass)
Detector configuration	16 × 0.625 (1st pass) 16 × 1.25 (2nd pass)
Rotation time (s)	0.5
Pitch	1.375
Table speed (mm/rotation)	13.75 (1st pass), 27.5 (2nd pass)
kVp	120 – 140 (dependent on body habitus)
mA	AutomA 3-D Noise index 14 (1st pass) Noise index 15.8 (2nd pass)
Reconstruction algorithm	Standard
Prospective slice thickness (mm)	0.625 (1st pass), 1.25 (2nd pass) 2.5 (workstation review)
Reconstruction interval (mm)	0.625 (1st pass), 1.25 (2nd pass) 2.5 (workstation review)
Oral contrast	Water
IV contrast concentration (mg/ml)	370
IV contrast volume (cc)	150
IV contrast injection rate (cc/s)	6
Scan delay (fixed or bolus tracking)	Time to peak on preliminary mini bolus in supra celiac aorta plus 4 s (1st pass) 100 s (2nd pass)
Saline chaser (cc)	50 ml (at 6 ml)
Comment	Double-pass examination 1st pass – arterial mapping (3-D imaging) 2nd pass – tumor delineation and staging Axial, sagittal- and coronal plane display

Name of the protocol	Kidney Mass
Vendor and detector rows	GE 64
Phase	Arterial, nephrogram (double pass)
Scan range	Diaphragm to mid pelvis (1st pass) Diaphragm to inferior pelvis (2nd pass)
Detector configuration	64 × 0.625
Rotation time (s)	0.5
Pitch	0.984
Table speed (mm/rotation)	40
kVp	120 – 140 (dependent on body habitus)
mA	AutomA 3-D Noise index 14 (1st pass) Noise index 15.8 (2nd pass)
Reconstruction algorithm	Standard
Prospective slice thickness (mm)	0.625 (3-D imaging) 2.5 (workstation review)
Reconstruction interval (mm)	0.625 (3-D imaging) 2.5 (workstation review)
Oral contrast	Water
IV contrast concentration (mg/ml)	370
IV contrast volume (cc)	150
IV contrast injection rate (cc/s)	6
Scan delay (fixed or bolus tracking)	Time to peak on preliminary minibolus in supraceliac aorta plus 4 s
Saline chaser (cc)	50 ml (at 6 ml/s)
Comment	Double-pass examination 1st pass – Arterial mapping (3-D imaging) 2nd pass – tumor delineation and staging Axial, sagittal and coronal plane display

Name of the protocol	Kidney Mass
Vendor and detector rows	Siemens 16
Phase	Noncontrast/cortical/nephrographic
Scan range	Above diaphragm to iliac crest*
Detector configuration	16 × 1.5/0.75/1.5
Rotation time (s)	0.5
Pitch	0.9
Table speed (mm/rotation)	22/11/22
kVp	120
Effective mAs	180
Reconstruction algorithm	Soft tissue (B20f)
Prospective slice thickness (mm)	3/3 & 1/3 **
Reconstruction interval (mm)	3/3 & 0.7/3 **
Oral contrast	None
IV contrast concentration (mg/ml)	370
IV contrast volume (cc)	125 (100<150 lbs; 150>250 lbs)
IV contrast injection rate (cc/s)	4
Scan delay (fixed or bolus tracking)	30 s/100 s
Saline chaser (cc)	30 (optional)
Other	* For cortical enhancement phase: above top of kidneys to below bottom of kidneys ** Noncontrast: 3 × 3 Cortical: 3 × 3 & 1 × 0.7 Nephrographic: 3 × 3

Name of the protocol	Kidney Mass
Vendor and detector rows	Siemens 64
Phase	Noncontrast/cortical/nephrographic
Scan range	Above diaphragm to iliac crest*
Detector configuration	64 × 0.6
Rotation time (s)	0.5
Pitch	1
Table speed (mm/rotation)	19.2
kVp	120
Effective mAs	240**
Reconstruction algorithm	Soft tissue (B20f)
Prospective slice thickness (mm)	3/3 & 1/3 ***
Reconstruction interval (mm)	3/3 & 1/3 ***
Oral contrast	None
IV contrast concentration (mg/ml)	370
IV contrast volume (cc)	125 (100<150 lbs; 150>250 lbs)
IV contrast injection rate (cc/s)	4
Scan delay (fixed or bolus tracking)	30 s/100 s
Saline chaser (cc)	30 (optional)
Other	* For cortical enhancement phase: above top of kidneys to below bottom of kidneys ** Use CARE Dose 4-D *** Noncontrast: 3 × 3 Cortical: 3 × 3 & 1 × 0.7 Nephrographic: 3 × 3

MDCT Protocols - Urography

Name of the protocol	CT Urography
Vendor and detector rows	Philips 16
Phase	Precontrast, nephrographic/excretory
Scan range	Diaphragm to ischium
Detector configuration	16×0.75
Rotation time (s)	0.75
Pitch	0.95
Table speed (mm/rotation)	11.4
kVp	120
mA	275 (average patient) with DoseRight™
Reconstruction algorithm	Filter kernel C
Prospective slice thickness (mm)	5 (noncontrast), 3 (neph/excret)
Reconstruction interval (mm)	5 (noncontrast), 2 (neph/excret)
Oral contrast	Water or VoLumen ™
IV contrast concentration (mg/ml)	370
IV contrast volume (cc)	100–130 lbs: 85 ml, 130–200: 115, 200–240: 140, >240: 175
IV contrast injection rate (cc/s)	Adjust rate to target duration of 30 s
Scan delay (fixed or bolus tracking)	100 s after injection begins
Saline chaser (cc)	40
Other	Administer 250 ml normal saline IV
	Administer additional ~1/5 iodine dose by hand, wait 10 min, then do neph/excret phase with remainder.
	Administer Lasix, 10 mg IV prior to contrast injection
	Contraindications: allergy to Lasix, sulfa drugs, BP < 90 systolic
	3-mm Coronals recon from 2.5-mm slices
	3-D Volume rendering

Name of the protocol	CT Urography
Vendor and detector rows	Philips 40 and 64
Phase	Precontrast, nephrographic/excretory
Scan range	Diaphragm to ischium
Detector configuration	40 × 0.625 or 64 × 0.625
Rotation time (s)	0.75
Pitch	1.375 (noncontrast), 1.17 (neph/excret)
Table speed (mm/rotation)	34.4–55 (40-64 slice noncontrast), 29.2–46.8 (40-64 slice neph/excret)
kVp	120
mA	275 (average patient) with DoseRight™
Reconstruction algorithm	Filter kernel C
Prospective slice thickness (mm)	5 (noncontrast), 3 (neph/excret)
Reconstruction interval (mm)	5 (noncontrast), 2 (neph/excret)
Oral contrast (pos or neg)	Water or VoLumen ™
IV contrast concentration (mg/ml)	370
IV contrast volume (cc)	100–130 lbs: 85 ml, 130–200: 115, 200–240: 140, >240: 175
IV contrast injection rate (cc/s)	Adjust rate to target duration of 30 s
Scan delay (fixed or bolus tracking)	100 s after injection begins
Saline chaser (cc)	40
Other	Administer 250 ml normal saline IV Administer additional ~1/5 iodine dose by hand, wait 10 min, then do neph/excret phase with remainder. Administer Lasix, 10 mg IV prior to contrast injection. Contraindications: allergy to Lasix, sulfa drugs, BP < 90 systolic 3-mm Coronals recon from 2.5-mm slices 3-D Volume rendering

Name of the protocol	CT Urography
Vendor and detector rows	GE 16
Phase	Pre, nephropyelogram phase
Scan range	Dome of liver through pubic bones
Detector configuration	16 × 1.25
Rotation time (s)	0.5
Pitch	1.375
Table speed (mm/rotation)	27.5
kVp	120 – 140 (dependent on body habitus)
mA	AutomA 3-D Noise index 15.8
Reconstruction algorithm	Standard
Prospective slice thickness (mm)	1.25 (reformations, 3-D) 2.5 (workstation review)
Reconstruction interval (mm)	1.25 (reformations, 3-D) 2.5 (workstation review)
Oral contrast	None
IV contrast concentration (mg/ml)	350 – 370
IV contrast volume (cc)	Split Bolus, 80 ml followed in 10 mins with 90 ml
IV contrast injection rate (cc/s)	4
Scan delay (fixed or bolus tracking)	100-s delay, see comment (2)
Saline chaser (cc)	
Comment (1)	Preliminary precontrast study for urolithiasis
Comment (2)	Nephropyelogram phase acquisition 80-ml contrast medium IV, 15-min injection delay, 90-ml contrast medium IV 100 s acquisition delay No oral or IV fluids or diuretics between 2 contrast injections
Comment (3)	Delayed CT digital radiographs of urinary tract

Name of the protocol	CT Urography
Vendor and detector rows	GE 64
Phase	Pre, nephropyelogram phase
Scan range	Dome of liver through pubic bones
Detector configuration	64×0.625
Rotation time (s)	0.5
Pitch	0.984
Table speed (mm/rotation)	40
kVp	120 – 140 (dependent on body habitus)
mA	AutomA 3-D Noise index 15.8
Reconstruction algorithm	Standard
Prospective slice thickness (mm)	0.625 (reformations, 3-D imaging) 2.5 (workstation review)
Reconstruction interval (mm)	0.625 (reformations, 3-D imaging) 2.5 (workstation review)
Oral contrast	None
IV contrast concentration (mg/ml)	350 – 370
IV contrast volume (cc)	Split Bolus, 80 ml followed in 10 min with 90 ml
IV contrast injection rate (cc/s)	4 ml/s
Scan delay (fixed or bolus tracking)	100 s; see comment (2)
Saline chaser (cc)	
Comment (1)	Preliminary precontrast study for urolithiasis
Comment (2)	Nephropyelogram phase acquisition 80-ml contrast medium IV, 15 min injection delay, 90-ml contrast medium IV 100-s acquisition delay No oral or iv fluids or diuretics between 2 contrast injections
Comment (3)	Delayed CT digital radiographs of the urinary tract

Name of the protocol	Urography (CTU)
Vendor and detector rows	Siemens 16
Phase	Noncontrast/nephrographic/excretory
Scan range	Above kidneys to lesser trochanters
Detector configuration	$16 \times 1.5/1.5/0.75$
Rotation time (s)	0.5
Pitch	0.9
Table speed (mm/rotation)	22/11/22
kVp	120
Effective mAs	200
Reconstruction algorithm	Soft tissue (B20f)
Prospective slice thickness (mm)	2/2/1*
Reconstruction interval (mm)	2/2/0.7*
Oral contrast	None
IV contrast concentration (mg/ml)	370
IV contrast volume (cc)	125 (100<150 lbs; 150>250 lbs)
IV contrast injection rate (cc/s)	3
Scan delay (fixed or bolus tracking)	100 s/10 min
Saline chaser (cc)	120 ml**
Other	* Noncontrast: 2×2 Nephrographic: 2×2 Excretory: 1×0.7 ** Patient drinks two 16-oz cups (or 1,000 ml) of water 15-30 min before study. 120 ml normal saline chaser administered IV immediately after contrast bolus
Comment	Patient should empty bladder shortly before study

Name of the protocol	Urography (CTU)
Vendor and detector rows	Siemens 64
Phase	Noncontrast/nephrographic/excretory
Scan range	Above kidneys to lesser trochanters
Detector configuration	64×0.6
Rotation time (s)	0.5
Pitch	0.9
Table speed (mm/rotation)	17.3
kVp	120
Effective mAs	240
Reconstruction algorithm	Soft tissue (B20f)
Prospective slice thickness (mm)	2/2/2*
Reconstruction interval (mm)	2/2/1*
Oral contrast	None
IV contrast concentration (mg/ml)	370
IV contrast volume (cc)	125 (100<150 lbs; 150>250 lbs)
IV contrast injection rate (cc/s)	3
Scan delay (fixed or bolus tracking)	100 s/10 min
Saline chaser (cc)	120 ml**
Other	* Noncontrast: 2×2 Nephrographic: 2×2 Excretory: 2×1 ** Patient drinks two 16-oz cups (or 1,000 ml) of water 15-30 min before study. 120 ml normal saline chaser administered IV immediately after contrast bolus
Comment	Patient should empty bladder shortly before study

MDCT Protocols - Adrenal

Name of the protocol	Adrenal
Vendor and detector rows	Philips 16
Phase	Noncontrast, portal venous, 15 min delayed, if necessary
Scan range	Diaphragm to mid-kidneys (noncontrast), diaphragm to ischium (PV), Diaphragm to mid-kidneys (15 min delayed)
Detector configuration	16×0.75
Rotation time (s)	0.75
Pitch	0.95
Table speed (mm/rotation)	11.4
kVp	120
mA	275 (average patient) with DoseRight™
Reconstruction algorithm	Filter kernel C
Prospective slice thickness (mm)	3 (noncontrast), 5 (PV), 3 (delayed)
Reconstruction interval (mm)	2 (noncontrast), 3 (PV), 2 (delayed)
Oral contrast	Positive
IV contrast concentration (mg/ml)	370
IV contrast volume (cc)	100–130 lbs: 85 ml, 130–200: 115, 200–240: 140, >240: 175
IV contrast injection rate (cc/s)	Adjust rate to target duration of 30 s
Scan delay (fixed or bolus tracking)	40 s after injection *completion*
Saline chaser (cc)	40
Other	Stop after noncontrast if no mass or mass <10 HU 3-mm coronals recon from 2.5-mm slices

Name of the protocol	Adrenal
Vendor and detector rows	Philips 40 and 64
Phase	Noncontrast, portal venous, 15 min delayed, if necessary
Scan range	Diaphragm to mid-kidneys (noncontrast), diaphragm to ischium (PV), Diaphragm to mid-kidneys (15 min delayed)
Detector configuration	40×0.625 or 64×0.625
Rotation time (s)	0.75
Pitch	1.17
Table speed (mm/rotation)	29.2 (40-slice), 46.8 (64 slice)
kVp	120
mA	275 (average patient) with DoseRight™
Reconstruction algorithm	Filter kernel C
Prospective slice thickness (mm)	3 (noncontrast), 5 (PV), 3 (delayed)
Reconstruction interval (mm)	2 (noncontrast), 3 (PV), 2 (delayed)
Oral contrast	Positive
IV contrast concentration (mg/ml)	370
IV contrast volume (cc)	100–130 lbs: 85 ml, 130–200: 115, 200–240: 140, >240: 175
IV contrast injection rate (cc/s)	Adjust rate to target duration of 30 s
Scan delay (fixed or bolus tracking)	40 s after injection *completion*
Saline chaser (cc)	40
Other	Stop after noncontrast if no mass or mass <10 HU 3-mm coronals recon from 2.5-mm slices

Name of the protocol	Adrenal
Vendor and detector rows	GE 16
Phase	Pre, hepatic (portal venous) and 15 min delayed
Scan range	Diaphragm to mid kidney (for each pass)
Detector configuration	16 × 1.25
Rotation time (s)	0.5
Pitch	1.375
Table speed (mm/rotation)	27.5
kVp	120 – 140 (dependent on body habitus)
mA	AutomA 3-D Noise index 15.8
Reconstruction algorithm	Standard
Prospective slice thickness (mm)	1.25
Reconstruction interval (mm)	1.25
Oral contrast	Water
IV contrast concentration (mg/ml)	350 – 370
IV contrast volume (cc)	150
IV contrast injection rate (cc/s)	4
Scan delay (fixed or bolus tracking)	Bolus tracking (smart prep) hepatic attenuation threshold of 50 HU
Saline chaser (cc)	
Comment (1)	? Adrenal adenoma – check after 1st pass, if clearly adenoma, stop. Otherwise proceed to parenchymal and delayed phase.
Comment (2)	Adrenal tumor staging – Arterial and parenchymal phase

Name of the protocol	Adrenal
Vendor and detector rows	GE 64
Phase	Pre, hepatic and 15-min delayed
Scan range	Diaphragm to mid kidney (for each pass)
Detector configuration	64 × 0.625
Rotation time (s)	0.5
Pitch	0.984
Table speed (mm/rotation)	40
kVp	120 – 140 (dependent on body habitus)
mA	AutomA 3-D Noise index 15.8
Reconstruction algorithm	Standard
Prospective slice thickness (mm)	1. 25
Reconstruction interval (mm)	1. 25
Oral contrast	Water
IV contrast concentration (mg/ml)	350 – 370
IV contrast volume (cc)	150
IV contrast injection rate (cc/s)	4
Scan delay (fixed or bolus tracking)	Bolus tracking (smart prep) hepatic attenuation threshold of 50 HU
Saline chaser (cc)	
Comment (1)	? Adrenal adenoma – check after 1st pass, if clearly adenoma, stop. Otherwise proceed to parenchymal and delayed phase.
Comment (2)	Adrenal tumor staging – Arterial and parenchymal phase

Name of the protocol	Adrenal
Vendor and detector rows	Siemens 16
Phase	Noncontrast/portal venous/15-min delay*
Scan range	Above diaphragm to mid-kidneys
Detector configuration	16 × 0.75**
Rotation time (s)	0.5**
Pitch	1
Table speed (mm/rotation)	12
kVp	120
Effective mAs	240*
Reconstruction algorithm	Soft tissue (B20f)
Prospective slice thickness (mm)	2
Reconstruction interval (mm)	2
Oral contrast	None
IV contrast concentration (mg/ml)	370
IV contrast volume (cc)	100 (75<150 lbs; 125>250 lbs)
IV contrast injection rate (cc/s)	3
Scan delay (fixed or bolus tracking)	60 s/15 min
Saline chaser (cc)	
Other	* In many cases, IV contrast is not necessary. If adrenal lesion is indeterminate on noncontrast imaging, obtain portal venous and 15-min delay images. ** For very large patients, increase rotation time to 1.0 s and increase effective mAs as needed. Can also increase slice thickness to 10 mm

Name of the protocol	Adrenal
Vendor and detector rows	Siemens 64
Phase	Noncontrast/portal venous/15-min delay*
Scan range	Above diaphragm to mid-kidneys
Detector configuration	64 × 0.6**
Rotation time (s)	0.5**
Pitch	1
Table speed (mm/rotation)	19.2
kVp	120
Effective mAs	280**; ***
Reconstruction algorithm	Soft tissue (B20f)
Prospective slice thickness (mm)	2**
Reconstruction interval (mm)	2
Oral contrast	None
IV contrast concentration (mg/ml)	370
IV contrast volume (cc)	100 (75<150 lbs; 125>250 lbs)
IV contrast injection rate (cc/s)	3
Scan delay (fixed or bolus tracking)	65 s****
Saline chaser (cc)	
Other	* In many cases, IV contrast is not necessary. If adrenal lesion is indeterminate on noncontrast imaging, obtain portal venous and 15-min delay images. ** For very large patients, increase detector collimation to 1.2, rotation time to 1.0, and mAs to 380 eff. *** Use CARE Dose 4-D **** Increase scan delay by 10 s for every 0.5 ml/s decrease in injection rate

MDCT Protocols - Thoracic Aorta

Name of the protocol	CTA Thoracic Aorta-dissection
Vendor and detector rows	Philips 16
Phase	Noncontrast, arterial
Scan range	Lower neck to costophrenic recess
Detector configuration	16 × 0.75
Rotation time (s)	0.5
Pitch	1.25
Table Sspeed (mm/rotation)	15
kVp	120
mA	250 (average patient) with DoseRight™
Reconstruction algorithm	Filter kernel C
Prospective slice thickness (mm)	5 (noncontrast), 1.5 (for 3-D, MPR from contrast series), 5 (for axial review)
Reconstruction interval (mm)	5 (noncontrast), 1.0 (for 3-D, MPR from contrast series), 5 (for axial review)
Oral contrast	None
IV contrast concentration (mg/ml)	370
IV contrast volume (cc)	80
IV contrast injection rate (cc/s)	4
Scan delay (fixed or bolus tracking)	Tracking descending aorta @ 100
Saline chaser (cc)	40
Other	3-mm coronal MIP recon

Name of the protocol	CTA Thoracic Aorta-dissection
Vendor and detector rows	Philips 40 and 64
Phase	Noncontrast, arterial
Scan range	Lower neck to costophrenic recess
Detector configuration	40 × 0.625 or 64 × 0.625
Rotation time (s)	0.5
Pitch	1.17
Table speed (mm/rotation)	29.2 (40-slice), 46.8 (64 slice)
kVp	120
mA	250 (average patient) with DoseRight™
Reconstruction algorithm	Filter kernel C
Prospective slice thickness (mm)	5 (noncontrast), 1.5 (for 3-D, MPR from contrast series), 5 (for axial review)
Reconstruction interval (mm)	5 (noncontrast), 1.0 (for 3-D, MPR from contrast series), 5 (for axial review)
Oral contrast	None
IV contrast concentration (mg/ml)	370
IV contrast volume (cc)	80
IV contrast injection rate (cc/s)	4
Scan delay (fixed or bolus tracking)	Tracking descending aorta @ 100
Saline chaser (cc)	40
Other	3-mm coronal MIP recon

Name of the protocol	Thoracic Aorta
Vendor and detector rows	GE 16
Phase	Arterial
Scan range	Thoracic inlet to diaphragm
Detector configuration	16 × 0.625
Rotation time (s)	0.5
Pitch	1.375
Table speed (mm/rotation)	13.75
kVp	120 – 140
mA	AutomA 3-D Noise index 14
Reconstruction algorithm	Standard
Prospective slice thickness (mm)	0.625 (3-D imaging) 2.5 (workstation review)
Reconstruction interval (mm)	0.625 (3-D imaging) 2.5 (workstation review)
Oral contrast	None
IV contrast concentration (mg/ml)	370
IV contrast volume (cc)	90, see comment (2)
IV contrast injection rate (cc/s)	5ml/s
Scan delay (fixed or bolus tracking)	Time to peak on preliminary mini bolus in ascending aorta plus 4 s
Saline chaser (cc)	50 ml, 5 ml/s
Comment	Nongated acquisition for known or suspected aneurysm of the thoracic aortic arch or descending aorta

Name of the protocol	Thoracic Aorta/Aneurysm, dissection
Vendor and detector rows	GE 64
Phase	Arterial
Scan range	Thoracic inlet to pelvis
Detector configuration	64 × 0.625
Rotation time (s)	0.5
Pitch	0.984
Table speed (mm/rotation)	40, see comment (2)
kVp	140
mA	AutomA 3-D Noise index 14
Reconstruction algorithm	Standard
Prospective slice thickness (mm)	0.625 (3-D imaging) 2.5 (workstation review)
Reconstruction interval (mm)	0.625 (3-D imaging) 2.5 (workstation review)
Oral contrast	None
IV contrast concentration (mg/ml)	370
IV contrast volume (cc)	72, see comment (2)
IV contrast injection rate (cc/s)	6
Scan delay (fixed or bolus tracking)	Time to peak on preliminary mini bolus in ascending aorta plus 4 s
Saline chaser (cc)	50 ml, 6 ml/s
Comment (1)	Non gated acquisition for known or suspected aneurysm of the thoracic aortic arch or descending aorta.
Comment (2)	Preliminary determination of arterial flow velocity. Table speed adjusted (by changing rotation time, pitch, and beam width in that order to equal flow velocity. Contrast injection time equals scan delay of 4 s plus acquisition interval

Name of the protocol	Thoracoabdominal Aorta
Vendor and detector rows	GE 16
Phase	Arterial
Scan range	Thoracic inlet to pelvis
Detector configuration	16 × 1.25
Rotation time (s)	0.5
Pitch	1.375
Table speed (mm/rotation)	27.5
	55
kVp	140
mA	AutomA 3-D
	Noise index 14
Reconstruction algorithm	Standard
Prospective slice thickness (mm)	1.25 (3-D imaging)
	2.5 (workstation review)
Reconstruction interval (mm)	1.25 (3-D imaging)
	2.5 (workstation review)
Oral contrast	None
IV contrast concentration (mg/ml)	370
IV contrast volume (cc)	90, see comment (2)
IV contrast injection rate (cc/s)	5
Scan delay (fixed or bolus tracking)	Time to peak on preliminary mini bolus in ascending aorta plus 4 s
Saline chaser (cc)	50 ml, 5 ml/s
Comment	Nongated acquisition for known or suspected aneurysm/dissection of the thoracoabdominal aorta

Name of the protocol	Thoracoabdominal Aorta
Vendor and detector rows	GE 64
Phase	Arterial
Scan range	Thoracic inlet to pelvis
Detector configuration	64 × 0.625 (standard) see comment (2)
Rotation time (s)	0.5 (standard) see comment (2)
Pitch	1.375 (standard) see comment (2)
Table speed (mm/rotation)	55 (standard) see comment (2)
kVp	140
mA	AutomA 3-D
	Noise index 14
Reconstruction algorithm	Standard
Prospective slice thickness (mm)	0.625 (3-D imaging)
	2.5 (workstation review)
Reconstruction interval (mm)	0.625 (3-D imaging)
	2.5 (workstation review)
Oral contrast	None
IV contrast concentration (mg/ml)	370
IV contrast volume (cc)	90, see comment (2)
IV contrast injection rate (cc/s)	5
Scan delay (fixed or bolus tracking)	Time to peak on preliminary mini bolus in ascending aorta plus 4 s
Saline chaser (cc)	50 ml, 5 ml/s
Comment (1)	Nongated acquisition for known or suspected aneurysm/dissection of the thoracoabdominal aorta.
Comment (2)	Preliminary determination of arterial flow velocity. Table speed adjusted (by changing rotation time, pitch, and beam width in that order) to equal flow velocity. Contrast injection time equals scan delay of 4 s plus acquisition interval

Name of the protocol	Thoracic Aorta Prospective Gating
Vendor and detector rows	GE 64
Phase	Arterial
Scan range	Thoracic inlet to diaphragm
Detector configuration	64 × 0.625
Rotation time (s)	0.350
Pitch	Cine freeze frame mode
Table speed (mm/rotation)	20, see comment (2) 20, heart rate 60, see comment (2)
kVp	120
mA	Thin 450 Average 550 Large 750
Reconstruction algorithm	Standard
Prospective slice thickness (mm)	0.625 (3-D imaging) 2.5 (workstation review)
Reconstruction interval (mm)	0.625 (3-D imaging) 2.5 (workstation review)
Oral contrast	None
IV contrast concentration (mg/ml)	370
IV contrast volume (cc)	100
IV contrast injection rate (cc/s)	6
Scan delay (fixed or bolus tracking)	Time to peak on preliminary mini bolus in ascending aorta plus 4 s
Saline chaser (cc)	50 ml, 6 ml/s
Comment (1)	Prospectively gated acquisition for evaluation of suspected or known ascending aortic aneurysm or dissection.
Comment (2)	Step and shoot technique with axial scanning. 40 mm beam width with each acquisition triggered at preset time after R wave of alternate heart beat. 40-mm table motion during other alternate heart beat between acquisitions

Name of the protocol	Thoracic Aorta Prospective Gating
Vendor and detector rows	GE 64
Phase	Arterial
Scan range	Thoracic inlet to diaphragm
Detector configuration	64 × 0.625
Rotation time (s)	0.350
Pitch	0.18 – 0.24 (varies with heart rate), see comment (2)
Table speed (mm/rotation)	8, see comment (2)
kVp	120
mA	Thin 350 -450 Average 450-550 Large 600-750 EKG based dose modulation
Reconstruction algorithm	Standard
Prospective slice thickness (mm)	0.625 (3-D imaging) 2.5 (workstation review)
Reconstruction interval (mm)	0.625 (3-D imaging) 2.5 (workstation review)
Oral contrast	None
IV contrast concentration (mg/ml)	370
IV contrast volume (cc)	84
IV contrast injection rate (cc/s)	6
Scan delay (fixed or bolus tracking)	Time to peak on preliminary mini bolus in ascending aorta plus 4 s
Saline chaser (cc)	50 ml, 6 ml/s
Comment (1)	Retrospectively gated acquisition for evaluation of suspected or known ascending aortic aneurysm or dissection.
Comment (2)	Pitch and thus table speed varies with heart rate, slower table speed with slower heart rate

Name of the protocol	Thoracic Aorta-dissection
Vendor and detector rows	Siemens 16
Phase	Noncontrast/arterial
Scan range	Above lung apex to lesser trochanters
Detector configuration	16×1.5
Rotation time (s)	0.5
Pitch	1
Table speed (mm/rotation)	24
kVp	120
Effective mAs	175
Reconstruction algorithm	Soft tissue (B20f)
Prospective slice thickness (mm)	5/2*
Reconstruction interval (mm)	5/2*
Oral contrast	None
IV contrast concentration (mg/ml)	370
IV contrast volume (cc)	90 (75<150 lbs; 115>250 lbs)
IV contrast injection rate (cc/s)	4
Scan delay (fixed or bolus tracking)	CARE Bolus**
Saline chaser (cc)	40 (optional)
Other	* Noncontrast: 5×5 Arterial: 2×2 ** Place ROI on descending thoracic aorta, out of aneurysm, if possible. Begin monitoring scans at 15 s Add 4 s delay after threshold (120 HU) is reached

Name of the protocol	Thoracic Aorta-dissection
Vendor and detector rows	Siemens 64
Phase	Noncontrast/arterial
Scan range	Above lung apex to lesser trochanters
Detector configuration	64×1.2
Rotation time (s)	0.5
Pitch	0.75
Table Speed (mm/rotation)	14.4
kVp	120
Effective mAs	200
Reconstruction algorithm	Soft tissue (B20f)
Prospective slice thickness (mm)	2
Reconstruction interval (mm)	2
Oral contrast	None
IV contrast concentration (mg/ml)	370
IV contrast volume (cc)	90 (75<150 lbs; 115>250 lbs)
IV contrast injection rate (cc/s)	5
Scan delay (fixed or bolus tracking)	CARE Bolus*
Saline chaser (cc)	40 (optional)
Other	* Place ROI on descending thoracic aorta, out of aneurysm, if possible. Begin monitoring scans at 15-s Add 5 s. delay after threshold (120 HU) is reached

MDCT Protocols - Aorto-Iliac

Name of the protocol	Aorto-Iliac
Vendor and detector rows	GE 16
Phase	Arterial
Scan range	Supraceliac aorta to proximal thigh
Detector configuration	16×0.625
Rotation time (s)	0.5
Pitch	1.375
Table speed (mm/rotation)	13.75
kVp	140 (dependent on body habitus)
mA	AutomA 3-D Noise index 14
Reconstruction algorithm	Standard
Prospective slice thickness (mm)	0.625 (3-D imaging) 2.5 (workstation review)
Reconstruction interval (mm)	0.625 (3-D imaging) 2.5 (workstation review)
Oral contrast	None
IV contrast concentration (mg/ml)	370
IV contrast volume (cc)	90 (standard), see comment
IV contrast injection rate (cc/s)	5
Scan delay (fixed or bolus tracking)	Time to peak on preliminary mini bolus in supra celiac aorta plus 4 s
Saline chaser (cc)	50 ml (at 5 ml/s)

Name of the protocol	Aorto-Iliac
Vendor and detector rows	GE 64
Phase	Arterial
Scan Range	Supra celiac aorta to proximal thigh
Detector configuration	64×0.625 (standard) see comment
Rotation time (s)	0.5 (standard), see comment
Pitch	0.984 (standard), see comment
Table speed (mm/rotation)	40 (standard), see comment
kVp	140
mA	AutomA 3-D Noise index 14
Reconstruction algorithm	Standard
Prospective slice thickness (mm)	0.625 (3-D imaging) 2.5 (workstation review)
Reconstruction interval (mm)	0.625 (3-D imaging) 2.5 (workstation review)
Oral contrast	None
IV contrast concentration (mg/ml)	370
IV contrast volume (cc)	60 (standard), see comment
IV contrast injection rate (cc/s)	6
Scan delay (fixed or bolus tracking)	Time to peak on preliminary mini bolus in supra celiac aorta plus 4 s
Saline chaser (cc)	50 ml (at 6 ml/s)
Comment	Preliminary determination of arterial flow velocity. Table speed adjusted (by changing rotation time, pitch, and beam width in that order) to equal flow velocity. Contrast injection time equals scan delay of 4 s plus acquisition interval

Name of the protocol	Aorto-Iliac
Vendor and detector rows	Siemens 16
Phase	Noncontrast/arterial
Scan range	Above diaphragm to lesser trochanters
Detector configuration	16 × 1.5
Rotation time (s)	0.5
Pitch	0.938
Table speed (mm/rotation)	18.75
kVp	120
Effective mAs	180
Reconstruction algorithm	Soft tissue (B20f)
Prospective slice thickness (mm)	5/2*
Reconstruction interval (mm)	5/2*
Oral contrast	None
IV contrast concentration (mg/ml)	370
IV contrast volume (cc)	100 (75<150 lbs; 125>250 lbs)
IV contrast injection rate (cc/s)	4
Scan delay (fixed or bolus tracking)	CARE Bolus**
Saline chaser (cc)	40 (optional)
Other	* Noncontrast: 5 × 5 Arterial: 2 × 2 ** Begin monitoring scans at 15 s. Add 4-s delay after threshold (120 HU) is reached

Name of the protocol	Aorto-Iliac
Vendor and detector rows	Siemens 64
Phase	Noncontrast/arterial
Scan range	Above diaphragm to lesser trochanters
Detector configuration	64 × 1.2
Rotation time (s)	0.5
Pitch	1
Table speed (mm/rotation)	19.2
kVp	120
Effective mAs	240
Reconstruction algorithm	Soft tissue (B20f)
Prospective slice thickness (mm)	5/2 *
Reconstruction interval (mm)	5/2 *
Oral contrast	None
IV contrast concentration (mg/ml)	370
IV contrast volume (cc)	100 (75<150 lbs; 125>250 lbs)
IV contrast injection rate (cc/s)	4
Scan delay (fixed or bolus tracking)	CARE Bolus**
Saline chaser (cc)	40 (optional)
Other	* Noncontrast: 5 × 5 Arterial: 2 × 2 ** Begin monitoring scans at 15 s. Add 7 s. delay after threshold (120 HU) is reached

MDCT Protocols - Runoff

Name of the protocol	CTA Abdomen-Pelvis Runoff
Vendor and detector rows	Philips 16
Phase	Arterial
Scan range	Diaphragm through feet
Detector configuration	16 × 0.75
Rotation time (s)	0.75
Pitch	1.25
Table speed (mm/rotation)	15
kVp	120
mA	250 (average patient) with DoseRight™
Reconstruction algorithm	Filter kernel C
Prospective slice thickness (mm)	1.5 (for 3-D, MIP), 5 (for axial review)
Reconstruction interval (mm)	1.0 (for 3-D, MIP), 5 (for axial review)
Oral contrast	None
IV contrast concentration (mg/ml)	370
IV contrast volume (cc)	115
IV contrast injection rate (cc/s)	4
Scan delay (fixed or bolus tracking)	Tracking descending aorta @ 100
Saline chaser (cc)	40
Other	Not recommended. Should use 40-64

Name of the protocol	CTA Abdomen-Pelvis-Runoff
Vendor and detector rows	Philips 40 and 64
Phase	Arterial
Scan range	Diaphragm through feet
Detector configuration	40 × 0.625 or 64 × 0.625
Rotation time (s)	0.75
Pitch	1.17
Table speed (mm/rotation)	29.2 (40-slice), 46.8 (64-slice)
kVp	120
mA	250 (average patient) with DoseRight™
Reconstruction algorithm	Filter kernel C
Prospective slice thickness (mm)	1.5 (for 3-D, MIP), 5 (for axial review)
Reconstruction interval (mm)	1.0 (for 3-D, MIP), 5 (for axial review)
Oral contrast	None
IV contrast concentration (mg/ml)	370
IV contrast volume (cc)	115
IV contrast injection rate (cc/s)	4
Scan delay (fixed or bolus tracking)	Tracking descending aorta @ 150
Saline chaser (cc)	40
Other	Alternative 1: dual phase - s slower injection phase Alternative 2: slower table feed Alternative 3: monitor and perform s scan series in lower legs if outrun bolus 10-mm slab × 3-mm increment coronal MIP 3-D Surface volume rendered

Name of the protocol	Runoff
Vendor and detector rows	Siemens 16
Phase	Arterial
Scan range	Above kidneys to below toes
Detector configuration	16 × 1.5
Rotation time (s)	0.5
Pitch	1
Table speed (mm/rotation)	24
kVp	120
Effective mAs	180
Reconstruction algorithm	Soft tissue (B20f)
Prospective slice thickness (mm)	2
Reconstruction interval (mm)	1
Oral contrast	None
IV contrast concentration (mg/ml)	370
IV contrast volume (cc)	125
IV contrast injection rate (cc/s)	4
Scan delay (fixed or bolus tracking)	CARE Bolus*
Saline chaser (cc)	40 (optional)
Other	* Begin monitoring scans at 15 s. Add-15 s delay after threshold (120 HU) is reached

Name of the protocol	Runoff
Vendor and detector rows	Siemens 64
Phase	Arterial
Scan range	Above kidneys to below toes
Detector configuration	64 × 1.2
Rotation time (s)	0.33*
Pitch	0.8*
Table speed (mm/rotation)	15.4
kVp	120
Effective mAs	190*
Reconstruction algorithm	Soft tissue (B20f)
Prospective slice thickness (mm)	2
Reconstruction interval (mm)	1
Oral contrast	None
IV contrast concentration (mg/ml)	370
IV contrast volume (cc)	100–125*
IV contrast injection rate (cc/s)	4*
Scan delay (fixed or bolus tracking)	CARE Bolus**
Saline chaser (cc)	40 (optional)
Other	* For large patients, increase rotation time to 0.5, injection rate to 5, and use 150 ml of contrast. ** Place ROI on aorta above kidneys. Begin monitoring scans at 15 s Add 15 s. delay after threshold (120 HU) is reached

MDCT Protocols - Trauma

Name of the protocol	Musculoskeletal Trauma
Vendor and detector rows	GE 16
Phase	Precontrast
Scan range	Dependent on body region imaged
Detector configuration	16×0.625
Rotation time (s)	0.5
Pitch	0.516
Table speed (mm/rotation)	5
kVp	120 – 140 (dependent on body habitus)
mA	AutomA 3-D Noise index 18
Reconstruction algorithm	Bone
Prospective slice thickness (mm)	0.625 (for image reformations) 1.25 (workstation review)
Reconstruction interval (mm)	0.625 (for image reformations) 1.25 (workstation review)
Oral contrast	
IV contrast concentration (mg/ml)	
IV contrast volume (cc)	
IV contrast injection rate (cc/s)	
Scan delay (fixed or bolus tracking)	
Saline chaser (cc)	
Comment	Targeted small FOV with additional 1.25-mm sagittal and coronal plane reformations

Name of the protocol	Musculoskeletal Trauma
Vendor and detector rows	GE 64
Phase	Precontrast
Scan range	Dependent on body region imaged
Detector configuration	64×0.625
Rotation time (s)	0.5
Pitch	0.516
Table speed (mm/rotation)	20
kVp	120 – 140 (dependent on body habitus)
mA	AutomA 3-D Noise index 18
Reconstruction algorithm	Bone
Prospective slice thickness (mm)	0.625 (for image reformations) 1.25 (workstation review)
Reconstruction interval (mm)	0.625 (for image reformations) 1.25 (workstation review)
Oral contrast	
IV contrast concentration (mg/ml)	
IV contrast volume (cc)	
IV contrast injection rate (cc/s)	
Scan delay (fixed or bolus tracking)	
Saline chaser (cc)	
Comment	Targeted small FOV with additional 1.25-mm sagittal and coronal plane reformations

Name of the protocol	Cervical Spine (Trauma)
Vendor and detector rows	GE 16
Phase	Pre contrast
Scan range	Mid clivus to cervicothoracic junction
Detector configuration	16 × 1.25
Rotation time (s)	0.5
Pitch	0.938
Table speed (mm/rotation)	18.75
kVp	120 – 140 (dependent on body habitus)
mA	AutomA 3-D Noise index 15.8
Reconstruction algorithm	Bone
Prospective slice thickness (mm)	1.25 (for image reformations and workstation review)
Reconstruction interval (mm)	1.25 (for image reformations and workstation review)
Oral contrast	
IV contrast concentration (mg/ml)	
IV contrast volume (cc)	
IV contrast injection rate (cc/s)	
Scan delay (fixed or bolus tracking)	
Saline chaser (cc)	
Comment	Targeted small FOV with additional 1.25-mm sagittal and coronal plane reformations

Name of the protocol	Cervical Spine Trauma
Vendor and detector rows	GE 64
Phase	Precontrast
Scan range	Mid clivus to cervicothoracic junction
Detector configuration	64 × 0.625
Rotation time (s)	0.5
Pitch	0.984
Table speed (mm/rotation)	40
kVp	120 – 140 (dependent on body habitus)
mA	AutomA 3-D Noise index 15.8
Reconstruction algorithm	Bone
Prospective slice thickness (mm)	0.625 (for image reformations) 1.25 (workstation review)
Reconstruction interval (mm)	0.625 (for image reformations) 1.25 (workstation review)
Oral contrast	
IV contrast concentration (mg/ml)	
IV contrast volume (cc)	
IV contrast injection rate (cc/s)	
Scan delay (fixed or bolus tracking)	
Saline chaser (cc)	
Comment	Targeted small FOV with additional 1.25–mm sagittal and coronal plane rerformations

Name of the protocol	Thoraco Lumbar Spine Trauma
Vendor and detector rows	GE 16
Phase	Arterial (thorax), parenchymal (abdomen, pelvis)
Scan range	Inferior neck to inferior pubic bones
Detector configuration	16 × 1.25
Rotation time (s)	0.5
Pitch	1.375
Table speed (mm/rotation)	27.5
kVp	120 – 140 (dependent on body habitus)
mA	AutomA 3-D Noise index 15.8
Reconstruction algorithm	Bone
Prospective slice thickness (mm)	1.25 (for image reformations) 2.5 (workstation review)
Reconstruction interval (mm)	1.25 (for image reformations) 2.5 (workstation review)
Oral contrast	None
IV contrast concentration (mg/ml)	350
IV contrast volume (cc)	150
IV contrast injection rate (cc/s)	5
Scan delay (fixed or bolus tracking)	Fixed 25 s
Saline chaser (cc)	Included as part of standard trauma protocol
Comment	Sagittal reformations generated from overlapped axial slices Additional small FOV axial and coronal images used selectively for spine trauma

Name of the protocol	Thoraco Lumbar Spine Trauma
Vendor and detector rows	GE 64
Phase	Arterial (thorax), parenchymal (abdomen, pelvis)
Scan range	Inferior neck to inferior pubic bones
Detector configuration	64 × 0.625
Rotation time (s)	0.5
Pitch	0.984
Table speed (mm/rotation)	40
kVp	120 – 140 (dependent on body habitus)
mA	AutomA 3-D Noise index 15.8
Reconstruction algorithm	Bone
Prospective slice thickness (mm)	0.625 (for image reformations) 1.25 (workstation review)
Reconstruction interval (mm)	0.625 (for image reformations) 1.25 (workstation review)
Oral contrast	None
IV contrast concentration (mg/ml)	350
IV contrast volume (cc)	150
IV contrast injection rate (cc/s)	5
Scan delay (fixed or bolus tracking)	Fixed 25 s
Saline chaser (cc)	
Comment (1)	Included as part of standard trauma protocol
Comment (2)	Sagittal reformations generated from overlapped axial slices Additional small FOV axial and coronal images used selectively for spine trauma

Name of the protocol	Torso Trauma
Vendor and detector rows	GE 16 Pro
Phase	Portal venous (65 s at liver)
Scan range	Above apices to below lesser trochander
Detector configuration	16×1.25
Rotation time (s)	0.5
Pitch	1.375
Table speed (mm/rotation)	27.5
kVp	120
mA	AEC (NI 11.57; range 150 – 500)
Reconstruction algorithm	Standard*
Prospective slice thickness (mm)	5*
Reconstruction interval (mm)	5
Oral contrast	Positive (as tolerated)
IV contrast concentration (mg/ml)	350
IV contrast volume (cc)	130 (split-bolus)***
IV contrast injection rate (cc/s)	3.5
Scan delay (fixed or bolus tracking)	55
Saline chaser (cc)	30
Other	* For Ortho, 2.5×2.5 retrospective bone & standard algorithm of location ** 5×5 mm coronal and Sagittal slices routinely *** 30 cc pre-bolus, 3 min delay, 100 cc bolus

Name of the protocol	Torso Trauma
Vendor and detector rows	GE 64 VCT
Phase	Portal venous (65 s at liver)
Scan range	Above apices to below lesser trochander
Detector configuration	64×0.625
Rotation time (s)	0.5
Pitch	1.375
Table speed (mm/rotation)	55
kVp	120
mA	AEC (NI 11.57; range 150 – 500)
Reconstruction algorithm	Standard*
Prospective slice thickness (mm)	5**
Reconstruction interval (mm)	5
Oral contrast	Positive (as tolerated)
IV contrast concentration (mg/ml)	350
IV contrast volume (cc)	130 (split-bolus)***
IV contrast injection rate (cc/s)	3.5
Scan delay (fixed or bolus tracking)	62
Saline chaser (cc)	30
Other	* For Ortho, 2.5×2.5 retrospective bone & standard algorithm of location ** 5×5-mm coronal and sagittal slices routinely *** 30 cc prebolus, 3-min delay, 100 cc bolus

Name of the protocol	Torso Trauma
Vendor and detector rows	Toshiba 16 Aquilion
Phase	Portal venous (65 s at liver)
Scan range	Above apices to below lesser trochander
Detector configuration	64×1
Rotation time (s)	0.5
Pitch	0.937
kVp	120
mA	AEC (SD 12; range 150 to 500)
Reconstruction algorithm	Standard*
Prospective slice thickness (mm)	5**
Reconstruction interval (mm)	5
Oral contrast	Positive (as tolerated)
IV contrast concentration (mg/ml)	350
IV contrast volume (cc)	130 (split-bolus)***
IV contrast injection rate (cc/s)	3.5
Scan delay (fixed or bolus tracking)	62
Saline chaser (cc)	30
Other	* For Ortho, 2×2 retrospective bone & standard algorithm of location ** 5×5-mm coronal and sagittal slices routinely *** 30 cc prebolus, 3-min delay, 100 cc bolus

Name of the protocol	Torso Trauma
Vendor and detector rows	Toshiba 64 Aquilion
Phase	Portal venous (65 s)
Scan range	Above apices to below lesser trochander
Detector configuration	64×0.5
Rotation time (s)	0.5
Pitch	0.828
Table speed (mm/rotation)	53
kVp	120
mA	AEC (SD 12; range 150 – 500)
Reconstruction algorithm	Standard*
Prospective slice thickness (mm)	5**
Reconstruction interval (mm)	5
Oral contrast	Positive (as tolerated)
IV contrast concentration (mg/ml)	350
IV contrast volume (cc)	130 (split bolus)***
IV contrast injection rate (cc/s)	3.5
Scan delay (fixed or bolus tracking)	62
Saline chaser (cc)	30
Other	* For Ortho, 2×2 retrospective bone & standard algorithm of location ** 5×5-mm coronal and sagittal slices routinely *** 30 cc prebolus, 3-min delay, 100 cc bolus

MDCT Protocols – Pulmonary Embolism

Name of the protocol	Pulmonary Embolism
Vendor and detector rows	Philips 16
Phase	Arterial
Scan range	Sternal notch to costophrenic recess
Detector configuration	16×0.75
Rotation time (s)	0.5
Pitch	1.25
Table speed (mm/rotation)	15
kVp	80
mA	250 (average patient) with DoseRight™
Reconstruction algorithm	Filter kernel C
Prospective slice thickness (mm)	3
Reconstruction interval (mm)	3
Oral contrast	None
IV contrast concentration (mg/ml)	370
IV contrast volume (cc)	95
IV contrast injection rate (cc/s)	4
Scan delay (fixed or bolus tracking)	Tracking ascending aorta @ 100
Saline chaser (cc)	40
Other	3-mm coronal MIP recon from 2-mm slices. 80 kVp causes 70% reduction of radiation dose, improved contrast, worse noise

Name of the protocol	Pulmonary Embolism
Vendor and detector rows	Philips 40 and 64
Phase	Arterial
Scan range	Sternal notch to costophrenic recess
Detector configuration	40×0.625 or 64×0.625
Rotation time (s)	0.5
Pitch	0.876
Table speed (mm/rotation)	21.9 (40-slice), 30.0 (64-slice)
kVp	80
mA	250 (average patient) with DoseRight™
Reconstruction algorithm	Filter kernel C
Prospective slice thickness (mm)	3
Reconstruction interval (mm)	3
Oral contrast	None
IV contrast concentration (mg/ml)	370
IV contrast volume (cc)	95
IV contrast injection rate (cc/s)	4
Scan delay (fixed or bolus tracking)	Tracking ascending aorta @ 150 (40-slice), 200 (64-slice)
Saline chaser (cc)	40
Other	3-mm coronal MIP recon from 2-mm slices. 80 kVp causes 70% reduction of radiation dose, improved contrast, worse noise

Name of the protocol	Pulmonary Embolism
Vendor and detector rows	GE 16
Phase	Arterial
Scan range	Lung apex, to diaphragm delayed indirect venography
Detector configuration	16 × 1.25
Rotation time (s)	0.5
Pitch	1.375
Table speed (mm/rotation)	27.5
kVp	120 – 140 (dependent on body habitus)
mA	AutomA 3-D Noise index 15.8
Reconstruction algorithm	Standard
Prospective slice thickness (mm)	1.25 (for image reformations) 2.5 (workstation review)
Reconstruction interval (mm)	1.25 (for image reformations) 2.5 (workstation review)
Oral contrast	None
IV contrast concentration (mg/ml)	370
IV contrast volume (cc)	120
IV contrast injection rate (cc/s)	4
Scan delay (fixed or bolus tracking)	Fixed 25 s
Saline chaser (cc)	50 ml, 6 ml/s
Comment (1)	Delayed indirect venography utilized in patients over 40 5-mm axial images every 20 mm from upper margin of acetabulum to distal popliteal vein.
Comment (2)	Sagittal and coronal plane thorax reformations standard

Name of the protocol	Pulmonary Embolism
Vendor and detector rows	GE 64
Phase	Arterial
Scan range	Lung apex to diaphragm delayed indirect venography
Detector configuration	64 × 0.625
Rotation time (s)	0.5
Pitch	0.984
Table speed (mm/rotation)	40
kVp	120 – 140 (dependent on body habitus)
mA	AutomA 3-D Noise index 15.8
Reconstruction algorithm	Standard
Prospective slice thickness (mm)	0.625 (for image reformations) 2.5 (workstation review)
Reconstruction interval (mm)	0.625 (for image reformations) 2.5 (workstation review)
Oral contrast	None
IV contrast concentration (mg/ml)	370
IV contrast volume (cc)	120
IV contrast injection rate (cc/s)	4
Scan delay (fixed or bolus tracking)	Fixed 25 s
Saline chaser (cc)	50 ml, 6 ml/s
Comment (1)	Delayed indirect venography utilized in patients over 40 5-mm axial images every 20-mm from upper margin of acetabulum to distal popliteal vein.
Comment (2)	Sagittal and coronal plane thorax reformations standard

Name of the protocol	Pulmonary Embolism (PE)
Vendor and detector rows	Siemens 16
Phase	Pulmonary arterial
Scan range	Lung bases to lung apices
Detector configuration	16 × 0.75
Rotation time (s)	0.5
Pitch	1
Table speed (mm/rotation)	12
kVp	120
Effective mAs	140
Reconstruction algorithm	Soft tissue (B20f); lung (B60f)
Prospective slice thickness (mm)	1 / 5 *
Reconstruction interval (mm)	1 / 5 *
Oral contrast	None
IV contrast concentration (mg/ml)	370
IV contrast volume (cc)	125
IV contrast injection rate (cc/s)	4
Scan delay (fixed or bolus tracking)	CARE Bolus**
Saline chaser (cc)	30 (optimal)
Other	* Soft tissue: 1×1 Lung: 5×5 ** Place ROI on main pulmonary artery Begin monitoring scans at 10 s Add 5-s delay after threshold (120 HU) is reached

Name of the protocol	Pulmonary Embolism (PE)
Vendor and detector rows	Siemens 64
Phase	Pulmonary arterial
Scan range	Lung bases to lung apices
Detector configuration	64 × 0.6
Rotation time (s)	0.5*
Pitch	1
Table speed (mm/rotation)	19.2
kVp	120
Effective mAs	180
Reconstruction algorithm	Soft tissue (B20f); lung (B60f)
Prospective slice thickness (mm)	1 soft tissue**/5 lung
Reconstruction interval (mm)	1 soft tissue/5 lung
Oral contrast	None
IV contrast concentration (mg/ml)	370
IV contrast volume (cc)	100
IV contrast injection rate (cc/s)	4**
Scan delay (fixed or bolus tracking)	CARE bolus ***
Saline chaser (cc)	30 (optimal)
Other	* Increase rotation time for large patients ** For large patients (>250 lbs) can increase injection rate to 5 ml/s and slice thickness to 2 or 3 mm in addition to increasing volume to 125 ml *** Place ROI on main pulmonary artery Begin monitoring scans at 10-s. Add 5-s. delay after threshold (120 HU) is reached

MDCT Protocols - Pediatrics

Name of the protocol	Pediatric Routine Chest
Vendor and detector rows	GE LightSpeed 16 slice
Phase	Consider arterial for all chest
Scan range	Apex through sulcus
Detector configuration	16 × 0.625 if reformations anticipated 16 × 1.25 for other
Rotation time (s)	0.5
Pitch	0.938 or 1.375 (see Chapter 26, Table 11)
Table speed (mm/rotation)	18.75 (lower pitch, 16 × 1.25) or 27.5 (higher pitch, 16 × 1.25)
kVp	Size adjusted (see Chapter 26, Table 11)
mA	Size adjusted (see Chapter 26, Table 11)
AEC	Optional (see Chapter 26, Table 13)
Reconstruction algorithm	Soft tissue
Prospective slice thickness (mm)	3.75 – 5.0 (see Chapter 26, Table 11)
Reconstruction interval (mm)	2.5 (favored) – 5.0
Oral contrast	None
IV contrast concentration (mg/ml)	300
IV contrast volume (cc)	1.5 ml/kg to adult dose as max
IV contrast injection rate (cc/s)	1.5-3.0 injector Manual: fast as possible
Scan delay (fixed or bolus tracking)	At end of injection (minimal delay) or CTA technique (see Chapter 26, Table 10)
Saline chaser (cc)	Optional
Other	5-mm-thick/2.5 spacing coronals for trauma, assessment, congenital malformations, airway depiction

Name of the protocol	Pediatric Routine Abdomen and Pelvis
Vendor and detector rows	GE LightSpeed 16
Phase	Portal venous*
Scan range	Diaphragm to symphysis pubis
Detector configuration	64 × 0.625 if reformations anticipated; otherwise 16 × 1.25
Rotation time (s)	0.5
Pitch	0.938 or 1.375 (see Chapter 26, Table 12)
Table speed (mm/rotation)	18.75 (lower pitch, 16 × 1.25) or 27.5 (higher pitch, 16 × 1.25)
kVp	Size adjusted (see Chapter 26, Table 12)
mA	Size adjusted (see Chapter 26, Table 12)
AEC	Optional (see Chapter 26, Table 13)
Reconstruction algorithm	Soft tissue
Prospective slice thickness (mm)	3.75 – 5.0
Reconstruction interval (mm)	2.5 (favored) – 5.0
Oral contrast	Positive
IV contrast concentration (mg/ml)	300
IV contrast volume (cc)	2.0 ml/kg to adult dose as max
IV contrast injection rate (cc/s)	1.5–3.0 injector Manual: fast as possible
Scan delay (fixed or bolus tracking)	25–30 s following *completion of injection*
Saline chaser (cc)	Optional
Other	*Delays for liver lesions, evaluation of renal collecting system 5-mm thick/2.5 spacing coronals for acute abdomen (e.g., appendicitis, obstruction), complex disorders including masses, trauma

Name of the protocol	Pediatric Routine Chest
Vendor and detector rows	GE VCT 64 slice
Phase	Consider arterial for all chest
Scan range	Apex through sulcus
Detector configuration	64 × 0.625
Rotation time (s)	0.4
Pitch	0.984 or 1.375 (see Chapter 26, Table 14)
Table speed (mm/rotation)	39.37 (for lower pitch) or 55 (for highes pitch) (see Chapter 26, Table 14)
kVp	Size adjusted (see Chapter 26, Table 14)
mA	Size adjusted (see Chapter 26, Table 14)
AEC	Optional (see Chapter 26, Table 13)
Reconstruction algorithm	Soft tissue
Prospective slice thickness (mm)	3.75 – 5.0 (see Chapter 26, Table 14)
Reconstruction interval (mm)	2.5 (favored) – 5.0
Oral contrast	None
IV contrast concentration (mg/ml)	300
IV contrast volume (cc)	1.5 ml/kg to adult dose as max
IV contrast injection rate (cc/s)	1.5-3.0 injector Manual: fast as possible
Scan delay (fixed or bolus tracking)	At end of injection (minimal delay) or CTA technique (see Chapter 26, Table 10)
Saline chaser (cc)	Optional
Other	5-mm thick/2.5 spacing coronals for trauma, assessment, congenital malformations, airway depiction

Name of the protocol	Pediatric Routine Abdominal and Pelvis
Vendor and detector rows	GE VCT 64 slice
Phase	Portal venous*
Scan range	Diaphragms to symphysis pubis
Detector configuration	64 × 0.625
Rotation time (s)	0.4
Pitch	0.984 or 1.375 (see Chapter 26, Table 15)
Table speed (mm/rotation)	39.37 (for lower pitch) or 55 (for highes pitch) (see Chapter 26, Table 15)
kVp	Size adjusted (see Chapter 26, Table 15)
mA	Size adjusted (see Chapter 26, Table 15)
AEC	Optional (see Chapter 26, Table 13)
Reconstruction algorithm	Soft tissue
Prospective slice thickness (mm)	3.75 – 5.0 (see Chapter 26, Table 15)
Reconstruction interval (mm)	2.5 (favored) – 5.0
Oral contrast	None
IV contrast concentration (mg/ml)	300
IV contrast volume (cc)	2.0 ml/kg to adult dose as max
IV contrast injection rate (cc/s)	1.5-3.0 injector Manual: fast as possible
Scan delay (fixed or bolus tracking)	35 s following *completion* of IV contrast
Saline chaser (cc)	NA
Other	* 5-mm thick/2.5 spacing coronals for acute abdomen (e.g., appendicitis obstruction), complex disorders including masses, trauma

Name of the protocol	Pediatric Routine Chest
Vendor and detector rows	Siemens definition
Phase	Consider arterial for all chest
Scan range	Apex through sulcus
Detector configuration	64 × 0.6
Rotation time (s)	0.5
Pitch	1.0 or 1.4 (see Chapter 26, Table 16)
Table speed (mm/rotation)	NA
kVp	Size adjusted (see Chapter 26, Table 16)
Note: mAs_{eff} not mA	Size adjusted (see Chapter 26, Table 16)
AEC	insufficient experience at this point
Reconstruction algorithm	Soft tissue (kernel B31f)
Prospective slice thickness (mm)	3.0 – 5.0 (see Chapter 26, Table 16)
Reconstruction interval (mm)	2.5 (favored) – 5.0
Oral contrast	None
IV contrast concentration (mg/ml)	300
IV contrast volume (cc)	1.5 ml/kg to adult dose as max
IV contrast injection rate (cc/s)	1.5-3.0 injector Manual: fast as possible
Scan delay (fixed or bolus tracking)	At end of injection (minimal delay) or CTA technique (see Chapter 26, Table 10)
Saline chaser (cc)	Optional
Other	5-mm thick/2.5 spacing coronals for trauma, assessment, congenital malformations, airway depiction

Name of the protocol	Pediatric Routine Abdomen and Pelvis
Vendor and detector rows	Siemens definition
Phase	Portal venous*
Scan range	Diaphragm to symphysis pubis
Detector configuration	64 × 0.6
Rotation time (s)	0.5
Pitch	1.0 or 1.4 (see Chapter 26, Table 17)
Table speed (mm/rotation)	NA
kVp	Size adjusted (see Chapter 26, Table 17)
Note: mAs_{eff} not mA	Size adjusted (see Chapter 26, Table 17)
AEC	insufficient experience at this point
Reconstruction algorithm	Soft tissue (kernel B31f)
Prospective slice thickness (mm)	3.0 – 5.0 (see Chapter 26, Table 17)
Reconstruction interval (mm)	2.5 (favored) – 5.0
Oral contrast	Positive
IV contrast concentration (mg/ml)	300
IV contrast volume (cc)	2.0 ml/kg to adult dose as max
IV contrast injection rate (cc/s)	1.5-3.0 injector Manual: fast as possible
Scan delay (fixed or bolus tracking)	35 s following *completion of injection*
Saline chaser (cc)	Optional
Other	*Delays for liver lesions, evaluation of renal collecting system 5-mm thick/2.5 spacing coronals for acute abdomen (e.g., appendicitis, obstruction), complex disorders including masses, trauma

Name of the protocol	Pediatric Routine CTA
Vendor and detector rows	GE VCT 64 and LightSpeed 16
Phase	Arterial
Scan range	Varies for indication
Detector configuration	16 × 0.625, 64 × 0.625
Rotation time (s)	0.5
Pitch	1.375
Table speed (mm/rotation)	55
kVp	Size adjusted (see Chapter 26, Table 18)
mA	Size adjusted (see Chapter 26, Table 18)
AEC	No recommendations
Reconstruction algorithm	Soft
Display slice thickness (mm)	1.25 – 5.0 (see Chapter 26, Table 18)
Reconstruction thickness (mm)	0.625
Reconstruction interval (mm)	0.5 – 1.0
Oral contrast	None
IV contrast concentration (mg/ml)	300–370
IV contrast volume (cc)	1.5 ml/kg to adult dose as max
IV contrast injection rate (cc/s)	1.5-5.0 injector Manual: fast as possible
Scan delay (fixed or bolus tracking)	Bolus tracking (SmartPrep); usual visual trigger for $\leq$ 7 years; adult HU trigger in older children
Saline chaser (cc)	Optional
Other	In small (e.g., < 1 year) children, begin bolus tracking (start contrast when first image displayed) *before starting contrast* so that peak bolus not missed. Can use test bolus (10% of total dose) even in infants

Printed in March 2008